POST COVID LIVING AT THE SHADOWS

POST COVID LIVING AT THE SHADOWS

RAMSIS F. GHALY, MD

Neurosurgeon and Anesthesiologist
Professor of Neurological Surgery and Anesthesiology
American Fully Trained and Board Certified in Quadruple Medical Specialties Neurological Surgery, Anesthesiology, Neurologic Critical Care and Pain Medicine

Library of Congress Control Number: 2022921732
ISBN: Hardcover 978-1-6698-5655-9
Softcover 978-1-6698-5654-2
eBook 978-1-6698-5653-5

Print information available on the last page.

Rev. date: 12/01/2022

To order additional copies of this book, contact:
Xlibris
844-714-8691
www.Xlibris.com
Orders@Xlibris.com
840244

CONTENTS

CHICAGO POST-COVID

I AM POOR AND NEEDY

FEAR NOT

MY LORD AND FATHER

KINGS AND QUEENS

POST COVID POLITICS

THE HUMAN BRAIN

POST COVID AGGRESSION

POST COVID RUSSIAN AGGRESSION

MEDICAL CARE POST COVID

WITH MY RESIDENTS AT POSTCOVID

PATIENTS STORIES AND COMMENTS POST COVID

BOOK AUTHORED BY DR RAMSIS F GHALY

RAMSIS F. GHALY, M.D., F.A.C.S.
PROFESSOR OF NEUROLOGICAL SURGERY AND ANESTHESIOLOGY

Board Certified in Neurosurgery, NeuroCritical Care, Anesthesiology & Pain Management & Independent Medical Examiner

BOOK AUTHORED BY DR RAMSIS F. GHALY

www.ghalyneurosurgeon.com

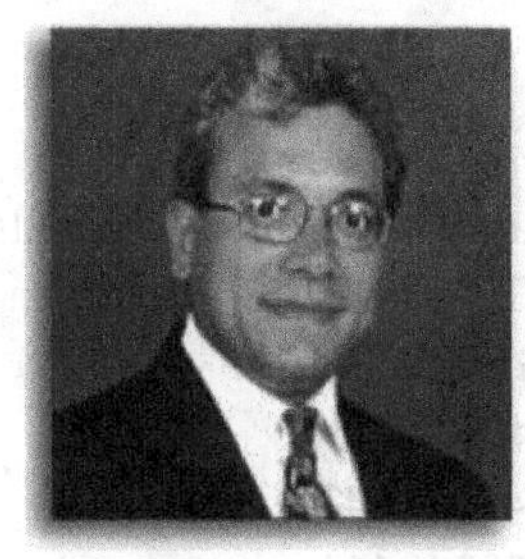

Books Authored by Dr. Ramsis F. Ghaly:

1- Christianity and The Brain: Faith and Medicine in Neuroscience
Christianity and the Brain: Volume I: Faith and Medicine in Neuroscience Care
ISBNs: Softcover: **9780595424931**
Hardcover : **9780595884940**
E-Book : **9780595868278**

Iuniverse
1663 Liberty Drive
Bloomington, IN 47403
P: 800.288.4677
customer.service@iuniverse.com

2- Christianity and The Brain: The Human Brain and Illness Journey Between Earth and Heaven
Christianity and the Brain Volume II: The Christian Brain and the Journey between Earth and Heaven
ISBNs: Softcover: **9780595424955**
Hardcover **9780595884957**

E-Book : **9780595868292**

Iuniverse
1663 Liberty Drive
Bloomington, IN 47403
P: 800.288.4677
customer.service@iuniverse.com

3- Christianity and The Brain: Last Hour Journey
Christianity and the Brain : Volume III
ISBNs: Softcover: **9780595424962**
Hardcover **9780595884964**
E-Book : **9780595868308**

Iuniverse
1663 Liberty Drive
Bloomington, IN 47403
P: 800.288.4677
customer.service@iuniverse.com

4- Christianity and The Brain: Stories of 100 Patients1. CHRISTIANITY AND THE BRAIN: PATIENTS STORIES : Subtitle: 100 STORIES OF HOPE, FAITH AND COURAGE
ISBNs: Softcover: **9781450240437**
Hardcover **9781450240420**
E-Book : **9781450240444**

Iuniverse
1663 Liberty Drive
Bloomington, IN 47403
P: 800.288.4677
customer.service@iuniverse.com

5- A Christian from Egypt, a Life Story of a Neurosurgeon Pursuing The Dreams For Quintuple Board Certifications: Volume I of III My Journey in Egypt
Ebook: 9781499080520, Softcover: 9781499080537, Hardcover: 9781499080544 PID 537164
XLIBRIS
1663 Liberty Drive
Bloomington, IN 47403
P: 888.795.4274
F: 610.915.0294 / 812.355.4079
www.Xlibris.com

6- A Christian from Egypt, a Life Story of a Neurosurgeon Pursuing The Dreams For Quintuple Board Certifications: Volume II of III My American Journey

Ebook: 9781503534551, Softcover: 9781503534568, Hardcover: 9781503538092 PID 704437
XLIBRIS
1663 Liberty Drive
Bloomington, IN 47403
P: 888.795.4274
F: 610.915.0294 / 812.355.4079
www.Xlibris.com

7- A Christian from Egypt, a Life Story of a Neurosurgeon Pursuing The Dreams For Quintuple Board Certifications: Healthcare Experiences, Views and Patients Testimonials
Ebook: 9781503521438, Softcover: 9781503521452, Hardcover: 9781503521445 PID 634031
XLIBRIS
1663 Liberty Drive
Bloomington, IN 47403
P: 888.795.4274
F: 610.915.0294 / 812.355.4079
www.Xlibris.com

8- The Persecuted Human Brains in the Way to The Cross
Ebook: 9781524543112, Softcover: 9781524543129, Hardcover: 9781524543136 PID749887
XLIBRIS
1663 Liberty Drive
Bloomington, IN 47403
P: 888.795.4274
F: 610.915.0294 / 812.355.4079
www.Xlibris.com

9- The Spirit of Christ in the Human Brain and Neurosurgery: Personal Views
Ebook: 9781543449099, Softcover: 9781543449105, Hardcover: 9781543449112 PID 766755
XLIBRIS
1663 Liberty Drive
Bloomington, IN 47403
P: 888.795.4274
F: 610.915.0294 / 812.355.4079
www.Xlibris.com

10- Divinity and Satanism in the Human Brain: A Reflection of a Coptic Christian Brain Surgeon

Ebook: 9781543449075, Softcover: 9781543449075, Hardcover: 9781543449082 PID 766757
XLIBRIS
1663 Liberty Drive
Bloomington, IN 47403
P: 888.795.4274
F: 610.915.0294 / 812.355.4079
www.Xlibris.com

11- The Spiritual Journey of a Coptic Christian Brain Surgeon: View and Reflections
ISBN: 1532059647, 9781532059643
2018
Iuniverse
1663 Liberty Drive
Bloomington, IN 47403
P: 800.288.4677
customer.service@iuniverse.com

12- Touching Stories of My Life in Journey to Christian Holiness and Hands on Patients Care in a Weeping Healthcare: Volume 1 (2019) Touching stories of my Life in Journey to Christian Holiness and Hands- on Patient Care in a Weeping Healthcare: The Brain of Man of God and the Hand of Man of God Reflection of a Coptic Christian Neurosurgeon (Volume I)
Ebook: 9781796035087, Softcover: 9781796035094, Hardcover: 9781796035100 PID 795541
XLIBRIS
1663 Liberty Drive
Bloomington, IN 47403
P: 888.795.4274
F: 610.915.0294 / 812.355.4079
www.Xlibris.com

13- Touching Stories of My Life in Journey to Christian Holiness and Hands on Patients Care in a Weeping Healthcare: Volume 2 (2019)
Touching stories of my Life in Journey to Christian Holiness and Hands-on Patient Care in a Weeping Healthcare: The Brain of Man of God and the Hand of Man of God Reflection of a Coptic Christian Neurosurgeon (Volume II) Ebook: 9781796038903, Softcover: 9781796038910, Hardcover: 9781796038927 PID 795542
XLIBRIS
1663 Liberty Drive

Bloomington, IN 47403
P: 888.795.4274
F: 610.915.0294 / 812.355.4079
www.Xlibris.com

14- My Journey Volume I (2020)
XLIBRIS
1663 Liberty Drive
Bloomington, IN 47403
P: 888.795.4274
F: 610.915.0294 / 812.355.4079
www.Xlibris.com

15- **My Journey Volume II xlibrius (2020)**
Ebook: 9781796081824, Softcover: 9781796081831, Hardcover: 9781796081848 PID 803494
XLIBRIS
1663 Liberty Drive
Bloomington, IN 47403
P: 877.775.7551 ext: 7117
F: 812.355.4079
tami.seno@authorsolutions.com

XLIBRIS
1663 Liberty Drive
Bloomington, IN 47403
P: 888.795.4274
F: 610.915.0294 / 812.355.4079
www.Xlibris.com

16- **Coronavirus the Pandemic of the Century and the wrath of God**
Xlibris (2020) 978-1-9845-8166-2
1663 Liberty Drive
Bloomington, IN 47403
P: 888.795.4274
F: 610.915.0294 / 812.355.4079
www.Xlibris.com
To order:
https://www.amazon.com/s?k=books+by+ramsis+ghaly&dc&qid=1567370930&ref=aw_s_fkmr0

Publishers:

www.amazon.com
www.xlibris.com +1 (888) 795-4274
www.iuniverse.com +1 (800) 288-4677

17- **The Roses of Love Bloom in my Christianity and Neurosurgery Patients**
Xlibris Published (2022)
1663 Liberty Drive
Bloomington, IN 47403
P: 888.795.4274
F: 610.915.0294 / 812.355.4079
www.Xlibris.com

To order:
https://www.amazon.com/s?k=books+by+ramsis+ghaly&dc&qid=1567370930&ref=aw_s_fkmr0

Publishers:
www.amazon.com
www.xlibris.com +1 (888) 795-4274
www.iuniverse.com +1 (800) 288-4677

18- **The Unfolding COVID-19: my Thoughts, Memoirs and Patient' Stories**
xlibris (Published 2022)
1663 Liberty Drive
Bloomington, IN 47403
P: 888.795.4274
F: 610.915.0294 / 812.355.4079
www.Xlibris.com

To order:
https://www.amazon.com/s?k=books+by+ramsis+ghaly&dc&qid=1567370930&ref=aw_s_fkmr0

Publishers:
www.amazon.com
www.xlibris.com +1 (888) 795-4274
www.iuniverse.com +1 (800) 288-4677

19- **The Little Wasn't The Least After All! COVID Last as Events Progress!**
xlibris (published 2022)
1663 Liberty Drive
Bloomington, IN 47403
P: 888.795.4274
F: 610.915.0294 / 812.355.4079

www.Xlibris.com

To order:
https://www.amazon.com/s?k=books+by+ramsis+ghaly&dc&qid=1567370930&ref=aw_s_fkmr0

Publishers:
www.amazon.com
www.xlibris.com +1 (888) 795-4274
www.iuniverse.com +1 (800) 288-4677

Preface

Will the world ever recover from COVID-19? As a practicing Neurosurgeon and anesthesiologist, I haven't stop or close my practice. In contrary, I was much busier and happy to be in the frontline saving lives. The book contains not only my review to events occurred as the world began to recover from COVID-19 but also many of my medical and surgical adventures including patients' stories during 2022 as COVID-19 slowing down! This is my fifth book since COVID-19 started! The fear is that COVID-19 has caused a lifetime impact and healed with visible permanent scar. Perhaps, the year 2022 is post-COVID. Living at the Shadows represents the New Era of "Hybrid Remote Living" for years to come! Indeed, COVID may be gone but not its shadow and the long-term impact of Lockdown!! Time has passed and the world hasn't yet looked at how COVID-19 was handled and what lessons have been learned! Instead of celebrating Thanksgiving, among many others, the world witnessed post-COVID aggression! This book presents the author's personal views, reflections and experiences during 2022 post-COVID-19 period covered over 178 chapters and 14 sections! The reader will reflect on what could be the new "norms" and events evolved as the world attempts to recover from the pandemic of "COVID-19"! In 14 sections over 153 chapters.

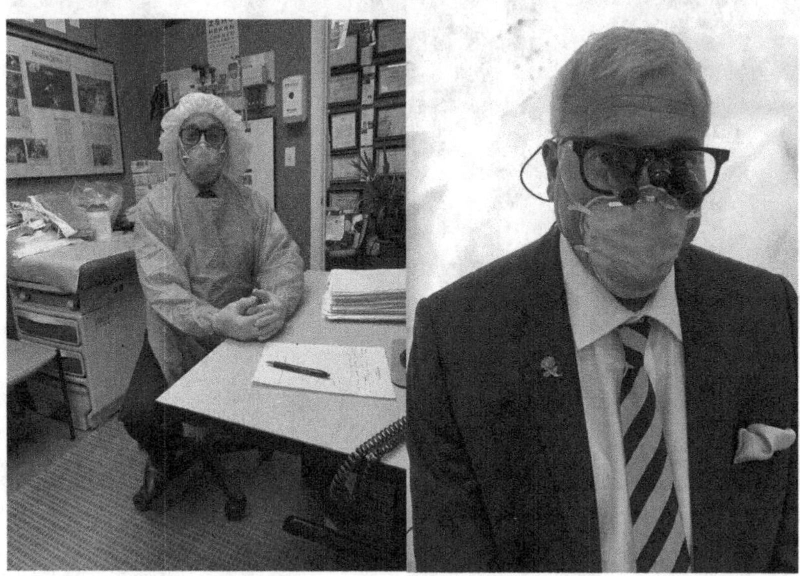

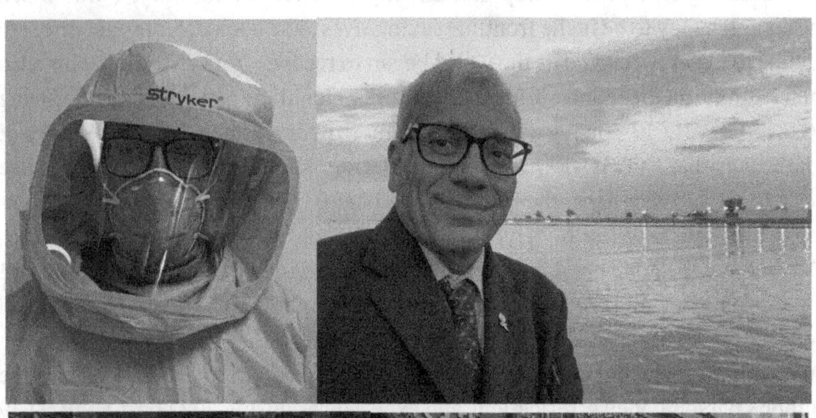
stryker

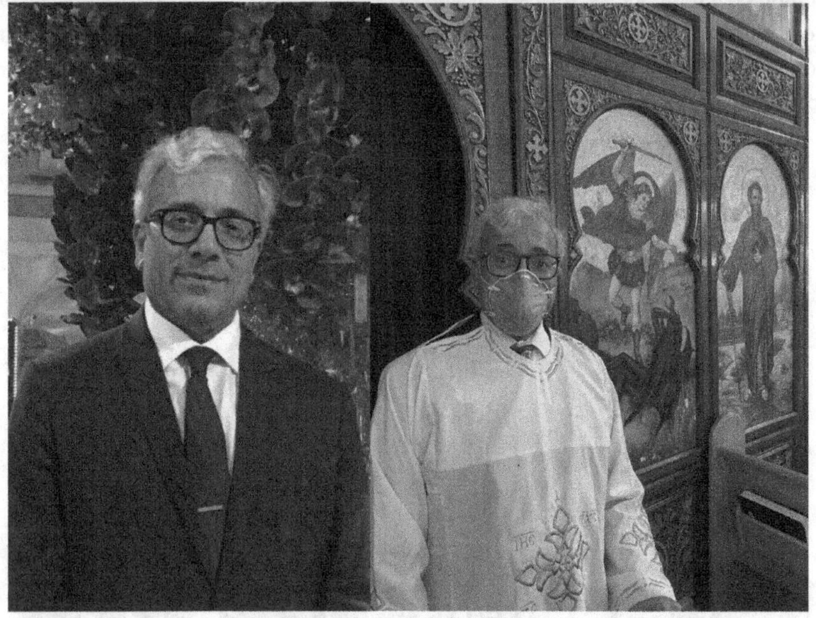

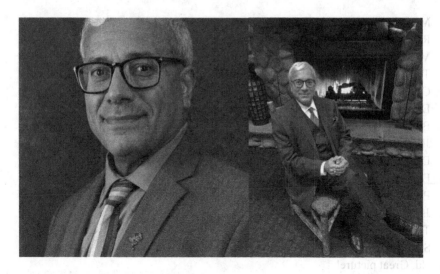

Ramsis Ghaly updated his cover photo.

CP, Very nice picture. :
Great picture
AK, Great picture
VA, Distinguished
SJ, Great picture
MA, Great picture
DE, That's a great picture!
LW, Looking good doctor....
MH, You look fabulous!
MW, Fabulous pic Dr Ghaly!
EL, Great picture Dr. Ghaly!!
CS, Yes he is
JV, Looking good
SKH, ou look amazing!
BM, Looking good
KO,Very nice picture Dr Ghaly
DM, Looks good
BV, Thankyou for who you are and what you do...sir....
DC, Very distinguished
SN, Great picture!
BV, Great picture
DK, Looking good, Dr. G!!!
Jb, Wonderful picture Dr.Ghaly. You look very distinguished!!
Jg, God Bless!
Mn, Looking good DrGhaly as always

Mn, That's a great picture!
Rh, You look great
Vw, Great picture!
Tw, Looking good, Dr. Ramsis Ghaly! You are a gift, my friend!
Cf, Great picture
Db, Such a wonderful picture…. Blessings to you Dr. Ghaly!
Bm, Very Handsome
Jk, Nice picture Doc.
Dn, Mk, Cg, That's a great picture!
Eo, Aren't you warm and cozy. Hugs and blessings.
Ph, Oh my. You look so charming. Quite a handsome man, as always.
Js, What a great picture!!
Tj, Professor, you look great.
Sm, I love this picture
Nd, Great picture!
Mc, Nice very nice.
Mh, Looking good My best doctor !!!
Th, Great photo
Vw, You look fabulous!
Jt, What a lovely picture!
Ya, NP, Awesome picture of a great man. Very blessed to know him.
BJ, Looking very presidential Dr.Ghaly!
LW, What a great photo!
KG, Very nice
BD, Blessing!!
ES, Great picture
ES, Love this picture.
JP, Lovely photo !
CG, So distinguished!!!
KE, Godly Doctor
Amen
KE, Love this picture
JC, Very nice!
KP, Great picture !
MH, One of my favorite pictures of you. Now that one belongs on a wall or desk.. absolutely stunning!
MH, A "Great Man!" Of God with an amazing talent for healing God's people.
CE, You sure look very respectable in this picture. I
feel privaleged to know you. You are such a great doctor!
MH, You should take another picture like this one. This time wear you rose pin on your jacket, then it will be perfect.
LL, Oh what a great picture!

HG, Yeah!!
Love this and you!
SS, Bella foto

TC, Looking good dr
LH, Very nice photo!
Have a beautiful weekend.
BCD, Love this picture you
CR, My dear doctor, you look so professional and good looking on this picture! Blessings and big hug.
BH, What a beautiful photo! You look healthy and happy! Excuse me though, don't you ever age dear Ramsis???!
DM, SE, Nice picture!
JM, "Excellent"
RM, Looking good G-Q look out
LH, Debonair, very handsome. Great photo!
TN, Nothing better than to be seated near a warm fire and looking so content with life.
EB, Nice picture Dr Ramsis
GK, Looking good Dr.Ramsis, may God bless you
PR, Good week beloved
GB, You look beautiful
HE, Very distinctive Professor!
KM, Great picture
RR, U handsome devil
JC, Great picture
RC, Great photo, superb physician!!
RP, MA, Love this picture
BV, JT, very handsome
JN, Great picture
VW, You're a class act, Dr. Ghaly!
CG, Love this picture
BC, Looking good
MM, Looking good
BM, ML, So handsome and scholarly looking .
KE, Love this picture
MH, Live the gray suite on you.
BH, So nice. Love the rose pin. Your smile is lovely. You love great. Frame this for your office.
JM, Wonderful Photo Dr. Ghaly
DW, RM, Looking good

Post COVID Living at the Shadows

Never Enough to Thank Our Lord Looking Back to COVID 19 Nightmare Time for Healing!

Written by Ramsis Ghaly

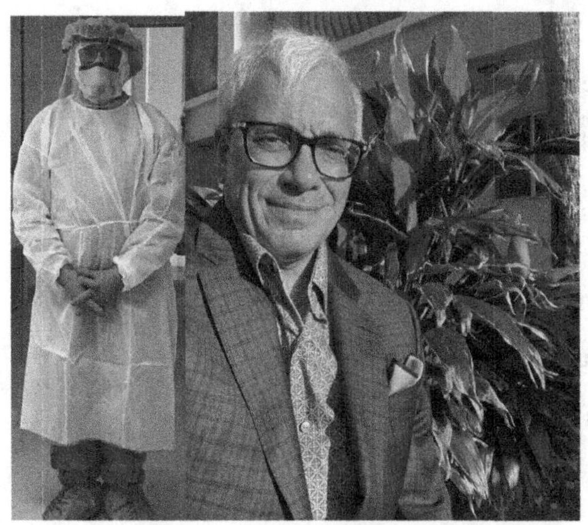

Never Enough to Thank Our Lord Looking Back to COVID-19 Nightmare!! Time for Healing!

In Comparison to orthodox Easter night of O4/23/2022 to that of 2020, Never Enough to Thank Our Lord!

Saturday morning Bright Saturday and Easter night 04/23/2023 a day to thank our Lord and Savior Jesus Christ from those two years of sickness and be completely gowned up, masked, isolated and distant away to return of life as our God always meant for mankind to live!!

It is the night to resurrection of our Savior who resurrected us from the world enemy COVID-19! Jesus rescued us from that evil virus !

Only you to thank O Lord and only You to praise Your Name Jesus. But not because of science of technology or wisdom but because of Your mercy and Grace, You brought us to this Free wide open day!!!

We shall never forgot those days of hell that imposed upon us throughout the world ! May God remember those lives were taken away and sufferers of COVID-19!

It is a time for Healing and ask for forgiveness and return to the Lord the Almighty!

“He sent out his word and healed them;

he rescued them from the grave.

Psalm 107:20

“Heal me, Lord, and I will be healed;

save me and I will be saved,

for you are the one I praise.”

Jeremiah 17:14

“Nevertheless, I will bring health and healing to it; I will heal my people and will let them enjoy abundant peace and security.” ~ Jeremiah 33:6

“The Lord gives sight to the blind,

the Lord lifts up those who are bowed down,

the Lord loves the righteous.”

Psalm 146:8

“So do not fear, for I am with you; do not be dismayed, for I am your God. I will strengthen you and help you; I will uphold you with my righteous right hand.” ~ Isaiah 41:10

“If you listen carefully to the Lord your God and do what is right in his eyes, if you pay attention to his commands and keep all his decrees, I will not bring on you any of the diseases I brought on the Egyptians, for I am the Lord, who heals you.”

Exodus 15:26

“if my people, who are called by my name, will humble themselves and pray and seek my face and turn from their wicked ways, then I will hear from heaven, and I will forgive their sin and will heal their land. Now my eyes will be open and my ears attentive to the prayers offered in this place.” ~ 2 Chronicles 7:14-15

“I have seen their ways, but I will heal them; I will guide them and restore comfort to Israel’s mourners, creating praise on their lips. Peace, peace, to those far and near,” says the LORD. “And I will heal them.” ~ Isaiah 57:18-19

Psalm 150

“Praise ye the Lord. Praise God in his sanctuary: praise him in the firmament of his power. [2] Praise him for his mighty acts: praise him according to his excellent greatness. [3] Praise him with the sound of the trumpet: praise him with the psaltery and harp. [4] Praise him with the timbrel and dance: praise him with stringed instruments and organs. [5] Praise him upon the loud cymbals: praise him upon the high sounding cymbals. [6] Let every thing that hath breath praise the Lord. Praise ye the Lord.”

“Come to me, all you who are weary and burdened, and I will give you rest. Take my yoke upon you and learn from me, for I am gentle and humble in heart, and you will find rest for your souls. For my yoke is easy and my burden is light.” ~ Matthew 11:28-30

“LORD, be gracious to us; we long for you. Be our strength every morning, our salvation in time of distress.” ~ Isaiah 33

JS, praise to LORD JESUS CHRIST

RF, God is good and so is Dr.Ghaly.

AV, Amen!

GH, Thank you Dr. Ghaly. I saved this post. Very healing verses, as I’m a Covid frontline worker as well.

KO, God bless your day and all front line workers

Bless us o Lord and hold those in your arms that passed on and unto the families that lost there loved ones, in JESES NAME.

Post COVID Living at the Shadows The New Era of "Hybrid Remote Living"

Written on 8/24/2022 by Ramsis Ghaly

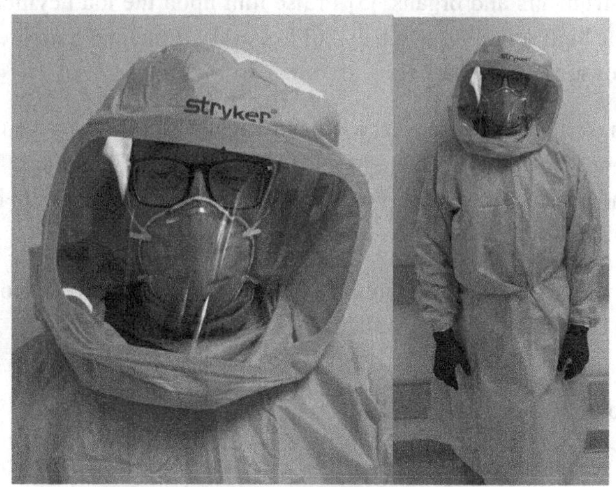

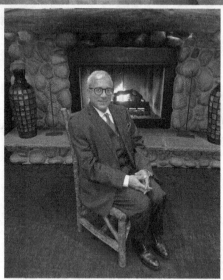

Post-COVID Living at the Shadows!! The New Era of "Hybrid Remote Living"

COVID may be gone but not it's shadow!! The Impact of Lockdown!!

Have those in-charge of worldwide lockdown asked themselves what the Implications of two-year straight Government and Science COVID Restrictions could Impose on the Longterm as a result of Side effects of Lockdown, Physical Distance, Outdoors Restrains and Social Isolation Might be??

Has COVID Lockdown Killed Return to Pre-COVID Open Living?

Pre-COVID Norm may Not be post-COVID Norm!!

Post-COVID NORMs:

- Minimal Hands on, Limited Hands Touch, Wireless, Paperless, Telecommunications and digital informatics are the foundations of the New Norm!

-Zoom Forever Telecom Work Technology is getting more and more widespread effective and innovative to the degree that it is so attractive to the new generations that lockdown social isolation and restricted in-person living were taken away and technology took over their thinking!!

- More self-independence and perhaps more efficient since it is based in the person's schedule, body needs and costumed accordingly to that specific person and not to HR human resource corporate doctrine: Take a break when needs, no eyes watching over, no ears listening over, conducting duties in a familiar environment non-threatening atmosphere and comfortable surrounding! All these can enhance very much satisfaction and productivity

-Pre-COVID Traditional Workplace transfigured to Post-COVID Zoom Workplace!

-Pre-COVID Traditional Full Suit, stir, Shirt, Cufflinks and shining shoes to Post-COVID upper body and face shorty suit attached to leg pajama and sandals !

-Pre-COVID Traditional Dress, Skirt and high heal shoes to Post-COVID upper dress attached to lower body kitchen cloth with slippers !

-Pre-COVID Traditional early awakening up and drive with luxury car or in time catching a train to Post-COVID In-House next door walk!

-Pre-COVID Traditional in-person standing before a crowd addressing the audience face-to-face to Post-COVID laptop communication with mute/unmute, video/ no video computer Camera Microsoft Team/ Zoom Telecommunication!

- Pre-COVID Traditional Hands-on Care to Post-COVID Hands-On Care!

- Pre-COVID Thousands of Years Traditional Human Touch living to Post-COVID Non-Human Touch living!

Mind Dazzling Thoughts??

- Remote work has proven to be table stakes to employees and the COVID pandemic has challenged the conventional thinking in other ways —perhaps permanently!

- Many see no issues of limited in-person social connections and being accustomed to the flexibility that comes with virtual reality from less time to commute to more time with family and pets, watching TV, Netflix and thousands of channels various virtual entertainments, listening to music and day and night in various social media!

- How Convenient has been to order anything a person needs on-Demand, anytime from anyplace to deliver at the home steps On-Line, going through thousands of choices and doesn't matter what ranging from shopping to remodeling to dining to processing applications —!

-Scared to return back to work, to school, to social gathering!

-Afraid to go back to Pre-COVID life to the open! Anxious to get out of thy shell !

-Concern about contracting more new strains of viruses or spread of new variants or more of evil man-made infectious Bioweapons!

-But perhaps, Thou might be so comfortable to live virtual at the Shadows of COVID-19!! Thou might be so happy to continue living behind the scenes operating through virtual reality and telecommunication!! What about you??? Are you feeling the same way??

-Why should thy go back and in live in person again?

-Why should thy go back to school?

-Why should thy go back to work?

-Why should thy go back to in person meeting?

-Why should thy join a crowd or concert or a party ever again?

-Why shouldn't thy be able to continue to work from home ?

-Why should thy get up get dressed and travel far from my comfort home?? How can I run away from my last two years of great lifestyle and perfect hone set up!! I am so content to have a working station in my bedroom, entertainment center next room with two huge 85-inch Television, play table in the basement, and secret Bar to my fulfillment at my private room and a gorgeous scenery at my balcony with a little telescope 🔭!!

- After two years of nationwide law of extreme restriction, thy love to be in my own and be with my family and don't have to his a Nanny or care giver!!

- In fact, it is pathetic to spend money in gasoline and drive miles away in traffic if I can work from home!! It just doesn't make sense and it never add on!!

- Who wants to return to old offices flock back to old building try to make it in time climbing up the stairs catching the elevators saluting unwelcoming faces and pushing through the traffic crossing busy intersections, waiting in lines, hurrying up before the signals turn red going downstairs for lunch break at the Subways, Portillo's or McDonald's??? Who and Why??

Thy so comfortable to live virtual at the Shadows!! Thy is so happy to continue living virtual away from the eyes and ears of others!

There are No worries about dad and mom and their generations!! They are going away and the new world will be all the younger generations and the New Breed!

Post-COVID Child Education

Almost 10 million children may never return to school following COVID-19 lockdown

World is facing a hidden education emergency

COVID-19 leaves estimated $77 billion gap in education spending for world's poorest children

Children in 12 countries are at extremely high risk of dropping out of school forever

In another 28 countries children are at moderate or high risk of not going back to school

Girls are at increased exposure to gender-based violence and risk of child marriage and teen pregnancy during school closures

Save the Children calls for increased funding of education, including conversion of debt liabilities into investment in children

https://reliefweb.int/.../almost-10-million-children-may...

https://hbswk.hbs.edu/.../covid-killed-the-traditional...

Where is the wisdom these days?

+ Let us stand together to fight for the future of our children and the premier existence of our life long live mankind!!

+Thou must stand strong to defend the freedom of living free and to the open!

+Thou must Neither be afraid Nor be threatened or intimidated to resume our forefather's way of living!

+ Thou must Not allow Industry, technology, corporate and government-imposed doctrine to take over our wellbeing as fearless children of God born in the Image of the Most High and He is greater than those against the established Godly Values!

+ Get engaged to design the future of our children to enjoy life as it was created since the beginning in the wide open to the nature to the people and to the world !

+ Thou be Instrumental to make a difference and stay in solidarity for the goodness of humanity for the post-COVID generation!

Jm, AGREE!!!

Cr, Thanks for being a truth teller. And dressing like a gentleman!!!

CG. Covid was about control and has affected so many lives and livelihoods. Our children have suffered because of covid and some schools are still requiring masks. Why???Our government has controlled everything for the last 2 years and continues to do so...

This one of my favorite pictures of you.

Ongoing COVID

Written on 9.4/22

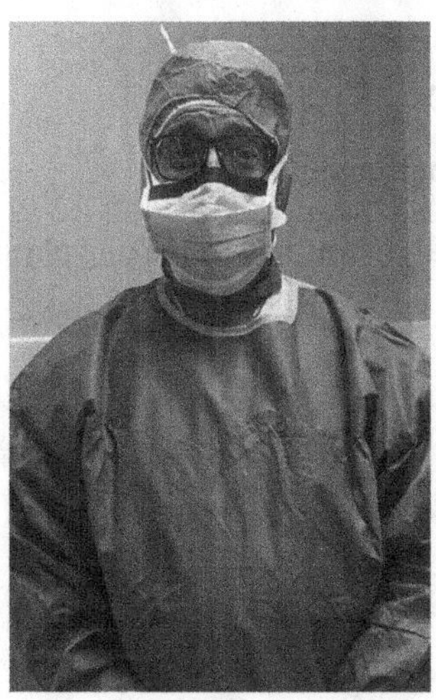

We still intubate and care for COVID patients yesterday a child and today an adult! I won't ease my PPE and Universal Precautions!!

So many years to care, teach and serve for years and years!! I consider it, my Lord Jesus honorable gift to me to serve His children!! Honored and privileged!!

Ramsis Ghaly

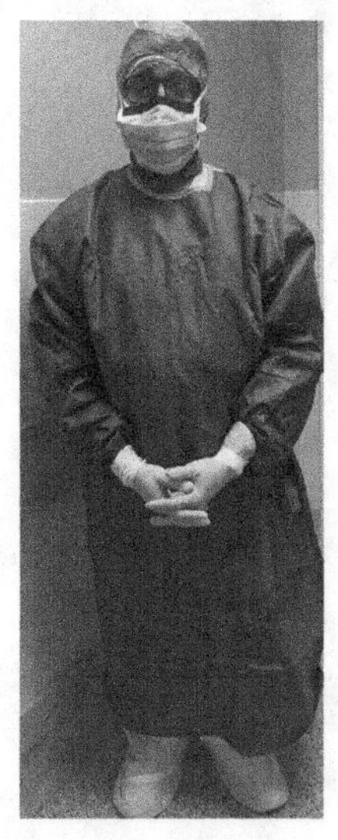

KO, Thank you for caring and love of all your patients you always give undivided love to them all,God bless you always Dr Ghaly

MS, Are you using zpac and ivermectin as protocols?

Hydrochloriquine?

V, God bless you Dr Ghaly.

SC, The doctor in action outstanding!

SR, God bless you Dr. Ghaly!! You are an amazing physician and teacher!! I miss working with you!

Post COVID Memorial Day!

Written on 5/30/22 by <u>Ramsis Ghaly</u>

As we all are going through hardest tines especially following COVID, Inflation and Recession and ongoing wars, today more than ever we remember those sacrificed their lives, efforts, times and whatever they have to others to make our country America great!!! It is the only country that serve the world to protect Freedom and the good cause of humanity!! Honor their Memory and Heroism!!!

I wish to share a Peom I wrote for you in the Memorial Day to celebrate you who sacrificed your lives for the USA and me, you and all:

In the Memorial Day, the American Flag is Up High and the Freedom of the Soul is Flying High and the Lord Jesus Blessing USA"

In peace I leave you, in love I let you go, in faith I will see you again, I did my part and you will do your part and in the Name of Lord, you remain one nation.

To you, I owe my life, to you I kneel with respect, to you I took off my hate and bow my head, your memories always alive and I will never forget you

FOR YOU THOSE SACRIFICED THEIR LIVES FOR OTHERS

Before you left me, I did not have a chance to say, I "Love You",

Before you departed, I did not express my gratitude,

Before they took your life, I did not show my appreciation,

I just wanted to say "You are my love and my pride"

Although I wanted to cry for the lives of those that sacrificed their lives for you, me and others,

Although I want to share my deep sadness of the lives that were taken away prematurely,

Although my heart is full of sorrows and condoles

Although my tears are running and my heart is broken with memories,

But today I will hide my tears and sadness,

But Today I will dress with the garment of joy,

I just wish to say "Thank You",

To you, I owe my life, to you I kneel with respect, to you I took off my gate and bow my head, your memories always alive and I will never forget you

To you all, I share my Poem written from my heart with fingers of love and wiped with tears of my eyes,

In the Memorial Day, the American Flag is Up High and the Freedom of the Soul is Flying High and the Lord Jesus Blessing USA"

In peace I leave you, in love I let you go, in faith I will see you again, I did my part and you will do your part and in the Name of Lord, you remain one nation.

To you, I owe my life, to you I kneel with respect, to you I took off my gate and bow my head, your memories always alive and I will never forget you

MEMORIAL IS LOVE AND LOVE IS MEMORIAL

LOVE LOVE LOVE LOVE

As God is Love so America is Love and so each of you is Love

"Greater love has no man than this, that a man lay down his life for his friends" (John 15:13)

"13Greater love hath no man than this, that a man lay down his life for his friends.
14Ye are my friends, if ye do whatsoever I command you. 15Henceforth I call you
not servants; for the servant knoweth not what his lord doeth: but I have called you
friends; for all things that I have heard of my Father I have made known unto you.
16Ye have not chosen me, but I have chosen you, and ordained you, that ye should
go and bring forth fruit, and that your fruit should remain: that whatsoever ye shall
ask of the Father in my name, he may give it you. 17These things I command you,
that ye love one another." (John 25:13-17)

They are my brothers, they are my sisters,

They are my parents, they are my children,

They are my siblings, they are my friends

For you all, I am ready to go and sacrifice my soul,

I can not be silent, I am no more silent,

I no longer could be quiet,

It is my time to stand up and defend them all,

This is life, people come and go

This is life souls live and die,

This is life, evilness and goodness together both grow,

This is life, love defeats hate and sacrifice brings victory

My Lord Jesus put His life for me and others, It is my time to do the same,

There is no love more than one put himself for others as Jesus said "Greater love has no man than this, that a man lay down his life for his friends" John 15:13

My friends, I am honored to lay down my life for you all,

It is the love I have for you and soon I will be with the Lord of Love, my Beloved Jesus our Almighty,

It will be tough and harsh, pain and torque to my physical body waiting for me, but to the Crucified My eyes are steadfast,

No matter how much I will suffer, for you all as my Lord Jesus taught me, I will look at Jerusalem soon it will be my eternal home,

CROSS CROSS CROSS CROSS

TODAY I AM CARRYING MY CROSS FOR YOU

"Then said Jesus unto his disciples, If any man will come after me, let him deny himself, and take up his cross, and follow me. 25For whosoever will save his life shall lose it: and whosoever will lose his life for my sake shall find it. 26For what is a man profited, if he shall gain the whole world, and lose his own soul? or what shall a man give in exchange for his soul? 27For the Son of man shall come in the glory of his Father with his angels; and then he shall reward every man according to his works." Matthew (16:24-27)

It is the time to go and carry my cross remembering My Lord Jesus as He said,

I was waiting for this moment to lay down my life for you,

For you I will die, for you I will deny myself,

Indeed for you I will not save my life, for you I will be the first to go,

You know I love you all so much and the live in me is from my Heavenly Father,

I could not just let it go, it will be selfish of me not to do so,

I know I left behind my newly born child and children,

I know I left behind my everything I have, my wife,

I know I left behind my lovely parents,

I know I left behind my sisters and brothers,

I know I left behind my friends and many more,

I am so sad, I am so sad,

The tears are shedding,

My heart is crying,

I had to keep it to myself,

I can not let you go but I must do,

You know I adore you,

You know I love you,

You know I do not want to leave you,

You my daughter, my son, my wife, my mother, my father, my sister, my brother and my friends

It was not easy to make the decision it my commitment to the Most High,

I know my Heavenly Father will be Your Father and one day He will put us all together again in His Heavenly Jerusalem,

What shall I say, today, in the steps of my crucified Lord, I am walking,

Tomorrow, I will rise again with my Lord Jesus Who denied His glory to redeem me the sinner of all,

For now there is nothing left for me her in the world, my call is at hand,

For you all I leave my love and you all keep the faith and strive to do the same for each other,

My Lord Jesus said "A new commandment I give unto you, That ye love one another; as I have loved you, that ye also love one another. By this shall all men know that ye are my disciples, if ye have love one to another." (John 13: 34-35),

In the Memorial Day, the American Flag is Up High and the Freedom of the Soul is Flying High and the Lord Jesus Blessing USA"

The Lord Jesus founded our home America and He is keeping it safe and prosperous for our coming children,

As my flesh is dying and my soul is ascending, I will pray for you saying

"May God Bless you all and May God Bless USA"

Goodbye to you all and in the Memorial Day remember me as I remember you before the Lamb of God,

You may not cry for me because of what I have done but know you all are worthy of my sacrifice and before my lord Jesus I commend my soul,

May the Lord accept my soul and the sacrifice and make me worthy to be with Him in eternity,

In peace I leave you, in love I let you go, in faith I will see you again, I did my part and you will do your part and in the Name of Lord, you remain one nation.

My blood is shed for you, my prayers always for you and may the Lord protect you

Rise and celebrate the Memorial Day,

By your home, by your neighbors, by your city, it is a feast day the day I died for you

AS GOD IS LOVE, SO ANERICA IS LOVE AND SO EACH OF YOU IS LOVE

As God is Love so America is Love and so each of you is Love

(1 John 4:7-21) God Is Love

"7 Beloved, let us love one another, because love is from God; everyone who loves is born of God and knows God. 8 Whoever does not love does not know God, for God is love. 9 God's love was revealed among us in this way: God sent his only Son into the world so that we might live through him. 10 In this is love, not that we loved God but that he loved us and sent his Son to be the atoning sacrifice for our sins. 11 Beloved, since God loved us so much, we also ought to love one another. 12 No one has ever seen God; if we love one another, God lives in us, and his love is perfected in us.

13 By this we know that we abide in him and he in us, because he has given us of his Spirit. 14 And we have seen and do testify that the Father has sent his Son as the Savior of the world. 15 God abides in those who confess that Jesus is the Son of God, and they abide in God. 16 So we have known and believe the love that God has for us. God is love, and those who abide in love abide in God, and God abides in them. 17 Love has been perfected among us in this: that we may have boldness

on the day of judgment, because as he is, so are we in this world. 18 There is no fear in love, but perfect love casts out fear; for fear has to do with punishment, and whoever fears has not reached perfection in love. 19 We love because he first loved us. 20 Those who say, "I love God," and hate their brothers or sisters, are liars; for those who do not love a brother or sister whom they have seen, cannot love God whom they have not seen. 21 The commandment we have from him is this: those who love God must love their brothers and sisters also.

Mh, Thank you to all military who served our country to protect us

Ma, Kg, And Thank You, Dr **Ramsis Ghaly**, for the greatest sacrifice of yourself that you give the world on a daily basis. You are truly an Angel, A Blessing on Earth.

God Bless all of our heroes for their ultimate sacrifices.

Dn, Beautifully said Praise God Amen

Av, Jm, THANK YOU TO ALL WHO HAVE PROTECTED US AND OUR COUNTRY

Dl, Praise the Lord Jesus Christ. May all their souls RIP.

Mn, Very well said DrGhaley

Cg, This is wonderful and I am sure it will touch the hearts of all who read it.

Our freedom isn't free. May we never forget those who gave up their freedom. For ours.

Rc, G9d blessall Who sacrifice ho and her lides for USA

Photo Comparison 2017/2020!

Ramsis Ghaly

As I was searching through memoirs of my personal photos, I realized the huge difference in the photo dated July 17, 2017, and that dated July 17, 2020!!!

2020: Indoors, locked down with facemask full of serious concerns terrorized by daily news snd politics!

Verses

2017: Outdoor, absolutely free running around with No facemask full of joy careless about politics!!

What a nightmare was COVID-19 Impact and restriction made in the worldwide!!

How many people worldwide have shared the nightmare of COVID-19 and Politics as displayed in photos!!

Modern medicine was defeated and so is pharmaceuticals and smartness of man. But yet in His glory, God rescued His children and saved the world from the evilness of man!

"Because the foolishness of God is wiser than men; and the weakness of God is stronger than men. [26] For ye see your calling, brethren, how that not many wise men after the flesh, not many mighty, not many noble, are called : [27] But God hath chosen the foolish things of the world to confound the wise; and God hath chosen the weak things of the world to confound the things which are mighty; [30] But of him are ye in Christ Jesus, who of God is made unto us wisdom, and righteousness, and sanctification, and redemption: [31] That, according as it is written, He that glorieth, let him glory in the Lord."1 Corinthians 1:25-27,30-31 KJV

But now all gone in prayers! As the world ease to norms and return back to free and open world as mankind was created for, May God the Almighty Lord of Healing who provided the entire world with Free natural immunity in each human being to fight the daily natural disasters but also man-made disasters, to continue to heal us, protect us and bless all His people worldwide!! Amen in Jesus Name!!

"It is of the Lord's mercies that we are not consumed, because his compassions fail not. [23] They are new every morning: great is thy faithfulness. [24] The Lord is my portion, saith my soul; therefore will I hope in him. [51] Mine eye affecteth mine heart because of all the daughters of my city. [52] Mine enemies chased me sore, like a bird, without cause. [53] They have cut off my life in the dungeon, and cast a stone upon me. [54] Waters flowed over mine head; then I said, I am cut off. [55] I called upon thy name, O Lord, out of the low dungeon. [56] Thou hast heard my voice: hide not thine ear at my breathing, at my cry. [57] Thou drewest near in the day that I called upon thee: thou saidst, Fear not. [58] O Lord, thou hast pleaded the causes of my soul; thou hast redeemed my life. [59] O Lord, thou hast seen my wrong: judge thou my cause."Lamentations 3:22-24,51-59 KJV

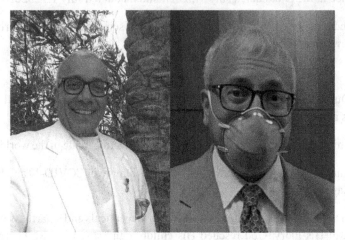

LK, A true heart shines bright inside and out. You will always be a beautiful soul. I miss you

CG, I thank God everyday that nightmare is over. With a smile or a mask you are still the same caring doctor.

First Convention Post COVID 2/23/2022: Back to Pre-Covid Slowly But Surely!

Attending the Spine Summit 2022 convention with renown neurosurgeon/ spine surgeon. I attended the last one in the immediate pre-COVID 2020 and this is the first pos-tCovid!! No masks, No boasts no testing!!

With the best spine surgeons and newest technology ranging from conventional navigation to robots to virtual reality and many more!!!

Ramsis Ghaly

Www.ghalyneurosurgeon.com

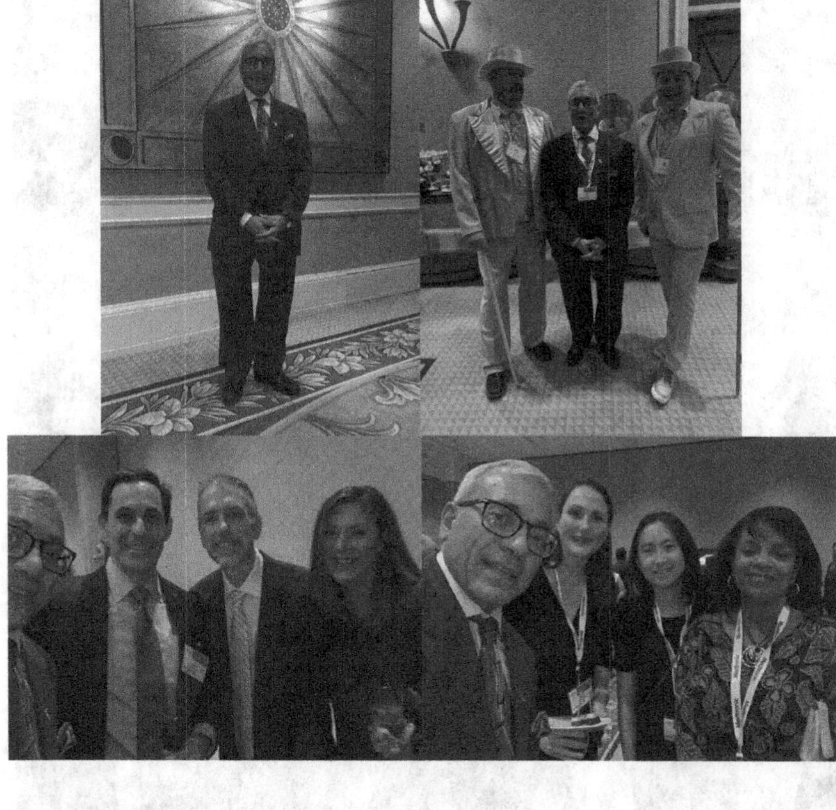

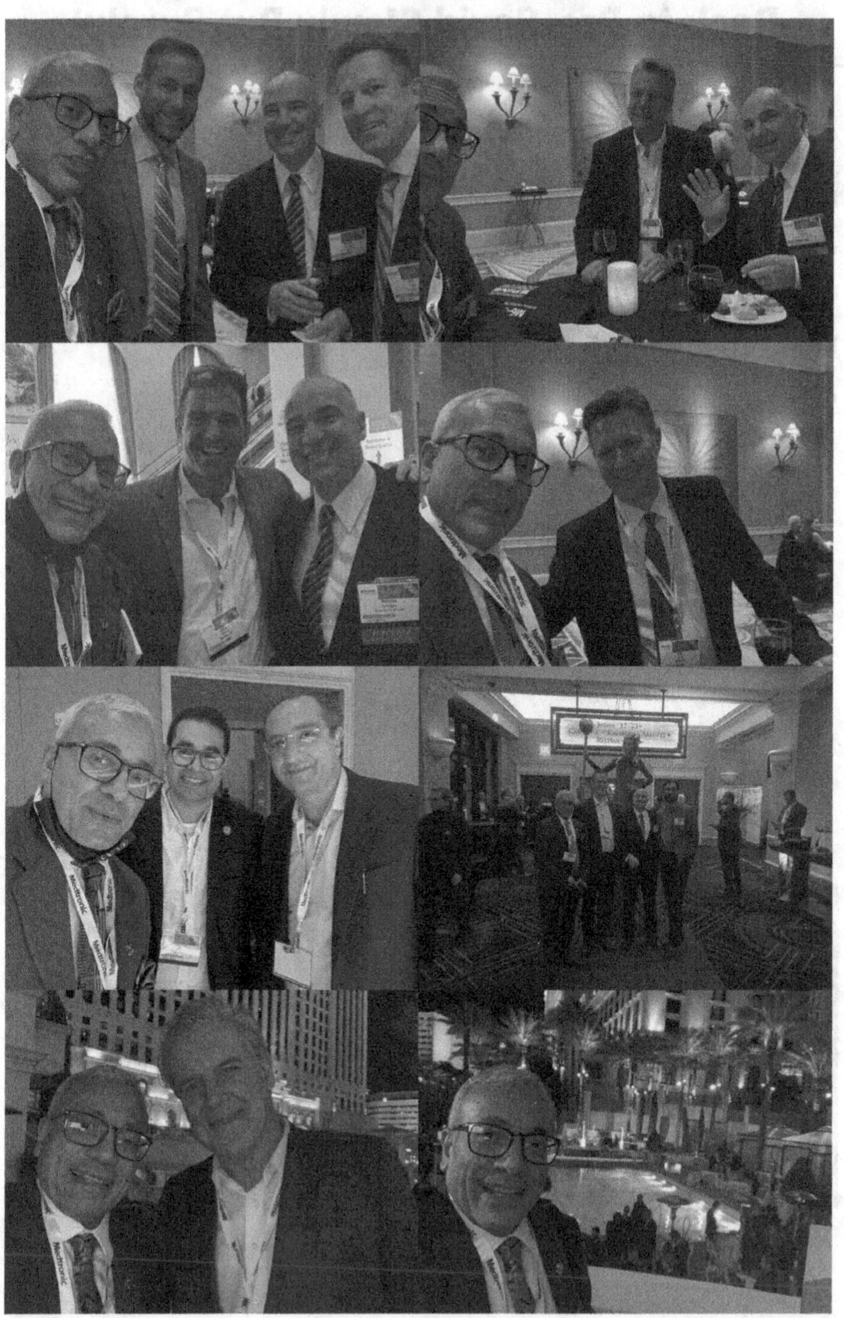

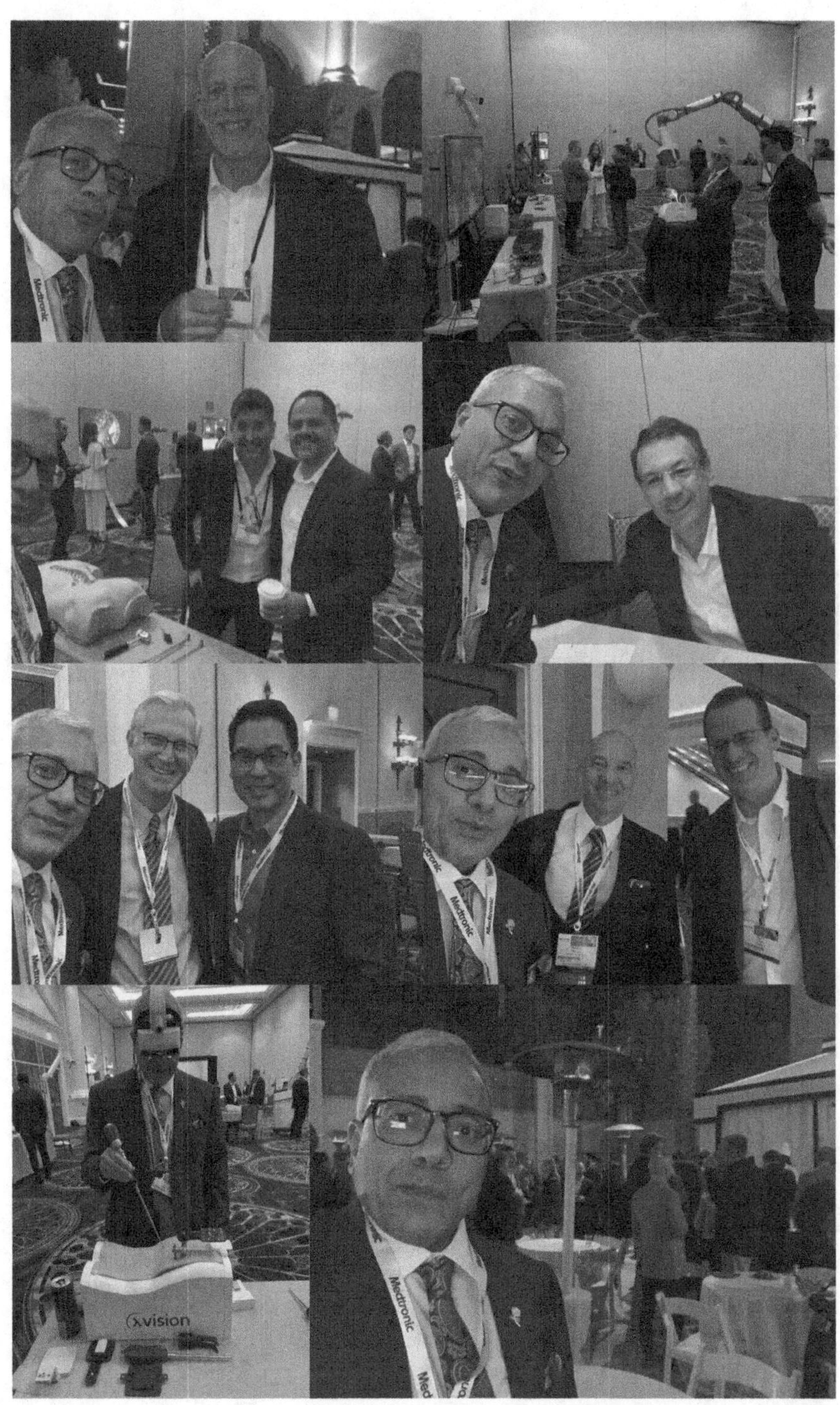
Medtronic
xvision

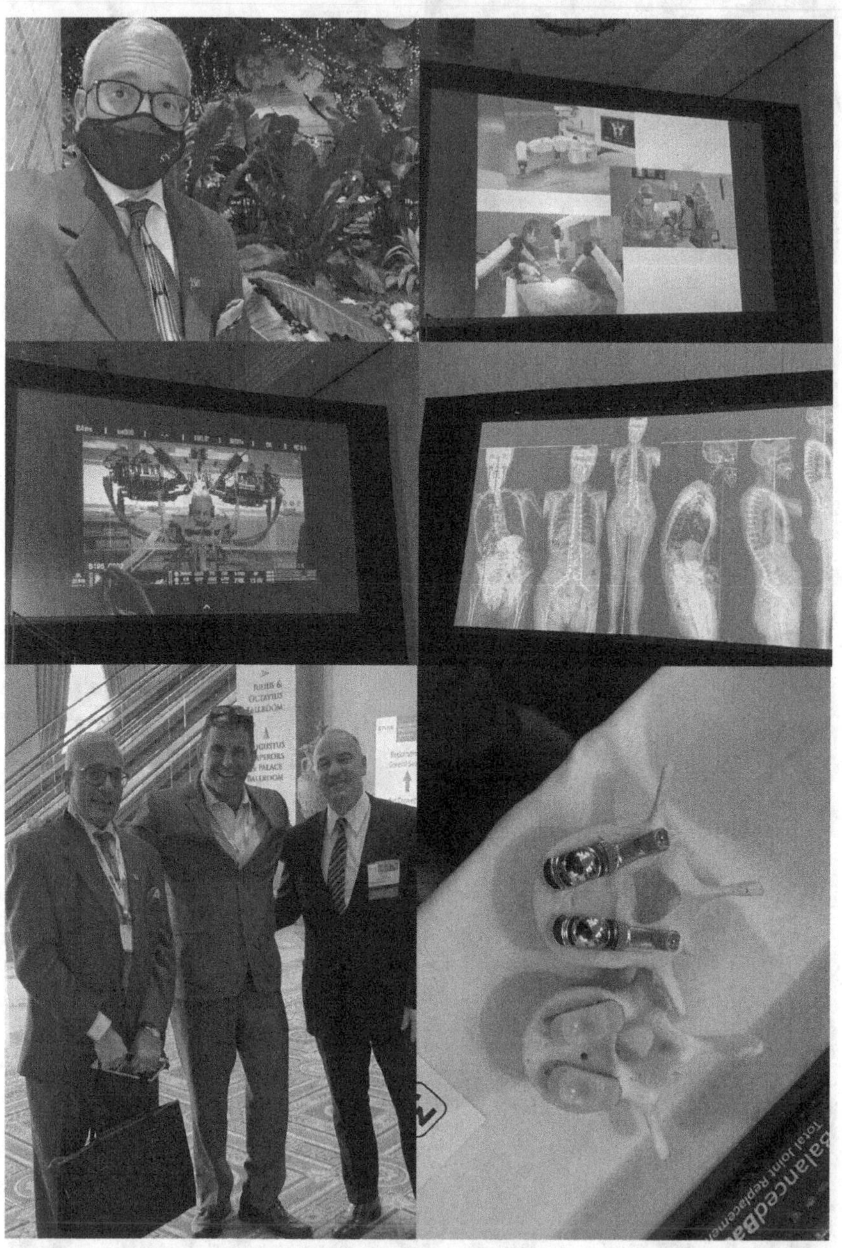
JULIUS &
OCTAVIUS
PALACE

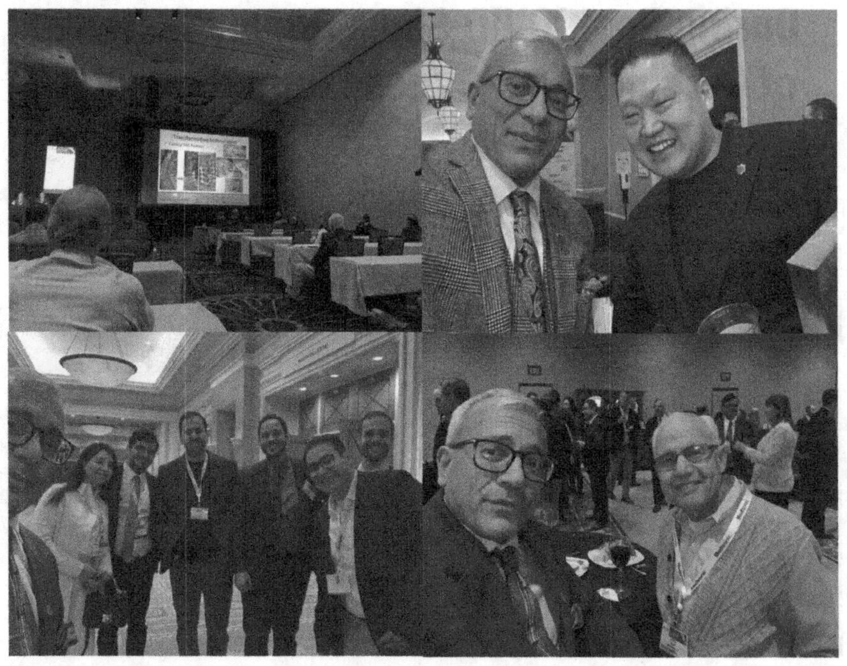

CG. Always learning to better help your patients. Blessings

SG. egas...Caesars Palace

<u>**JC.**</u> Love your work Ramsis

DH, Amazing stuff Dr Ghaly, you sure know alit of doctors

I NEED HELP TO WORK RIGHT AGAIN SO I CAN MAKE IT WALKING TO MAILBOX

JT, we need to get back to normal...enough with all this masking and mandatory shots and restrictions for everyone...natural immunity works....it is time to let people decide for themselves now!!!

DR, Great looking bunch of docs! Thank you all for everything you do! Masks off, only in the OR!

AV, Fantastic! God Bless you!

MH, Finally we can breath again, no more wearing our mask. Thank you Jesus praise the Lord. What a glorious day. You all look “Great!”

During PostCOVID Short Supply Instead of Cursing the darkness light a candle!

Written by Ramsis Ghaly

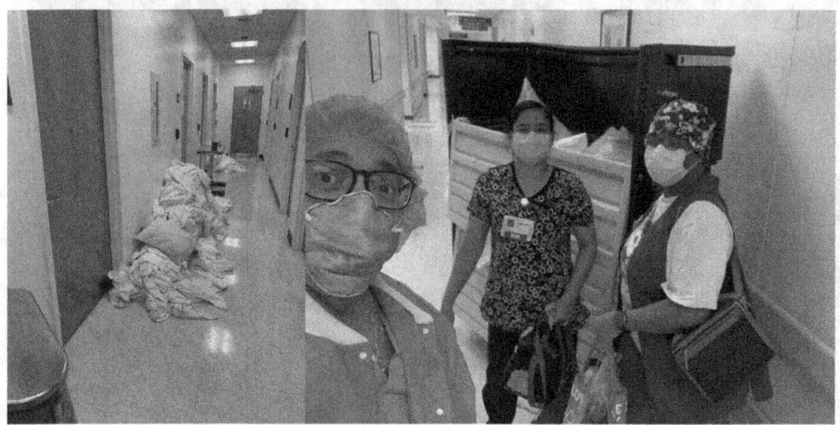

There was so many complaints about short of supplies and resources at JSH of Cook County hospital! Cook county hospital is one of the best public service to all people, all races, all socioeconomic classes from extreme poverty to the wealthy. Cook county hospital save lives regardless who they are and whatever the cost was or us or will be! It is the best charity organization ever exist for hundreds of years and it's mission never changed.

For more than week, the on call rooms were piled up with dirty linen by the hallway and they are complaining but no one took to himself or herself and clear the hallway and recycle the dirty linens. They all had been sending emails with complaints!!

I arrived this morning with a task to do. I found Felicia and Aisha from PACU ready to go home. I asked if they can volunteer with me. Both were so delighted to go so!

Three of us went to the on call room and cleaned the hallway. We pulled all the linen in the cart. The dirty linen are in way to be cleaned.

We love cook county and we are honored to be part of such a magnificent organization. For thirty six years, day and night I am proud to be part of it and to serve! I will never ever make fool out of the most living, giving charity helping organization serving our patient and greater metropolitan area!

I learned the British saying: “Instead of Cursing the darkness, light a candle”

Thank you for your service. Happy Father’s Day and June 20 Juneteenth celebrating the end of slavery!!

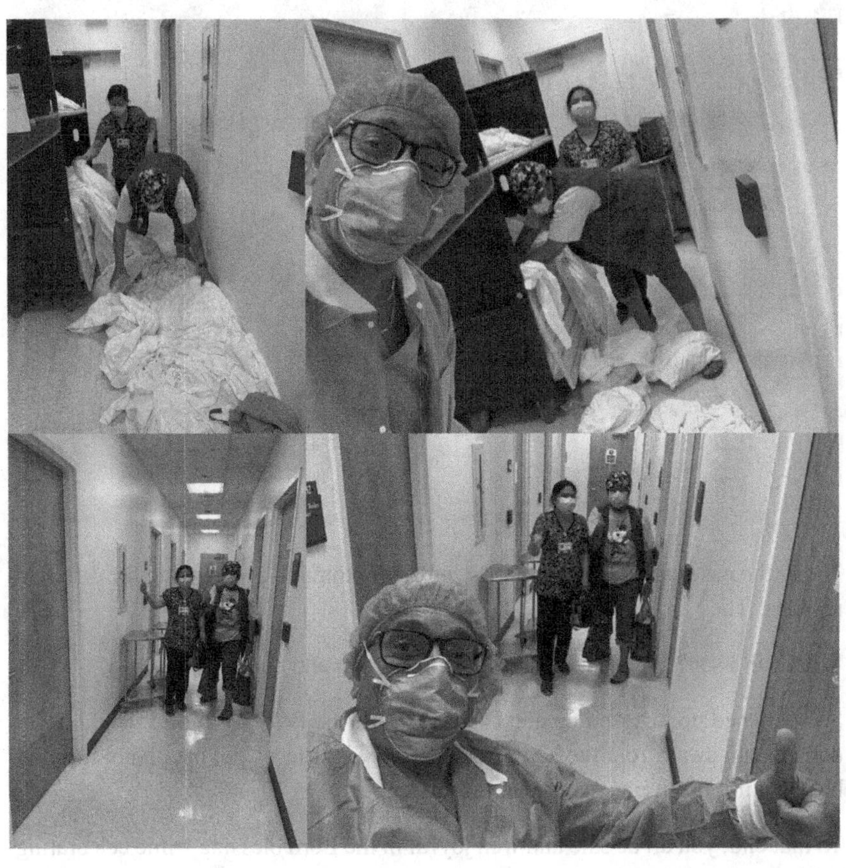

Mild COVID in the Rise!

Written By Ramsis Ghaly on 5/8/2022

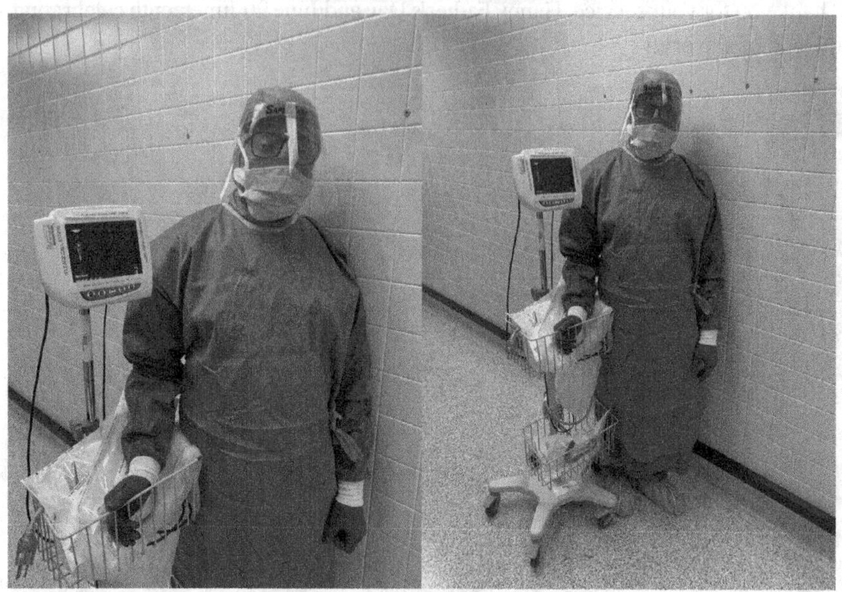

Today the cases are COVID positive but asymptomatic and coming for different reasons! They are on the rise!!

What can I say? We must keep going! Be caution and continue to serve!

So I gowned up, masked up and cared for patients. But one thing I would never do is to run away from the battlefield that my Lord Jesus put me on not turn my back from it or give an excuse not to participate!

To that end, you all be safe and well joyful in the Lord blessing while celebrating Mother's Day! Amen!

Ramsis Ghaly

CG, You never would turn your back on anyone who needs help. Bless you!!

DH, You are the kindest, God is with you Dr Ghaly

DL, I have a question...are the positive cases you are seeing Vaxxed patients ?

Post COVID Lockdown Continues until 2024!

Written on 06/03/2022 by Ramsis Ghaly

Lockdown Continues until 2024 due to Man-made disasters!

For two years 2019-2022, nations are forced to stay home because of man- made pandemic and forced social isolation and physical distancing!!

For coming two years 2022-2024, nations are forced to stay home because of man-made gasoline Oil crises and sky high prices as economy is crashing!

Just think: man-made Gas prices overtake man-made COVID crises!!

Every day passes by, supplies are getting expensive and reaching unheard of dollars!! The cost of living is skyrocketing and so is the prices of even basic living!!

The first two year lockdown was to prevent the spread of virus COPVID-19 and the current next two year lock down is because of the rise in cost, save money and inability to afford going out!

Businesses are moving away from hands-on in-person to virtual and distance away to save money in oil prices and decrease expenditure. The wars especially Russia/ Ukraine and fear of more wars such as China/ Taiwan are worsening the world condition increasing the poverty. Furthermore, the ongoing fear of more virus strains and new viruses such Monkey box is scarring so many. And as opportunistic self serves money hungry corporates and individuals use these circumstances to make money and serve themselves, the forced lockdown secondary to extreme poverty conditions and save money will continue!!

The entire world is in turmoil, stumbling and their heads are spinning. These lockdowns had drastically changed their routine and life living. Many have lost their life some due to sickness, others through mental health crisis and many more through aggression, hostility, violence, crimes, enraging and frustration with loss of hope and find themselves lonely with no support and no reason to living!!

Through these man-made atrocities, it must be clear, God is so innocent from all those man-made atrocities and lockdowns!!

Every good things are from God coming from above!! As it is written; "Let no man say when he is tempted, I am tempted of God: for God cannot be tempted with evil, neither tempteth he any man: [14] But every man is tempted, when he is drawn away of his own lust, and enticed. [15] Then when lust hath conceived, it bringeth forth sin: and sin, when it is finished, bringeth forth death. [16] Do not err, my beloved brethren. [17] Every good gift and every perfect gift is from above, and cometh down from the Father of lights, with whom is no variableness, neither shadow of turning."James 1:13-17 KJV

https://www.cnbc.com/.../gas-prices-and-inflation...

https://www.cbsnews.com/.../gas-prices-return-to-office/

https://www.kbb.com/.../gas-prices-plummet-as-drivers.../

https://www.timesunion.com/.../With-gas-prices-up...

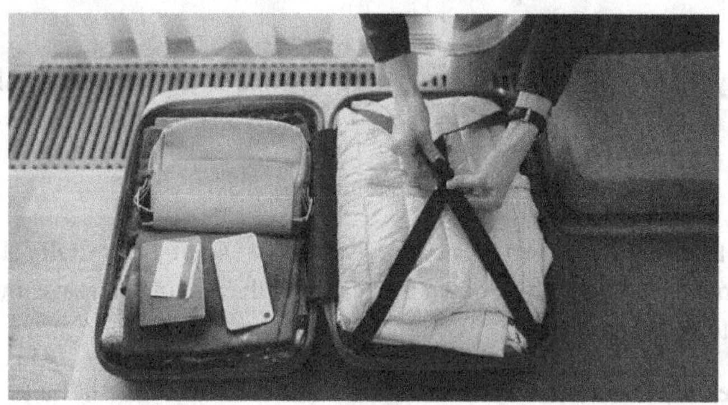

CNBC.COM

Rising gas prices and inflation top travel concerns, overtaking Covid, survey finds

Most Americans plan to travel this summer, but rising gas prices and inflation now top their list of concerns, overtaking Covid.

CG, We suffered for 2 long years.

We can't let the cost of gas stop us from traveling. We need to travel for our mental health.

DL, not if we don't have the money.

CG I know it's hard but it is possible to set aside a little money each week for a trip. You don't need to travel far.

Why China is seeing COVID Surge!!

Written on 4/9/2022 by Ramsis Ghaly

You will think that the most vulnerable region for COVID surge is the Region at war by Eastern Europe (Ukraine, Poland, Belarus, Moldova, Russia, Romania, ——overcrowded, no vaccine, travelling, camps, no good ventilation, no masks, no screen——NOT IN CHINA country at peace with restricted laws of screening, vaccination and lockdown!!!

It made me very curious as what is the scientific reason as among all the countries of the world, China is standing alone with the real COVID surge and Lockdown!!

China is the only country that has been so restricted, proactive and has zero tolerance nationwide to Leniency or exception to get out of control surge subvariant of omicron, BA.2 as follows: "In Shanghai, a city of 26 million, people are confined to their homes, able to go out only for essential supplies. Regular tests are mandatory. Officials throughout China check color-based "health code" systems to monitor people's movements. Everyone has a smartphone app that shows their personal QR health code: green for healthy, yellow for close contacts and red for confirmed or suspected cases. If someone tests positive for COVID-19 — even if they don't have symptoms — they must isolate in large temporary facilities set up in stadiums and convention centers. They can't leave until they test negative twice. Pets are even sent to other centers for monitoring. Public health officials cordon off the person's home and disinfected everything."

Perhaps because China is very aggressive in testing and lockdown!! But if this is the case China should be much better than any country and Surge free by now!!

- Perhaps because China aggressive vaccination! But again, this should make China surge free by now after two years already! Unless it is related to defective vaccine used??

- Perhaps it is another variant originates from the same region as COVID-19 and locally spreading before it makes its way to other countries!

- Perhaps it is related to the level of immunity of the Chinese population that makes it susceptible to such a variant since immunity varies among countries!

It has also been speculated the following: "The increase in the number of cases reflects a combination of factors. Your population that's immunologically naive, they haven't seen much of the virus in the past and because they haven't been vaccinated effectively to resist them," China has mostly used the Chinese-made

Sinovac and Sinopharm vaccines. Both companies said their vaccines were more than 78% effective against COVID-19, but studies suggested otherwise. Late-stage trials of the Sinovac candidate in Brazil showed an efficacy rate of 50.38%, barely above the World Health Organization threshold for approval. Other studies have suggested that immunity from two doses of these vaccines wanes rapidly and that the protection may be limited, especially among older people and especially compared with mRNA vaccines used in the U.S. And against omicron, all vaccines have been found to offer less protection."

What else?? Anyone curious insight??

https://www.wdsu.com/.../covid-19-surge-like-the.../39600998

https://apnews.com/.../coronavirus-pandemic-health...

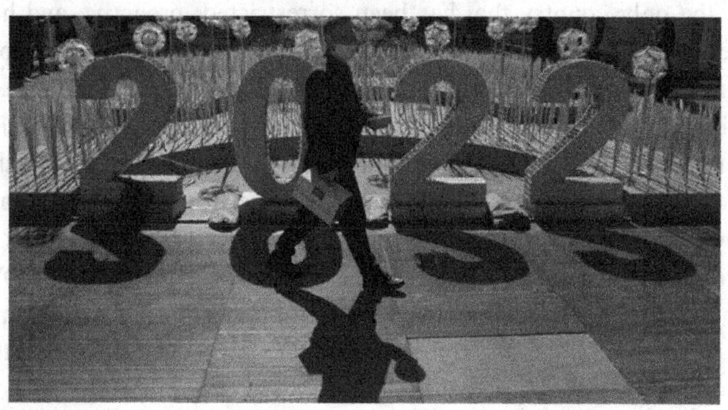

APNEWS.COM

China seeing new surge in cases despite 'zero tolerance'

BEIJING (AP) — China is seeing a new surge in COVID-19 cases across the vast country, despite its draconian "zero tolerance" approach to dealing with outbreaks. The mainland on Monday reported 214 new cases of infection over the previous 24 hours, with the most, 69, in the southern province of...

Do you think oil will be replaced by electricity?

Cg, Maybe their surge is because they have everyone in lockdown too long.

COVID Made Us Go Back to Our Ancient Times!

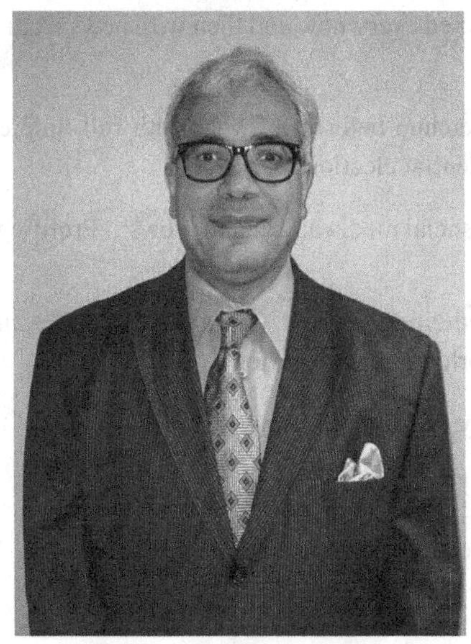

News update

Written on 5/10/2022

By Ramsis Ghaly

News update

Ramsis Ghaly

News update

Ramsis Ghaly

To overcome the rising crises; It is a time to do what my mom did 100 years ago in Egypt raise home chicken, duck and rabbits and if you are rich get cows and grow vegetables and fruits!!!! And buy a Kerisone lamp and stove and stay at home and walk cloth!!!

Social media News are grantees to keep it interesting and job security as follows

It used to be COVID crises--!

Then It is all about COVID Vaccine!!

Then followed by rise in gasoline price!

Soon rise in price of chicken, eggs and milk!

And news be interrupted every now and then with news from Putin, abortion and January 6!!

Now, they need to catchup before next year with full time coverage 24/7 more exciting about presidential election for 2024!!!!

Good business to be social media and anchor news!!! Prolific for the kids future!!

HH, Mein Bester Mediziner der Welt. Gratulation Pr.-Dr. Ramsis Ghaly.!!......My best doctor in the world. **Congratulations**

Pr.-DR. Ramsis ghaly. !!.

CK, YOU NAILED IT.

CG, Absolutely correct. Can't wait for November elections. You look dapper in that suit

The Lord Lovingkindnesses!

Ramsis Ghaly

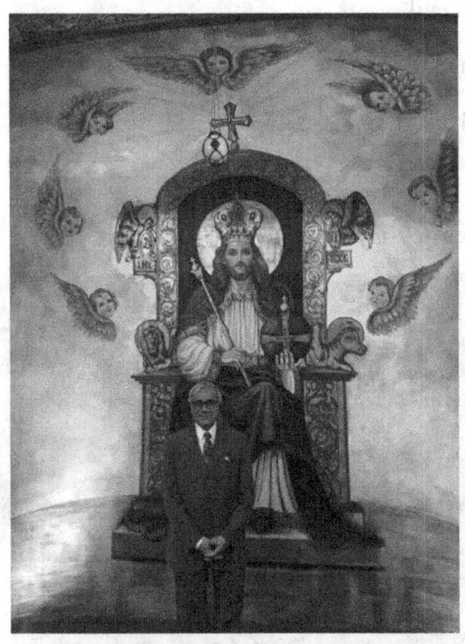

As COVID-19 terrified the world, yet God' Lovingkindness always has been remembered. In the beginning of each day and in the times of hardships, remember the Lovingkindness of the Lord and Prayers!!

"The Lord's lovingkindnesses indeed never cease, for His compassions never fail. They are new every morning; great is Your faithfulness." Lamentations 3:21-23

The Lord's Prayer

Our Father who art in heaven,

Hallowed be thy Name.

Thy kingdom come.

Thy will be done,

On earth as it is in heaven.

Give us this day our daily bread.

And forgive us our trespasses,

As we forgive those who trespass against us.

And lead us not into temptation,

But deliver us from evil.

For thine is the kingdom,

and the power, and the glory,

for ever and ever.

~ Amen as (Matthew 6:9-14)

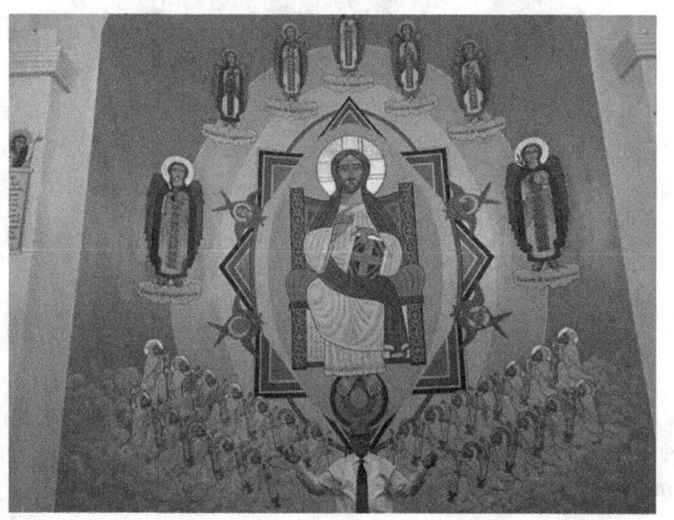

JS, AMEN

CG,God Be the Glory Forever and Ever, Amen

BM, Amen!

SS, Amen

The Past Glorify God and Strength the Future!

Wherever we look at the past years of COVID, we glorify GOD for His blessing and saved us during the horrific death by the virus. As we look at COVD in the past and God help, we glorify God and it gives more hope for the future.

Whenever, I look at past and see my abundant achievements, it makes me go for the future and gives me more and more strength giving my Lord the glory praising His Name always, Jesus our Lord and Savior and Premier Mentor!!

Psalm 29:1-3

Ascribe to the Lord, O heavenly beings, ascribe to the Lord glory and strength. Ascribe to the Lord the glory due his name; worship the Lord in the splendor of holiness. The voice of the Lord is over the waters; the God of glory thunders, the Lord, over many waters.

Psalm 19:1

To the choirmaster. A Psalm of David. The heavens declare the glory of God, and the sky above proclaims his handiwork.

1 Corinthians 10:31

So, whether you eat or drink, or whatever you do, do all to the glory of God.

Matthew 24:30

"Then will appear in heaven the sign of the Son of Man, and then all the tribes of the earth will mourn, and they will see the Son of Man coming on the clouds of heaven with power and great glory."

Philippians 2:11

And every tongue confess that Jesus Christ is Lord, to the glory of God the Father.

Romans 11:36

For from him and through him and to him are all things. To him be glory forever. Amen.

Www.ghalyneurosurgeon.com

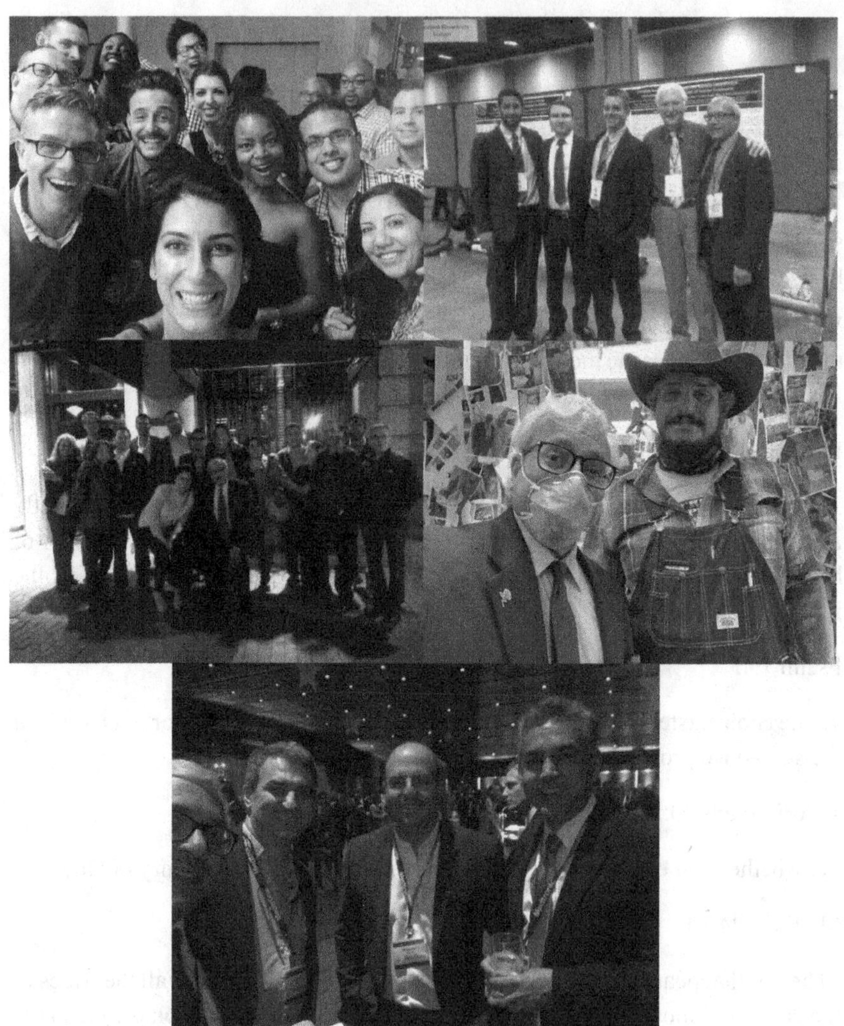

JT, Amen

CG, You have so many achievements to be proud of through the years. The Lord has been by your side the whole time. Blessings!

Flash Back to COVID Crises!

Written 10/20/2022

Praise our Lord those times are over. Not because of science or man intervention but because of our Lord Jesus and His mercy and the Natural immunity He created. It was horrific experience, many lost lives, exhausted frontliners and absolutely painful experience.

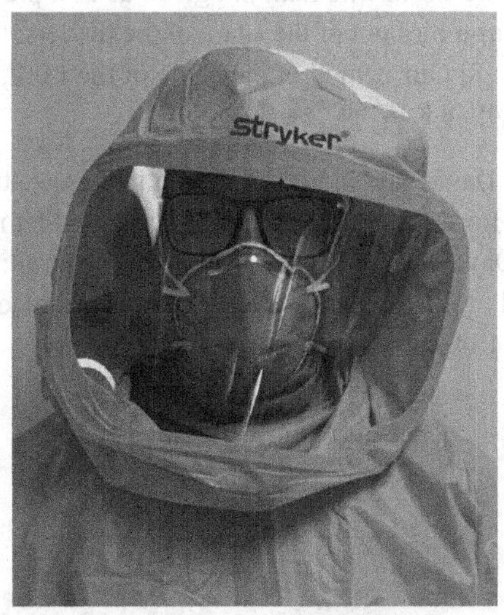

Ramsis Ghaly Post 10/20/2020

If It hadn't been For Our Lord Jesus who was in our side, COVID and Men would have swallowed us!!

Ramsis Ghaly

COVID Infectivity is high yet it isn't as lethal and frightening as used to be!

In my calls nowadays, only few COVID needed any serious interventions and ICUs are of few COVIDs and ventilators are not in use and by no means as it was!

Thank you our Lord Jesus for the Natural Immunity You have created in each of us and shielded us from our enemies! With that it is not only mankind conquers these corona viruses but also weakens their stings!

If You let us Lord under the mercy of man and science, they will continue to restrain, isolate and mask us all our lives!!

Yes indeed, if it wasn't for God, we all would been destroyed by the COVID and men but Our soul is escaped as a bird out of the snare of the fowlers: the snare is broken, and we are escaped. [8] Our help is in the name of the Lord, who made heaven and earth as the psalmist said: "If it had not been the Lord who was on our side, now may Israel say; [2] If it had not been the Lord who was on our side, when men (AND COVID) rose up against us: [3] Then they (COVID AND MEN) had swallowed us up quick, when their wrath (MEN AND COVID) was kindled against us: [4] Then the waters (OF MEN AND COVID) had overwhelmed us, the stream had gone over our soul: [5] Then the proud waters had gone over our soul. [6] Blessed be the Lord, who hath not given us as a prey to their teeth. [7] Our soul is escaped as a bird out of the snare of the fowlers: the snare is broken, and we are escaped. [8] Our help is in the name of the Lord, who made heaven and earth.' Psalm 124:1-8 KJV

Indeed as our father David said in his days: I am in a great strait: let us fall now into the hand of the Lord ; for his mercies are great: and let me not fall into the hand of man: "And David said unto Gad, I am in a great strait: let us fall now into the hand of the Lord ; for his mercies are great: and let me not fall into the hand of man." 2 Samuel 24:14 KJV

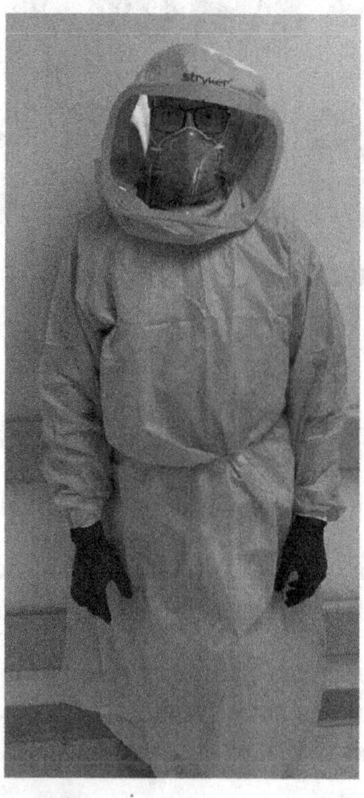

Post COVID: My Sincere Appreciation

My Earthly Heaven!!

Ramsis Ghaly

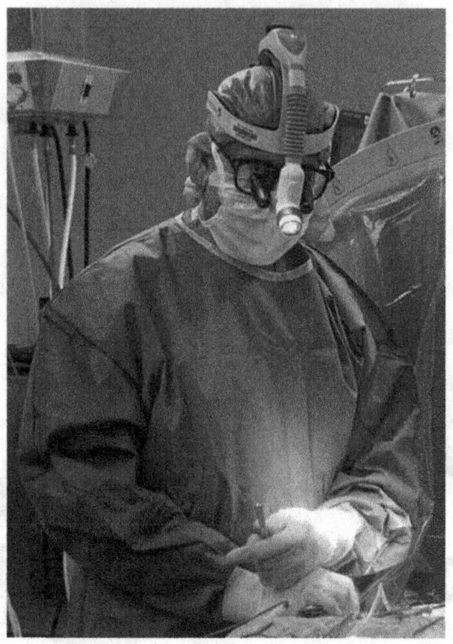

A Joy to operate on the human nervous system; Brain, Spinal Cord and nerves from the start to the end.

The nervous system can't handle any physical pressure or injury or interruptions from blood, blood pressure and oxygen!!

Nothing thus far can repair or regenerate the nervous system. But as a neurosurgeon, I take the pressure and secure the place fir the affected part of the nervous system.

Nothing worse than the affliction of a pinched nerve or headache or stroke or coma!

During surgery, I praise our Lord Jesus for creating the best ever self-sufficient, comprehensive, self-operated, minded, creative, autonomous and gifted system with specific highly respective and complex order as the human Brain being the only center station with so many branches, subspecialties, and wiring!!!

Psalm 8 "O Lord our Lord, how excellent is thy name in all the earth! who hast set thy glory above the heavens. [2] Out of the mouth of babes and sucklings hast thou ordained strength because of thine enemies, that thou mightest still

the enemy and the avenger. [3] When I consider thy heavens, the work of thy fingers, the moon and the stars, which thou hast ordained; [4] What is man, that thou art mindful of him? and the son of man, that thou visitest him? [5] For thou hast made him a little lower than the angels, and hast crowned him with glory and honour. [6] Thou madest him to have dominion over the works of thy hands; thou hast put all things under his feet: [7] All sheep and oxen, yea, and the beasts of the field; [8] The fowl of the air, and the fish of the sea, and whatsoever passeth through the paths of the seas. [9] O Lord our Lord, how excellent is thy name in all the earth!"

Song of Songs 8:7,14 "Many waters cannot quench love, neither can the floods drown it: if a man would give all the substance of his house for love, it would utterly be contemned. [14] Make haste, my beloved, and be thou like to a roe or to a young hart upon the mountains of spices."

SM, Your the best Dr G!!!

JT, our nervous system reminds me of this tree...

CG, You are an amazing doctor and God has truly given you a gift. He blessed you with the knowledge and compassion that you possess as a doctor. May he continue to guide and bless you.

RH, Your prayer is MIND blowing!!! And you say this while you're operating. I give thanks for your genius. God has given you some amazing gifts. you were so humble about it. You are loved doctor

DM, Lord Jesus Thank you for giving us Dr Ramsis Ghaly who submit himself totally to your authority.Bless him with strenght and wisdom which come only from you for the benefit of humanity.

Apostolic Blessing 2006!

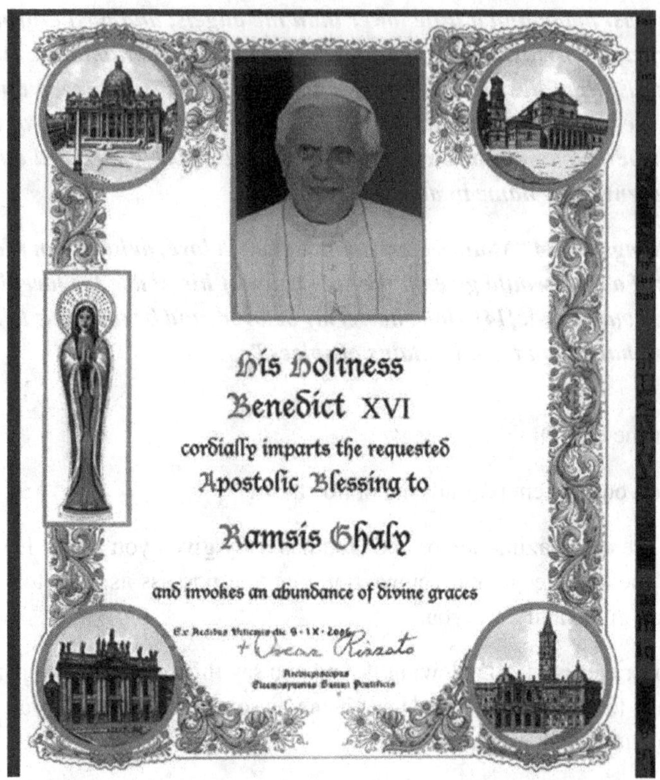

His Holiness
Benedict XVI
cordially imparts the requested
Apostolic Blessing to
Ramsis Ghaly
and invokes an abundance of divine graces

+ Oscar Rizzato

One of the Best Ever Blessing Award I have received as an unworthy servant is from Pope of Vatican his holiness Benedict XVI in 2006!!

Ramsis Ghaly

www.ghalyneurosurgeon.com

SC, as you are so in deservance of this!

MD, WOW what an honor!!

SL, Wow!

Congratulations

My mother actually grow up with his siblings and himself. They were neighbors in Germany

America Most Honored Doctors 2022!

www.ghalyneurosurgeon.com

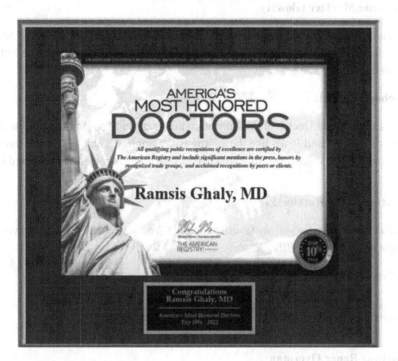

Dina Arvanitakis

Blessed to know Dr Ghaly and to call him my friend. Congratulations Dr. Ramsis Ghaly !!!!!! You are doing God's work and healing and restoring many people.

Emily Linn

My Neurosurgeon. My Hero.

If you need a neurosurgeon, this is the man you want to see. He's Quadruple Board certified: NeuroSurgery, Neuro-Critical Care, Anesthesiology & Pain Management. And the accomplishments only just start there. His bedside manner is one that I've never experienced in my life & I've been a nurse for 17 years. He cares.

Sebee Michael

You are amazing Dr. GHALY! I might be needing you soon after all these years of nursing.

Charlene Mentzer Glowaty

You are truly a great doctor and surgeon. You are personable, great listener, and empathetic to the concerns of your patients. God has truly blessed your patients when they found you

Michael Plunkett

You are an Angel Doctor of the Lord with the heart and soul in the right place. Awesome story, and looks like the airway is not impinged any longer and those vertebra are spaced and not crunching nerves making inflammation. You fixed it!

Cristina Rojas-Rutkowski

OMG!!!! So happy for you my favorite doctor!!!! You leave traces of love on every single patient's hearts!!!!!

CONGRATULATIONS!!!

Christie Loftin Well deserved! You perform God's Miracles!

Jillianne Renee Overman·

Dr Ramsis Ghaly is a man of faith and his hands work as God's tools. There is no doubt. He's my neurosurgeon and I wouldn't trust anyone else.

Sandi Benedict Crites

Congratulations

Sandi Benedict Crites

job well done my friend! proud of u!

Roksolana Zhuravchak

Congratulations!

Annette Cozzi

Most well deserving.

Darcie Francois

Well deserved !! One of the best !!

Congratulations Dr Ghaly !!

Harout Art Kaskanian

Congratulations

Angie Stanford

Congratulations!!!!

Rada Dosen

Well deserved !!!

Lisa Bertone Zizas

Congratulations!! You certainly deserve the honor!

Sima Aprahamian-Hovhannessian

congratulations

Lana Wania-Galicia

Congratulations

Ching Piamonte-Mission

Gordon Simms

Congrats Doc!!!!

Violet Besada

Congratulations!

Jori Christensen

Congrats Dr Ghaly!!

Carole Pasteris

Congratulations.

Kathy Manthei Sitar

Well deserved.

Kathy Marie

Congratulations! A well deserved honor!

Abraham Varghese

Congratulations

Ekhlas Bichai

Congratulations

Tonya Jackson-Cavanaugh

Well deserved Dr Ghaly!!

Congrats!!!

Carol Grant

Congratulations

Ian Wharton

Congratulations Well done

Brenda Linquist

You are amazing in the medical field and equally amazing and beautiful as an accomplished, dedicated, loving, human being.

CONGRATULATIONS Dr Ramsis Ghaly!

Diane Nelson

Congradulations

Kim Ann

Congratulations

Coey Baker Podraza

Yes you are!!!

Kathy O'Brien

Congratulations that's for sure, God bless

Hilda Harrell

Congratulations!

Sarah T. Marcus

Congrats!!!

Winnie Patricoski

Congrats

Elizabeth Fragoso Oliver

Congratulations. You are a blessed man as you have honored our Lord and your profession to bless all who are in your care. Have a wonderful day.

Rita Castillo

Proud of your recognition!

Stephanie Mickelson Decker

Congratulations

Joseph Johnson

Congratulations! Dr . Ghaly

Yvonne Drew Reddoch

Congratulations

Mary Khalil

Congratulations and a much deserved award!

Michelle Brcik

Congratulations

Sharon Strons Ledbetter

Well done

Well deserved

May God continue to bless the work of your hands all for His Glory

Janet Conger

Congratulations, you deserve that

Melinda Withers

What a wonderful gift you are to all of us. You have the biggest heart I've ever seen in my life

Belen Montenegro

Congratulations, Dr Ghaly!!!!

Kathy Stephens

Congratulations

! An award well deserved!

Debbie Lund Hewitt Million

Congratulations Dr. Ghaly

Olezia Comsulea

Congratulations

Mary Sturm

Congratulations

Sally Brady

Wonderful honor for a great doctor.

Congrats

Debbie Loomis-Earles

Congrats

Mague García

Congratulations Dr. Ghaly

Flor De Andocutin

Congratulations Dr Ghaly

Brenda Cooky Dickerson

Awesome, **congratulations**

Sandy Shadle

Congratulations

Mischa Doyel

This is fantastic. You deserve it. **Congratulations**

Annette Valtman

Congratulations praying for you!

Carolyn Prochazka-Campbell

Well deserved

Charlene Mentzer Glowaty

Congratulations! You work so hard every day to achieve this accomplishment, and I can't think of anyone who deserves it more. .You set an amazing example for other doctors and your students.

Charlene Mentzer Glowaty true THAT CHAR

Angel Schultz

Congratulations

Julie Soucy

Congratulations

Susan Lardi Esparza

Congratulations!!!

Heda Rechnitz-Kijner

Congratulations

Lori Schlage Malczewski

Much deserved you are Awesome **Congratulations**!!!

Maja Canak

Gratulation

Linda Mata

May God continue to bless you in your healing!!

Congratulations!!

Jack Jane Cole Duvick

Well deserved !!!

Julie Grandgeorge

AWESOME Dr. Ghaly!

Congratulations!

John Pisha

Congratulations

Stacey OBrien

Wonderful! **Congratulations**

Kathleen MacGregor Grace

Be sure, when I need surgery one day on my back..You are the ONLY Doctor I'll trust to do it.

Congratulations and God Bless you! A true Hero to all! Sending love from Egypt

Diane Swanstrom

You are the BEST!! **Congrats!**

Karen Boland Geheber

You are top shelf, Dr. Ghaly!

Zenaida Capul

You are the best Dr.Ghaly,

Congratulations

.

Tammie Ruesenberg

You deserve this and more!!

Chuck Bishop

Congratulations!

Chita Bello

Congratulations Dr. Ghaly! You deserved it.

Emily Linn

Of course!. **Congrats** Dr **Ramsis Ghaly**

Shelly Sypien

Well deserved!

Deborah Whitaker Queen

Congratulations

Barbara Calvert Grant

Congratulations

Janice Moss

"**ongratulations** Dr. Ghaly

Judy Ron Conderman

Congratulations! You are so deserving of this award Dr Ghaly.

Jane Wills

Congratulations Dr. Ghaly! Well deserved

Cheryl Hollmier

Congrats!!! That's awesome!!

Joan McGrath Pocius

Well deserved

Kathy Petrucci

Big **congrats**

Liliana Gentile

Congratulations

Dottie Lopez

Awesome. **Congratulations**. Well deserved.

Phil Valera

Congratulations Dr. Ghaly

Val Wolfe

Congratulations!

Carol Rambo

Of course you are! **Congrats**

Joyce Hairald Riley

Congratulations

Kristyn Joy

Congratulations

Aleksandra Stojanovic

Congratulations! Well deserved!

Mansour Khalil

Congratulations

Mary Nixon

Vantastic and we'll deserved. **congrats**

Romeo Hermiz Shoshoo

Congratulations

Steve Gill

You are an amazing Doctor……Dr Ghaly!

Jessica Graham

Love this and so very deserving!

Shannon Campbell-Cangiano

Congratulations

Mansour Khalil

Congratulations

Bird Bvs

Congratulations

Mary Siegel

So Very True. **Congratulations**

Amy Stapleton Conderman

Congratulations Dr. Ghaly on your latest well-deserved award!

Flori Manalo

Congratulations Dr Ghaly

Christie Loftin

Well deserved! You perform God's Miracles!

Carrie Weber

Much deserved. **You're the best** there is!

Myrna Macaso

Congratulations Dr.Ghaly

Cristina Rojas-Rutkowski

OMG!!!! So happy for you my favorite doctor!!!! You leave traces of love on every single patient's hearts!!!!!

CONGRATULATIONS

Daisy SLusinski

Congratulations

Well deserved

Mary Ellen

Congratulation

Thomas J. McGrath

Well deserved!

Teresa Martinez

Congratulations God bless

Tiet Gorsak

Congratulations well deserved you doing God will !

Louise Keane

Congratulations Dr Ghaly!

Chandur Piryani

Congratulations

Sota Omoigui

Congratulations Ramsis!!!

A Hero! Gift Drawing from My patients!

Cindy Kuykendall Rice

August 22 at 11:36 PM ·

#HEROESDONTALLWEARCAPES

Someone posted this hashtag and I absolutely loved seeing it! Life is hard and LOVE is the only way to get through it

Dr Ramsis Ghaly I snapped this off your wall of pictures! So thought if you when I seen this hashtag!

My Sincere Unconditional Love to My Patients and the Children!

Written by Ramsis Ghaly

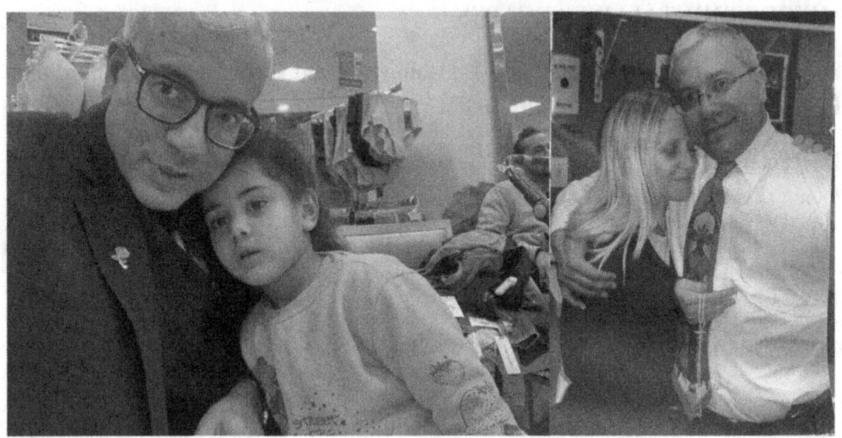

Childhood and suffering including illness are the most moving in the depth of human hearts and Heaven!!

The inward hearts of those Childhood and suffering including illness are full of love and unselfishness!

The most innocent stages of human journey are childhood and suffering including illness!

Childhood and suffering including illness are also the most vulnerable stages in human nature!

Childhood and suffering including illness are most periods of dire need, dependence and high demand!

Childhood and suffering including illness are most appreciative and thankful!

Childhood and suffering including sickness are the most purity stage of human life!

Childhood and suffering including sickness are the most humbly and tearful part of human lifespan!

Childhood and suffering including illness are the simplest nature in human bloodstream!

Childhood and suffering including illness are the meekest close to heartfelt emotions!

Childhood and suffering including illness are the least envious!

Childhood and suffering including illness are the most periods where evil men take advantage!

Childhood and suffering including illness are the lands of use, misuse and abuse!!

Childhood and suffering including illness are prayerful and very close to the face of God!

Jesus our God is visible in Childhood and suffering including illness!

The Childhood and suffering including illness are the victimized helpless souls in human race that their cries close to the Ears of the Heavenly Father!

"And said, Verily I say unto you, Except ye be converted, and become as little children, ye shall not enter into the kingdom of heaven. [4] Whosoever therefore shall humble himself as this little child, the same is greatest in the kingdom of heaven. [5] And whoso shall receive one such little child in my name receiveth me. [6] But whoso shall offend one of these little ones which believe in me, it were better for him that a millstone were hanged about his neck, and that he were drowned in the depth of the sea."Matthew 18:3-6 KJV

"Blessed are the poor in spirit: for theirs is the kingdom of heaven. [4] Blessed are they that mourn: for they shall be comforted. [5] Blessed are the meek: for they shall inherit the earth. [6] Blessed are they which do hunger and thirst after righteousness: for they shall be filled. [7] Blessed are the merciful: for they shall obtain mercy. [8] Blessed are the pure in heart: for they shall see God. [9] Blessed are the peacemakers: for they shall be called the children of God. [10] Blessed are they which are persecuted for righteousness' sake: for theirs is the kingdom of heaven. [11] Blessed are ye, when men shall revile you, and persecute you, and shall say all manner of evil against you falsely, for my sake. [12] Rejoice, and be exceeding glad: for great is your reward in heaven: for so persecuted they the prophets which were before you." Matthew 5:3-12 KJV

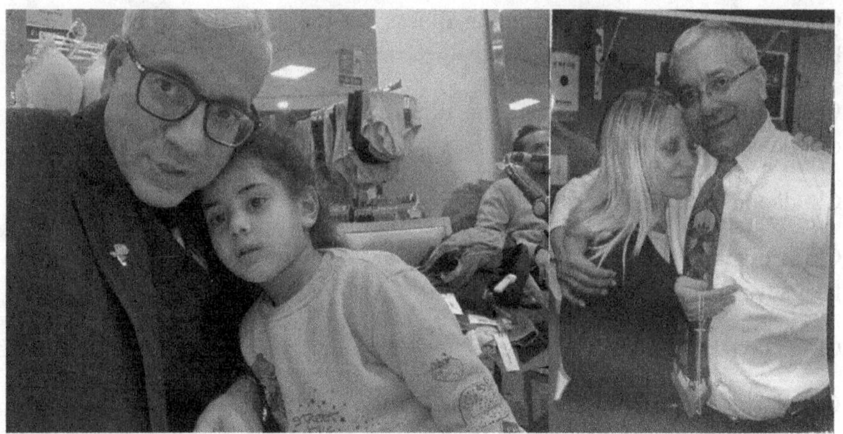

JM, AMEN

LM, You are a man with a pure heart. God bless you abundantly and exceedingly with love, peace and joy in doing with what God has wanted you to do.

CG. Well said doctor

Childhood is the most precious years. To see or hear that a child has an illness is so heartbreaking. Bless the children.

My Mom Always Special to Me!

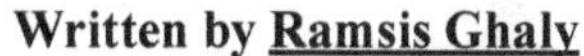

Written by Ramsis Ghaly

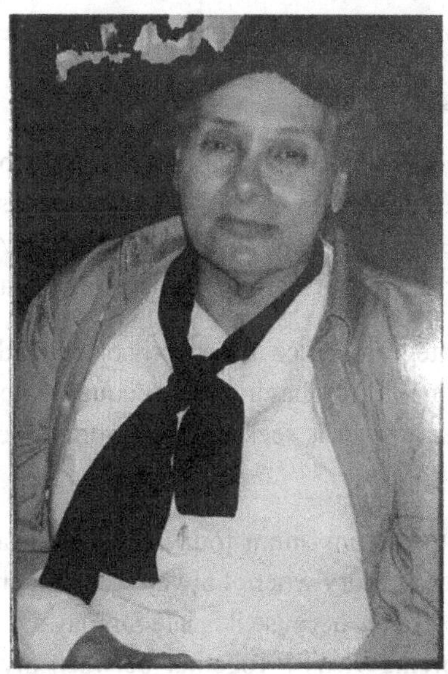

My mom always special to me!

My identity is attached to her since I was in her womb!

When she departed, I felt that deep part of me was taken away!

My mom was my being, and she passed away, my being was shacked, and it has never been the same since!

My mom knew me from inside out and my belongings were hers. And since her death, my belongings are so lonely!

Somehow, I still feel I am connected to my mom although she isn't with me physically but spiritually, she is, and the connection has never been separated even after her death!

However, I live to that day to unit with my source to regain my originality again!

Indeed, humanity is the continuity from the very first mother and father by the breath of life created from God with no parents until the end of times!

For now, I shall continue to live in her memory wondering how wonderful the life will be when that time to come eternity with my Lord Jesus my Heavenly Father and my mom and dad again!!

Ramsis Ghaly

Tonight I Thought of My Mom and the Topic was about the Virus!

Written by Ramsis Ghaly

"Science is True Science if with Honesty, Integrity and Good Well to Man" My quote I wrote, Ramsis Ghaly 1981, very early in my career as a passionate medical neuroscientist restrained in Egypt and inspired to come to America to follow my dreams! It was my words to the American Consulate, in Cairo, Egypt!

Indeed an honest and integral science is perfectly okay to admit not having a well tested management plan and not having the adequate knowledge in a "Novel" virus ! Perhaps the best answer is seek wisdom from the elders and forefathers ——-

It wasn't coincidence to call my mom today! It is the feast celebration of the ascension of our Mother St Mary where I always remember my mom and I write a post! But tonight was strange because it is late Sunday night and the Topic about how to handle the evolving virus ! Together between my parents and myself, over 120 years since the turn of 1900, we went through many illnesses of various pathogens and do many infectious endemics and pandemics! We made through!!!! Never ever witnessed such nonsense and erratic management!!

Sometimes it is good to leave things to the nature when you deal with NOVEL enemy so that does not anger and not to make things worse. Perhaps at this situation is good seek advice from the wise ancient elders and ask ourselves what our forefathers and ancestors would have done!! It is time not to put our ancestor wisdom down and believe science is much so superior! Science can be faulty and the natural wisdom not written in books much superior!

Despite being illiterate and poor raising 8 children in the villages of Egypt with extreme poverty and hunger, my mom kept us all safe, prevented any harm and illnesses! Therefore tonight I decided to remembered her and call her in Heaven: "Mom I need you: I keep reflecting to how you dealt with viruses when we were little children vulnerable and we had nothing. As you remember we were very poor and everything was so polluted and unclean but despite all of these, you kept us so healthy! I miss your wisdom and guidance. All around me is so confusing and doesn't make sense! Help me to figure this out!"

My Illiterate Egyptian Christian Mom from upper Egypt, Decades ago once told me when I was a little boy scared of getting sick of the virus like my brother just had, she said: "Don't be afraid to get sick of the virus and get fever and skin rashes all over and look Buffy, because your body will develop lifetime natural immunity"

It is strange looking around and I keep hearing almost every day, many different variants developing in the same time in different regions of the world and spreading so fast!

I couldn't help it but tonight I called my Gorgeous mom in Heaven and I asked her what she thinks?? I miss my mom more than she miss me for sure! I always consulted with her and the older I got, the more I did until God took her home. Yet whenever I get unto analysis inquiry, I call her and I know she with my dad"

And these are the thoughts——. The worldwide development of various variants in the same time in different countries makes my mind wonders if the measures science had taken are firing back since the world has been for a while a huge free laboratory!!

It appears each country is suffering from a different variant and that particle is different from one region to another! It almost make me believe hundred percent one size doesn't fit all and each person respond differently and be treated differently. Each body has his own defense system to handle the virus and hence is susceptible differently to different variants based in his biology and immunity. Vaccines might actually produce different responses and different immunities that viruses can easily outsmart!

Face masking might also be hindering the widespread development of natural immunity, the normal occurrence of daily fights between the viruses and hosts that usually result in weakening of the viruses and opportunities to be defeated after the first blast. Both observations may explain the inability to defeat the virus and keep returning of viruses with different shapes and forms!

But viruses have hard time outsmart the body natural immunity that stood the times before the birth if do called "modern science"

Can the reason of seeing the come back of all these viruses of different variants in various regions of the world in the same time and instead of one time only, one type deal only and one variant only is the premature administration of weak non-inclusive vaccine!

In addition, the spread of vaccination may actually limits the development of the much inclusive comprehensive natural immunity and therefore gives the chance to the virus to mutate to a variants resistant to the restricted vaccine-mediated immunity but would have been sensitive to the much powerful comprehensive Naturally- mediated immunity!

When I was a child my mother told me, if you get sick of the childhood virus and your body will develop lifetime strong natural immunity that will sustain you all your life! It is okay to get sick for a short time and yet look for the benefit in the long run! Sure enough, since we were 6 sibling living in a small studio and we got sick of the virus with rashes and aches but since then we developed natural immunity and the virus never ever came back. Exactly as my mom said!

My mom never went to school but she was a smart woman with so much naturally learned intuition and acquired skills. She did know how to read or write but her communication skills and knowledge were much more that any doctor or PHD especially those modern graduates with limited hands on experience and lessons learned in life!

It wasn't much time left with mom! Thank you I miss you very much mom! Pray for all of us and the world before our Heavenly Father and Savior of the world Jesus our God with intercession of St Mary the mother of God.

Mom Rest In Peace and Thank you for always be!!!!

I leave all with my quote:

"Science is True Science if with Honesty, Integrity and Good Well to Man" My quote I wrote, Ramsis Ghaly 1981, very early in my career as a passionate medical neuroscientist inspired to come to America!

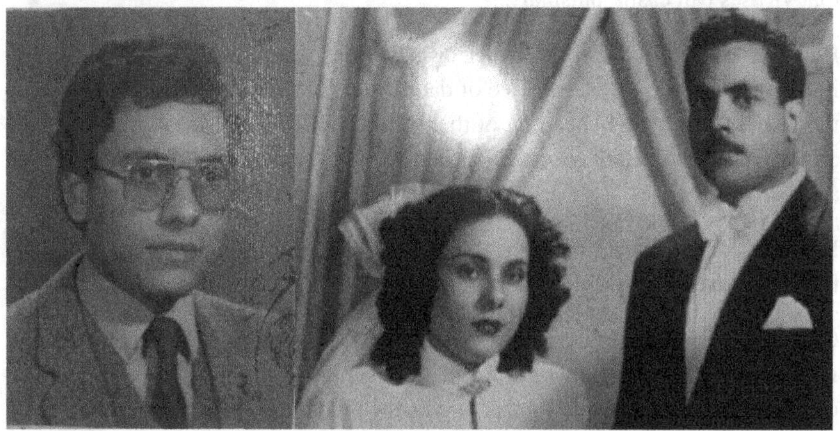

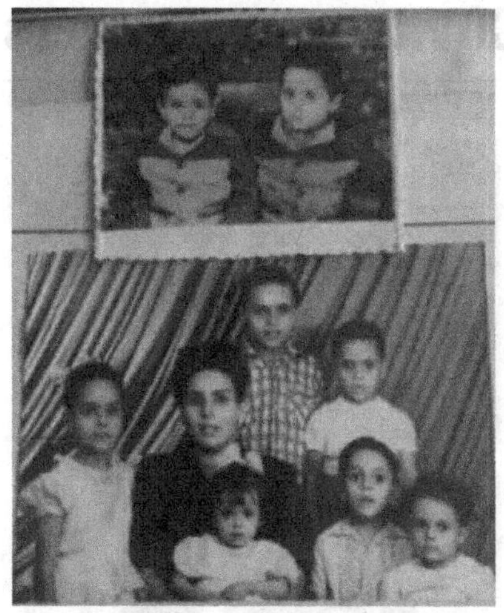

Mk, She looks like a movie star , so lovely....

Js, Love this!!

Post COVID Happy Mothers Day!

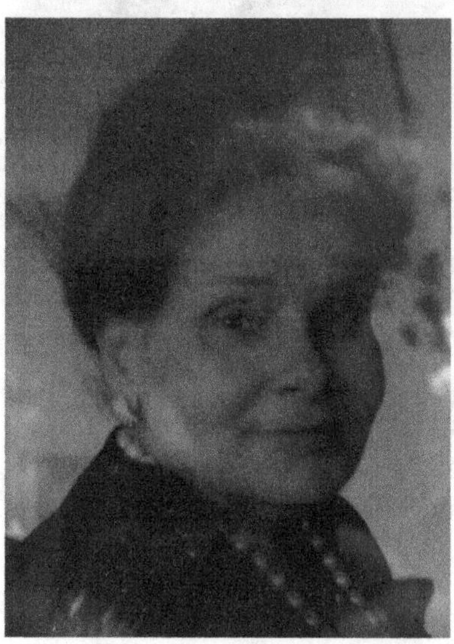

“Mothers never die” as Love never fails!!

Dedicated to the living and heavenly Mothers and my mother Sania Fouad Michael

Written by Ramsis Ghaly

Mothers have special place in Jesus’s Heart ! He knows their hearts and they are are His sheep! Hear their voice no matter where, when, what and how!! They are true angels of love living among us!

History repeat itself as with a man named Putin aggression and murders entered the region, with mother true love, prosperity peace enter the earth! And mothers are restoring life and building what man’s aggression had done! Mothers are a true testimony of love shall always prevail and never fails!

When you see a mom stop, take your hate off and with a smile, appreciation and gratitude saying: “Happy Mother’s Day” in sincerity utter the heartfelt genuine words! Show love and This day isn’t just about an outing, a brunch, a dinner or a gift but about believing and paying back! Do act of love and kindness!! I hope, It isn’t just a brunch, it wasn’t just a word. It wasn’t just an act when a man say “Happy Mother’s Day”

Let every mankind, let all human beings say: “Happy Mother’s Day” as “Mothers never die”

I watched all the beautiful photos celebrating the "Happy Mother's Day"; Thank you you all

I wish to remind you all; "Mothers never die";

"Happy Mother's Day" to the billions of the mothers!!!

Mothers are of divinity dressed in the flesh as the pure image of God. Despite the first woman came from God and the rib of a man, yet Mothers across thousands of years superseded man in nobility, loyalty and unconditional love!

As Love never fails so is Mother's love ever fails. "Charity never faileth: but whether there be prophecies, they shall fail; whether there be tongues, they shall cease; whether there be knowledge, it shall vanish away." (1 Corinthians 13:8). It is because Mother's love is "4Charity suffereth long, and is kind; charity envieth not; charity vaunteth not itself, is not puffed up, 5Doth not behave itself unseemly, seeketh not her own, is not easily provoked, thinketh no evil; 6Rejoiceth not in iniquity, but rejoiceth in the truth; 7Beareth all things, believeth all things, hopeth all things, endureth all things." (1 Corinthians 13:8)

If you lost your Mother please be comforted since "Mother's never die" so join the living and wish your heavenly Mother "Hapoy Mother's Day".

To the living and to the heavenly mothers and to the present, the past and future mothers: from our hearts of the living and the heavenly, in earth and in heavens in one voice we say: "Happy Mother's Day" as "Mothers never die"

The mothers are the hearts of love and the wombs of every newborn coming to the world since the first Eve to the very last Eve before our world comes to an end: "Happy Mother's Day" as "Mothers never die";

The love with tears in joy as Love with joy in tears because it is the love from the heart that never dies say: "Happy Mother's Day" as "Mothers never die";

God has given the breath of life to Mother's no matter where they are. As there is no life in the world with no Mothers so there is no generations with no mothers as there is no future without mothers: "Mothers never die" as Love never fails". So let us all say: "Happy Mother's Day" as "Mothers never die";

Why: "Mothers never die" as Love never fails" as follows:

-Mothers have made possible to save the world so the Incarnated of Baby Jesus in our Mother Mary.

-Mothers have kept Satan away from terminating the human race.

- Mothers have kept the love in the dangerous world we live in.

-Mother's have kept the life in the deadly world we live in.

-Mothers have kept the open gates in the shattered world we live in.

-Mothers have kept the peace in the world of animosity and aggression.

-Mothers have kept the light in the the dark world we live in.

-Mothers have kept the hope in the hopeless world we live in.

-Mothers have kept the help in the helpless world we live in.

-Mothers have kept the faith in the faithless world we live in.

-Mothers have kept the human race walking through the roads of the tortuous world we live in.

-Mothers have rescued the human race from the tribulations of the world we live in.

-Mothers are the pillars of mankind through the shaky grounds of the world we live in.

-Mothers have kept the sanity and promote dignity over generations in the degrading world we live in.

-Mothers have maintained values and morals in the immoral world we live in

-Our Lord Jesus remembered the mothers at the days of terrors in the world we live in: "28But Jesus turning to them said, "Daughters of Jerusalem, stop weeping for Me, but weep for yourselves and for your children. 29"For behold, the days are coming when they will say, 'Blessed are the barren, and the wombs that never bore, and the breasts that never nursed.' 30"Then they will begin TO SAY TO THE MOUNTAINS, 'FALL ON US,' AND TO THE HILLS, 'COVER US.' 31"For if they do these things when the tree is green, what will happen when it is dry?" (Luke 23:28-31)

-And Jesus our Lord and Savior remember the Mothers at the end of days of the world we live in: "But woe to those who are pregnant and to those who are nursing babies in those days! 20 And pray that your flight may not be in winter or on the Sabbath. 21 For then there will be great tribulation, such as has not been since the beginning of the world until this time, no, nor ever shall be. 22 And unless those days were shortened, no flesh would be saved; but for the elect's sake those days will be shortened." (Matthew 24:20-22)

So let us all say: "Happy Mother's Day" as "Mothers never die";

At that day, each human soul love in earth will be measured against the Mother's Love as the human race love is scaled by the Mother's love

Nothing will ever express our appreciation and gratitude to Mothers as nothing will ever compensate the mothers of what they had and continue to do: we bow with respect and love saying "Mothers never die" as Love never fails

As from the Mothers the first breath of Newborn comes so is the last breath of each human soul goes.

Mothers gives a man identity. Mothers are sealed stamp in mankind!

We love you all Mothers: So let us all say: "Happy Mother's Day" as "Mothers never die";

Only Mothers do!

Whatever I write —Whatever I say—- Whatever I do— Nothing will ever come close to describe mothers and what mothers do!

Mothers are the holiness within our human race! Mothers are the wholeness among mankind! Mothers never die and so is mothers' Love!

Mothers are made of divine Love and their glory is within

Just know the mother was the only race found worthy in the eyes of God to give birth to the Most High, her creator, baby Jesus, the savior of the world.

(Proverbs 17:6) "6] Children's children are the crown of old men; and the glory of children are their fathers."

(Isaiah 66:13-14) "[13] As one whom his mother comforteth, so will I comfort you; and ye shall be comforted in Jerusalem. [14] And when ye see this, your heart shall rejoice, and your bones shall flourish like an herb: and the hand of the Lord shall be known toward his servants, and his indignation toward his enemies."

(Proverbs 31:28) "[28] Her children arise up, and call her blessed; her husband also, and he praiseth her."

Mothers are so special. The unconditional love, sacrifice and care are beyond human limits. Why???

When our Lord try to find a closer love, he said "if the mother forget her baby, I will not" because a mom will never leave her child. So Christ love and sacrifice to His children is so eternal and unimaginable.

Mother's heart is pure, eternal and heavenly. Even in earth where mothers are surrounded with wars of men, hate, selfishness, and ruddiness, mothers spread heavenly love.

It is not a coincidence and it is not hormonal as many think. But it is integral part of the mothers hearts of the brains. It is the breath of God and the love of His Son that handed specially to mothers from generation to generation

I wrote so many stories of mothers of my patients in my books II and III “”Christianity and the brain” I dedicated my third book to my mother story and her life journey as mother of ten children.

It is so amazing to me that my mother unconditionally loved the ten children equally and much love went to her miscarriage and my little sister that died at the age of one years old. She could no separate herself or drop thinking about both of them. She always said, both are pure angels in heaven and I am going to be with them in Heaven. She loved St Mary, the pure mother of God. I owe my life to my mom and dad, may God repose their souls

Since I was——

Since I was a baby, I fell in love with my mother!

Since I was a child, I fell in love with my mother and all the mothers!

Since I was a young man, I adored my wife, my mother and all the mothers!

Since I was an adult, there was no one to relay to but to the mother of my chikdren, to my mother and to all the mothers!

Since I was an old man, it wasn't enough to say thank you to the mother of my children, to my mother and to all mothers!

Since I was—- since I am—- Since I shall be—- I always praise my Lord Jesus for the mother of my children, my mother and all the mothers regardless!

It is through the mothers' unconditional love, by the mothers' unquestionable Love and for the mothers' unquenchable Love, what mothers do!

Have You——

Have you ever stopped for a moment and considered what mothers do for mankind?

Have you ever asked yourself why only mothers do what mothers do in a daily basis?

Have you ever stopped for a moment and considered what mothers do for mankind?

It is through the mothers' unconditional love, by the mothers' unquestionable Love and for the mothers' unquenchable Love, what mothers do!

It is not only—but also—-

It is not only every twenty four hours, not every shift, not every hour but also it is every moment all day long what mothers do for humanity!

It is not only every daytime, not every nighttime, not every sun rise, not every sun set, but also it is all day long 24/7 what mothers do for human race!

It is not only every day or every week or every month or every quarter or every year, but also it is all years what mothers do for mankind!

It is not only in the winter or the summer or the spring or the fall, but also it is all seasons what mothers' do for human creation!

It not only one decade, one century, one era but also it is across the generations since the beginning of the world until the end of ages, what mothers do for the world!

It is through the mothers' unconditional love, by the mothers' unquestionable Love and for the mothers' unquenchable Love, what mothers do!

It is not only as newborn girl, a growing child, a daughter, a student, a career woman, a wife, a mother, and grandmother and great grand mother but also it is in every role what mothers do!

It is not only during the daughterhood, wifehood, household, motherhood, work-hood but also it is everywhere what mothers do!

It is not only in house, in school, in community college, in a city university, in works, in community, city, state and country but also it is worldwide what mothers do!

It has never been interrupted, not only in the good times, or the comfort hours or the peaceful times, but it is unrelenting and unforgettable what mothers have done, been doing and continue to do until their last breath for human beings!

It is through the mothers' unconditional love, by the mothers' unquestionable Love and for the mothers' unquenchable Love, what mothers do!

It is the day and day out and beyond mothers' sacrifice, service, cheerful giving, give their life away, production, patience, tolerance, endurance, perseverance, protection, joy, peace-makers, keeping life, maintaining life and keeping balance to the human race in the hostile world and its foundation and much much more what mothers do!

It is not only what mothers do, but also what mothers single-handed go through during their lifespan throughout their lifetime including but not limited to the pains and aches, bloodshed, hardship, inequality, persecution, injustice, humiliation, victimized to physical and verbal violence, taking advantage of, denisle of their human rights, and many many more what mothers bear and do!

It is through the mothers' unconditional love, by the mothers' unquestionable Love and for the mothers' unquenchable Love, what mothers do!

Mothers are noble and so what mothers do!

Mothers are novel and so what mothers do!

Mothers are unprecedented and so what mothers do!

Mothers are unmatched and so what mothers do!

Mothers are unparalleled and so what mothers do!

Mothers are exceptional and so what mothers do!

Mothers are groundbreaking and so what mothers do!

It is through the mothers' unconditional love, by the mothers' unquestionable Love and for the mothers' unquenchable Love, what mothers do!

To everyone —— Let us——

To every nostril breather worldwide, let us —-

Let us praise our Lord Jesus for mothers!

Let us bless mothers!

Let us give thanks to mothers!

Let us provide true Love to mothers!

Let us bring bouquet of Roses to mothers!

To everyone born of a woman worldwide, let us —

Let us reach out to all mothers across the globe!

Let us acknowledge mothers!

Let us appreciate mothers!

Let us award mothers!

Let us celebrate mothers!

To everyone related and unrelated, let us —-

Let us be kind to mothers!

Let us be sensitive to mothers!

Let us be empathetic to mothers!

Let us be just to the mothers!

Let us stand by the mothers!

To everyone male or female, let us—-

Let us carry some of the burden of mothers!

Let us share the greatness in mothers!

Let us respect mothers!

Let us take our hates off for mothers!

Let us kneel to mothers!

Let us pray for all mothers worldwide!

(Proverbs 31:10-31) "10] Who can find a virtuous woman? for her price is far above rubies. [11] The heart of her husband doth safely trust in her, so that he shall have no need of spoil. [12] She will do him good and not evil all the days of her life. [13] She seeketh wool, and flax, and worketh willingly with her hands. [14] She is like the merchants' ships; she bringeth her food from afar. [15] She riseth also while it is yet night, and giveth meat to her household, and a portion to her maidens. [16] She considereth a field, and buyeth it: with the fruit of her hands she planteth a vineyard. [17] She girdeth her loins with strength, and strengtheneth her arms. [18] She perceiveth that her merchandise is good: her candle goeth not out by night. [19] She layeth her hands to the spindle, and her hands hold the distaff. [20] She stretcheth out her hand to the poor; yea, she reacheth forth her hands to the needy. [21] She is not afraid of the snow for her household: for all her household are clothed with scarlet. [22] She maketh herself coverings of tapestry; her clothing is silk and purple. [23] Her husband is known in the gates, when he sitteth among the elders of the land. [24] She maketh fine linen, and selleth it ; and delivereth girdles unto the merchant. [25] Strength and honour are her clothing; and she shall rejoice in time to come. [26] She openeth her mouth with wisdom; and in her tongue is the law of kindness. [27] She looketh well to the ways of her household, and eateth not the bread of idleness. [28] Her children arise up, and call her blessed; her husband also, and he praiseth her. [29] Many daughters have done virtuously, but thou excellest them all. [30] Favour is deceitful, and beauty is vain: but a woman that feareth the Lord, she shall be praised. [31] Give her of the fruit of her hands; and let her own works praise her in the gates"

Therefore, today, When you see a mom stop, take your hate off and with a smile, appreciation and gratitude saying: "Happy Mother's Day" in sincerity utter the heartfelt genuine words! Show love and This day isn't just about an outing, a brunch, a dinner or a gift but about believing and paying back! Do act of love and kindness!! I hope, It isn't just a brunch, it wasn't just a word. It wasn't just an act when a man say "Happy Mother's Day"

We love you all Mothers: So let us all say: "Happy Mother's Day" as "Mothers never die";

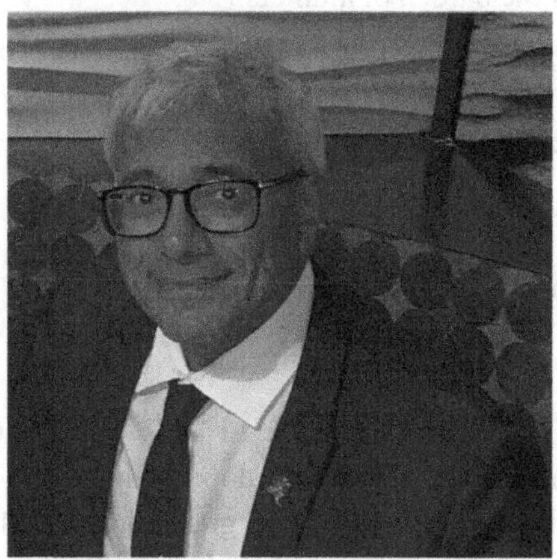

RY, So tender and so loving. Very eloquent words my friend as I am thinking of my mom and Leslie's girls today. Without a mother's love we are nothing. Thank you for writing this and May God bless all mothers in heaven and those that are still among us.

LY, Beautiful Dr. **Ramsis Ghaly**!

JT, you have your beautiful mama's smile Ramsis...

ES, So beautifully said.

Dl, My momma is 81 & I'm so thankful I still have her !

BCD, So true.

JC, Happy heavenly Mother's Day to your beautiful Mother

CG, These words touch my heart So beautiful! You are correct that mother's never die, those that have transitioned are alive in our memories every single day. Happy Mother's Day to all.

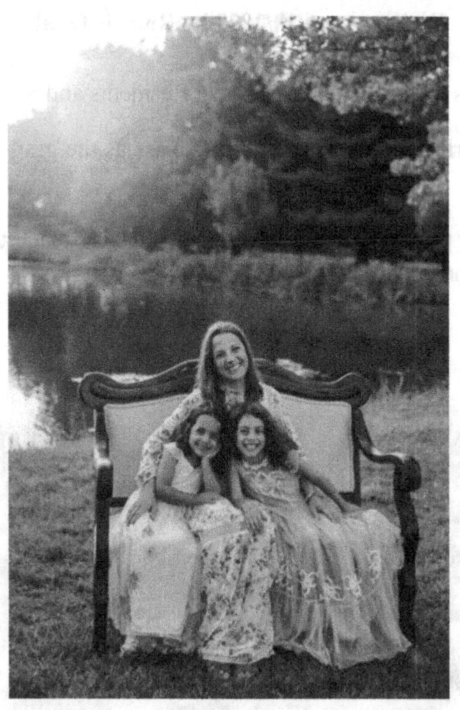

Mandy

Thank you Dr Ghaly!

I worked last night and I only want to share this with you because it's why we do what we do...a 39 year old woman of 2 young children had an emergency brain surgery at 1am on Mother's Day! The best gift of Mother's Day for me was her waking up and saying Im thirsty my head hurts and moving all her extremities

Dr Ghaly, I know your heart and why you live, we share that and always will, and I know that we want to give the world what God has given us. You inspire me to be the best version of myself for my children and the world. Im honored not only know you but call you my friend.

Emily Coley

Taking my tumor out Thank you Dr. Ghaly. Best Mother's Day ever thanks to you

Post COVID Happy Father's Day!

Written on 6/18/2022 by Ramsis Ghaly

My Father's Day is Joyful with my Patients, Residents and Students!

First month to work with the new resident's class as the graduate class is going away to practice!

It is an honor and privilege to continue to mentor and teach the new class and generations you come since 1991!!!

Ramsis Ghaly

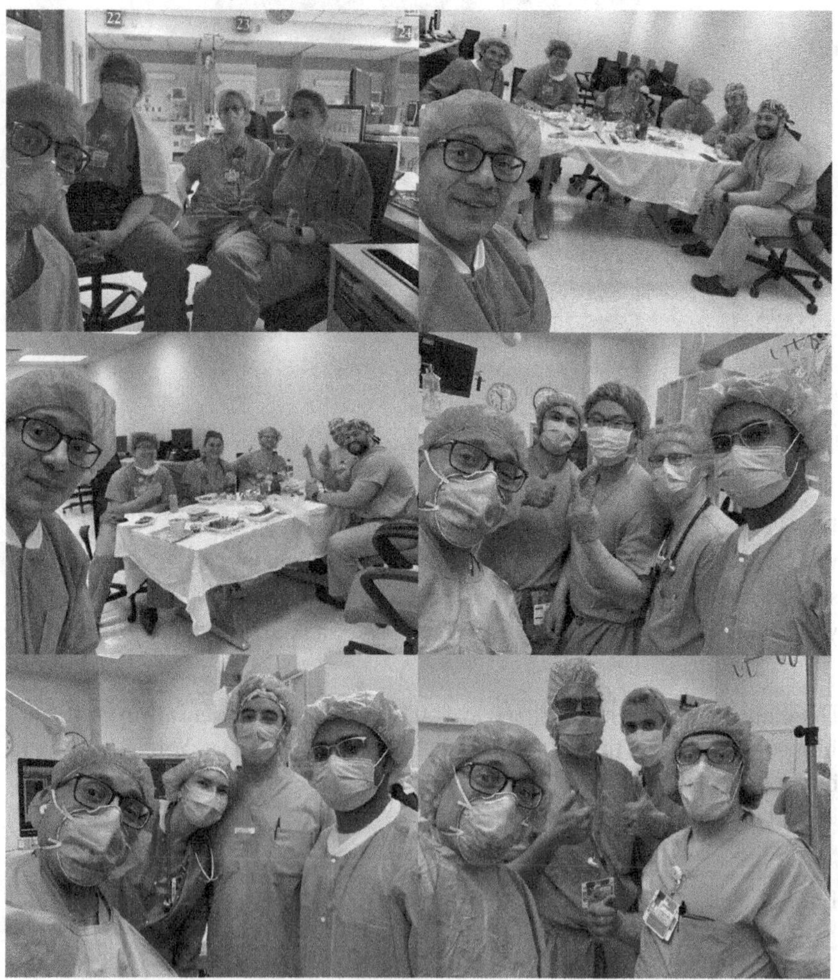

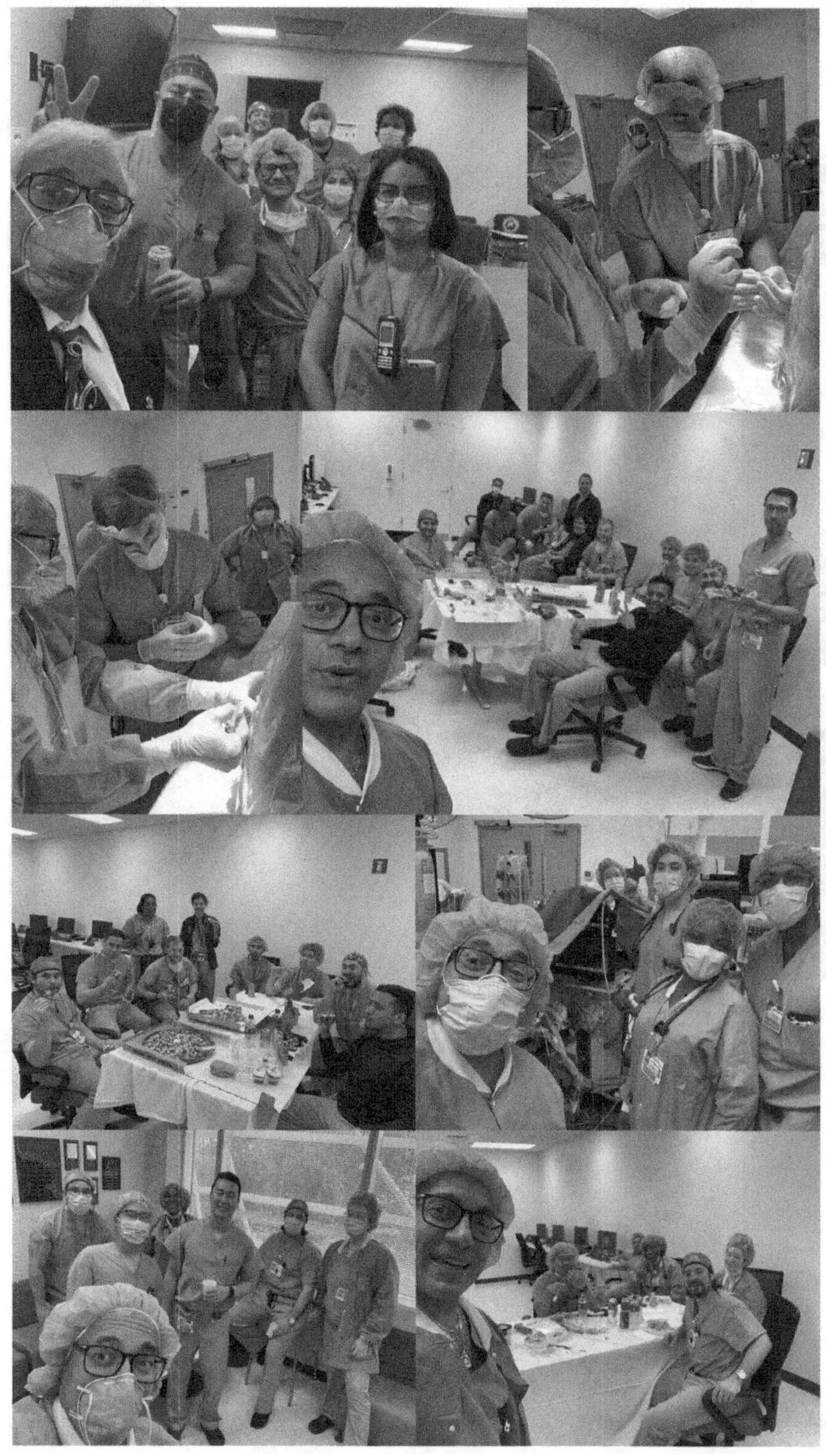

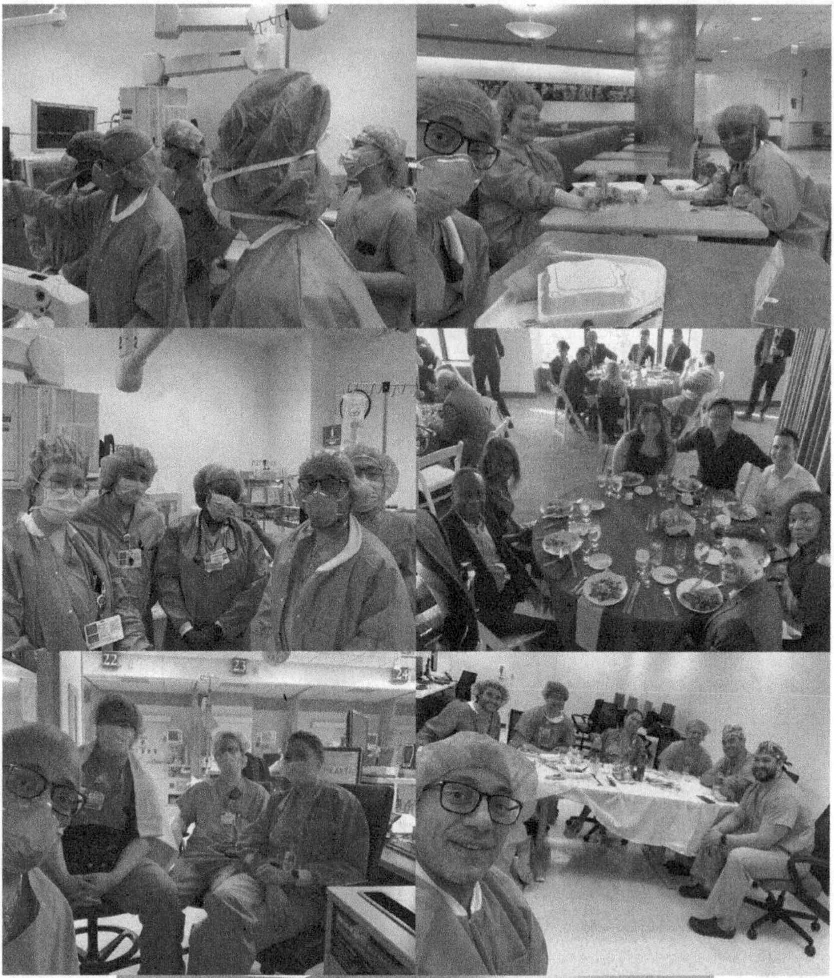

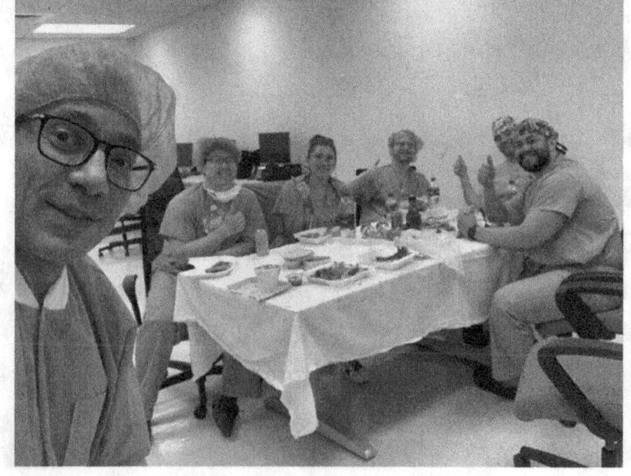

Happy Father's Day

Written by Ramsis Ghaly

Happy Father's Day. Thank you all for who you are and all what you do

It is a journey where it begins it shall end,

But the life you endure, the love you give, the heroic steps you undertake, and the sacrifice you leave behind, it will all last forever and ever more

It is a journey where it begins it shall end,

But the life you endure, the love you give, the heroic steps you undertake, and the sacrifice you leave behind, it will all last forever and ever more

Happy Father's Day. Thank you all for who you are and all what you do

Respectfully

Ramsis Ghaly

cg, They are fortunate you are their teacher. Wishing them all a great year.

Kg, **Congratulations** and Keep.up the great work!.Awesome! Happy Father's Day

Dh, **Congratulations** Dr Ghaly! Keep up all of the Great work you do, you are awesome! Wishing all of your students much success ! Happy Father's Day!

dh, Thank you Dr Ghaly, may God Bless you, so inspirational, the Love of a Father

May God Bless you sir, may our God keep you safe, keep his hedge of protection over you and all of those sacrificing and giving their all for our country. Thank you for your service .

My Love Journey to Exceptionalism!

Written by Ramsis Ghaly

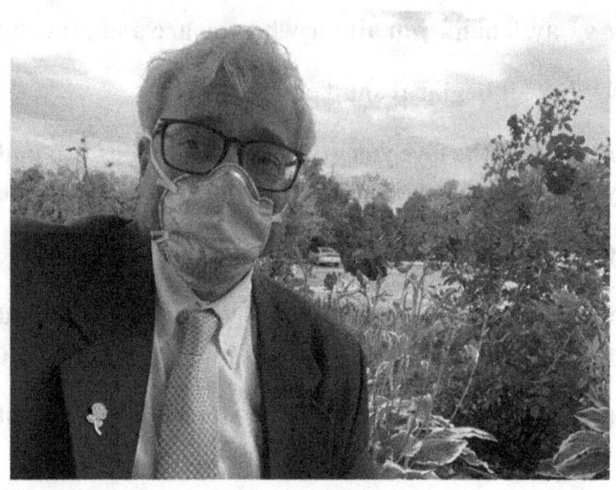

Lord Jesus Love to Humanity leads to adoption!

Adoption leads to sons and daughters of God!

God leads to Spiritual Gifts!

Faith leads Gifts!

Love creates Talents!

Humility results in Appreciation!

Appreciation mixed with Love and Humility leads to Dedication!

Dedication with Faith Flourishes More Talents!

Talents come with Passionate!

Passionate comes with Talents!

Talents require Commitment!

Commitment requires Patience!

Patience leads to Perseverance!

Perseverance requires Sacrifice!

Sacrifice leads to Excellence!

Excellence leads to Quality!

Quality leads to Exceptionalism!

Exceptionalism crowns Love!

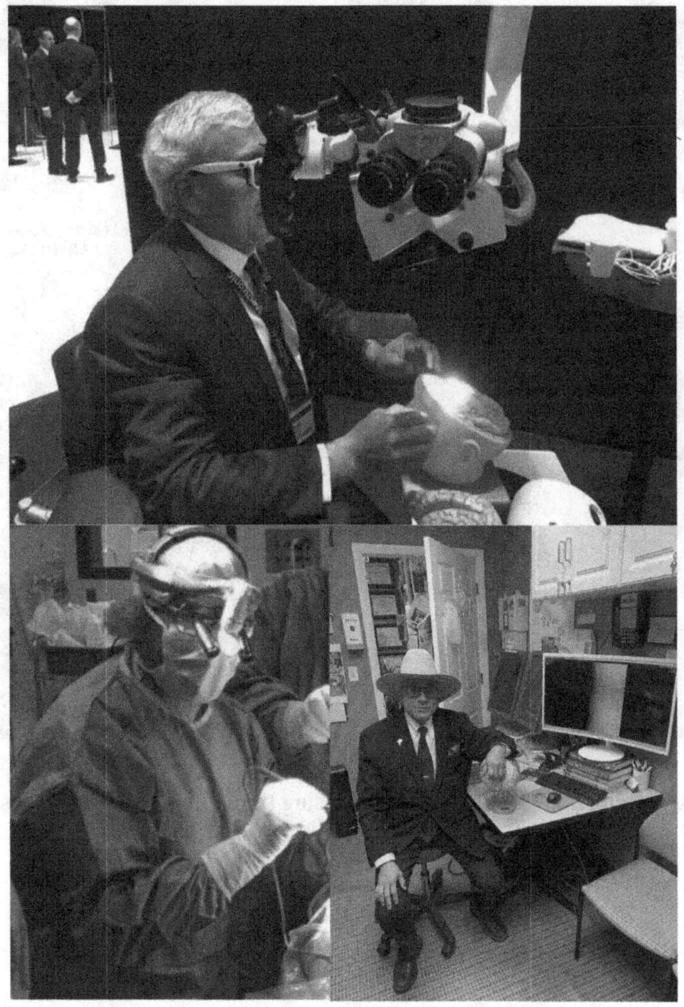

Personal Selected Photos!

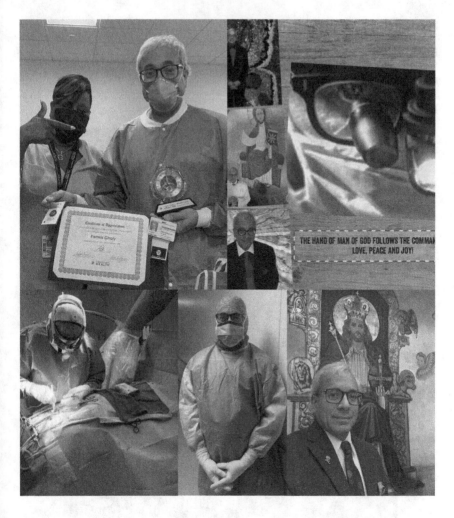

CG, You certainly have a knack for expressing through your writing. Bless you!

Lord Jesus Do So Much Good Through Human Hands While They May Never Know!

Written on 3/18/2022 by Ramsis Ghaly

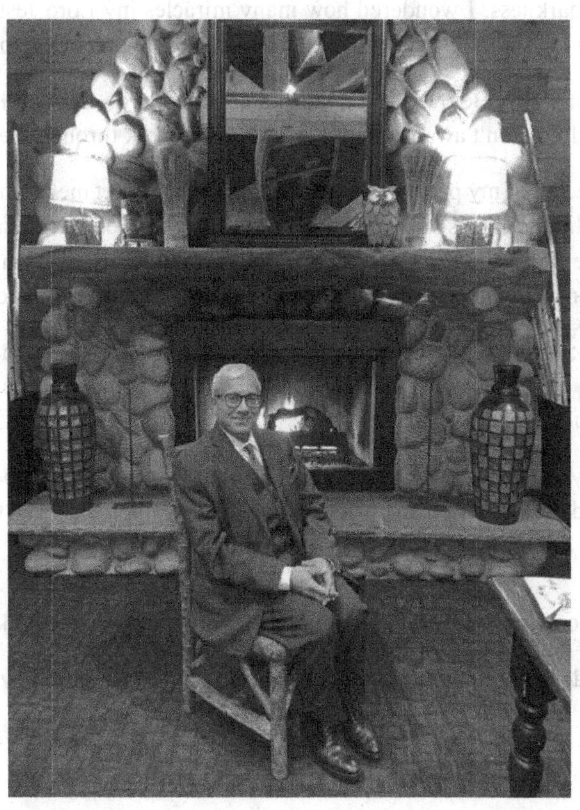

I was down in my knees and saddened with the lives lost in Ukraine and those children, mothers and civilians are dying shot-dead and bombed!

I looked at my Lord Jesus photo and asked Him: "Why O my Lord You allow this atrocity! The Ukrainians are too Your children and they do believe in You and You are too their Savior"

And then I received a message and a phone call from a previous patient long ago! I called and He surprised me in the phone as if he knew me very well and said: "Hi Dr Ghaly I am the nation champion you operated on me 1998 and because of you and your surgery, I had the best career winning so many awards! I moved on to be a very successful heavy Olympic weightlifter champion and made it through the years of lifting heavy weights and entered into so many competitions and won national awards more than 70 competitions —-!

I was shocked with my patient's words and felt so guilty that I didn't know and I was ashamed of my self that all these years I haven't give thanks to my Healer my lord Jesus!

Despite the darkness, I wondered how many miracles my Lord Jesus had done thus far and I fell short of giving Him thanks and show appreciation to my Savior?

How many more my Beloved had done and continue to do through His children and His children aren't aware for all His unceasing work through their hands???

I felt that the call of my patient is from God Almighty to let me see more of Him and He is telling me He is still in control regardless of the dark News around!! He has the entire world and all His children in the Palm of His Hand even if the world is trying to snash them from His hand! The Lord is indeed In-Control!

I said to him; "O my Lord Jesus for all these years, I didn't know that You used my hands to do miracles to Your children!!!"And How many of me You do the same and much more??

Indeed, today I realized that How many times Lord Jesus do for His people all over the world and the world in turn do not acknowledge or appreciate His Great work!

++

Lord Jesus does so much good in human hands and they may never know!

Lord Jesus does so many miracles through human hands and they may never know!

++

Lord Jesus does so much good in human hands and they may never recognize!

Lord Jesus does so many miracles through human hands and they may never recognize!

++

Lord Jesus does so much good in human hands if they just believe!

Lord Jesus does so many miracles through human hands if they just believe!

++

Lord Jesus does so much good in human hands if they just open our eyes!

Lord Jesus does so many miracles through human hands if they just open our eyes!

++

Lord Jesus does so much good in human hands if they just look around!

Lord Jesus does so many miracles through human hands if they just look around!

Look at generosity of our Savior in every day and every minute of human lives!

Yet, the human side of human nature is seeing the negatives, hearing the negatives, overwhelming by the negatives and talking about the negatives! And they are ignoring the miracles of God and He is in Control!

And our Lord savior is still working and so His Father despite the human side of our nature, as He said: John 5:17 KJV "But Jesus answered them, My Father worketh hitherto, and I work."

Ephesians 3:19-21 KJV "And to know the love of Christ, which passeth knowledge, that ye might be filled with all the fulness of God. [20] Now unto him that is able to do exceeding abundantly above all that we ask or think, according to the power that worketh in us, [21] Unto him be glory in the church by Christ Jesus throughout all ages, world without end. Amen."

2 Corinthians 9:8,11,15 KJV "And God is able to make all grace abound toward you; that ye, always having all sufficiency in all things, may abound to every good work: [11] Being enriched in every thing to all bountifulness, which causeth through us thanksgiving to God. [15] Thanks be unto God for his unspeakable gift."

John 16:23-24 ESV "In that day you will ask nothing of me. Truly, truly, I say to you, whatever you ask of the Father in my name, he will give it to you. Until now you have asked nothing in my name. Ask, and you will receive, that your joy may be full."

Malachi 3:10 KJV "Bring ye all the tithes into the storehouse, that there may be meat in mine house, and prove me now herewith, saith the Lord of hosts, if I will not open you the windows of heaven, and pour you out a blessing, that there shall not be room enough to receive it."

Deuteronomy 11:14 "that He will give the rain for your land in its season, the early and late rain, that you may gather in your grain and your new wine and your oil."

Job 5:10 "He gives rain on the earth

And sends water on the fields,"

Acts 14:17 KJV "Nevertheless he left not himself without witness, in that he did good, and gave us rain from heaven, and fruitful seasons, filling our hearts with food and gladness."

Psalm 147:7-9 KJV "Sing unto the Lord with thanksgiving; sing praise upon the harp unto our God: [8] Who covereth the heaven with clouds, who prepareth rain for the earth, who maketh grass to grow upon the mountains. [9] He giveth to the beast his food, and to the young ravens which cry."

Colossians 3:14-17 KJV "And above all these things put on charity, which is the bond of perfectness. [15] And let the peace of God rule in your hearts, to the which also ye are called in one body; and be ye thankful. [16] Let the word of Christ dwell in you richly in all wisdom; teaching and admonishing one another in psalms and hymns and spiritual songs, singing with grace in your hearts to the Lord. [17] And whatsoever ye do in word or deed, do all in the name of the Lord Jesus, giving thanks to God and the Father by him."

1 Thessalonians 5:16-24 KJV "Rejoice evermore. [17] Pray without ceasing. [18] In every thing give thanks: for this is the will of God in Christ Jesus concerning you. [19] Quench not the Spirit. [20] Despise not prophesyings. [21] Prove all things; hold fast that which is good. [22] Abstain from all appearance of evil. [23] And the very God of peace sanctify you wholly; and I pray God your whole spirit and soul and body be preserved blameless unto the coming of our Lord Jesus Christ. [24] Faithful is he that calleth you, who also will do it."

Philippians 4:5-8 KJV "Let your moderation be known unto all men. The Lord is at hand. [6] Be careful for nothing; but in every thing by prayer and supplication with thanksgiving let your requests be made known unto God. [7] And the peace of God, which passeth all understanding, shall keep your hearts and minds through Christ Jesus. [8] Finally, brethren, whatsoever things are true, whatsoever things are honest, whatsoever things are just, whatsoever things are pure, whatsoever things are lovely, whatsoever things are of good report; if there be any virtue, and if there be any praise, think on these things."

Amen Thank you Lord Jesus!

Come to Grandpa Arms My Little Baby Girl! Let me Hug You! I was Just Waiting for that Moment!

A Poem dedicated to the Patricoski's
Written on 10/2/22 by Ramsis Ghaly

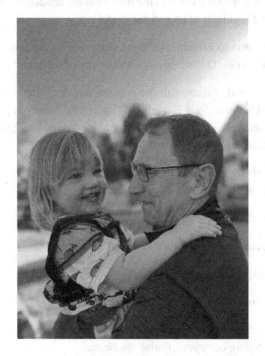

What should I say as I am humbly looking at this adorable picture!!!

From outside, the arms of grandpa is carrying a little angel as her arms around his shoulders but what is inexpressible is the unseen but heartfelt unceasing river of love and cohesiveness pouring between them!

Grandpa and grandma love like no one else to their grandchild! Juniper you are the crown of Patricoski's! Welcome to our family!

I just can't find a word to express but all what I can say and feel is this: "Love and Humanity" as God Almighty created in its purity and innocence!! The children and grandchildren be blessed and multiply in God's glory and good will to man as it is in heaven so it is on earth!!

This what humanity is and should be in the image and likeness of God the Love ! May I carry thee up high in my arms! The world can't fill our hearts as our grandchild Juni have done to ours!!

I pray that if just everyone look at this photo and praise God in His children, admire the unconditional love, the peace and joy from the hearts of fathers to the children and grandchildren!

I shall never forget the moment you were born and that day I carried thee in my arms! You stole our hearts forever as the world has never been the same since that time! You are the highlight of us and our pride!

O little Juniper come to grandpa, little me carry you in my arms! Look at you! Your eyes, your cheeks, O little sweetheart and ray of sunshine!

My name is Mark and you can call me grandpa and my wife is name is Winnie and you may call her grandma! But tell us What is your name our grandchild little baby girl! You are from our bones, hearts and blood! God has gifted us by theel and filled our hearts exceedingly that day you were born!

O my love Juni if you just know how much you filled our hearts and souls when thee came to the world since the day you get born!

The sweetest little face melting grandpapa and grandma away!!!

Aren't you gorgeous cutie pie junior Patricoski!

Grandpa admires you little precious soul!

How adorable you are baby girl!!! Thou close to my heart!

I thank God for letting grandpa and grandma live to the day to see our seeds grow more and more before our eyes!! Praise thy Name!

I just hope for you little ones to live up to our heritage and values and be blessing wherever you go! Come often we will watch over you, babysit thee and teach you all about thy heritage!

Look at you little cute, the joy, the smile and confidence filling the world around thee, you have acquired from your grandpa!

I just love you much and grandpa and grandma always here for you! And so our endless love to mommy and daddy and all our family, children and grandchildren!

So thankful to our daughter Kate and our son in law to bring thee to our life! The Patricoski's can't be more proud!!!

Our family is blessed and to that we give our thanksgiving! Wait little Juni, we have much surprises coming your way at the Halloween, Thanksgiving and Christmas!!!

May our Lord keep you and your parents forever, protect you and bless you all more and more!! Amen !

Come to Grandpa Arms My Little Baby Girl!! Let me Hug You! I was Just Waiting for that Moment!

Pertinent Biblical Verses

Proverbs 17:6 "Children's children are a crown to the aged, and parents are the pride of their children."

Psalm 92:14 "They will still bear fruit in old age, they will stay fresh and green."

Proverbs 16:31 "Gray hair is a crown of glory; it is gained in a righteous life."

Psalm 103:17 "But from everlasting to everlasting the Lords love is with those who fear him, and his righteousness with their children's children.

Proverbs 13:22 "A good person leaves an inheritance for their children's children, but a sinner's wealth is stored up for the righteous."

Deuteronomy 5:16 "Honor your father and your mother, as the Lord your God commanded you, that your days may be long, and that it may go well with you in the land that the Lord your God is giving you."

Proverbs 4:1-5 "Hear, O sons, a father's instruction, and be attentive that you may gain insight, for I give you good precepts; do not forsake my teaching. When I was a son with my father, tender, the only one in the sight of my mother, he taught me and said to me, 'Let your heart hold fast my words; keep my commandments, and live. Get wisdom; get insight; do not forget, and do not turn away from the words of my mouth."

Psalm 71:9 "Do not cast me off in the time of old age; forsake me not when my strength is spent."

Proverbs 1:8-9 "Hear, my son, your father's instruction, and forsake not your mother's teaching, for they are a graceful garland for your head and pendants for your neck."

Proverbs 16:31 "Grey hair is a crown of splendor; it is attained in the way of righteousness."

Isaiah 46:4 "Even to your old age I am he, and to gray hairs I will carry you. I haves made, and I will bear; I will carry and will save."

Psalm 37:25 "I have been young, and now am old, yet I have not seen the righteous forsaken or his children begging for bread."

Psalm 92:14-15 "They still bear fruit in old age; they are ever full of sap and green, to declare that the Lord is upright; he is my rock, and there is no unrighteousness in him."

Isaiah 40:28-31 "Have you not known? Have you not heard? The Lord is the everlasting God, the Creator of the ends of the earth. He does not faint or grow weary; his understanding is unsearchable. He gives power to the faint and to him who has no might he increases strength. Even youths shall faint and be weary, and young men shall fall exhausted; but they who wait on the Lord shall renew their strength; they shall mount up with wings like eagles; they shall run and not be weary; they shall walk and not faint."

Psalm 100:5 "For the LORD is good. His unfailing love continues forever, and his faithfulness continues to each generation."

Psalm 73:26 "My flesh and my heart may fail, but God is the strength of my heart, my portion forever."

Hebrews 13:8 "Jesus Christ is the same yesterday and today and forever."

26. Psalm 145:4 "One generation commends your works to another; they tell of your mighty acts."

2 Timothy 3:14-15 "But as for you, continue in what you have learned and have firmly believed, knowing from childhood you have been acquainted with the sacred writings, which are able to make you wise for salvation through faith in Christ Jesus."

Deuteronomy 6:1-2 "Now this is the commandment, the statutes and the rules that the Lord your God commanded me to teach you, that you may do them in the land to which you are going over, to posssess it, that you may fear the Lord your God, you and your son and your son's son, by keeping all his statutes and his commandments, which I command you, all the days of your life, and that your days may be long."

Genesis 45:10 "You shall dwell in the land of Goshen, and you shall be near me, you and your children and your children's children, and your flocks, your herds, and all that you have."

Deuteronomy 32:7 "Remember the days of old; consider the generations long past. Ask your father and he will tell you, your elders, and they will explain to you."

Proverbs 13:1 A wise son accepts his father's discipline, But a scoffer does not listen to rebuke.

Matthew 19:19 Honor your father and mother; and You shall love your neighbor as yourself."

Colossians 3:20 Children, be obedient to your parents in all things, for this is well-pleasing to the Lord.

Ephesians 6:2 Honor your father and mother (which is the first commandment with a promise),

Proverbs 3:12 For whom the Lord loves He reproves, Even as a father corrects the son in whom he delights.

Malachi 4:6 He will restore the hearts of the fathers to their children and the hearts of the children to their fathers, so that I will not come and smite the land with a curse."

Proverbs 1:8 Hear, my son, your father's instruction

And do not forsake your mother's teaching;

Proverbs 15:20 A wise son makes a father glad,

But a foolish man despises his mother.

Proverbs 4:10 Hear, my son, and accept my sayings

And the years of your life will be many.

Ephesians 6:3 so that it may be well with you, and that you may live long on the earth.

Proverbs 23:22 Listen to your father who begot you, And do not despise your mother when she is old.

Proverbs 19:14 House and wealth are an inheritance from fathers, But a prudent wife is from the Lord.

John 3:1 See how great a love the Father has bestowed on us, that we would be called children of God; and such we are. For this reason the world does not know us, because it did not know Him.

Proverbs 22:6 Train up a child in the way he should go, Even when he is old he will not depart from it.

Proverbs 13:24 He who withholds his rod hates his son, But he who loves him disciplines him diligently.

Come to Grandpa Arms My Little Baby Girl!! Let me Hug You! I was Just Waiting for that Moment!

With love and blessings!

Ramsis Ghaly

Mp, Dr. Ghaly

Thanks so much and so beautifully written. It describes the way we feel about Juni and her parents.

Mark

Wp, Doc- that is beautiful and we are so grateful for not only Juniper in our lives but all our family. And you my friend are a wonderful part of our family. Thank you for all you do, for us, your patients and to all those you meet.

Dp, That is precious. Incredible poem.

Dn, So beautifully written

Cg, Such s sweet poem for a beautiful little girl.

Rc, Beautiful poem!!!

My Birthday 2022 Meditation!

Ramsis Ghaly

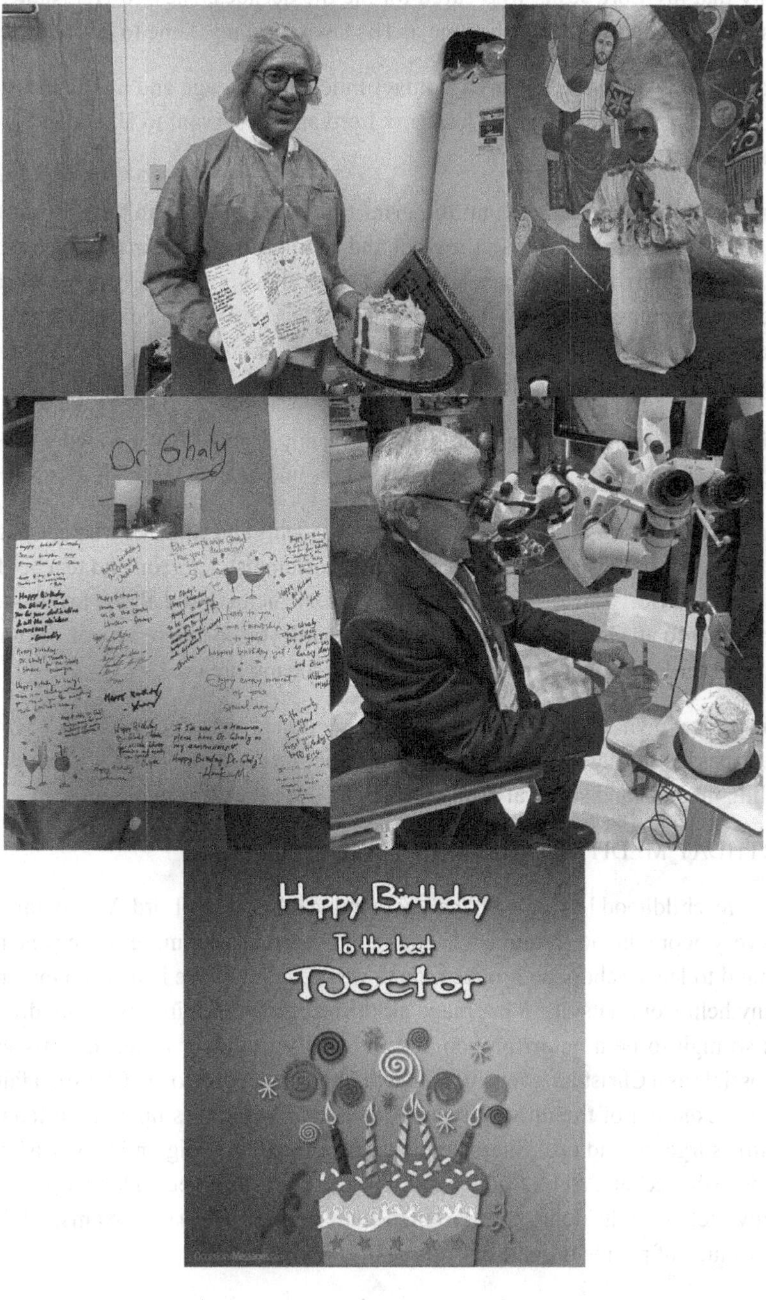

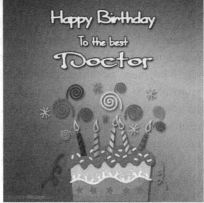

In my Birthday I Prayed to my Lord to do what I am always do which is to continue to fulfill my cause at the center of my core! And thankfully this is what I will do! My patient does not know that he was sent and he actually my precious birthday gift!

I pray that my Lord Jesus who cared for me the decades, Blessed His Name, to bless him and continue to utilize me as His Own until my Time to go!

I was asked what I want for my birthday! Indeed, in my age and all the blessing God has given me, nothing but Jesus my Lord and be servant to His people who He send in my way!

That particular patient that I am to perform his surgery, he can't even wait for another days. He is crawling in the floor and laying at the trunk in the back of the car from the horrific nerve pains. He can't sit or stand or walk or sleep 24/7! He is totally decompensating! And yet God put me in a position to heal and cure and be source of comfort to others! What an honor and privilege to be in and I always be grateful to the gifts that I am not worthy!

I will never ever ask God for more!! Indeed, many nights I feel unworthy to For God to grant me the gifts and endurance to serve and heal and teach in His Name!

In my birthday, I thank so much my patients, residents and students who entrusted me to be their neurosurgeon, physician, anesthesiologist, surgeon and teacher for more than 45 (forty-five) years! To my mentors and helpers and all the loved ones, thank you. To all God had placed in my way, thank you so much! I thank so much America for let me in and be in the land to pursue my dreams!

Many of my own, God had taken them, many others retired or quit early while others passed through unfortunate circumstances to force them away from their healing medical and surgical profession!

BIRTHDAY MEDITATION

Since my childhood I dreamed to be a doctor and to serve my Lord. Yet my family was very poor with no resources. In addition, I was one out 7 more sibling and the demand to leave school and make money was very high. We had no connection or any help from outside. What made all things worse back in Egypt, my dream was so high to be a neurosurgeon and university professor to teach. This was impossible as a Christian minority with extreme persecution to my Christian faith. I was kicked out of the university, and I was told I am "so stupid" by a fanatic Islamic surgeons and examiners that they were trained in England by Christians and Jewish teachers. At that time, I felt it was my end and I see no longer purpose for my life! I shut the doors and started to study hard for American exams. I didn't know much of people or have any valuable connections!

Through every step of my life, I saw all the doors were closing and I worked hard to look for more doors and even those were also closing! Yet there was always a tiny hidden road wide open and only one that missed and somehow God let me see it and it was my pass.

In my journey, there was never plain B for me because of my demand in myself that I must pursue plan A regardless. How many times, I was rejected, infuriated, belittled, discriminated, humiliated and I was left in the streets hungry, thirst and ashamed of my repeated failures. And every time I felt a relief was in the way, the entire thing crumbled to the degree that I always knew "It was my luck, and nothing would be ever easy before me! To the degree when I saw light, I immediately made it look dark so that I won't lift my hopes up!! God knows how many times my hopes were up and my soul landed all the way down unto the pit! I became a close friend to the failures and the infamous!

And at the eleventh hour, I closed my eyes and prayed in secret to my God in tears! I reflected deeply, analyses my daily events and let the past hours rewind before my brain! And I cried and said repeatedly to Him "for how long my Lord".

Next minute I did I drifted into the night with heavy burden and all of a sudden, I woke up with a heavenly reply accompanied with hope! My Lord was always with me and inside me, but I didn't see Him and I was busy with the outside world not listening to His voice and seeing His hands!! He was knocking in my door, and I didn't notice because I was so busy carrying my burden all alone!

Jesus my Lord snd God said: "Behold, I stand at the door, and knock: if any man hear my voice, and open the door, I will come in to him, and will sup with him, and he with me. [21] To him that overcometh will I grant to sit with me in my throne, even as I also overcame, and am set down with my Father in his throne. [22] He that hath an ear, let him hear what the Spirit saith unto the churches."Revelation 3:20-22 KJV

Soon, my life was loaded by disappointments and much of failures and osses1 I was told; "Why are you here, get your bags and go where you came from. You don't belong here" I called my dad and my mom and said: "They don't want me here in US, I am coming back!" My mom and dad replied: "Where you are coming, there is nothing for you here in Egypt. Your dreams are high, we have no money, and you are Christian! I hang up as my soul is torn and no one from my own empathetic or reached out!

Yet I heard my Lord words: "Come unto me, all ye that labour and are heavy laden, and I will give you rest. [29] Take my yoke upon you, and learn of me; for I am meek and lowly in heart: and ye shall find rest unto your souls. [30] For my yoke is easy, and my burden is light."Matthew 11:28-30 KJV

Anyhow, I realized early on, I was meant to struggle, and I wasn't anyone important! Therefore, I hardly heard any words of hope for many around me. I even asked to do work for free as a volunteer just let me in and put among the medical books. Nonetheless, I realized I wasn't worthy, and I shouldn't had expected any miracles or easy ways!

I have kept going and the truth to be said: "I never knew how" I worked in restaurants, cleaned tables, scammed repeatedly, mocked frequently, spitted upon, laughed at my face, climbed walls, hid in closets, and always watched over my shadows!

Yet, my life radically changed after a brief dream back in high school where God said: "He shall never leave me and He will always be the blessing", I have never slowed down or deviated from the mission He had put before me. My enthusiasm and energy 24/7 were thought by the surrounding that it is very hard to be explained and can't be humanly!!

The fact was and is and will be, my eyes were fixated unto that High Mountain and I ran through hills and walked through valleys and my vision never departed from my dream and mission. I went through steadfast whatever barriers. My Beloved shined up high and picked me up to His arms. He is my Savior and always here for me! I perhaps don't see Him and He doesn't speak to me in spoken words, yet He lives within my soul, spirit, heart, mind and thoughts and to Whom I will always be loyal to and report to! At the end my day, I sat by His feet at the cross as His precious droplets of blood soaked my face and my flesh and told me, how much He loved me!

My Lord came so many times to save me! Jesus always came at the heat of the storm as it bombarded me, lean down, wrote with His fingers. And gradually peace and quiescence surrounded and then He raised His head and looked at my worrisome feeble soul saying: "When Jesus had lifted up himself, and saw none but the woman, he said unto her, Woman, where are those thine accusers? hath no man condemned thee? [11] She said, No man, Lord. And Jesus said unto her, Neither do I condemn thee: go, and sin no more. [12] Then spake Jesus again unto them, saying, I am the light of the world: he that followeth me shall not walk in darkness, but shall have the light of life."

John 8:10-12 KJV

Through my journey abroad I lost my parents that I have missed so much. They were with me in struggles and have never seen my successes! To the patients past, present and future, you always be in my heart ! To my residents and students, I will always pray for your success!

In my birthday, I kneel to my Savior saying: "Thank you for all the years and another year"! To my Heavenly Father: " O Father when You are ready for me to come home? My parents were taken away to early and their families, my early peers of my own are too gone! Please, at Your time, take me to your garden and let us walk together by the valley.

O my God, You have given me abundantly! Let the world know with Your abundant mercy! Praise our Lord Hod Jesus the Savior of the world! O God forgive me; I have done the least for You and Your children!! I could have done better! Perhaps You are giving my soul another year to be much more faithful than the previous years! Promise me, this year as all the years in the past, You shall never leave me!! There is no life away from You as it is written: "Lord, to whom shall we go? thou hast the words of eternal life. And we believe and are sure that thou art that Christ, the Son of the living God." John 6:68-69 KJV

Thank you all for letting me part of your life and thank you for all your birthday wishes!!!

Amen

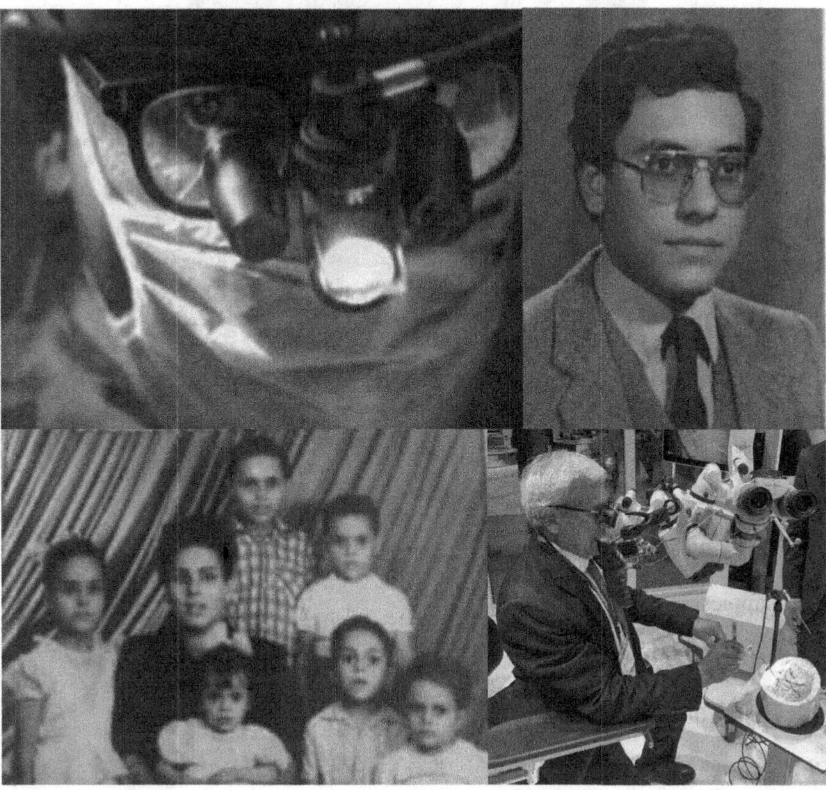

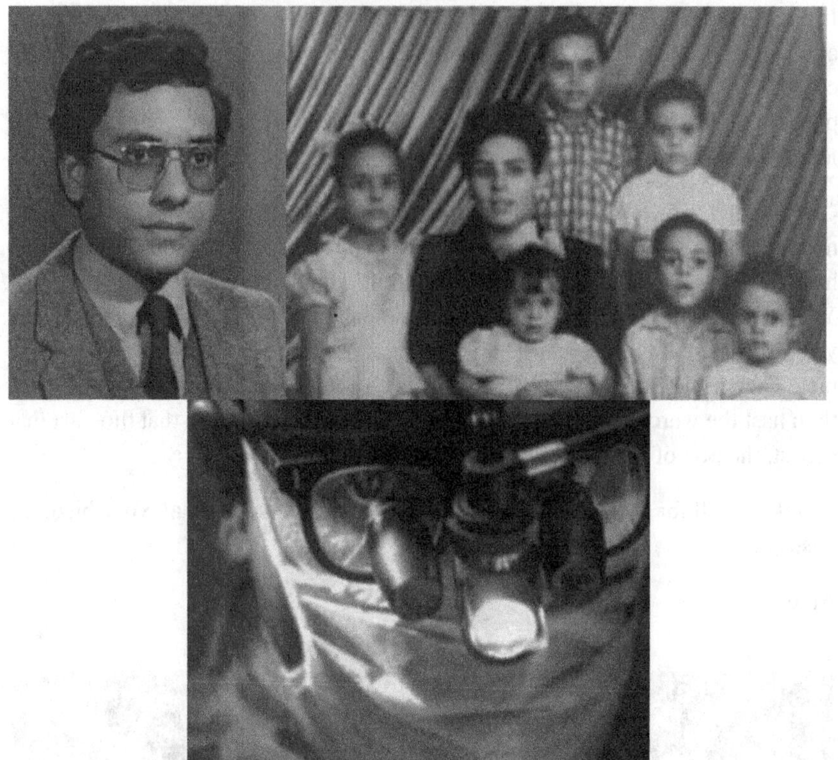

FL, Happy birthday

AL, Happy birthday

BS, Happy birthday!

CS, Happy Birthday, Dr. Ghaly!

VS, Happy birthday Dr Ghaly! Many blessings to you on your day and always.

JV, Happy birthday

LM, Blessings to you

GL, Happy birthday Dr

LR, Happiest Birthday Dr. Ghaly

LA, Happy Birthday!

GR, Happy birthday

Cheri Polich

May God continue to bless you in all your work & for a healthy & happy future. You are a miracle worker and have helped so many people. I am grateful to all you have done for me. Happiest of Birthdays to you Dr. Ghaly!

Kathy Manthei Sitar

Happy Birthday, Dr. Ghaly. I remember when you were in Joliet and the Herald News had a great article on you. You saved a classmate of mine by removing a tumor from her brain and she made a magnificent recovery . May God bless you today and every day.

SY, Happy Birthday Dr. Ghaly! May the Lord bless you and keep you always!

CP, Happy Birthday dear sir

BD, Happy Birthday

CR, Happy Happy Birthday

PH, Happy birthday!

RC, It is wonderful to see how God has brought you through all of these years. I'm glad you remained faithful to your calling/dream. Happy birthday to you!

SA, Happy Birthday Dr. Ghaly! Thank you for all you do for your patients, including me! I hope you had a wonderful day today!

BV, Happy Birthday God Bless you

NW, Happy Birthday!

WM, Happy birthday

AL, Que el señor lo siga bendecido grandemente, que tenga un feliz cumpleaños

SJ, Happy birthday, Dr. Ghaly

SN, Happy Birthday, Dr. Ghaly! I hope you have a great day

PR, Most excellent prayer, much work ahead and enjoy the night, hope you have some celebration for yourself, thank you for sharing

RS, Happy Birthday

CS, Happy Birthday!

BP, Happy Birthday Dr. Ghaly!!!

RA, Hope you had a blessed birthday Dr. Ghaly.

JP, Happy Birthday Dr. GHALY

Annette Cozzi

A Blessed & Happy Birthday to you Dr Ghaly. We who have been blessed by your gift in this lifetime are eternally thankful for the day you were born. God had such a beautiful plan for your life. We are grateful to be part of it.

MG, Happy birthday dear Dr. **Ramsis Ghaly** - God bless

MJ, Happy birthday, God Bless you

BL, Happy Bday, wishing you all the best

RP, Happy birthday doctor god Bless You

TJ, Happy birthday

Karen Boland Geheber

Happy happy Birthday Dr. Ghaly. Your story is an inspiration to all of us to never give up, pray hard, and always believe that God hears us and answers our prayers

DM, Happy Birthday Dr. Ghaly

DE, Happy birthday

JG, Happy Birthday, Dr. Ghaly!

JW, Happy birthday, Dr. **Ramsis Ghaly**! Hope all is well.

YB, Happy Birthday

VW, Happy happy birthday!

GS, Happy Birthday

JE, Happy Birthday Dr. **Ramsis Ghaly**!

LG, Happy birthday, Dr. Ghaly! God bless you!

JW, Happy Birthday to You Dr. **Ramsis Ghaly** Hope you had a great day

DC, Happy Birthday

TN, Happy Birthday Ramsis

JP, Happy Birthday Dr. Ghaly!! God bless you.!

Tanya Rand

Dr. **Ramsis Ghaly**, you are not only a healer, you are an inspiration, reminding us that God will always show us the way if we allow it. Happy birthday

LM, Happy Blessed Birthday

SH, All the best for your birthday and always!

BZ, Happy Birthday! God is good!

SP, Happiest Of Birthdays Ramsis

JF, Happy Birthday Dr. Ghaly!

Darrius Washington

Happy birthday Dr. Ghaly God bless I know your parents are watching over you from Heaven with so much joy, you are their gift to the world and you help heal the world and we are so grateful for you. Hope you enjoy your birthday

RC, Great words! Happy birthday to you!

SK, Happy Birthday!

DM, Happy birthday!! My family is truly blessed you fulfilled your dreams in the US. God bless you

TD, Happy Birthday to a Great Man!

TN, Happy birthday Dr. Ghaly

AF, عيد ميلاد سعيد وعمر مديد لحضرتك يا د.رمسيس كل سنه وانت طيب وبخير وفى كامل الصحه والسعاده . رحلة كفاح مشرفه . ربنا يبارك حياتك ويفرح قلبك دايما .

JC, Happy Birthday

BB, Happy Birthday!

DM, Happy birthday!

KF, Happy birthday

SS, Happy birthday!

KG, Happy Birthday! Thank you for sharing

SA, Happy Birthday

Terry Lee Ebert Mendozza

Happy birthday to my special friend, Healer and Anointed of Christ our Lord, to whom I am so grateful for your caring friendship. I cry when I read your stories, but I am always inspired by them. May the Lord's blessings always fall upon you, Ramsis. Happy birthday to you, my dear friend

Giza Salas Happy birthday to a great man! May God bless you today on your special day and always..

I will forever be thankful for everything you did for my father. You rock!

JP, Happy birthday ! May your day be filled with joy and Gods' greatest blessings.

TH, Happy Birthday Dr Ghaly

WP, Happy Birthday Doc!

LL, Happy Birthday!!!

WS, Happy birthday!!

LS, Happy birthday!

Gabriela Miller Have a blessed birthday, you are a living inspiration and your words… full of wisdom for those who (including myself) at times, forget God and all his call and love every day

SC, Happy birthday beautiful soul

KM, Happy birthday. May god continue to keep you safe as always

ML, Many happy returns of the day Dr. Ghaly!

NH, "Happy Birthday Dr. Ghaly!"

MP, Happy Birthday Dr Ghaly

BCD, You are very gifted and BLESSED

Angel Schultz

Happy happy birthday you are a wonderful person . Everyone in my son-in-law's family told me what a wonderful doctor you are . I hope you have a beautiful birthday enjoy

Michael Plunkett

May you always have God's Blessings. You are a faithful one, Amen . You are the special healer. I see you everyday enjoying the Present, life offers. You share and help others enjoy their present 's too. You are a special human. Enjoy the Present !

GW, HAPPY BIRTHDAY DR GHALY-

SH, Happy Birthday!

DM, HAPPY HAPPY BIRTHDAY GREETINGS from ARIZONA. May God continue to Bless and keep you.

DL, Happy Birthday Dr. Ghaly

RF, Happy Birthday my friend.

TM, Happy Birthday Dr. Ghaly

LS, Happy Birthday

Deanna Brockman Johnson

Happy Birthday Dr Ghaly, you have been a gift of healing to so many, your compassion and care of your patients and their families is very rare indeed God bless you always

KE, Happy Birthday Dr. Ghaly!!!

LM, Have a wonderful birthday Dr.Ghaly

GR, HAPPY BIRTHDAY !!!

Terry Falconhawke

Happy Birthday

Because today's so special, it really wouldn't do to send one simple birthday wish to last the year through.

So this wishes happy moments, a day when dreams come true and a year filled with all the things that mean the most to you.

DL, Happy Birthday. God bless you Dr. **Ramsis Ghaly**. Wishing you many more wonderful birthdays.

GC, Happy Birthday! Cheers to you and many more!

ES, Happy birthday Ramsis! Love you

KH, Happy birthday

VG, Best wishes on your birthday, Dr. Ghaly!

SO, Happy birthday Ramsis !!

MO, Happy birthday!! God bless this special day and every other day as well!!

SA, Happy Birthday Dr Ghaly

Judy Dzurko Sargent

May GOD'S BLESSINGS SURROUND YOU WITH A FEELING OF PEACE HAPPY BIRTHDAY DR GHALY RICH & JUDY

DS, Happy Birthday! Dr. Ghaly May the Peace of The Lord be with you and keep you safe

NV, Happy Birthday and God Bless you Doctor Ghaly

RV, Happy Birthday!

SA, Dr. Ramsis may God bless you and be with you all the time & to help you continue your great work which you do with so much love and care, may this year be filled with love & joy and all God's blessings showers you

SS, Happy Birthday Many many more blessed ones!

ER, Happy birthday! Best wishes

RH, Happy Birthday

FA, Happy birthday Dr Ghaly

MR, Such an amazing story! God Bless you & Happy Birthday

YCM, appy birthday, Dr. Ghaly! God's blessings be upon you.

BM, Happy birthday Dr Ghaly!!!

JS, Happy birthday Dr Ghaly!

GS, Happy Birthday

SH, Happy birthday Dr. Ghaly!

Blessed is the man who makes the Lord his trust.

~ Psalm 40:4

Celebrating life, celebrating blessings, celebrating God's workmanship, celebrating YOU!

Praying that on this special day, you'll know the fullness of God's joy, the goodness of His grace, and the blessing of His love.

Anna Kay Thompson

CD, Happy Happy Birthday!! Enjoy your special day.

DH, Happy Birthday

Enjoy your day

God's Blessings for the year to come!

GF, Happy Birthday and many blessings to you!!!!

AH, Happy Birthday

KM, Happy birthday young man. God bless you. Hope you have a day as amazing as you are.,

DM, Happy blessed birthday

MW, Happy Birthday god bless you

LS, Happy Birthday Sir !

SJ, Happy birthday

F,Happy Birthday Dr.Ghaly! More blessings ..Good health & more birthdays for you to celebrate!

DK, Wishing you a very Happy Birthday!

JJ, Happy birthday many blessings your way

Jk, Happy Birthday may God bless you with many more years to come so you can help others.

CM, Happy birthday

JT, Happy Birthday!!!!!

EB, Happy Birthday

RP, Happy Happy Happy birthday Doc.

GA, Happy birthday doctor ghaly

Sally Brady

Happy Birthday, Dr. . Ghaly. Thank the Lord you never gave up. Your Faith kept you going and He never lets us down so long as we focus on Him and thank him continually for all our blessings. You are one fantastic doctor and our family loves you. Thanks for being there for us when we were so in need for you. May our Heavenly Father continue to bless you.

DR, Happy Birthday!

KM, Wishing YOU a VERY ...

Bretonya Phillips-Johnson

Happy birthday Dr.Ghaly! You are unmatched, truly a gift to us all, a gift to the world!

KC, Happy Birthday!!

DC, Happy Birthday!

TC, Happy Birthday Dr Ghaly!

Violeta Dato Morrison

HAPPY HAPPY BIRTHDAY MY GENIUS KIND DEDICATED HARD WORKING FRIEND . THE BEST NEUROSURGEON PAIN MANAGEMENT PHYSICIAN. MORE BIRTHDAYS AND BLESSINGS TO CELEBRATE

AS, Happy birthday Dr Ghaly!

God blessings!

JC, Happy Birthday Dr Ghaly!!! Wishing you many blessings!

JJ, Happy Birthday

CH, Happy Birthday!

KK, Happy birthday Dr.Ghaly!!!

JM, Happy birthday!

DD, A very inspirational story Ramsis! God is great! Happy birthday! Keep'em coming!

CR, Your writings this morning touched my heart. I left my job yesterday. I was working with a precious little girl with Mitochondrial Disorder after 3 of her 4 years. I am 75 and like you look forward to where God will use me now. There is plenty to d...

SC, Happy birthday sir

DB, Blessings on your birthday Dr Ghaly!

LZ, Happy birthday!!! Have a most wonderful day!!

JJ, Happy Birthday

Jennifer L. Johnston

Happy Birthday! God had big plans to use you and He did!!! I am so thankful you were born and are a great blessing to many. Have fun celebrating today!!!

GG, By the way, October birthdays are the best!

SJ, Happy Birthday Dr.Ghaly

BV, Many many more Dr Ghaly!!!

OR,

Happy happy birthday Dr Ghaly!

JC,Happy birthday Dr Ghaly

JG, God Bless you Dr Ghaly!

Violeta Dato Morrison

HAPPY HAPPY BIRTHDAY MY GENIUS KIND DEDICATED HARD WORKING FRIEND . THE BEST NEUROSURGEON PAIN MANAGEMENT PHYSICIAN. MORE BIRTHDAYS AND BLESSINGS TO CELEBRATE

KE, Happy Blessed Birthday Great Doctor Lifesaver!

Amen

CR, Happy Birthday, Dr Ghaly!!

DC, Happy Birthday

CE, Happy birthday!

DK, Happy Birthday, Dr. Ghaly!!!

SM, Happy Birthday

NL, Happy Birthday Dr Ghaly!!

JD, Happy Birthday Dr. Ghaly !!!! May you have many,many more !!!

MR, Happy birthday!

MW, Happy Birthday and many more have a blessed day

SA, Happy Birthday!!!

PI, Happy birthday Dr Ghaly

DU, May God grant you many more happy and blessed years.

CG, Happy Birthday Enjoy!

RC, Happy Birthday!

MR, Happy Birthday

NT, Happy Birthday, Dr. Ghaly!

VH, Happy birthday sweetie

CD, Happy happy birthday! God bless you and all that you do.

DN, Beautiful birthday message Dr. Ghaly happy birthday and many more

MK, Happy Birthday.

MN, Happy birthday Dr. Ghaly. Enjoy your day

EO, May the Lord's blessings continue to hold you in His arms. Hugs.

JY, Happy Birthday Dr Ghaly!! Much love and Blessings!!!

LS, Happy Birthday!

JP, Happy Birthday Doctor; enjoy your special day.

KH, Happy birthday 🎂

SA, Happy birthday Dr. Ghaly

Valerie Williams

Happy Birthday Dr Ghaly, you are one of those chosen ppl that you never want to forget. You are such a blessing. I've learned so much from reading this excerpt of your life and through the Grace Of God you still kept your FAITH. You are one of the best.

Norma Jean

Happy Birthday Dr. Ghaly! May God continue to bless you and your hands so that you can continue to do more good and save more lives! Wishing you all the very best!!

DW,

Happy Birthday Ramsis!

MM, Happy birthday Dr.Ghaly, GodBless

MN, Happy birthday DrGhaly to the best doctor the lord placed on this earth have a great day miss you

DH, Happiest of Birthdays to you Dr. Ghaly!

Thanking all you have done helping people, God has truly given you a gift of being a successful surgeon, you do Good works thru our Lord & Savior

CE, Happy Birthday Dr Ghaly!! Many blessings for u and I pray for many more years of ur wonderful gift

JS, Happy Birthday! We haven't met but i can tell your a fabulous dotcor!

JM, AMEN! Happy Birthday Dr. Ghaly

EB, Happy happy birthday

RB, Happy Birthday !!

MP, Happy birthday Ramsis! May God bless you always.

NS, Happy birthday

CR, Thank you for never giving up on God or yourself. Your story is beautiful. Happy birthday and may the Lord continue to bless you and use you in miraculous ways in His faithful service.

JC, Happy birthday Dr, hope you had a wonderful day

CS, Happy birthday Dr**Ghaly**

JW, Hi Doctor Ghaly!! Happy birthday!!! Hope you have an amazing year!!!!

Charlene Mentzer Glowaty

You write from your heart,about something you're passionate about. Your heart, your passion, and your emotions are what you share with us. Bless you on your birthday and everyday.

KO, Happy birthday Dr Gahly

DC, Happy birthday Dr.

LM, Happy birthday to you!

RY, Happy birthday to you

EM, Happy birthday dear Dr **Ramsis Ghaly** . God bless

AP, Happy birthday and may be blessed with many more

AU, Happy birthday Dr G. Hope your birthday is as wonderful as you are

SS, Happy boy dr Ghaly

JT, Happy birthday!

KP, Happy Belated Birthday Wishes your way

CR, Cristina Rojas-Rutkowski

My dear favorite doctor, a little bit late but HAPPY BIRTHDAY!!! Hugs.

KH, Happy Birthday!

SS, Happy birthday a little late

Id, **Happy Birthday to an amazing human!**

Tammi Ciciora Dr Ghaly, I read every word of your birthday wish. You truly are a gift to the world and of course anyone who's ever met you. Your faith, perseverance and drive are unmatched by anyone I've ever known. Wishing you as much as you have given and beyond in your birthday year!

Mike Nutoni

Happy birthday DrGhaly to the best doctor the lord placed on this earth have a great day miss you

Norma Jean

Happy Birthday Dr. Ghaly! May God continue to bless you and your hands so that you can continue to do more good and save more lives! Wishing you all the very best!!

Valerie Williams

Happy Birthday Dr Ghaly, you are one of those chosen ppl that you never want to forget. You are such a blessing. I've learned so much from reading this excerpt of your life and through the Grace Of God you still kept your FAITH. You are one of the best.

Shelley Peyton Alexander

Happy Birthday Dr. Ghaly! Thank you for all you do for your patients, including me! I hope you had a wonderful day today!

GL, Happy birthday Dr. Ghaly and many more BLESSINGS.

KB, Happy birthday Dr.Ghaly!!

Spydie Rider

Happy birthday Dr. Ghaly!! Blessings to you and all throughout the year! Thank you for all you do for your patients!

LS, Happy birthday

LK, Happy birthday Dr Ghaly! Thank you for all that you do

CL, "Happy Birthday Dr Ghaly!" May God bless you.

RC, Happy Birthday Dr. Ghaly

JH, Happy birthday Dr. Ghaly.

CM, Happy birthday uncle **Ramsis Ghaly** God bless your life

TS, Happy birthday Dr.Ghaly

KC, Thank you for sharing your story, hope you have the best birthday and many more!

RS, Happy birthday!!

Heidi Walker

Happy Birthday Dr. Ghaly!God Bless you and all you do for others

EB, Happy birthday Ramsis, enjoy your day and have a blessed year

Edwina Bator-Swanson

Happy Birthday Dr Ghaly. May you have many many more years ahead of you. You are loved by so many and you have a large family of friends and many patients that are so grateful for your skills.

AL, Happy birthday Dr. Ghaly 🎂. God made you to have the Will power to Help people, God bless🙏

BS, Happy birthday Dr Ghaly

YR, Happy Birthday Dr Ghaly!

Jackie Mitchell Martin

Happy Birthday Dr Ghaly! And thank you for your faith that shines like a beacon for the lost

JH, Happy Birthday Dr Ghaly!

LW, Happy birthday!

JL, Happiest of birthdays birthdays Dr Ghaly

AS, Happy happy birthday Dr.

GV, Happy birthday! Enjoy your special day!!

KS, Happy birthday Dr. Ghaly

KW, Happiest of Birthdays to you. Dr Ghaly

SS, Happy happy birthday Doc!

AM, HAPPY BIRTHDAY

Dr. **Ramsis Ghaly**.

Wishing you Always best wishes, and good health....

SA, Happy birthday Dr. Ghaly wish you an amazing one!

CH, Parabens. Many Happy Returns young Dr Ramsis Ghaly

MI, Happy happy happy birthday !!!!

CL, Happy Birthday! God has blessed you in so many ways. In turn, it blesses us too!

LS, Happy birthday

Sandi Benedict Crites

Happy birthday my friend $ many many more your work here is far from finished the good lord is gonna keep you here to save many more lives

JM, "Happy Birthday" Dr. Ghaly

SC, Good news my friend i have an up& comming nurse traing to come& work with you

MH, Your an amazing Dr. Hope you have an amazing birthday

BCD, Bless you. Your Birthday message made me cr

Christie Loftin

Happy Birthday! God has blessed you in so many ways. In turn, it blesses us too!

Arsho Mahserejian

HAPPY BIRTHDAY

Dr. **Ramsis Ghaly**.

Wishing you Always best wishes, and good health.

I always follow your successful stories and I like your spiritual soul, humanitarian heart and clever mind.

Thanks for always sharing your beautiful writings.

Please pray for peace to this world and in the meantime pray for my people and for their land in Armenia .

Thanks and God bless you and your family

Amelia Molina-lucena

Happy birthday Dr. Ghaly . God made you to have the Will power to Help people, God bless

John Peter Solimon

Happy Birthday to you Doctor Ramsis Ghaly For many many more

Blessings May The Lord Our God rewards you Abundantly. Enjoy your day.

Judy Conderman

Happy Birthday Dr. Ghaly!! May you enjoy many more healthy happy years. You are a gift from God and the most caring, compassionate, admired and gifted doctor. Our family loves you and appreciates all that you have done for us. Enjoy this beautiful day.

Sarah Popp

Happy birthday to the best doctor

Mammaponio

Compassionate knowledgeable doctor and beautiful soul!

Ilene Davis

Happy Birthday to an amazing human!

Aldrete

Happy Birthday Ramsis- we love you and are so grateful you are in our lives - you are the most amazing person and doctor and friend and we love you- much love Retta

Ausra Cibiene

Dear Dr. Ramsis Ghaly, Your birthday is a moment to spread Your love for all. May You too find the grace of fulfilment and wisdom. Happy Birthday. I send You roses from my home

Cecilia Gonzalez

Happy birthday blessings to an amazing Doctor.

Gill Boland, Susan Trinth and Kevin

Happy Birthday to the legendary Dr Ghaly!! Hope you have a great day!

CL, Happy Birthday and God Bless you!!!

MD, Very Happy Birthday Ramsis from Richmond Virginia.

MB, Happy Birthday wish you all the best

MK, Happy birthday filled with love faith and joy

DL, appy blessed birthday !

DH, Happy Birthday Dr Ghaly

MN, Happy Birthday

MH, Your an amazing Dr. Hope you have an amazing birthday

BD, Bless you. Your Birthday message made me cry.

SL, Happy Birthday!!!!!

VL, Happy birthday

<u>**Milena Paunovic**</u>

Your life story impresses and inspires. Nothing happens without a clear goal, without faith in yourself, and without faith in God. Your life and dedication to your profession and to the Lord is admirable.

Happy Birthday! Happy birthday!

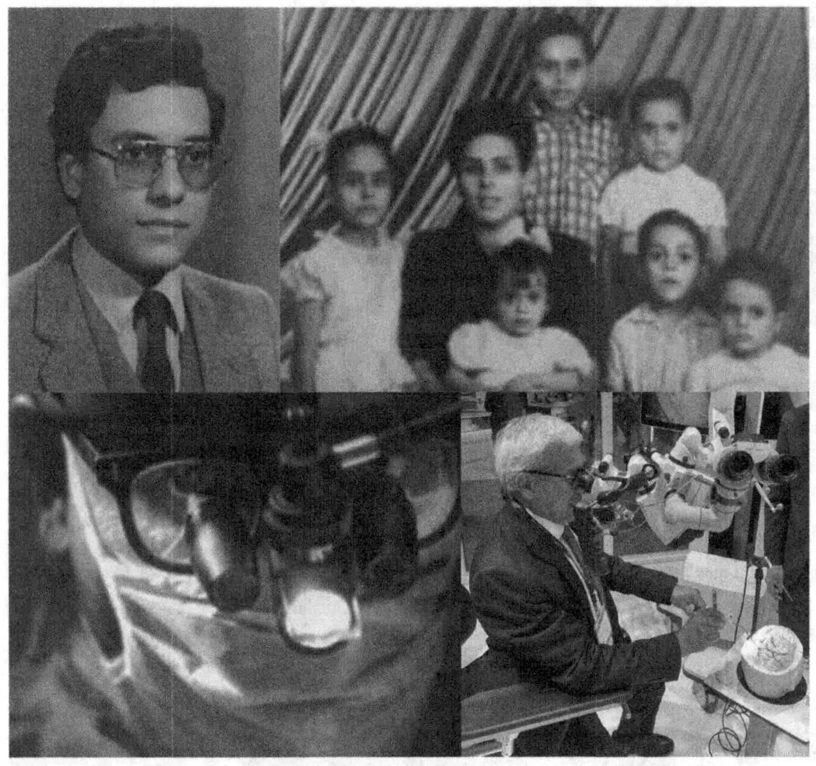

SL, Happy Birthday!!!!!

VL, Happy birthday

LR, Happy birthday!

EL, Happy belated Birthday Dr. Ghaly!!

My family is my residents and patients!!

What a surprise! My residents made a great party for my belated birthday with much of emotions snd love !!! A delicious birthday cake and Polaroid Camera with self automatic prints.

You all touched my heart and you all my family and friends forever. What an honor to be a mentor and teacher for generations and generations and work have in hand night and day to save lives and prepare generations for years to come.

Thank you so much!

Ramsis Ghaly

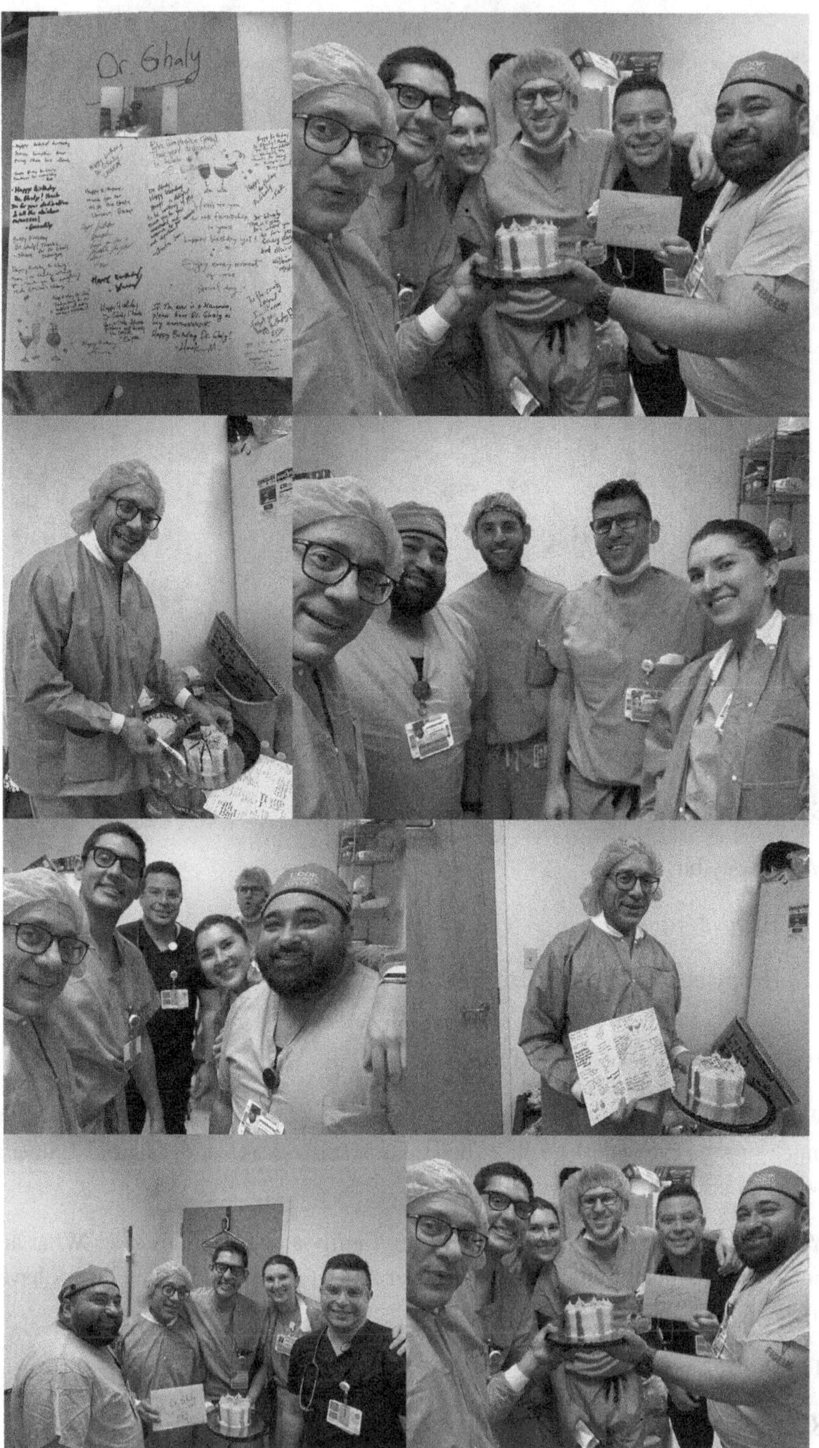
Dr. Ghaly

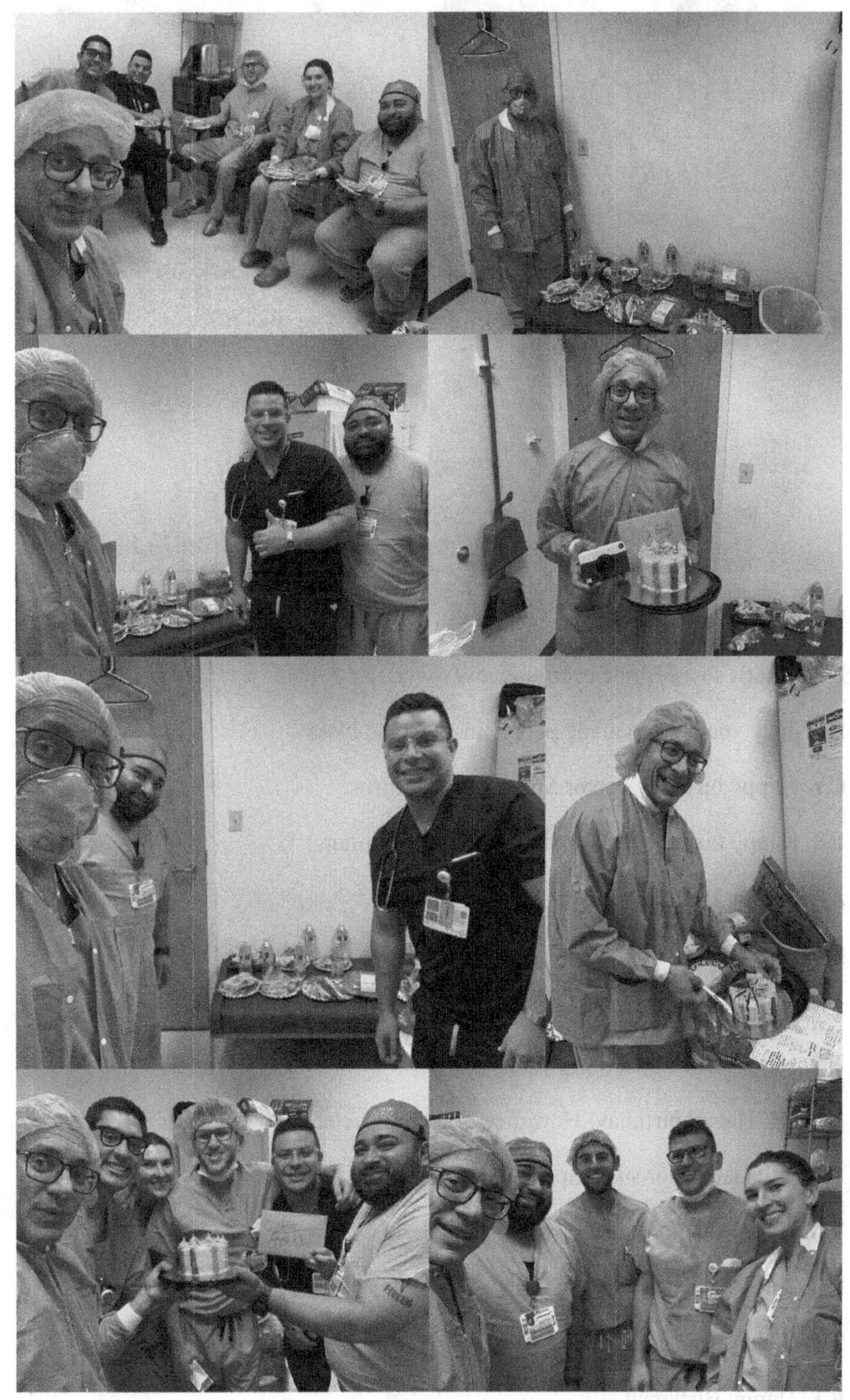

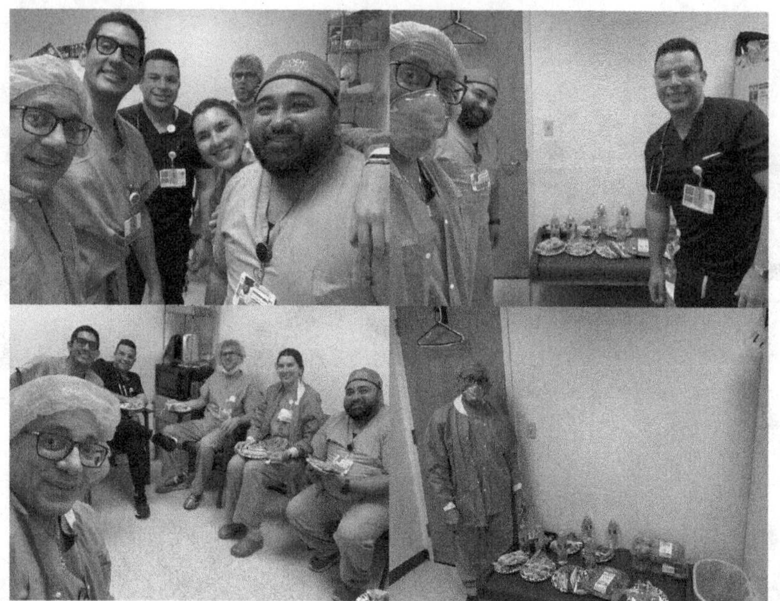

KC, How sweet!!

KO, That's so awesome everyone loves you

Dr Ghaly you help so many people in life, God bless

CY, Happy birthday doctor Many happy returns

BB, Happy birthday Dr. Ghaly! Enjoy every minute!

AN, Happy Birthday

CG, You are so loved by your students. Great pictures!

JW, Happy birthday doc!!!

TN, Happy Birthday!!

KL, JZ, Happy birthday! How nice of them to celebrate with you!

LP, Felicidades por su cumpleaños docto

VG, Happy birthday

LW, Happy Birthday!!!

SH, Happy belated Birthday!

KY, Happy Birthday!

DK, Happy belated birthday Dr. You are such a blessing from God to everyone!!!

BB, Happy birthday Dr. Ghaly!

PP, Happy belated Birthday! God bless you.

YW, You deserve it all

AH, Happy Birthday

JJ, Happy Birthday ! Ramsis and many more . Enjoy ! Your very special day . Cheers !

TJ, Happy birthday Dr. Ghaly

TL, Happy Birthday Dr. Ghaly

EL, Happy Birthday Dr. Ghaly

JF, Happy Birthday!!

LM, Happy belated birthday!

DU, May God grant you many more happy and blessed years!

SR, Happy birthday Dr. Ghaly!!! God bless you!!

ER, Happy birthday

MB, Happy Birthday wish you happiness,good health and success

OZ, Happy Birthday, Dr Ghaly! All the best to you!

LK, Happy birthday bless you Dr. Ghaly!

SA, Happy birthday Dr.Ghaly

LR, Happiest Birthday Dr. Ghaly

Mf, Happy birthday Dear Doctor... God bless you and your beautiful family

Lanette Yingling: **Happy Birthday to the most amazing doctor on the planet!!!**

ZC,Happiest Birthday Dr,Ghaly.

CP, Happy blessed birthday to you Dr. Ghaly. Wishing you much happiness & continued good health and working miracles

BH, appy Birthday

JB, Happy Birthday Dr. Ghaly

KA, Happy birthday

JB, Thanks to all healthcare workers. You'll always be my heroes

KW, Happy Birthday Dr. Ramsis!

CS, Happy birthday

SA, كل سنه وحضرتك طيب د. رمسيس وسنه حلوه مع يسوع مليئه بالفرح والسلام

SJ, Happy birthday Dr. Ghaly!!!! Thank you for your miracle work you do. That work saved my dad **Rick Malina** so any years a go. Now get hold and see all his grandchildren grow up.

DC, Happy Birthday!

DW, May God grant you many years!

MM, Happy Birthday Dr. Ghaly!!

JS, Happy Birthday

JR, All the best to you Dr. Ghaly. Happy birthday !!

CR, Happy Birthday! You deserve a party and celebration. I'm so glad that you are appreciated for being such a great ctor and instrument of the Lord.

BJ, Happy birthday Dr, Ghaly! You are a true blessing!

JH, Happy birthday Dr. Ghaly!

KE, Happy Blessed Birthday Dr

Ghaly Amen

JM, **Congratulations** Dr. Ghaly

RM, Happy Birthday Sir God bless you Dr Ghaly

PH, Happy Birthday

KG, Happy Birthday Dr. Ghaly

They're lucky to have you!!!

LM, Happy birthday

JT, smiles smiles smiles!

BM, Happy birthday Dr.Ghaly

The Cycle of Heartfelt Love and Passionate as the Core of Success!

Written by Ramsis Ghaly

Heartfelt Love and Passionate

lead to

Success

Lead to

Perseverance and Determination

Lead to

Quality

Lead to

Dedication

Lead to

Excellence

Lead to

More Love and Passionate

Respectfully

Ramsis Ghaly

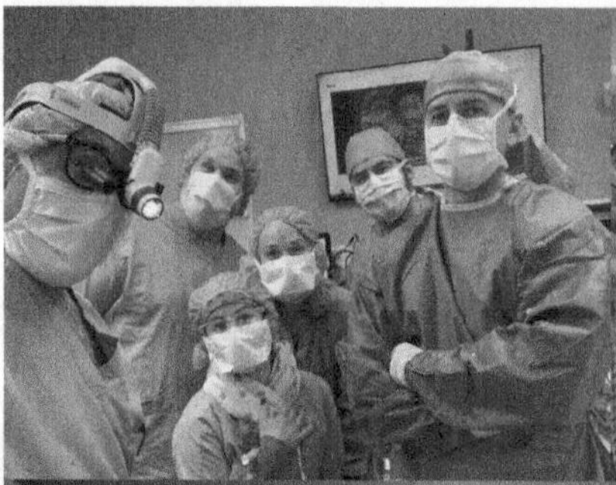

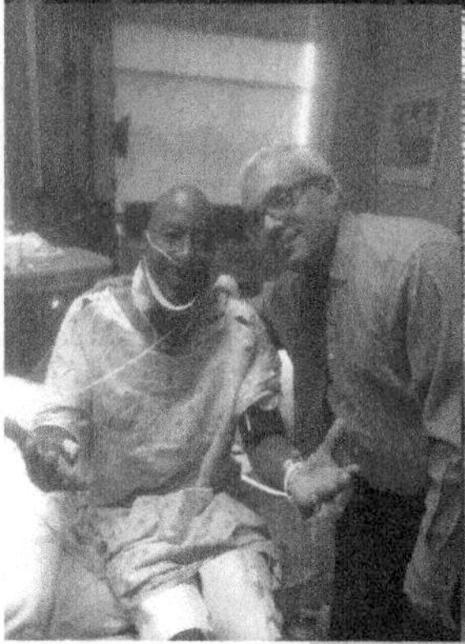

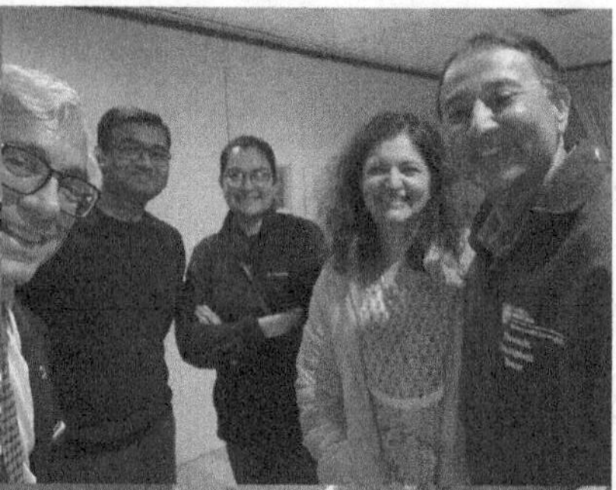

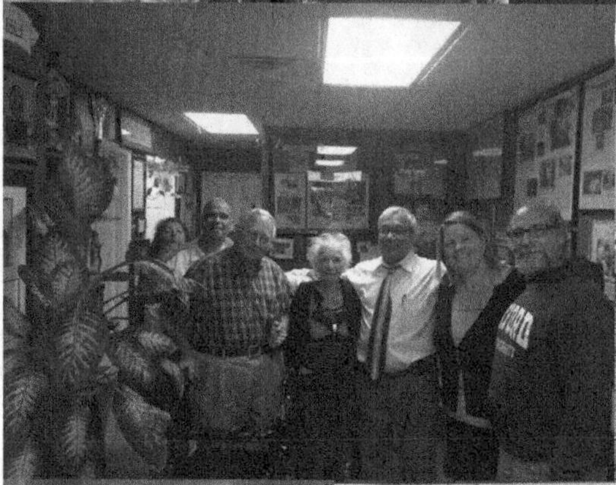

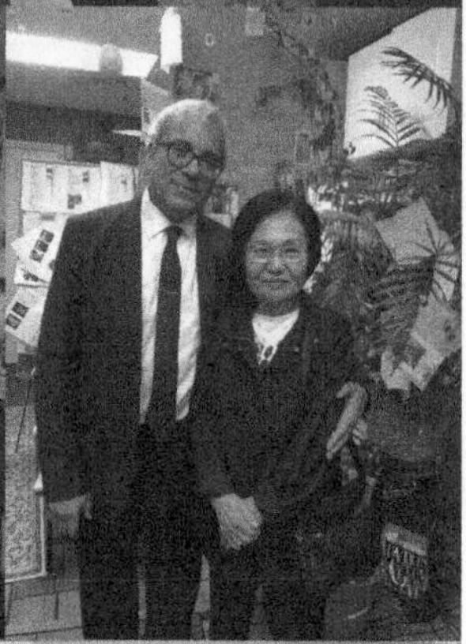

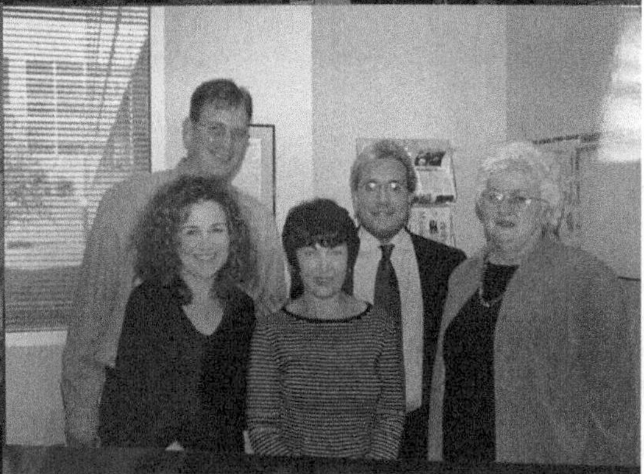

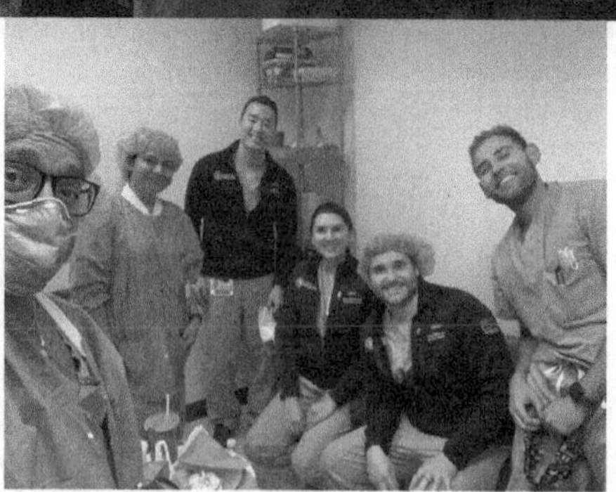

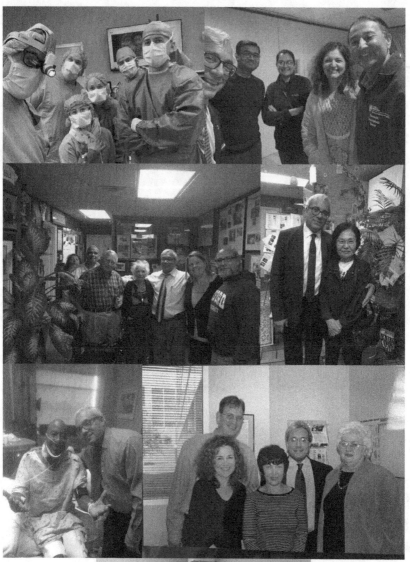

The Monastery is My life!

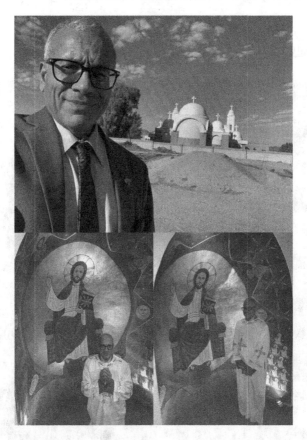

It is a worshiper place praising the Most High, praying day and night in the desert where not much of the world there. It is a place I routinely visit and spend much time since childhood. Unity, Sharing, Love, Faith, quiescence, serenity, humility and practice Christianity are fulfilled. Our church encourages visiting the monasteries in a routine basis. It is part of the church, the silent prayers. Jesus Cross is elevated so high and is the sign of salvation in every corner of the monastery.

Therefore, Come and visit and join my soul unto the solitude life of the Holy Monks of Coptic Orthodox Church of Egypt, the Ancient orthodoxy following St Mark the Apostle of our Lord and Savior Jesus Christ:

My visit to St Antony Monastery, Coptic Orthodox in the depth of Mojave Desert: 43725 Bragdon Rd, Newberry Springs, CA 92365 https://saintantonymonasteryus.org/

The fathers are praying for all of us and the world unceasing.

Amen

Ramsis Ghaly

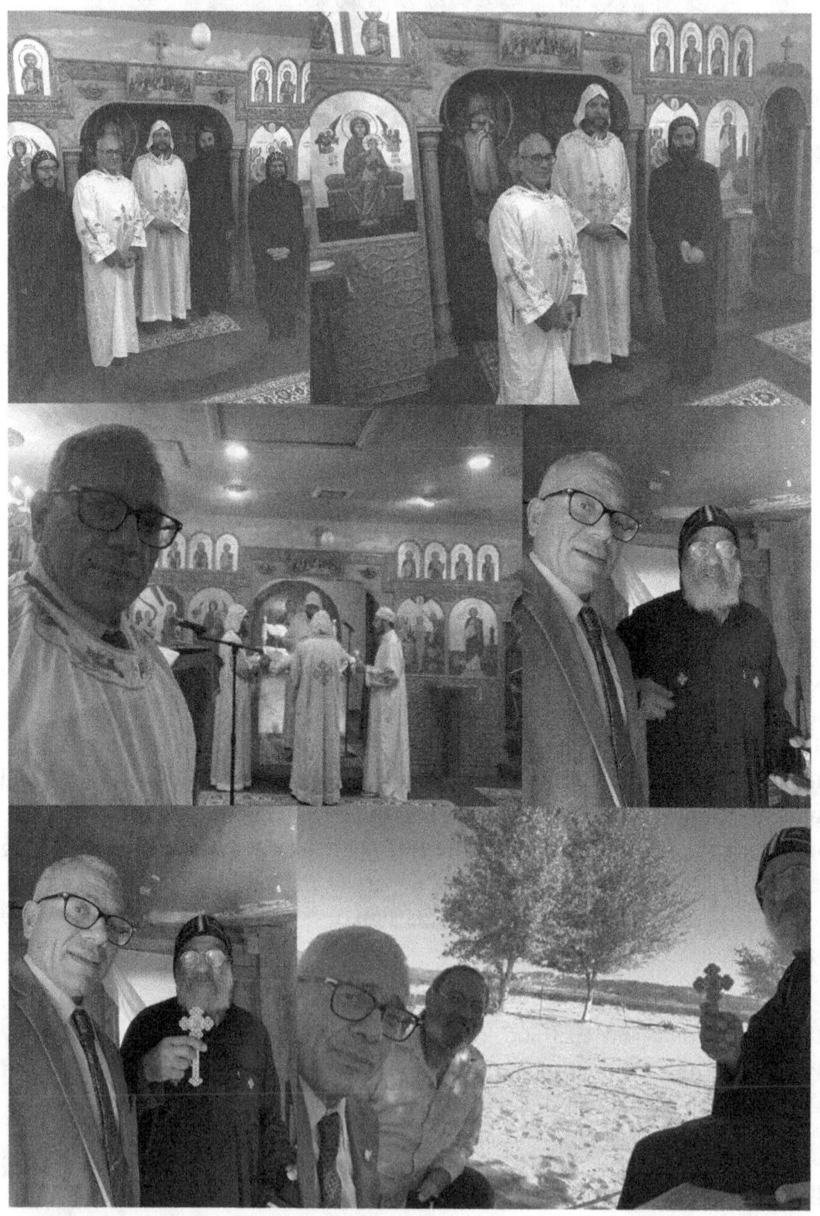

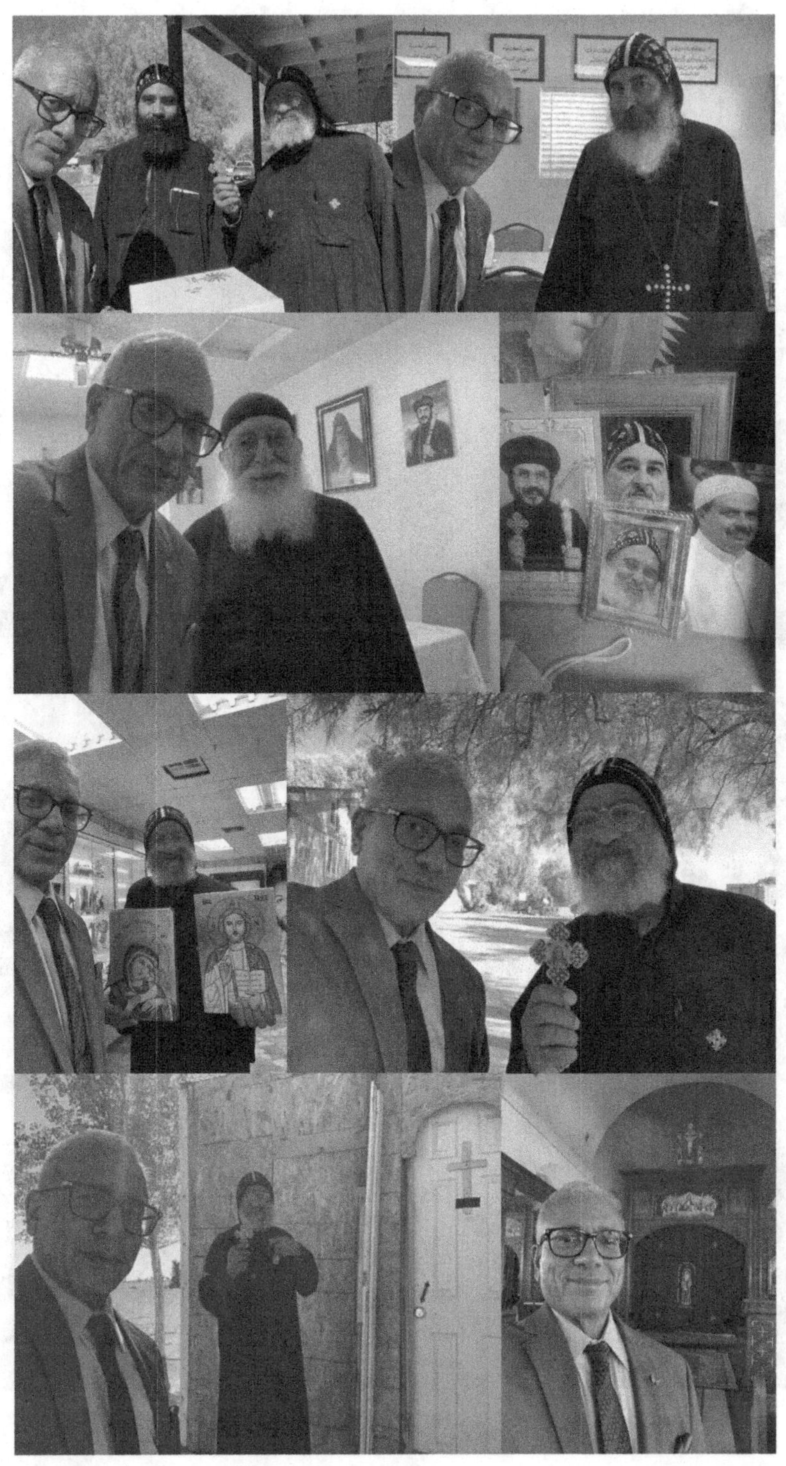

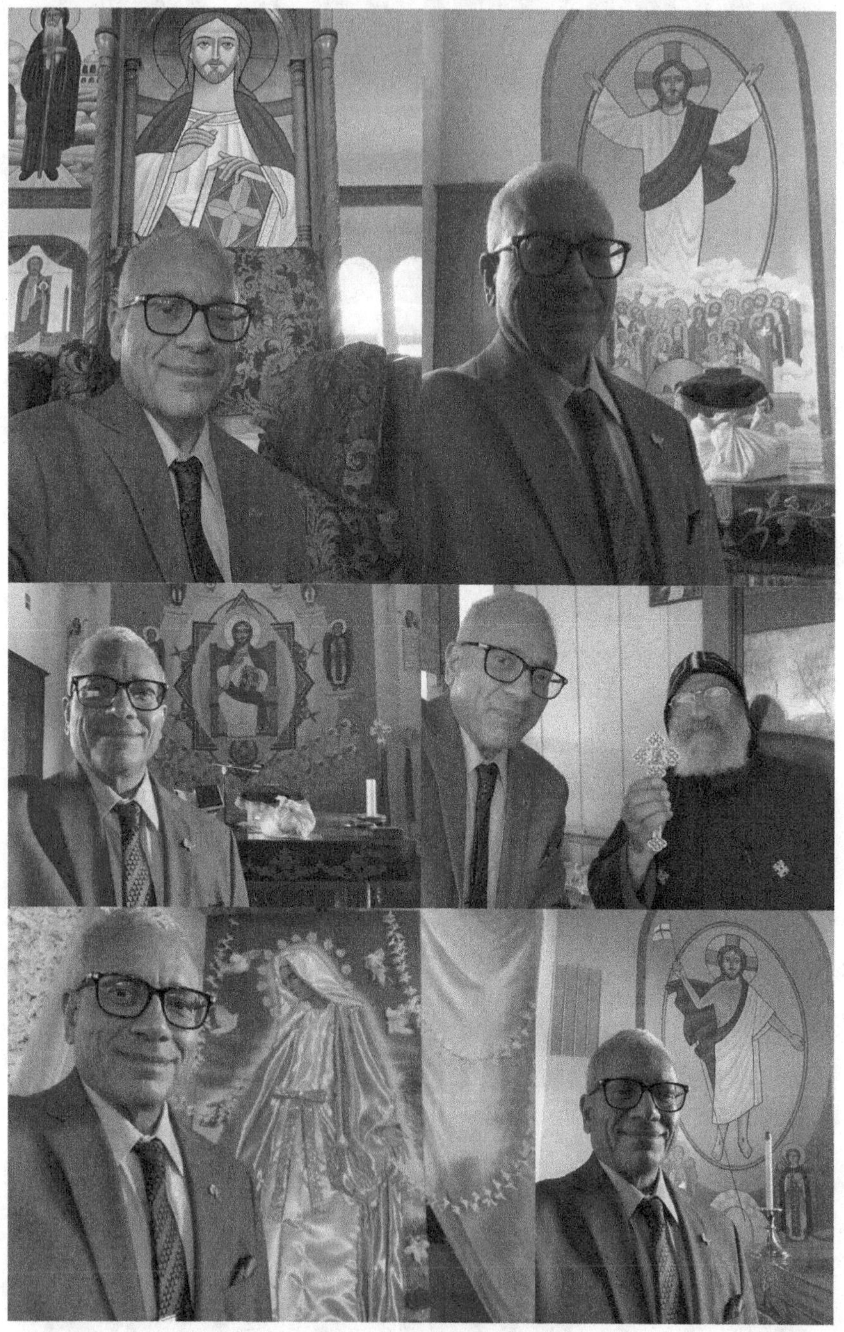

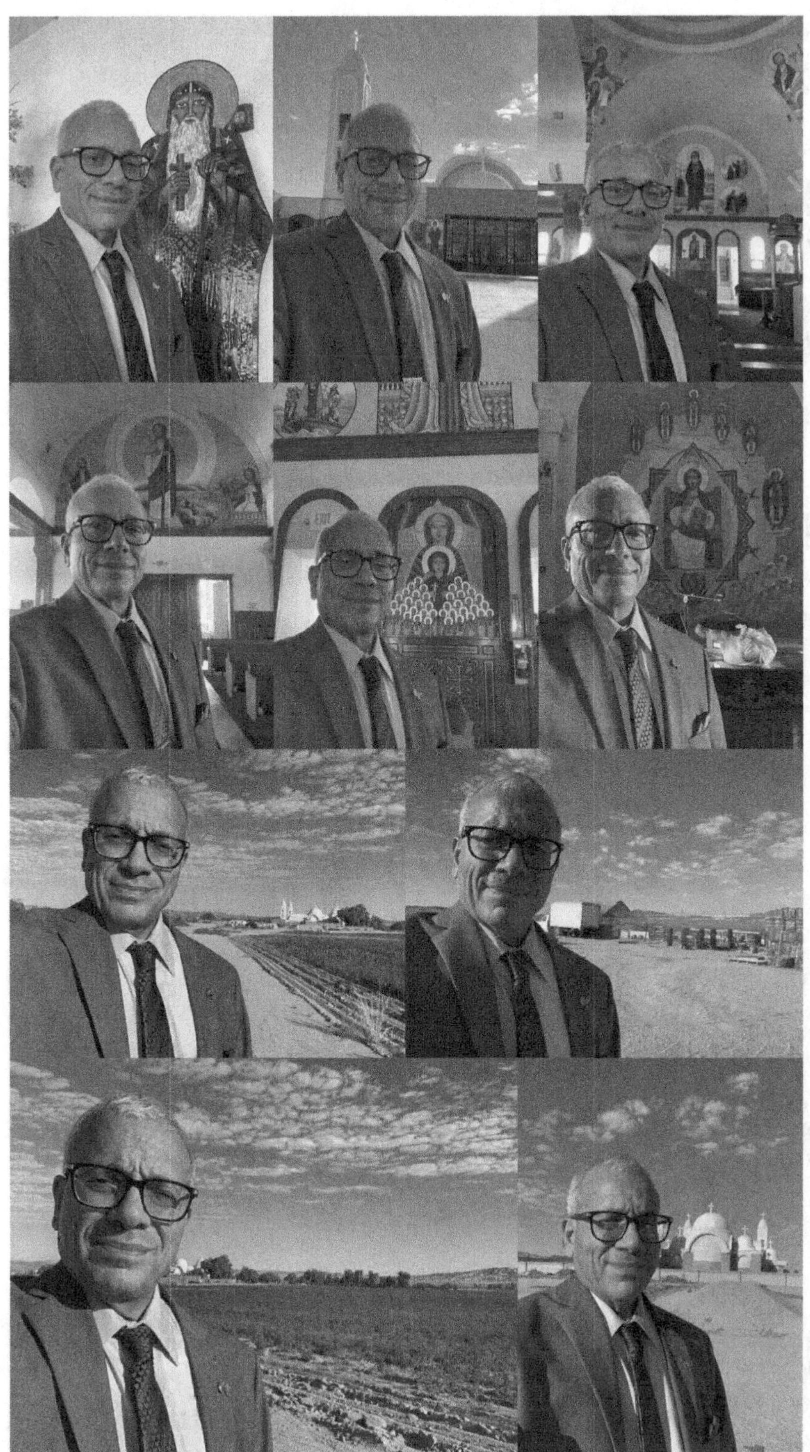

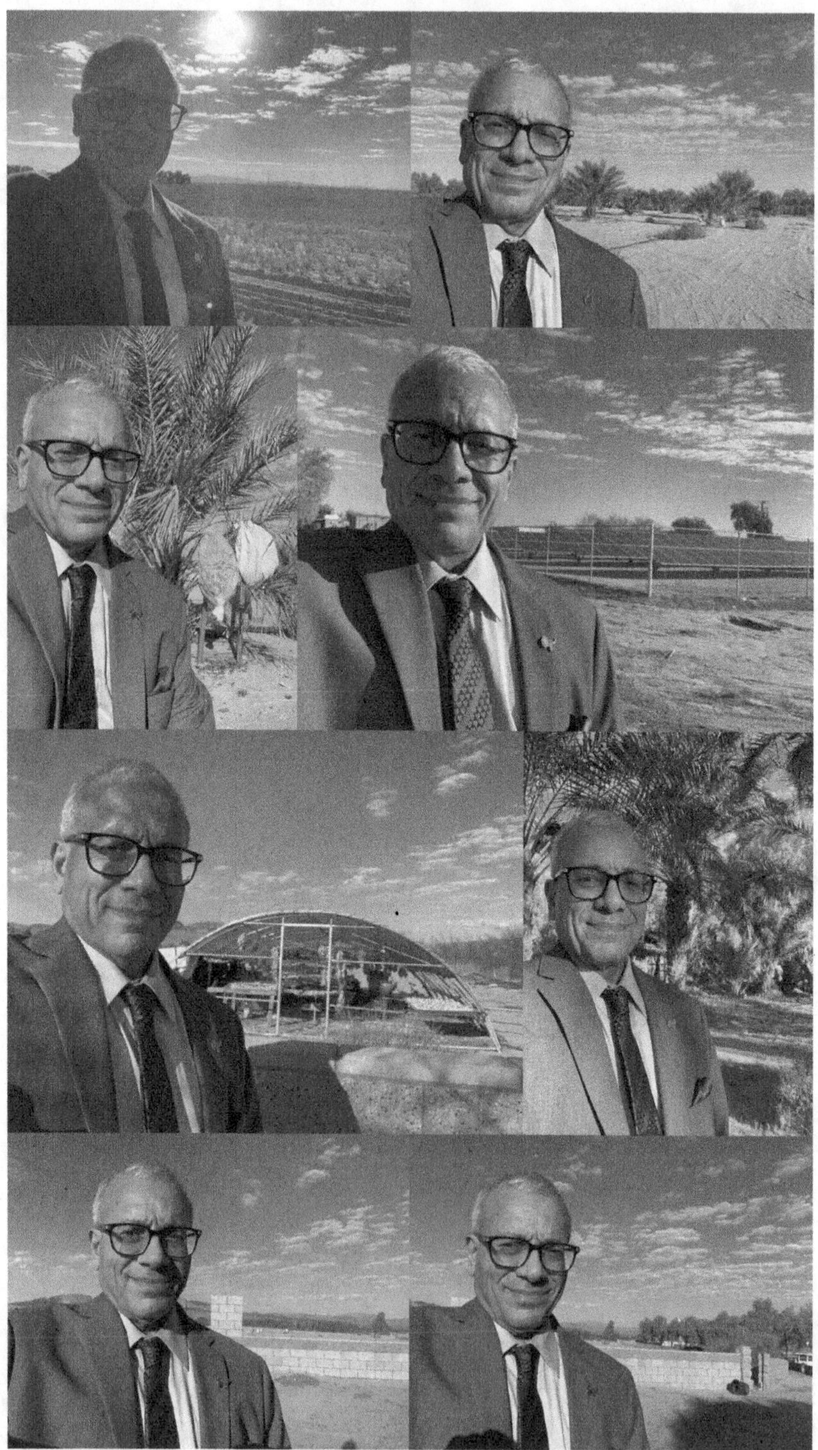

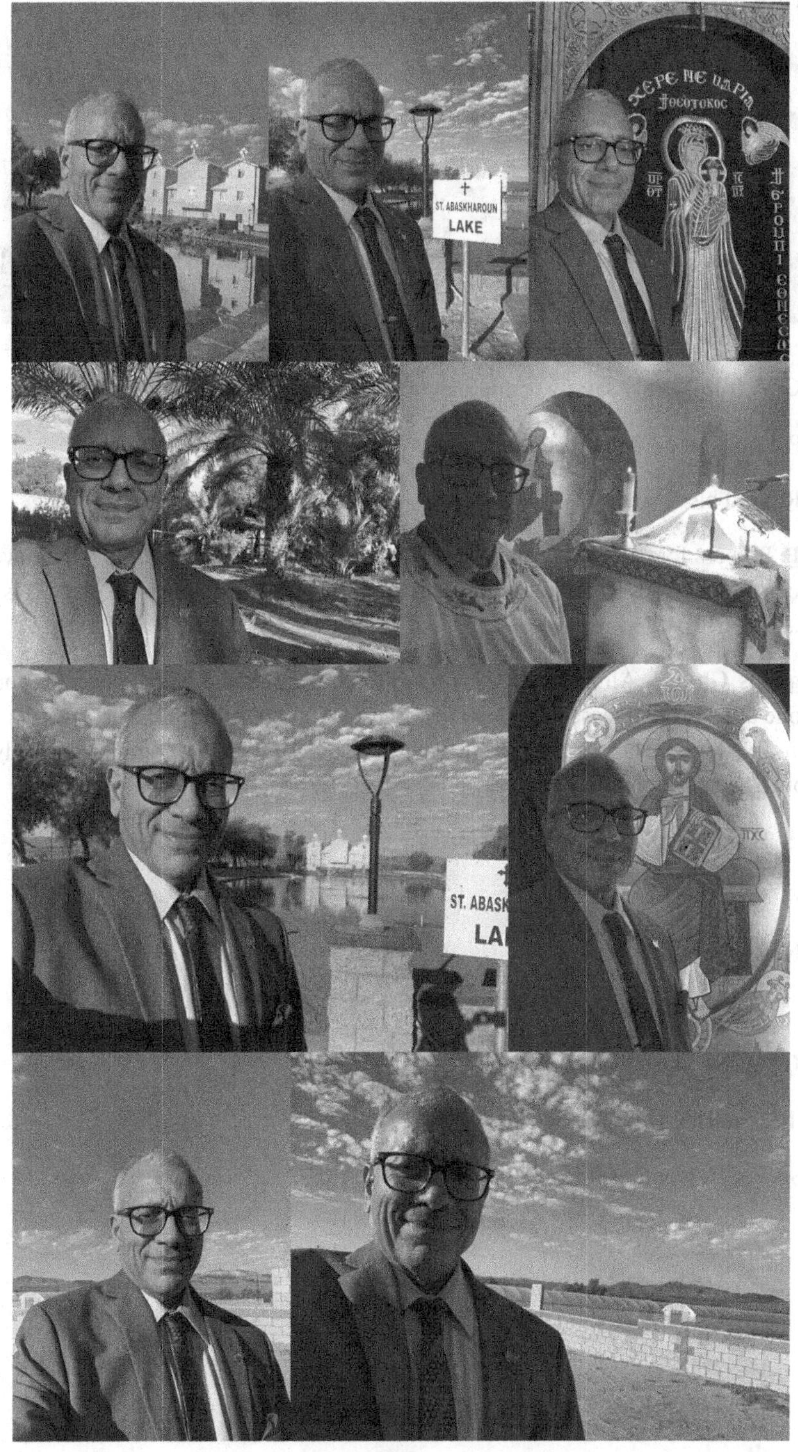
ST. ABASKHAROUN
LAKE

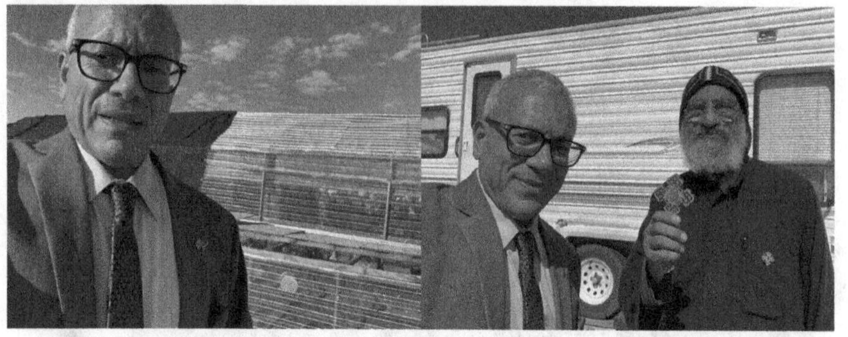

HG, A true earthly saint worshiping amongst the saints. Perfection.

CP, Looks like a beautiful place.

LR, God bless you!

AP, Prayers for the Monks and guests through the intercessions of all who have received blessings from the saintly Bsp Karas- in whose memory we give praise to Jesus Christ!

Ramsis Ghaly - Almighty God, you are to be praised and worshipped for you alone are worthy. Please bless my friends at St Antonys and fill the heart of your son and servant Dr Ramses. In the name of the Father, the Son and the Holy Spirit. Amen

MS, Beautiful place to worship God.

JM, AMEN!!!

DN, Beautiful picture

SL, Pray for my soul

CG, Looks like a beautiful place.

MB, God Bless you brother

ES, What a wonderful experience!!!!!

In So Many Ways---

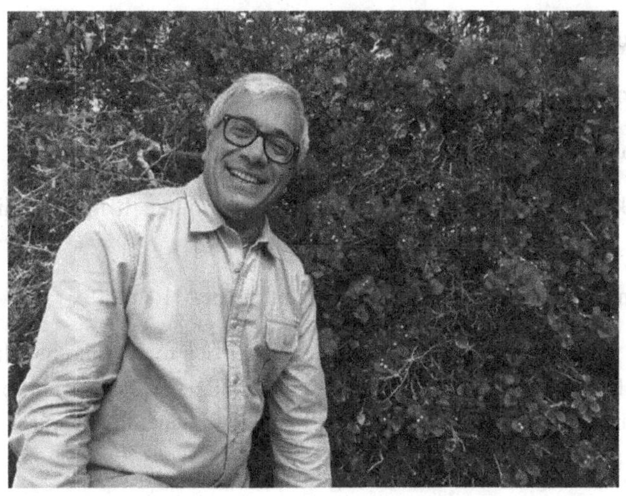

Written By Ramsis Ghaly

In so many ways, we share what we go through in our journeys.

Let us live together the life worthy in love and service one to another----

The good that we do, the bad that we do not mean to do and the ups and downs that we always face in our days.

Our minds wonders of when we began, where are we going and why should it be this way???

Friends, what matters are what we do for others and the fruits we leave behind.

In the meanwhile, we continue living, learning from the past and stronger we get and wiser we become.

In the morning, we renew our vows to the God of goodness and looking up to heavens for a better day ahead.

So my friends, today is coming to an end, yesterday is behind and tomorrow is at hand together we shall share.

Let us live together the life worthy in love and service one to another----

Respectfully

Ramsis Ghaly www.ghalyneurosurgeon.com

SP, EO, Dr., you do so much for others. You work so many hours healing so many with our Lord's hands guiding. Yet, you find the time to write so many beautiful thoughts of encouragement. Blessings to you.

DM, One of a kind .nice knowing you

AC, Awesome mood and smile

CP, Very nice picture.

RC, Thank you for the love and service for the other. It make a difference. Blessings!

NP, Not only handsome but brilliant! Best of the best11

CG, Jesus is the perfect example of love and service to one another. In His life on earth, He cared for the poor, He healed the blind, He welcomed little children. You are our living example of Jesus in all you do day in and day out.

MA, Keep up the good work!I Sending love

DN, JC, Very nice picture

SS, You look better every day Mr.Dapper

LM, Love of God and service to others are very important and wonderful

Chicago Post-COVID

The Famous Chicago River Walk in Photos!

Written by Ramsis Ghaly on 5/30/22

This is Chicago and yes, it is my very First time in 35 years to explore "Chicago River Walk".

With my precious green suit and the green festival char tie!!

I am not unto the crowed and smash burgers with draft beers!!

But I am rather to wander in meditation reflecting deep as the Spirit roves over the waters!!!!

Ramsis Ghaly

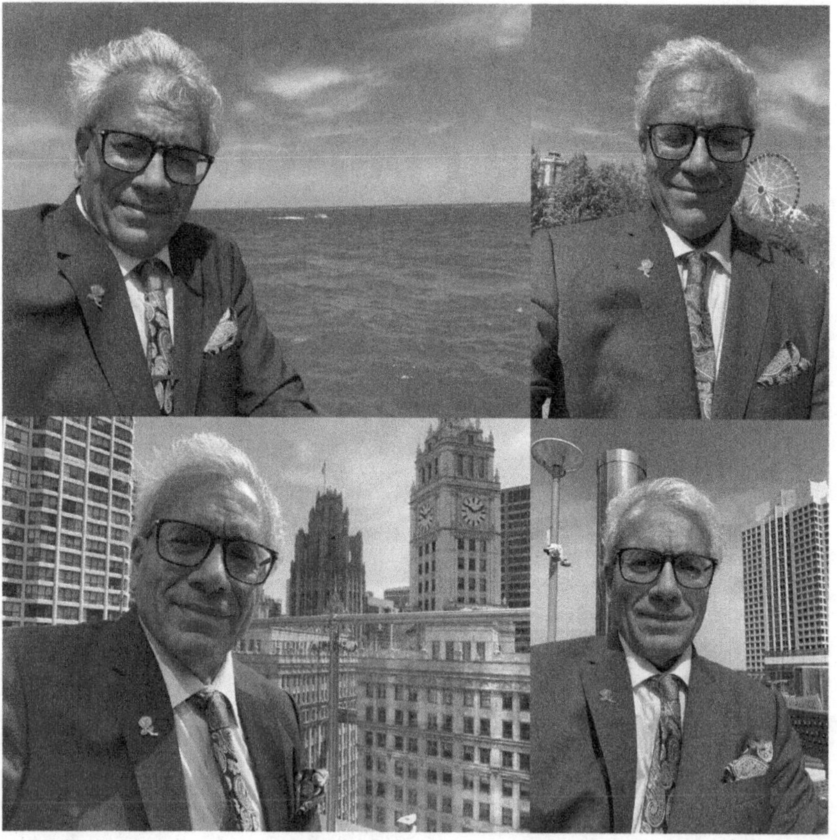

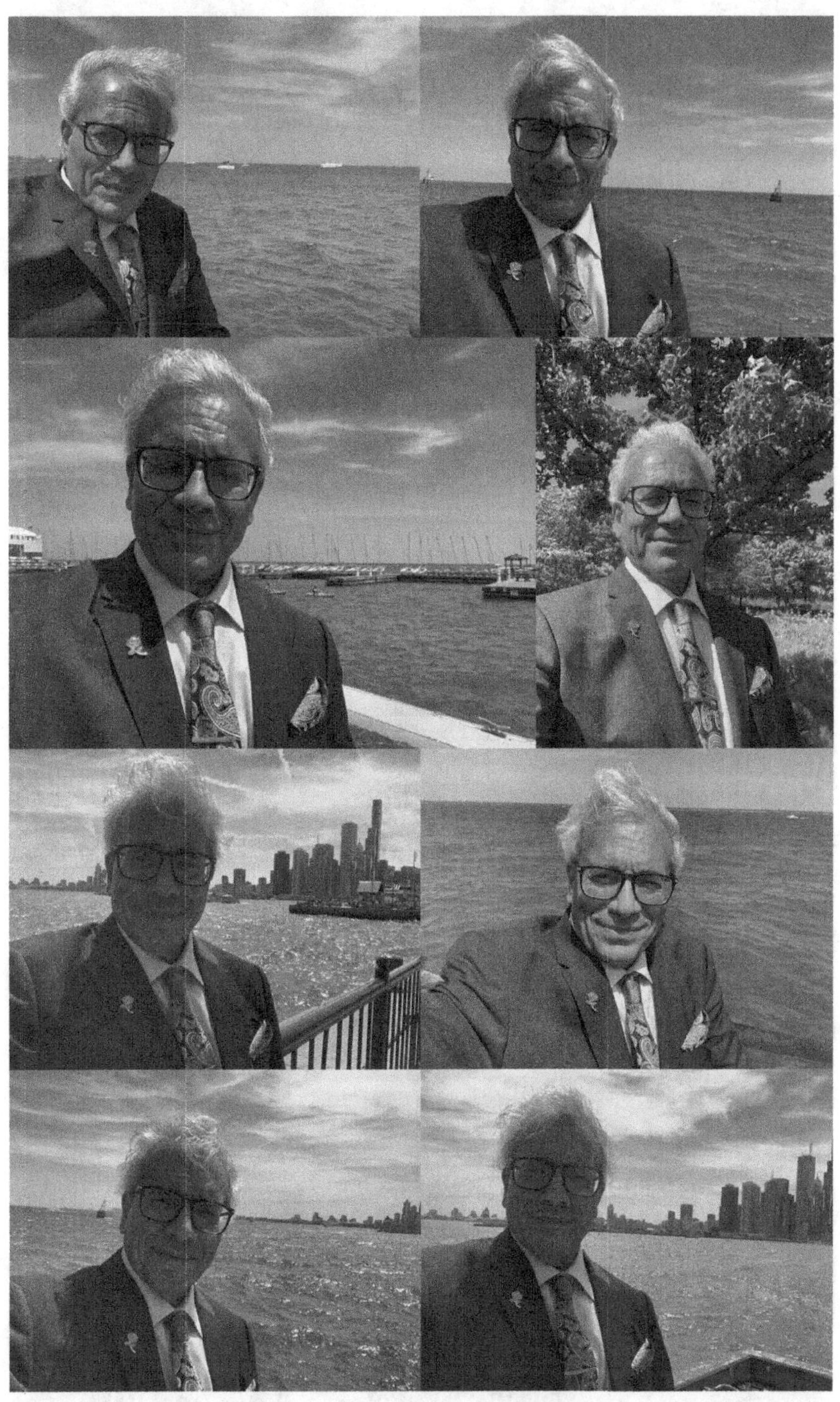

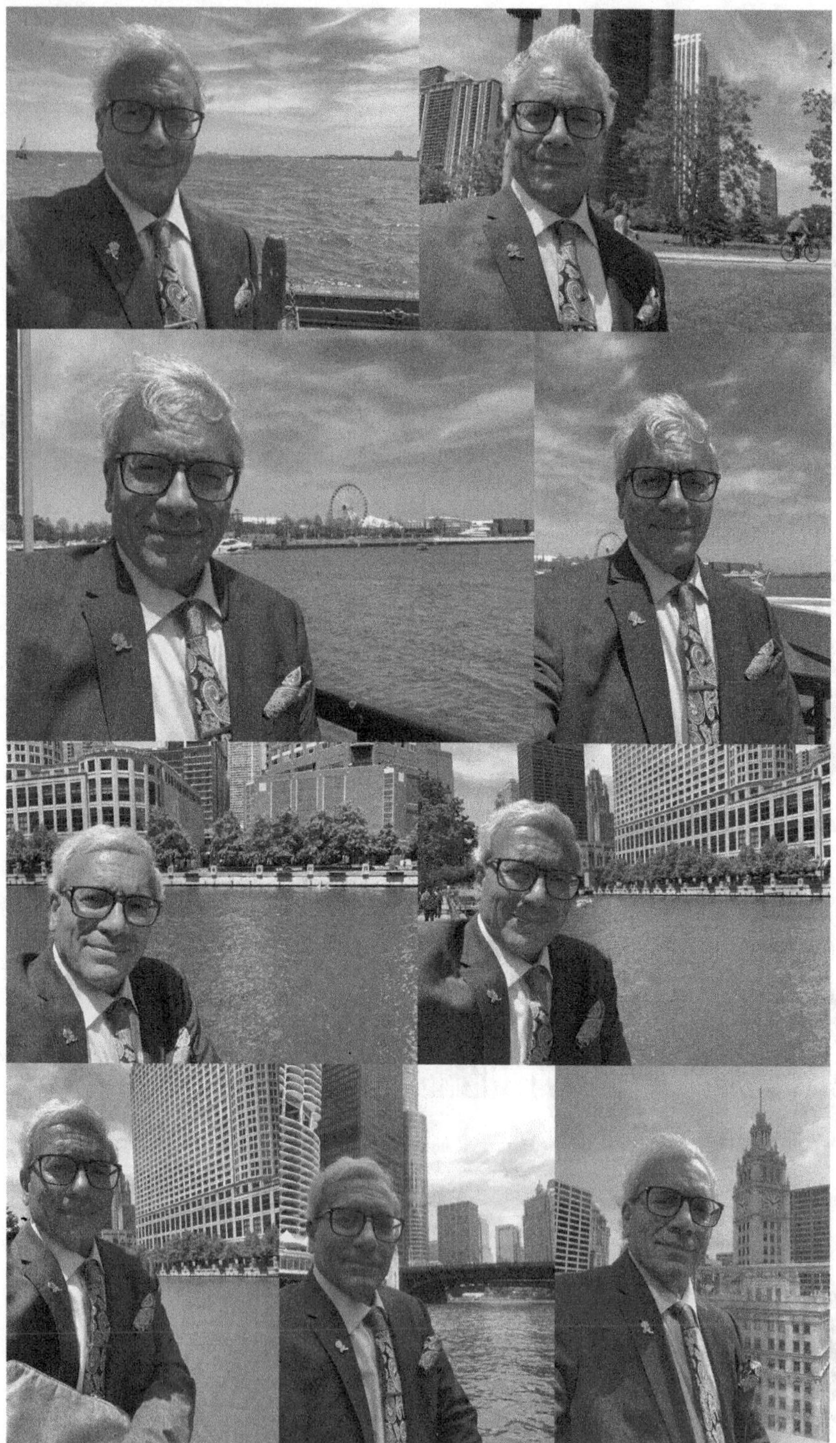

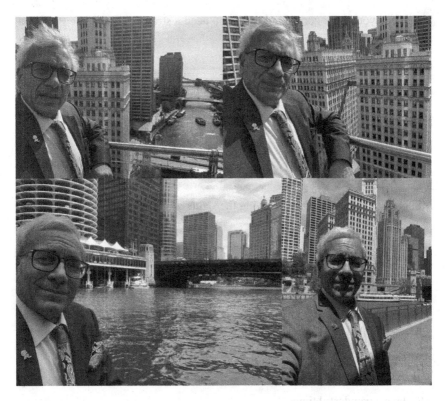

DC, Absolutely love the Chicago river walk and hope you enjoyed the day. I'm sure it was a great day to walk and explore the Riverwalk areas

CP, Looking good, great day to be in the beautiful City of Chicago!

CG, Hope you enjoyed seeing all the sights of your beautiful city. Next time you should wear sunglasses.

PF, You look awesome!

MA, Awesome pictures!F

MN, Looking good DrGhaly.

LW, Wonderful pics and a beautiful day. We'll be in Chicago very soon.

KG, Absolutely gorgeous!!!Love Chicago! Hope you had a fabulous adventure exploring and enjoying the beautiful day. God Bless you, Dr Ramsis Ghaly. You always lighten and brighten everyone's day. Thank you so much! Blessings from Egypt.

LM, I hope you enjoyed yourself

SM, Hope you had a good day Dr G! You need a straw hat and some Bermuda shorts!!

RC, Have a

wonderful time

EP, Have a

wonderful time

! Love the pictures

MS, Nice to see you out and enjoying the sights

DS, Great picture

SP, What a great picture!! If its still there Shaws Crab House sooooo good food

LW, You look great and the colors of your shirt and tie are perfect with the water!

PI, Looking great Dr Ghaly

JD, My friend!

CR, Very elegant!!!!

AP, Have a wonderful time

JP, God's tapestry is such a masterpiece. I'm glad you have the opportunity to enjoy it.

CS, How wonderful and exciting! The green is perfect!

CG, Looking Good!

JM, Great Photos Dr. Ghaly

TG, What a great picture . Have a wonderful day

CR, Beautiful place to meditate.

CC, Take the Architectural Boat Tour the next time you're downtown. It's great and so informative

SJ, Enjoy

JJ, Good man!

MH, Did you get to see the bean also.

TN, Try to visit the Peninsula Hotel for its beauty and Chinese cuisine. You are looking very handsome!!!

ET, JT, you photos are so wonderful

FL, Looks like a beautiful day . Nice suite !

KG, Absolutely gorgeous!!!Love Chicago! Hope you had a fabulous adventure exploring and enjoying the beautiful day. God Bless you, Dr Ramsis Ghaly. You always lighten and brighten everyone's day. Thank you so much! Blessings from Egypt.

LM, I hope you enjoyed yourself

SM, Hope you had a good day Dr G! You need a straw hat and some Bermuda shorts!!

SM, and a cool pair of sunglasses

RC, Have a wonderful time

EP, Have a wonderful time

MS, Nice to see you out and enjoying the sights

Walk by Chicago River to Know thyself!!

Written by Ramsis Ghaly

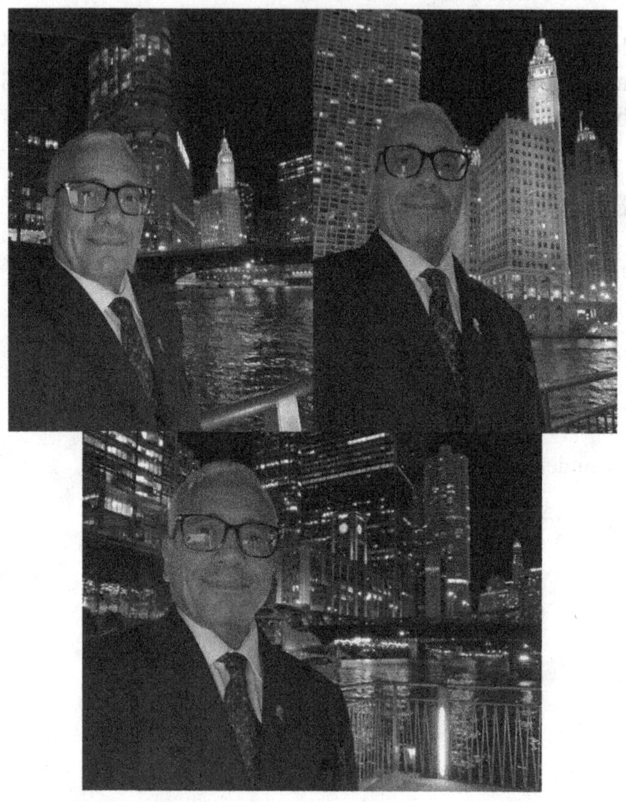

I walked by the Chicago river late at night after a heavy day performing surgery and caring for my neurosurgery patients! I felt a relief and started to pray and sang a God praise!

I kept looking at the waters and staring unto what was beyond the little waves on the surface! The waters became like mirror glancing lights and I could see myself image!

My self image was roving on the waters and began to float bouncing from side to side. I was motivated to keep walking by the River starting at the waters and I said to my mind: "What a better way to get know myself!" Yet the great Chicago architecture didn't take my mind away! The view of the beautiful Chicago skyscrapers and the surrounding loud songs, music, laughs, and the bright Lit lightening of the most attractive city didn't blow my mind or distract my mind!

As I started to take a deep breath of fresh air by the famous Chicago River, the heavy burden of my day events began to come out one by one before my critical and analytical mind! It was almost as if I was standing before a judge giving an account of what I had done today, good or bad and in between!!

I thought it was a time at the end of day for my mind, soul and body to take a detour and come here to the Chicago magnificent River to cool down, to take a break and to enjoy the surrounding! And it wasn't supposed to overwhelm my mind with thoughts, fill my heart with guilt and provide report of sequence of events and details of what had transpired at each event!!

I couldn't helped but continue to review my other past events and various performances! My mind opened for more and more! Even my subconscious mind started to vent the hidden thoughts and deeds!! And to my surprise, not shameful, many struggling thoughts and difficult memories didn't shy to come out and instead poured like rivers with their stored emotions that I couldn't stopped them from coming!!

Thought by thought, event by event, action by action, deed by deed like a record rewinding with no end! My mind was displaying each event before the non-lenient and critical mind acting as a judge scrutinizing, searching, reflecting, dreaming, judging and coming with "problem solving" and "lessons learned" for tomorrow"

It turned out that Chicago River walk at the end of the day was to examine my actions, get to know myself and be critical of my doing. To do so, put myself in a judgment seat started as a fun River walk for rest of mind and a break of my heavy workday load!

Those honest talks and reviews provides "self-examination" and "self-disciplined" to oneself at the end of the day are so crucial in self-discipline and progress!!! Many call them: "Summary of the day", "Synoptic review of the day events" or Examining thyself" "get to know thyself" at the end of each day and write a memoir for each day living and review those memoirs at later age of life!!

A person is required to discipline himself and criticizes oneself honestly and harshly for better self! Judge thyself before thy get judged! It was time for humility and forgiveness and thanksgiving renewing our oath to our Savior God the Lord Jesus!

The end of my Chicago River walk!

Intermittently, my eyes drifted to people watching and attempt to read faces of those around me of what were going unto their minds? What they are talking to each other about?

As midnight was approaching, I noticed the surrounding changed and people looked different some drunken, others high in street drunks, police cars, ambulance Sirens—-!

This is Chicago the most violent city of the national! I looked at myself and realized I was the only one dressed with a suit and tie and no one else around! It was the time to get back home and continue my thoughts at my closet!!

Biblical Verses on "Examining thyself"

Job 13:23 "How many are my iniquities and sins?

Make known to me my rebellion and my sin.

Psalm 4:4 "Tremble, and do not sin;

Meditate in your heart upon your bed, and be still. Selah."

Psalm 32:3-5 "When I kept silent about my sin, my body wasted away. Through my groaning all day long. For day and night Your hand was heavy upon me; My vitality was drained away as with the fever heat of summer. Selah.

I acknowledged my sin to You,

And my iniquity I did not hide;

I said, "I will confess my transgressions to the Lord"; And You forgave the guilt of my sin. Selah."

Psalm 77:6 "I will remember my song in the night;

I will meditate with my heart,

And my spirit ponders:"

Psalm 119:59 "I considered my ways

And turned my feet to Your testimonies."

Jeremiah 31:19 "For after I turned back, I repented;

And after I was instructed, I smote on my thigh;

I was ashamed and also humiliated

Because I bore the reproach of my youth.'"

Lamentations 3:40 "Let us examine and probe our ways, And let us return to the Lord."

Ezekiel 18:27-28 "Again, when a wicked man turns away from his wickedness which he has committed and practices justice and righteousness, he will save his life. Because he considered and turned away from all his transgressions which he had committed, he shall surely live; he shall not die."

Haggai 1:5-7 "Now therefore, thus says the Lord of hosts, "Consider your ways! You have sown much, but harvest little; you eat, but there is not enough to be satisfied; you drink, but there is not enough to become drunk; you put on clothing, but no one is warm enough; and he who earns, earns wages to put into a purse with holes." Thus says the Lord of hosts, "Consider your ways!"

Luke 15:17-24 "But when he came to his senses, he said, 'How many of my father's hired men have more than enough bread, but I am dying here with hunger! I will get up and go to my father, and will say to him, "Father, I have sinned against heaven, and in your sight; I am no longer worthy to be called your son; make me as one of your hired men."'

Corinthians 11:27-31 "Therefore whoever eats the bread or drinks the cup of the Lord in an unworthy manner, shall be guilty of the body and the blood of the Lord. But a man must examine himself, and in so doing he is to eat of the bread and drink of the cup. For he who eats and drinks, eats and drinks judgment to himself if he does not judge the body rightly."

2 Corinthians 13:3-5 "since you are seeking for proof of the Christ who speaks in me, and who is not weak toward you, but mighty in you. For indeed He was crucified because of weakness, yet He lives because of the power of God. For we also are weak in Him, yet we will live with Him because of the power of God directed toward you. Test yourselves to see if you are in the faith; examine yourselves! Or do you not recognize this about yourselves, that Jesus Christ is in you—unless indeed you fail the test?"

Galatians 6:4 "But each one must examine his own work, and then he will have reason for boasting in regard to himself alone, and not in regard to another."

1 John 1:9 "If we confess our sins, He is faithful and righteous to forgive us our sins and to cleanse us from all unrighteousness."

1 John 3:20-21 "in whatever our heart condemns us; for God is greater than our heart and knows all things. Beloved, if our heart does not condemn us, we have confidence before God;"

Matthew 7:5 "You hypocrite, first take the log out of your own eye, and then you will see clearly to take the speck out of your brother's eye."

1 Corinthians 11:28 "But a man must examine himself, and in so doing he is to eat of the bread and drink of the cup."

2 Corinthians 13:5 "Test yourselves to see if you are in the faith; examine yourselves! Or do you not recognize this about yourselves, that Jesus Christ is in you—unless indeed you fail the test?"

Biblical Verses "Know thyself"

Lamentations 3:40 "Let us test and examine our ways, and return to the Lord!

1 John 3:20 ESV "For whenever our heart condemns us, God is greater than our heart, and he knows everything."

Romans 12:3 ESV "For by the grace given to me I say to everyone among you not to think of himself more highly than he ought to think, but to think with sober judgment, each according to the measure of faith that God has assigned."

1 Corinthians 13:1-13 ESV "If I speak in the tongues of men and of angels, but have not love, I am a noisy gong or a clanging cymbal. And if I have prophetic powers, and understand all mysteries and all knowledge, and if I have all faith, so as to remove mountains, but have not love, I am nothing. If I give away all I have, and if I deliver up my body to be burned, but have not love, I gain nothing. Love is patient and kind; love does not envy or boast; it is not arrogant or rude. It does not insist on its own way; it is not irritable or resentful; ..."

Acts 1:8 ESV "But you will receive power when the Holy Spirit has come upon you, and you will be my witnesses in Jerusalem and in all Judea and Samaria, and to the end of the earth."

Psalm 119:105 ESV "Your word is a lamp to my feet and a light to my path."

Romans 8:27 ESV "And he who searches hearts knows what is the mind of the Spirit, because the Spirit intercedes for the saints according to the will of God."

John 14:1-31 ESV "Let not your hearts be troubled. Believe in God; believe also in me. In my Father's house are many rooms. If it were not so, would I have told you that I go to prepare a place for you? And if I go and prepare a place for you, I will come again and will take you to myself, that where I am you may be also. And you know the way to where I am going." Thomas said to him, "Lord, we do not know where you are going. How can we know the way?" ...

Psalm 139:23-24 "Search me, O God, and know my heart! Try me and know my thoughts! And see if there be any grievous way in me, and lead me in the way everlasting!"

John 4:24 "God is spirit, and those who worship him must worship in spirit and truth."

John 3:16 "For God so loved the world, that he gave his only Son, that whoever believes in him should not perish but have eternal life."

Psalm 25:14 "The friendship of the Lord is for those who fear him, and he makes known to them his covenant."

2 Timothy 3:16 "All Scripture is breathed out by God and profitable for teaching, for reproof, for correction, and for training in righteousness,"

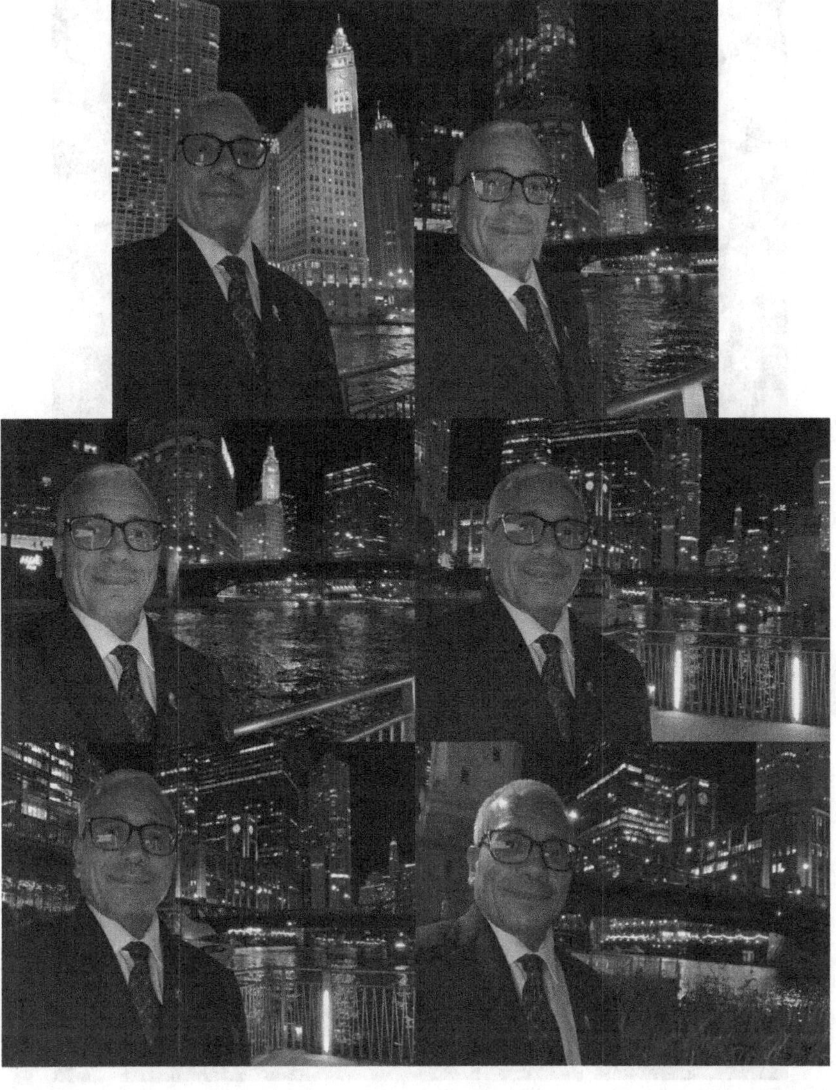

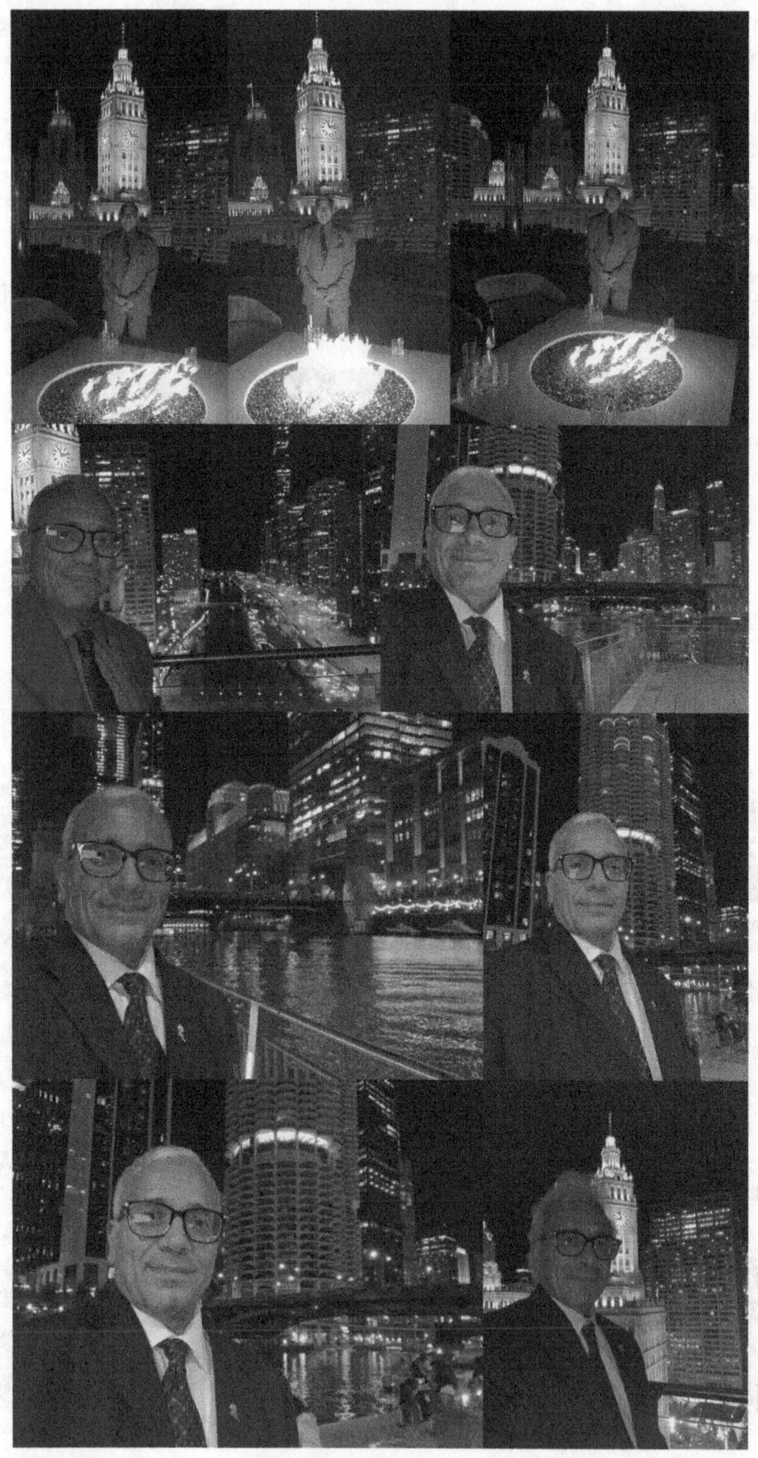

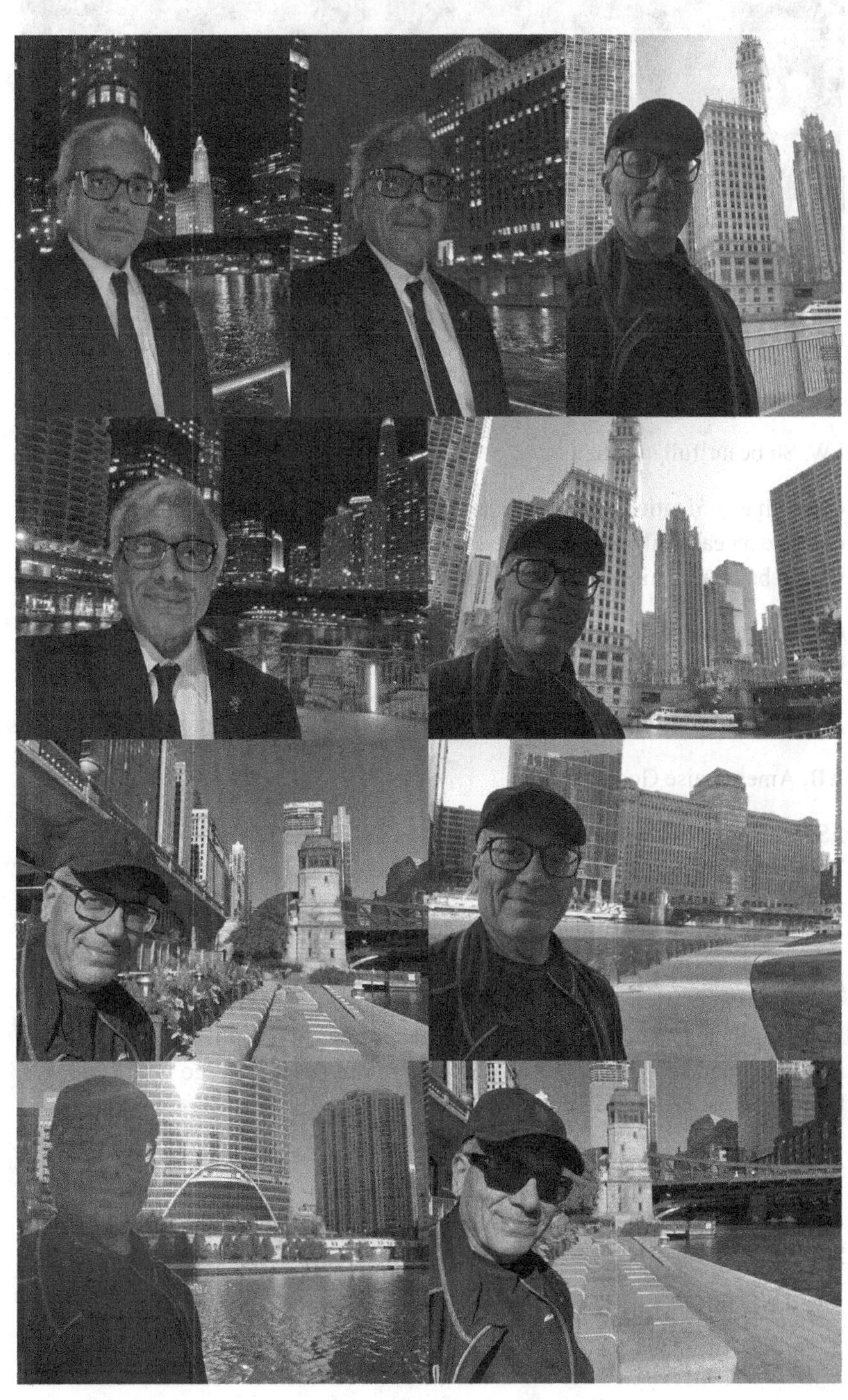

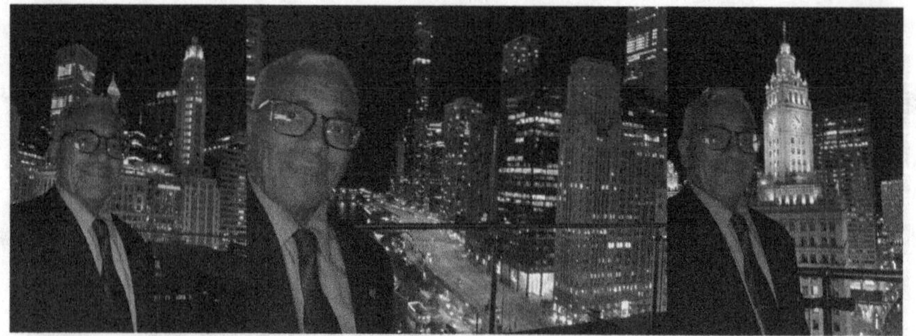

CR,Thank you for sharing your honest thoughts with us with such humility.

JT, your words ... gave me the chills...

LW, So beautifully written.

CG, Self examination is good becuase you learn how you are unique. There is no one else on earth like you. You have your own thoughts and ideas on how things should be done. This is something we all should do sometime.

CH, It's sad that such a beautiful city has gone down so bad. Being born and raised in the city I miss going downtown, just seem to be a safe place to be these days

JF, Beautiful words! I would love to walk with you there! **#PastorJeff90210**

AB, Amen praise God

ES, Such wise words Dr. G but please, don't walk the street at such late hours. They aren't safe. You are loved by so many people and we want you to be safe.

TN, Beautiful. My husband was born and raised in Chicago.

Arthur Almassy Bro Ramsis…

You continue to amaze me. You are handsome, accomplished, exceedingly intelligent and very much more. Your waters run deep. Chicago needs you. It's been my great pleasure knowing you!

Bro Arthur

AL, The best M.D. …. Fathered patients in giving excellent medical care for many years & counting. Happy Father's day Doc

VW, Love this picture Happy Father's Day!

RC, Great picture

Causal Sporty Unuform

Causal sporty

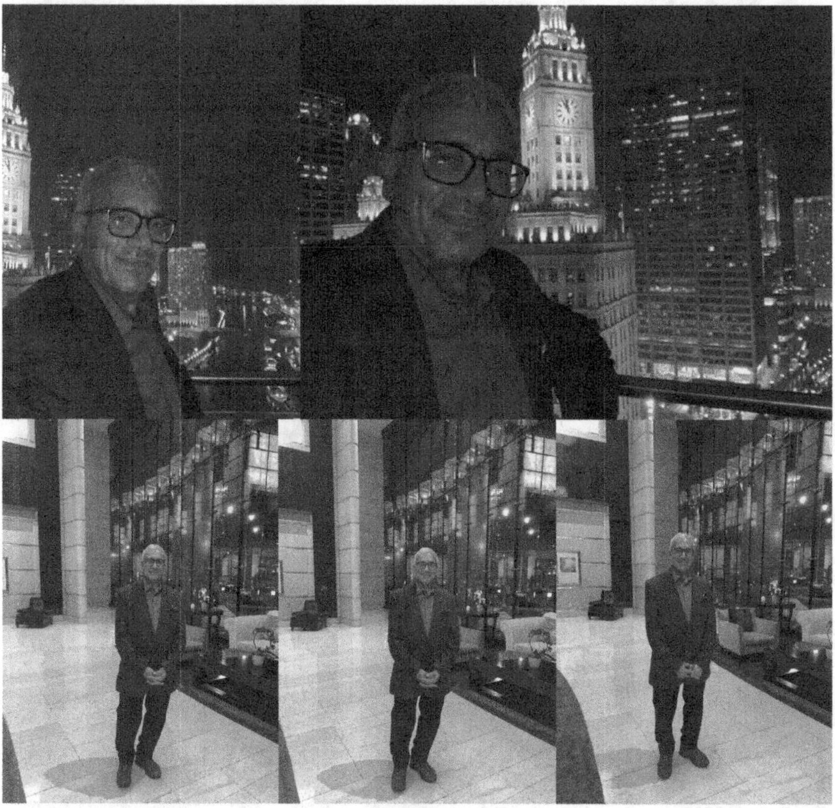

Chicago River photos

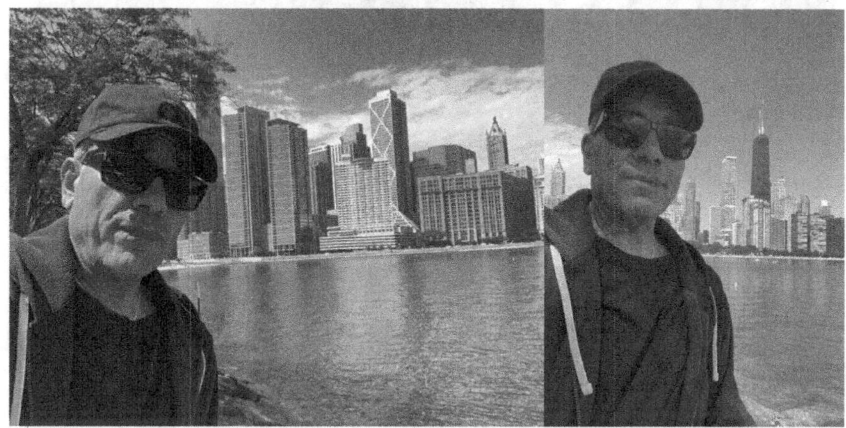

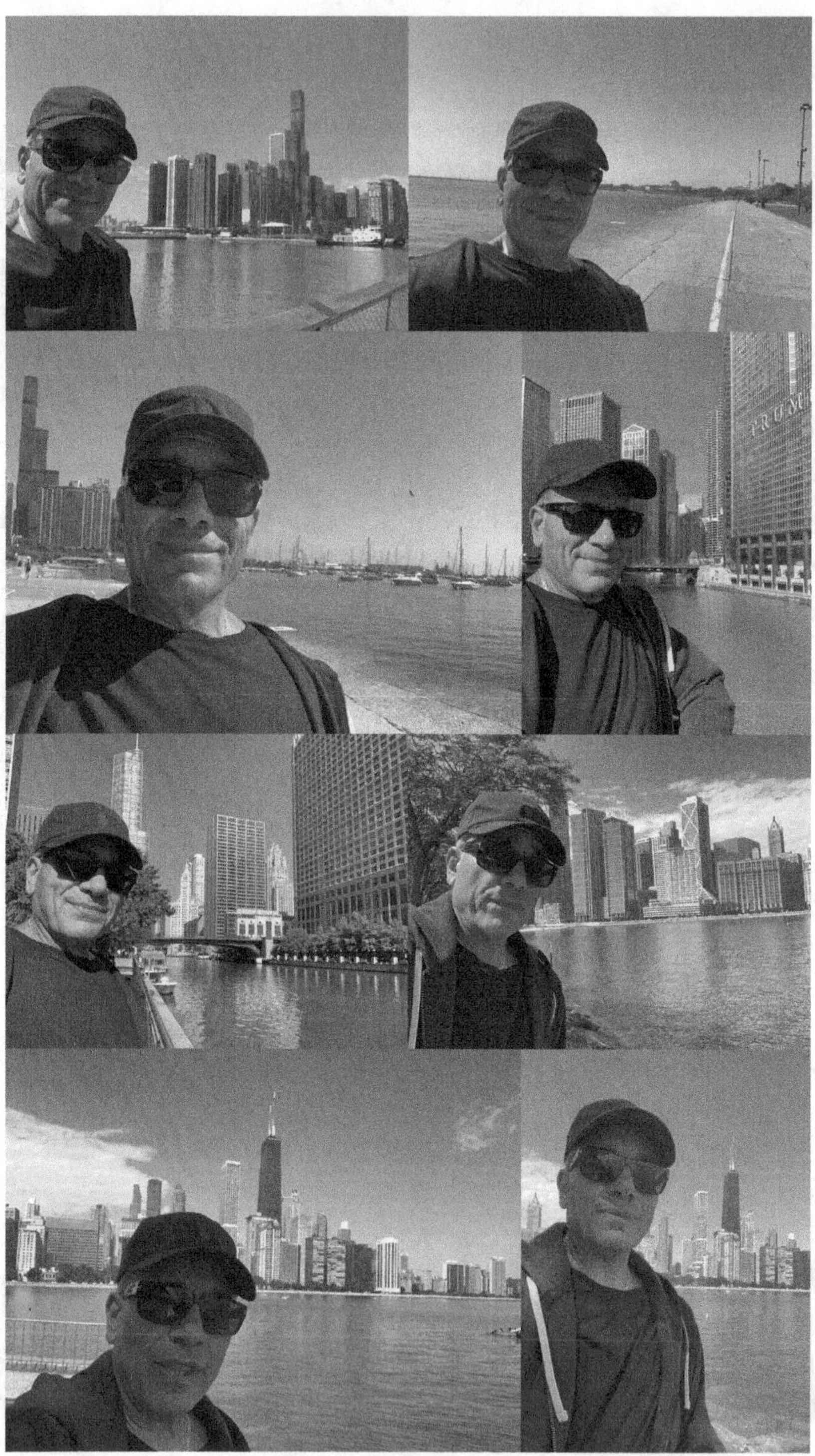

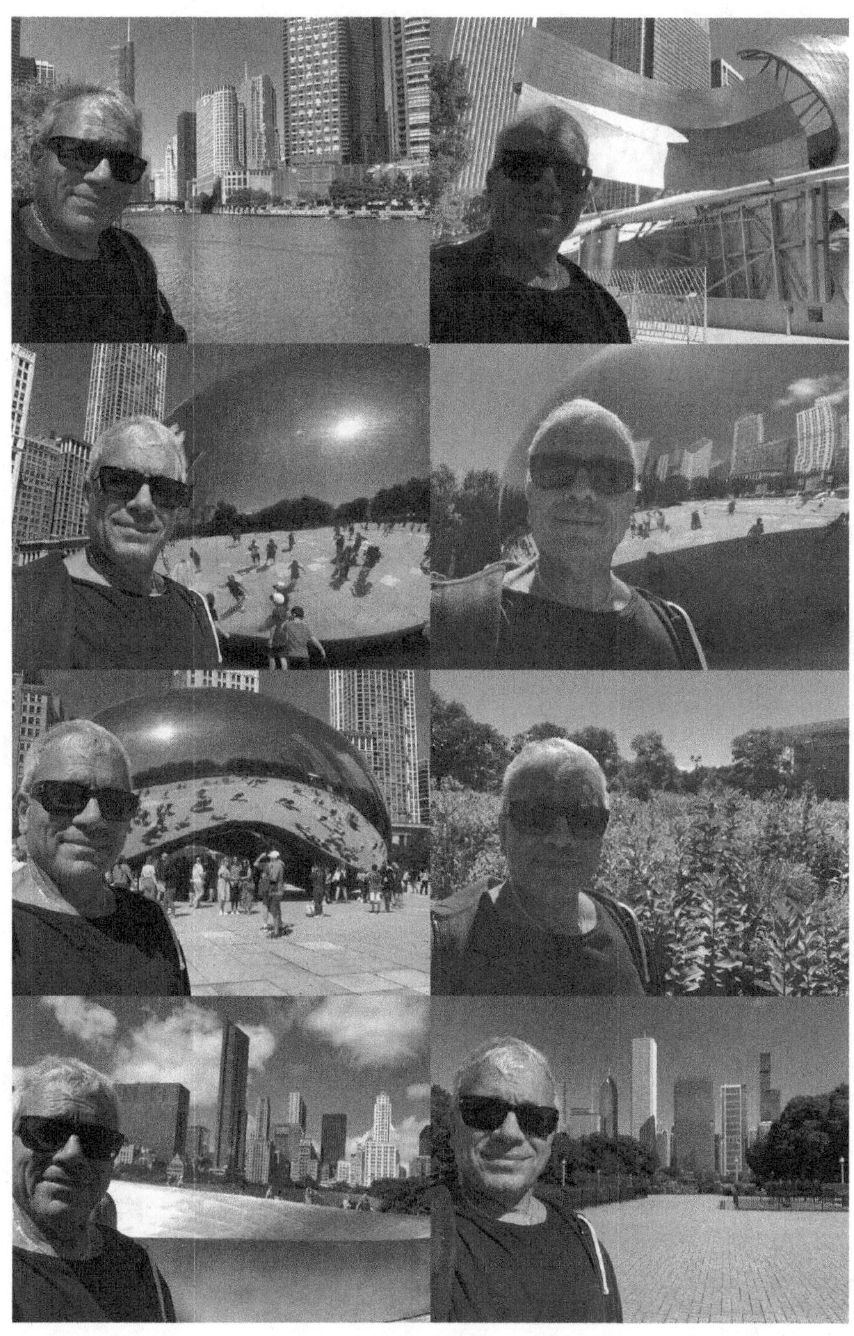

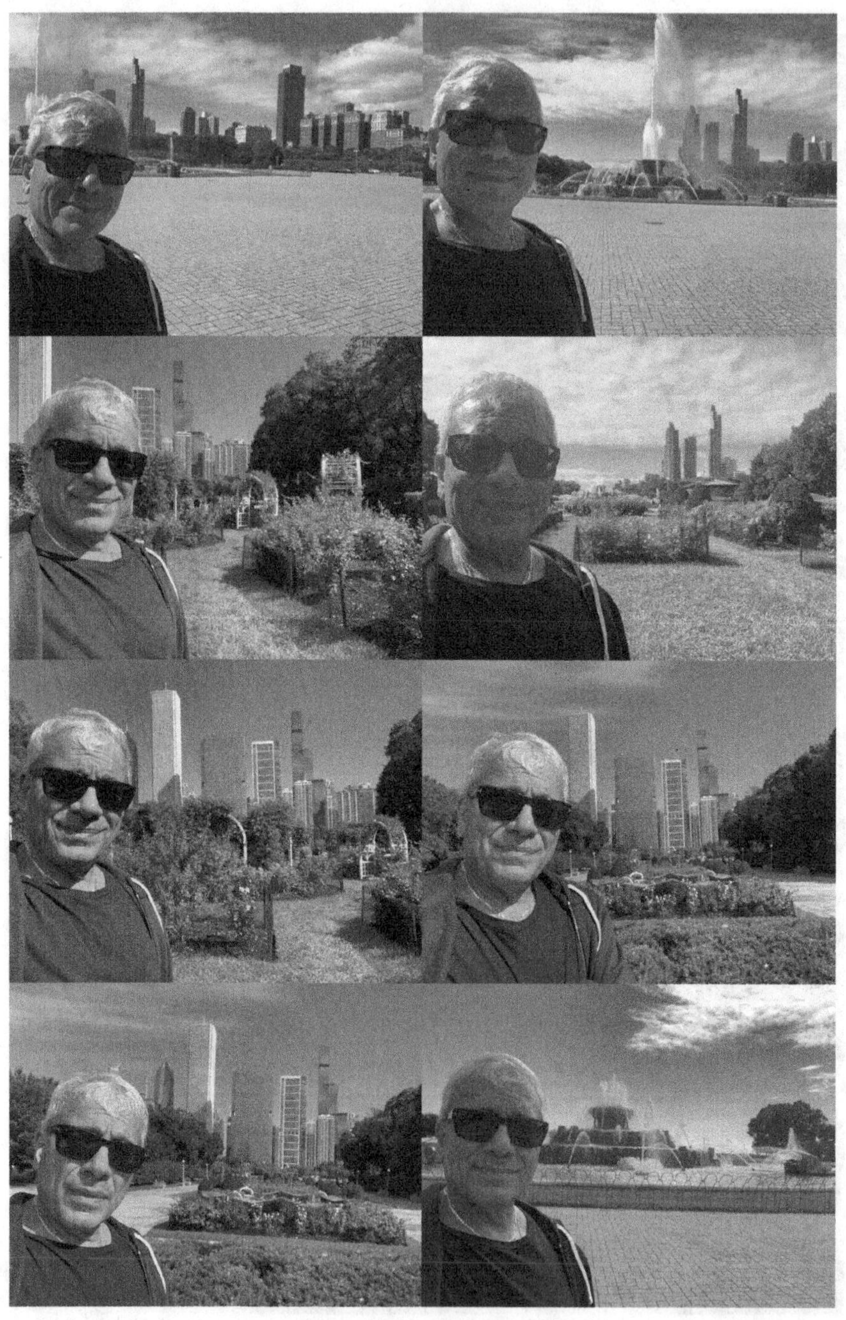

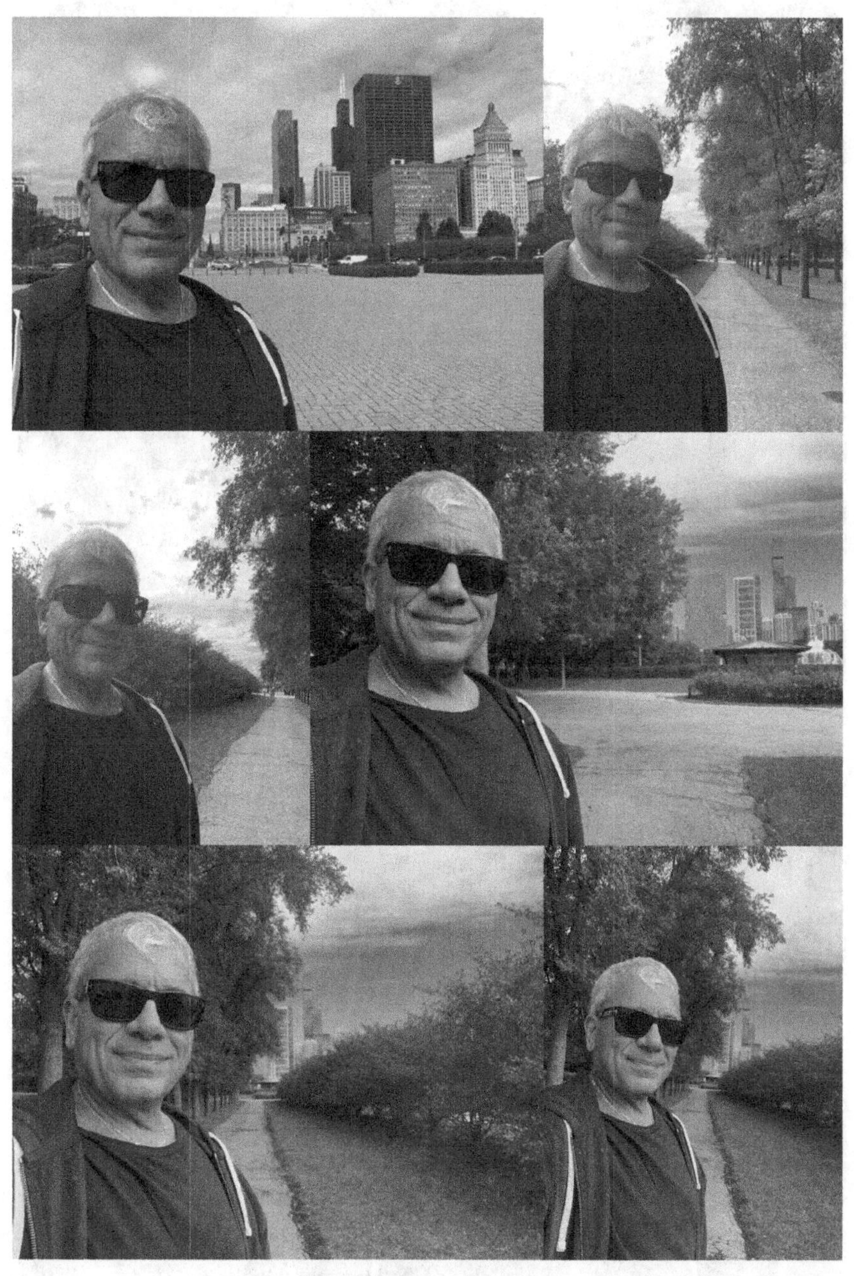

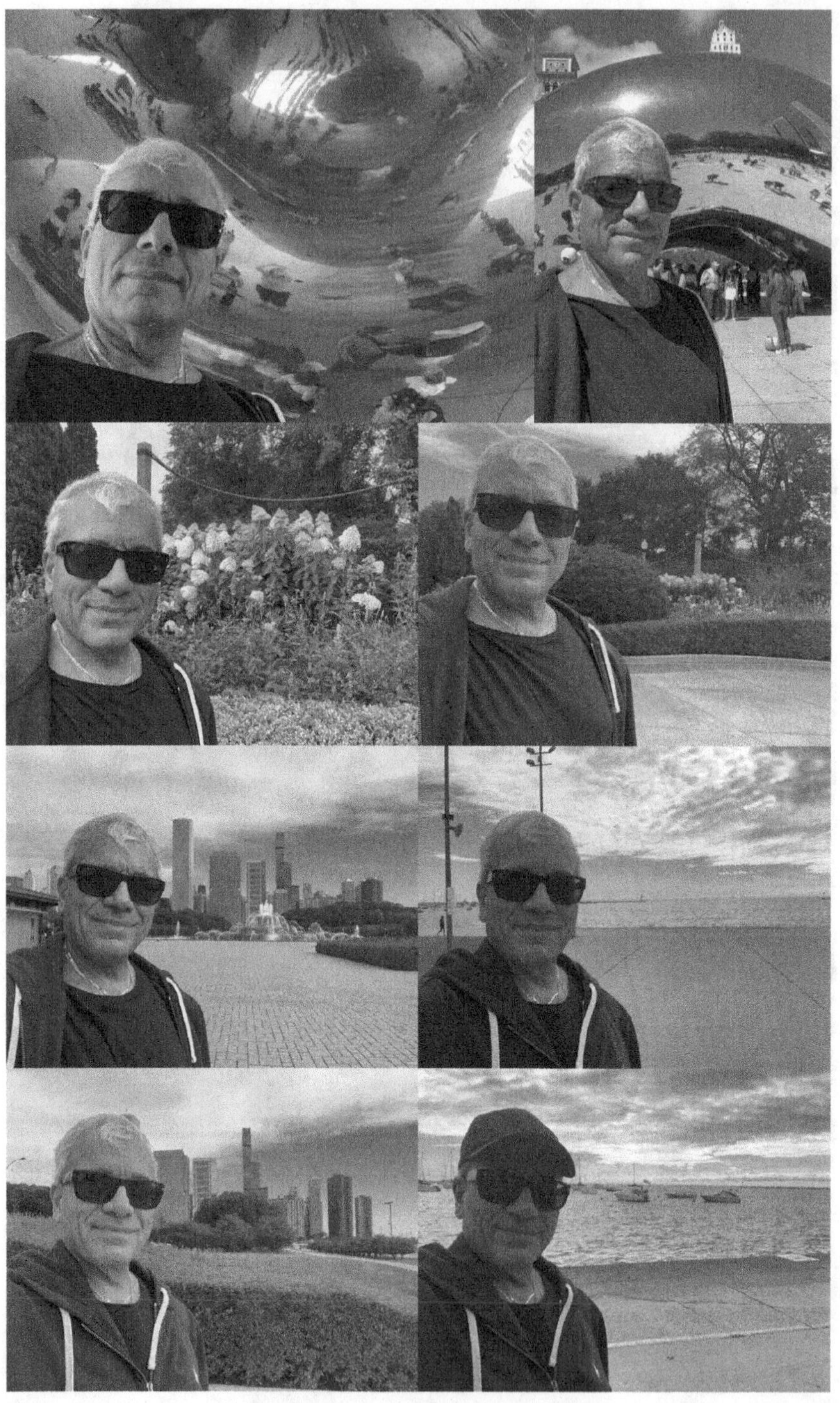

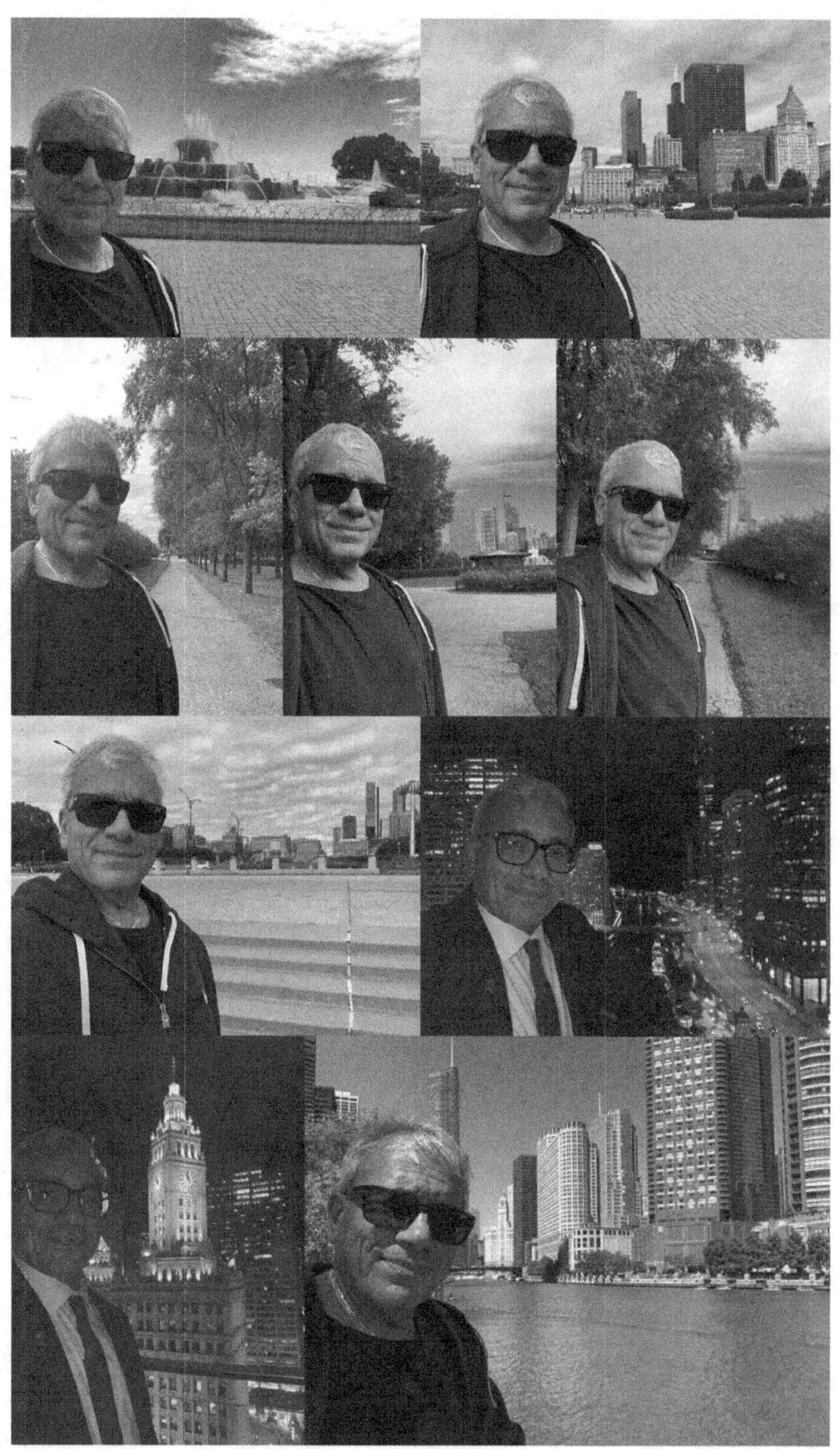

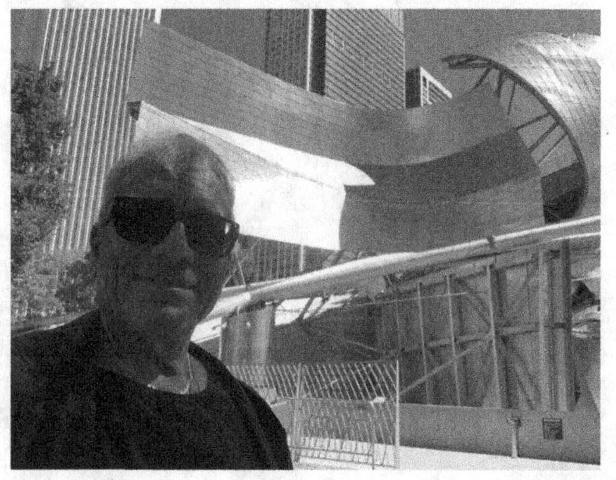

The Founder of Chicago!

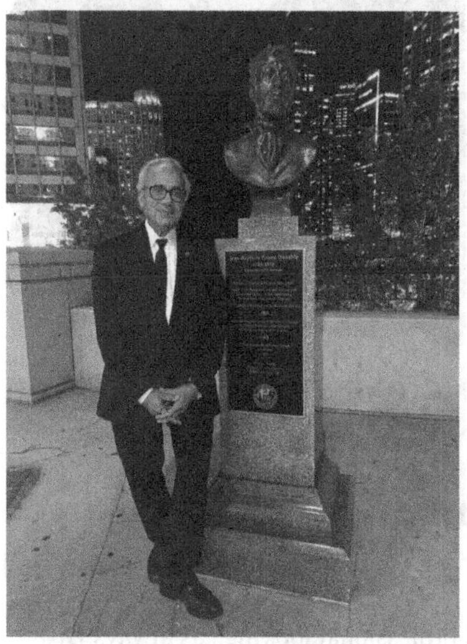

The Founder of Chicago, An Haitian Indignant Settler Native African and French-Canadian origin!

Jean Baptiste Pointe DuSable 1745-1818

Jean Baptiste Point du Sable (also spelled Point de Sable, Point au Sable, Point Sable, Pointe DuSable, Pointe du Sable[n 1]; before 1750[n 2] – 28 August 1818) is regarded as the first permanent non-Indigenous settler of what would later become Chicago, Illinois, and is recognized as the "Founder of Chicago".[7] A school, museum, harbor, park, bridge, and road have been named in his honor. The site where he settled near the mouth of the Chicago River around the 1780s is identified as a National Historic Landmark, now located in Pioneer Court.

https://en.m.wikipedia.org/wiki/Jean_Baptiste_Point_du_Sabl

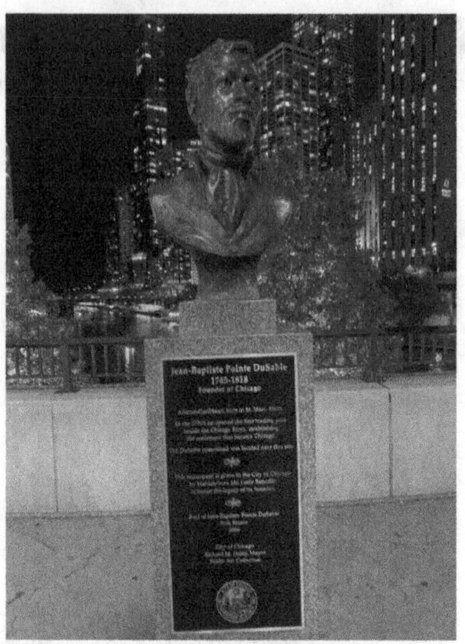

SC, Very nice photo

DL, So handsome & professional looking...as always Dr !

CG, Just noticed the other day on one of my many trips to the city that Lake Shore Drive has been renamed Jean-Baptiste Pointe DuSable Lake Shore Drive.

MA, Great picture

DN, Very nice

JM, “Fascinating” Dr. Ramsis

I found the Next President as I Waked By Lack Michigan and Chicago River!!!

Written by Ramsis Ghaly 5/30/2022

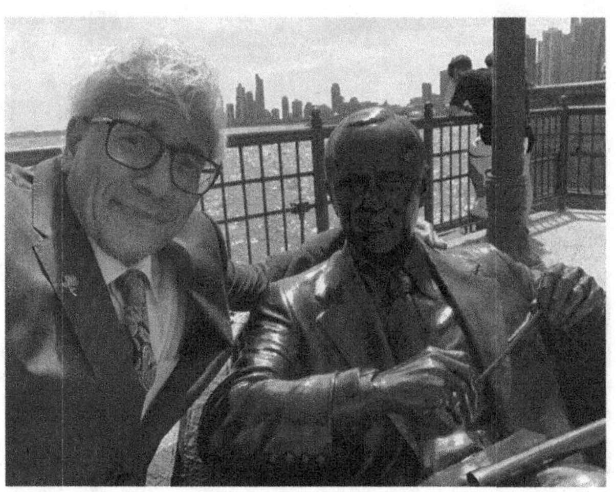

As I walked by Chicago River and Lack Michigan, I found the Next President! I Shaked his hand and put my arm around to salute him and what he is about to do as he shall take nation one more time to prosperity according to the book of times!! It was the only time that I came close wishing him farewell. He, however, didn't know what is about to follow! It was hidden from him! It was his last!

As the suffering of people continues, that earth shall bring that man up from an unknown land!

With a full surprise, he shall find his way up with the kings and the vote shall be his!

He is Wise, calm, thinker and genius!!! A brave and hero to say the least! No one has ever thought he would be the one!!

He doesn't talk much and calculate each step of the way!!

And most importantly, he does what he has promised to do!

He is neither politician nor experienced in how the government works, but he is for the people. He is determined to do a great job! And to the degree that during his time, the world shall flourish again as God the Almighty shall bless the world through his hands!

He was among us and in an instant, he was gone! Tears were pouring in the streets raising concerns of why he taken so soon! He left an everlasting legacy!

At his prime, that life soon shall be taken away!! And After his time, it shall be the last as the horses shall flip one against the other!!!

Ramsis Ghaly

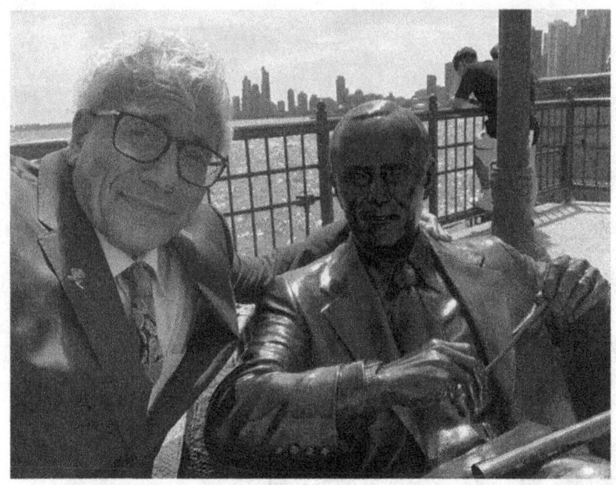

Sc. anout what we have now lol

cg, Sounds like he would be a great president if only he wasn't a statue. Great picture!

MH, What a great tribute to a wonderful man too bad he was taken from us. Have a happy Memorial Day.

By the waters!

So much of the author writing were by the waters, the mountains, and daily meditations. The daily events and provoking thoughts seasoned my writing!

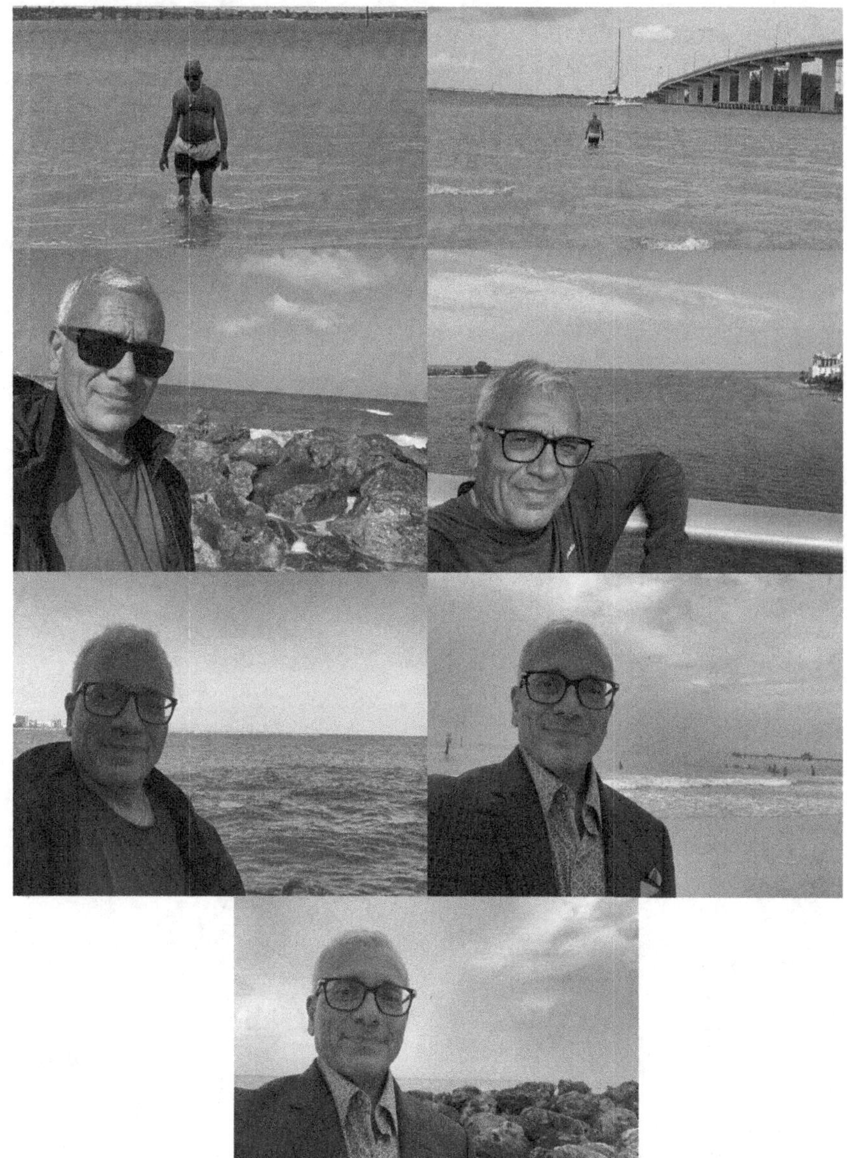

I am Poor and Needy

I am Poor and Needy!!

"But I am poor and needy: make haste unto me, O God: thou art my help and my deliverer; O Lord, make no tarrying." Psalm 70:5 KJV

Ramsis Ghaly

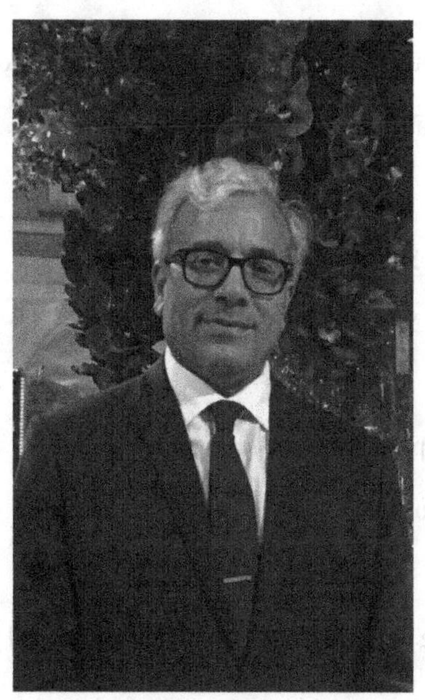

AC, Wonderful smile

MB, Blessed day Dr.Ghaly .

VG, God Bless you Dr Ghaly!!!

SC, smashing doctor you look amazing

KG, Nice picture, Dr. Ghaly!

GH, Beautiful verse also photo Dr.

AS, God bless you

MN, Looking good DrGhaly God bless you buddy.

DH, You are a Talented and Brilliant man Dr. GHALY, May God Contine to Bless You

JT, my favourite colour of flower...my favourite flower and my favourite doctor

KN, This should be FRAMED GREAT PHOTO of an AMAZING MAN

PI, Amen. Looking good Dr Ghaly

TG, Looking great!

God Blessed you as always.

CG, Amen! Bless you!

MA, God Bless you you are an excellent Dr keep up the good work

EO, Amen. Greetings and best wishes. Blessings.

JM, Amen!

FR GG, Very proud of you dear Dr **Ramsis Ghaly**

LW, Amen . God bless you.

TN, Amen.

DS, Amen Wonderful picture God Bless you Dr. Ghaly

SL, Amen! Great photograph

DM, God Bless

MH, You are a blessing to many, the lord definitely blessed you with a great talent to help others.

BCD, I loved seeing this post first thing this morning. Thank you Sir

I am Green Olive Tree!

Written by Ramsis Ghaly

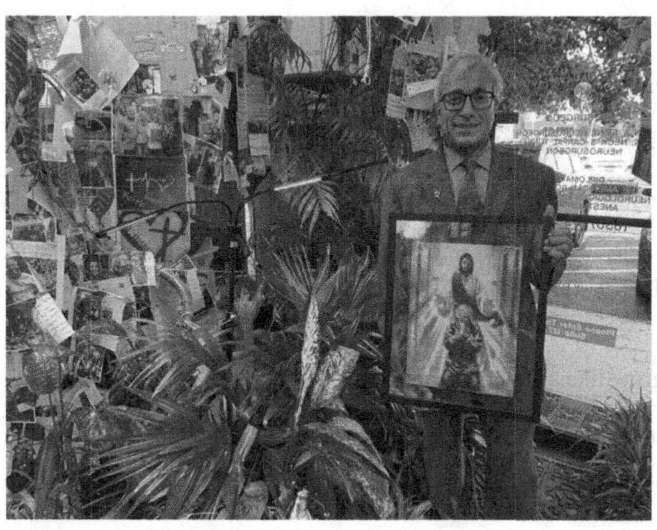

“The Lord called your name,

“A green olive tree, beautiful in fruit and form”;

With the noise of a great tumult

He has kindled fire on it,

And its branches are worthless. “Jeremiah 11:16

The signal light has just turned green and I am going in my way! I am green and tattooed with a green lively olive tree ! I am a green olive tree in the house of God; “But as for me, I am like a green olive tree in the house of God; I trust in the lovingkindness of God forever and ever.” Psalm 52:8

I am dressed in green and so is my way! Therefore, I am racing to the green valley so as long as I have given the green yield! I am laying down by the green pasture beside a still water: “He makes me lie down in green pastures; He leads me beside quiet waters.” Psalm 23:2

Those in green shall always give fruits and shall not age: They will still yield fruit in old age;

They shall be full of sap and very green,” Psalm 92:14

The servant of God is given roots to spread by the stream and leaves of green even in drought and shall not cease to yield fruit : "For he will be like a tree planted by the water,

That extends its roots by a stream

And will not fear when the heat comes;

But its leaves will be green,

And it will not be anxious in a year of drought

Nor cease to yield fruit. "Jeremiah 17:8

I saw a cedar tree planted in the house of God and within and a righteous man like a palm tree full of sap and very green: "The righteous man will flourish like the palm tree,

He will grow like a cedar in Lebanon.

Planted in the house of the Lord,

They will flourish in the courts of our God.

They will still yield fruit in old age;

They shall be full of sap and very green," Psalm 92:12-15

It is written that any green and those with the seal of God in their forehead won't hurt: "They were told not to hurt the grass of the earth, nor any green thing, nor any tree, but only the men who do not have the seal of God on their foreheads." Revelation 9:4

Yet, I heard an alarm sound followed by voice, Be in the watch as the signal about to turn Red and shall no longer be Green and thy must cease and come to full stop !

I replied: "Who are you?? I am green and I shall always be green and the signal shall turn green before me and always gives the yield to me!!"

I heard a reply: "Only in the Lord, by the Lord and for the Lord, as it is written in Ezekiel 17:24 "All the trees of the field will know that I am the Lord; I bring down the high tree, exalt the low tree, dry up the green tree and make the dry tree flourish. I am the Lord; I have spoken, and I will perform it."

My soul was elated Up high and my pride went above the roof and I felt I am above the clouds!!

I heard the reply: "Not with thy pride! Only if in one promise!!"

I replied: "And what shall that promise be?"

The voice with a smile: "If thy **"Be Down to Earth and Neither High Nor Down On Thyself"**

Since then, I chose to be level headed and **"Be Down to Earth and Neither High Nor Down On Thyself".** And never lost my Green signal yield my way!!

I love the Green and the bd around the green trees . I kept walking and walking by the valleys and all around me is full of green!!

Indeed, Life is an existence to serve and share love ! Life passes by so quickly and no time to waste before thy know it will be gone and thy will no longer to be around to make a difference! Life is just a few, so let us compete to serve one another! Life is just immeasurable, so let us do much more to help one another! Life is just a vapor soon shall fade away, let us spread love all around! Life is just blossoming flower for few, so let us be the Good Samaritan to others!

So I carried my cross and kept walking! I told myself: "Life is too short to slow down! So let us race to do good!" I kept uttering the words: **"Be Down to Earth and Neither High Nor Down On Thyself".**

I went to sleep, I closed my eyes and I heard a voice saying: "Don't Be Down On Thyself But Be Down to Earth"

We are all equal so might as well be servant to each other "Don't Be Down On Thyself, But Be Down to Earth" Indeed life is too short so let us race to do good!

"Why are you cast down, O my soul?

And why are you disquieted within me?

Hope in God;

For I shall yet praise Him,

The help of my countenance and my God" (Psalms 43:5)

I have been walking with high heal shoes at the daytime and getting weary! I'm would rather be causal and prefer to be natural barefooted down to earth!! I learned Looking Up all the time, hurts my neck, puffs me up and could be harmful!! And who knows while I am walking looking up all the time, I may not pay attention and inadvertently, I may hit whoever is in my way endangering myself and others!! So I would rather be at even level, lowly and looking steadily at my level. Yet inspired in my dreams to reach the top and strive to beyond what seems impossible!!

I am green and lowly, obedient and servant following my Master and Savior words: "Ye call me Master and Lord: and ye say well; for so I am. [14] If I then, your Lord and Master, have washed your feet; ye also ought to wash one another's feet. [15] For I have given you an example, that ye should do as I have done to you. [16] Verily, verily, I say unto you, The servant is not greater than his lord; neither he that is sent greater than he that sent him."John 13:13-16 KJV

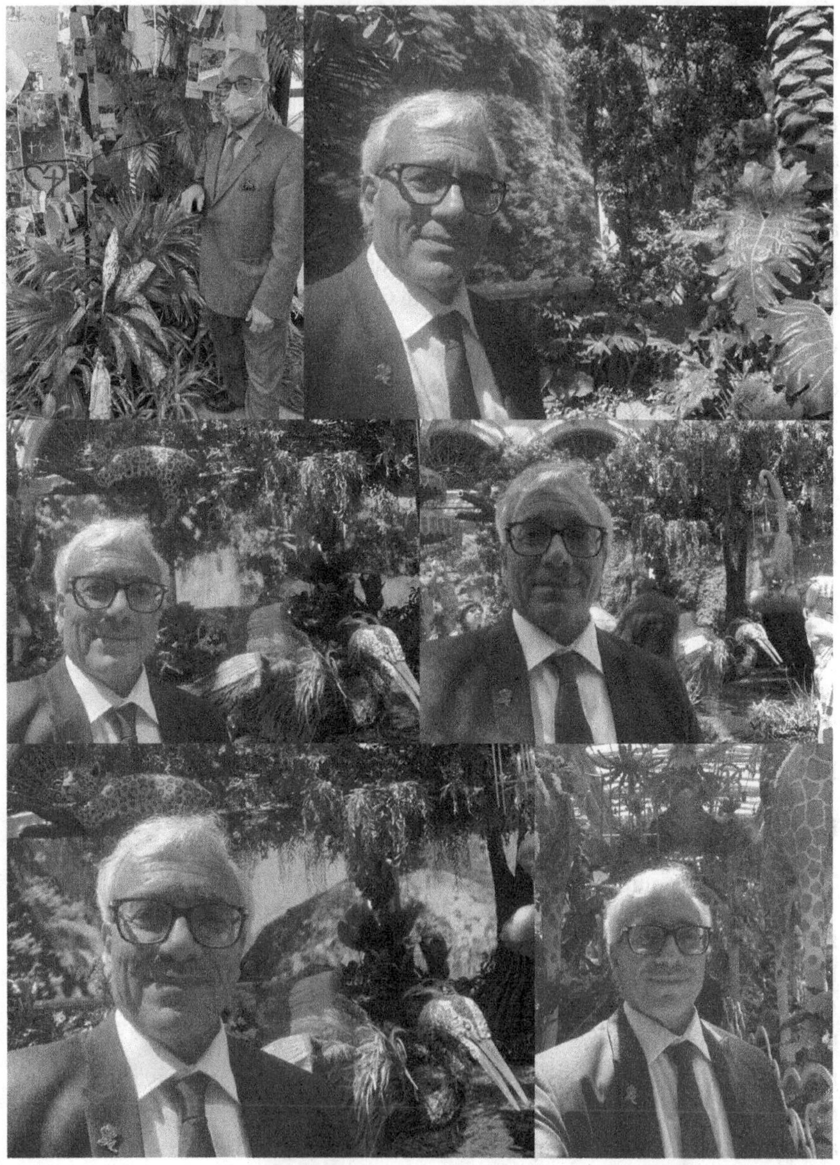

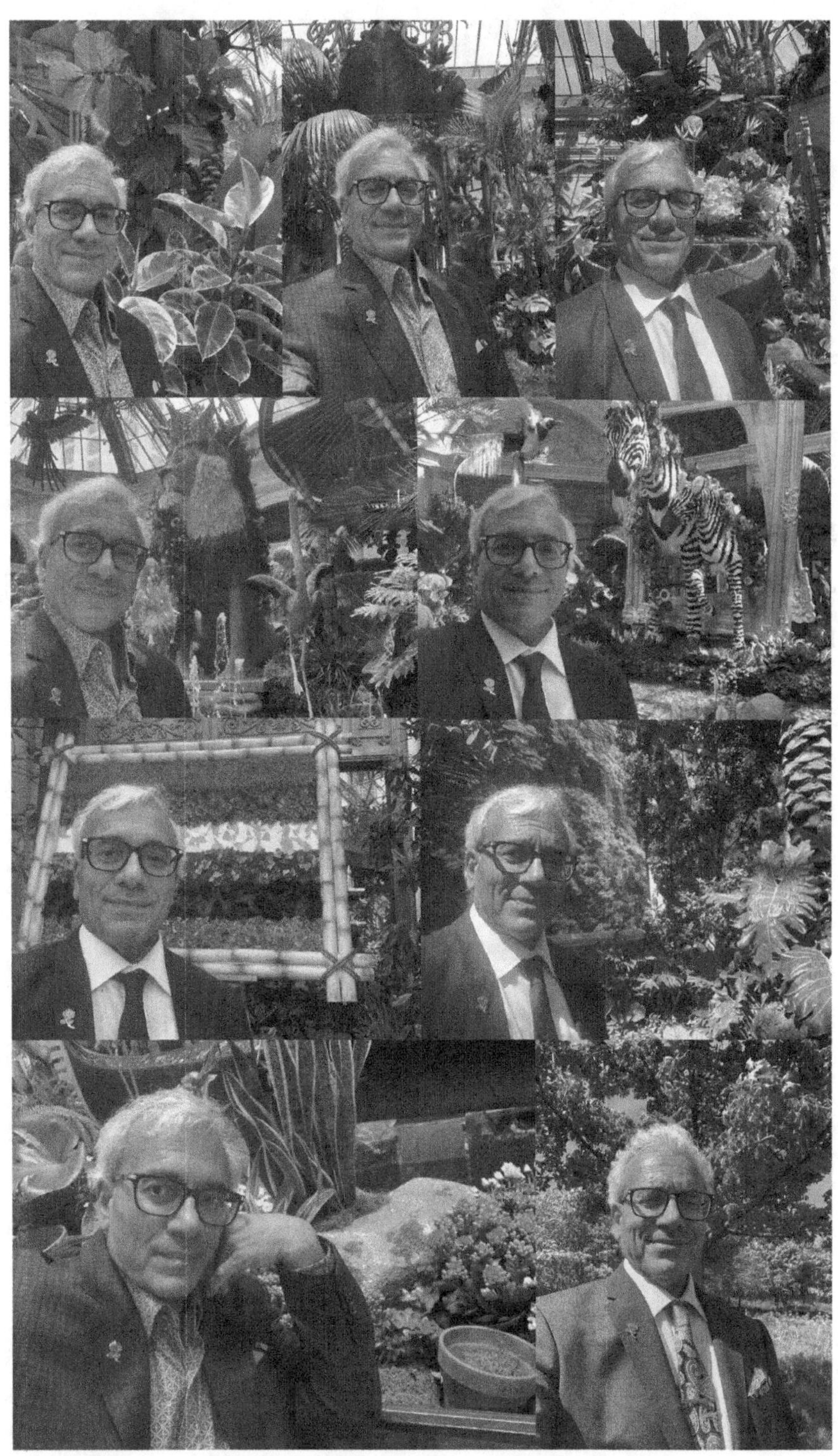

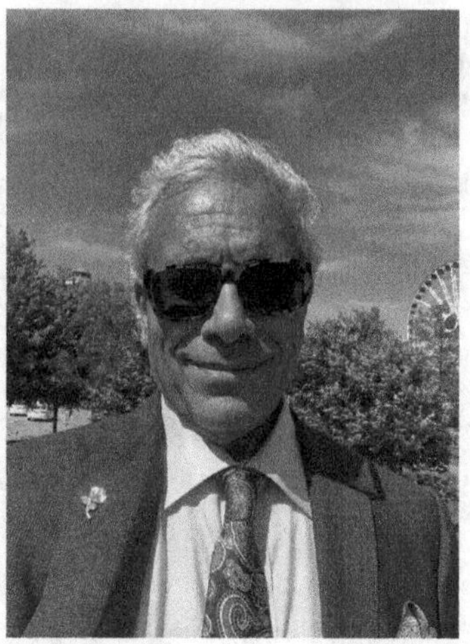

tr, Very deep and thought provoking

JT, i am forever buying plants and filling my house with growing things

DN, Very beautiful

It Is A Life Worth Living!!

Written by Ramsis Ghaly

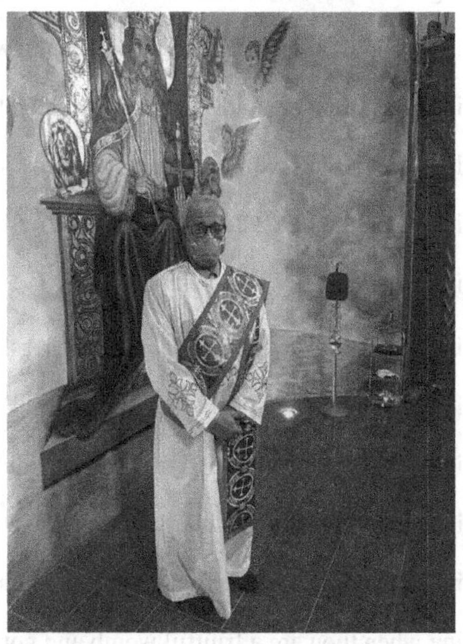

It is a life worth living when thou lay thy life for others!

It is a life worth living when thou are a true follower to the Savior of the world!

It is a life worth living when thou are a servant to the Truth!

It is a life worth living when thou are loving to thy enemy and those against thy!

It is a life worth living when thou are hungry and thirst for others sake!

It is a life worth living when thou are merciful and meek and not ashamed of thyself!

It is a life worth living when thou are spiritual in the lust world!

It is a life worth living when thou are seeker of the life eternity in the kingdom of God!

It is a life worth living when thou are testimony of the righteousness!

It is a life worth living when thou aren't offense to the little ones!

It is a life worth living when thou are poor in the spirit!

It is a life worth living when thou are persecuted against for sake of God and goodness!

It is a life worth living when thou are a faithful in a faithless crowd!

It is a life worth living when thou are living in abstinence in world full of lusts!

It is a life worth living when thou are a love among the haters!

It is a life worth living when thou save Love and not destroy love !

It is a life worth living when thou are a Rose among the lilies!

It is a life worth living when thou are the blossom flower in a withered land!

It is a life worth living when thou are a light in a darkness!

It is a life worth living when thou are a fruit in a dry ground!

It is a life worth living when thou give rise to fruits 30, 60 and hundred!

It is a life worth living when thou are a fountain of spring waters in a drought!

It is a life worth living when thou are a fertile ground in a famine time!

It is a life worth living when thou are a fruitful womb and not a barren womb!

It is a life worth living when thou are an eagle by the desert!

It is a life worth living when thou are a bird nest for the flying birds!

It is a life worth living when thou are a dove with a green leave after a fatal flood!

It is a life worth living when thou say hello to someone to cheer his day!

It is a life worth living when thou say hello to someone to cheer his day!

It is a life worth living when thou render a smile in a sorrowful soul!

It is a life worth living when thou love spread to others indiscriminately!

It is a life worth living when thou pray for someone!

It is a life worth living when thou bring life to dying soul!

It is a life worth living when thou bring joy to a doomed soul!

It is a life worth living when thou bring a comfort to a broken heart !

It is a life worth living when thou are a Physician to a sick!

It is a life worth living when thou are a Healer to a terminal!

It is a life worth living when thou alleviate someone's pain!

It is a life worth living when thou soak the wounds!

It is a life worth living when thou stop the bleeding in a atrocity!

It is a life worth living when thou are an eye to a blind, an ear to a deaf and a tongue to a mute!

It is a life worth living when thou are a defense to the defeat!

It is a life worth living when thou are a shield to the unprotected!

It is a life worth living when thou are a peacemaker in violence!

It is a life worth living when thou a distinguisher in a fire rage!

It is a life worth living when thou be watchful and fill thy lamp with the eternal oil that never go out!

It is a life worth living when thou are a forgiving among the revengers!

It is a life worth living when thou cover for the shortcoming of others and thou not criticizing thy brothers!

It is a life worth living when thou don't look down at others and elevate thou in the bottom!

It is a life worth living when thou lift up the broken, walk behind the crippled, motivate the discouraged, strengthen the fearful and hug the lowly!

It is a life worth living when thou bring up positivity and not negativity!

It is a life worth living when thou are a true witness against the false accusatory!

It is a life worth living when thou are an innocent among criminals!

It is a life worth living when thou are a solution and not the problem!

It is a life worth living when thou are a quiescence in disputes and not a stirring!

It is a life worth living when thou are a builder and not a destructor!

It is a life worth living when thou are doer and not a talker!

It is a life worth living when thou are worker of good deeds and not of evil!

It is a life worth living when thou give to someone in need!

It is a life worth living when thou donate to an entity in dire need!

It is a life worth living when thou give hope to someone in despair!

It is a life worth living when thou a giver and not a taker!

It is a life worth living when thou are a shoulder for others to lean!

It is a life worth living when thou bring that lost sheep to be with the sheep!

It is a life worth living when thou are the body guard for the drown!

It is a life worth living when thou creditor for the discredit-or!

It is a life worth living when thou visit the sick and the prisoner!

It is a life worth living when thou are kind to the underprivileged!!

It is a life worth living when thou are Compass to the sailors!

It is a life worth living when thou provide a shelter to a homeless soul!

It is a life worth living when thou adopt an orphan!

It is a life worth living when thou support the feeble!

It is a life worth living when thou teach an illiterate!

It is a life worth living when thou rescue someone from the falls!

It is a life worth living when thou volunteer to help out regardless!

It is a life worth living when thou do without nothing in return!

It is a life worth living when thou host strangers!

It is a life worth living when thou reject not the uncomfortable!

It is a life worth living when thou raise the little and praise the least!

It is a life worth living when thou be the last!

It is a life worth living when thou live the life of a hidden treasure!

It is a life worth living when thou clear those stand in the way of the giant waves!

It is a life worth living when thou are neither opportunistic nor parasitic in action!

It is a life worth living when thou do an everlasting contribution that liveth on for so long after thou gone!

It is a life worth living when thou leaves behind an eternal legacy commemorating Thou existence!

It is a life worth living when thou make a difference and thou impact made the world a better place!

It is a life worth living when thou dark but comply, poor but rich, disregarded but regarded, persecuted but not excused!

It is a life worth living when thou are a victim for righteousness but not the source of darkness!

It is a life worth living when thou remain honest and endure to the end!

It is a life worth living when thou not condemned at that day and found with no inequities and not at fault before the Divine Judge!

It is a life worth living when thou— walketh not in the counsel of the ungodly, nor standeth in the way of sinners, nor sitteth in the seat of the scornful. [2] But his delight is in the law of the Lord ; and in his law doth he meditate day and night. [3] And he shall be like a tree planted by the rivers of water, that bringeth forth his fruit in his season; his leaf also shall not wither; and whatsoever he doeth shall prosper. [4] The ungodly are not so: but are like the chaff which the wind driveth away. [5] Therefore the ungodly shall not stand in the judgment, nor sinners in the congregation of the righteous. [6] For the Lord knoweth the way of the righteous: but the way of the ungodly shall perish."Psalm 1:1-6 KJV

It is a life worth living when thou strive to be perfect and holy!

It is a life worth living when thou persevere and sweat in labor in truth!

It is a life worth living when thou interior is full and exterior is empty!

It is a life worth living when thou flew from evil and those attraction and doubtful of faith!

It is a life worth living when thou kingdom is inward and not outward!

It is a life worth living when thou are seeking awards in heaven and building treasures in the unseen world not working for the seen!

It is a life worth living when thou are an uncommon to the world but common to God and unknown to many but known to the Almighty!

It is a life worth living when thou conquer Satan temptations and ordain thy life for Jesus!

It is a life worth living when thou succeed over the world's tribulation and keep thyself pure!

It is a life worth living when thou overcome the world as thou Savior and thy name is written in the kingdom of God!

Matthew 5:3-11 KJV "Blessed are the poor in spirit: for theirs is the kingdom of heaven. [4] Blessed are they that mourn: for they shall be comforted. [5] Blessed are the meek: for they shall inherit the earth. [6] Blessed are they which do hunger and thirst after righteousness: for they shall be filled. [7] Blessed are the merciful: for they shall obtain mercy. [8] Blessed are the pure in heart: for they shall see God. [9] Blessed are the peacemakers: for they shall be called the children of God. [10] Blessed are they which are persecuted for righteousness' sake: for theirs is the kingdom of heaven. [11] Blessed are ye, when men shall revile you, and persecute you, and shall say all manner of evil against you falsely, for my sake."

Matthew 5:44-48 KJV "But I say unto you, Love your enemies, bless them that curse you, do good to them that hate you, and pray for them which despitefully use you, and persecute you; [45] That ye may be the children of your Father which is in heaven: for he maketh his sun to rise on the evil and on the good, and sendeth rain on the just and on the unjust. [46] For if ye love them which love you, what reward have ye? do not even the publicans the same? [47] And if ye salute your brethren only, what do ye more than others ? do not even the publicans so? [48] Be ye therefore perfect, even as your Father which is in heaven is perfect."

Romans 12:9-21 KJV "Let love be without dissimulation. Abhor that which is evil; cleave to that which is good. [10] Be kindly affectioned one to another with brotherly love; in honour preferring one another; [11] Not slothful in business; fervent in spirit; serving the Lord; [12] Rejoicing in hope; patient in tribulation; continuing instant in prayer; [13] Distributing to the necessity of saints; given to hospitality. [14] Bless them which persecute you: bless, and curse not. [15] Rejoice with them that do rejoice, and weep with them that weep. [16] Be of the same mind one toward another. Mind not high things, but condescend to men of low estate. Be not wise in your own conceits. [17] Recompense to no man evil for evil. Provide things honest in the sight of all men. [18] If it be possible, as much as lieth in you, live peaceably with all men. [19] Dearly beloved, avenge not yourselves, but rather give place unto wrath: for it is written, Vengeance is mine; I will repay, saith the Lord. [20] Therefore if thine enemy hunger, feed him; if he thirst, give him drink: for in so doing thou shalt heap coals of fire on his head. [21] Be not overcome of evil, but overcome evil with good."

Ephesians 6:10-18 KJV "Finally, my brethren, be strong in the Lord, and in the power of his might. [11] Put on the whole armour of God, that ye may be able to stand against the wiles of the devil. [12] For we wrestle not against flesh and blood, but against principalities, against powers, against the rulers of the darkness of this world, against spiritual wickedness in high places. [13] Wherefore take unto you the whole armour of God, that ye may be able to withstand in the evil day, and having done all, to stand. [14] Stand therefore, having your loins girt about with truth, and having on the breastplate of righteousness; [15] And your feet shod with the preparation of the gospel of peace; [16] Above all, taking the shield of faith, wherewith ye shall be able to quench all the fiery darts of the wicked. [17] And take the helmet of salvation, and the sword of the Spirit, which is the word of God: [18] Praying always with all prayer and supplication in the Spirit, and watching thereunto with all perseverance and supplication for all saints;"

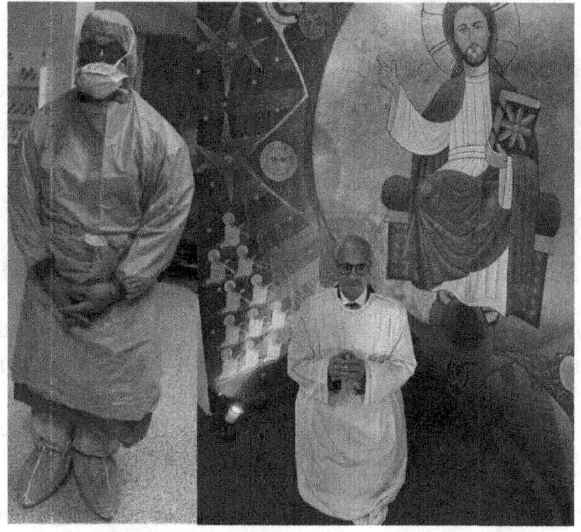

CR, Thank you for this most excellent post to which we all say amen!
MA, Amen
CG, Well said. All the above experiences and choices we make are what makes our lives worth living.
RC, Life is worth! Thank you for triste post. Amén!
TJ, Very well written. Thanks for sharing.
JM, "Beautiful" AMEN

I am the Unknown to thy My gratitude and Appreciation!

Written by Ramsis Ghaly

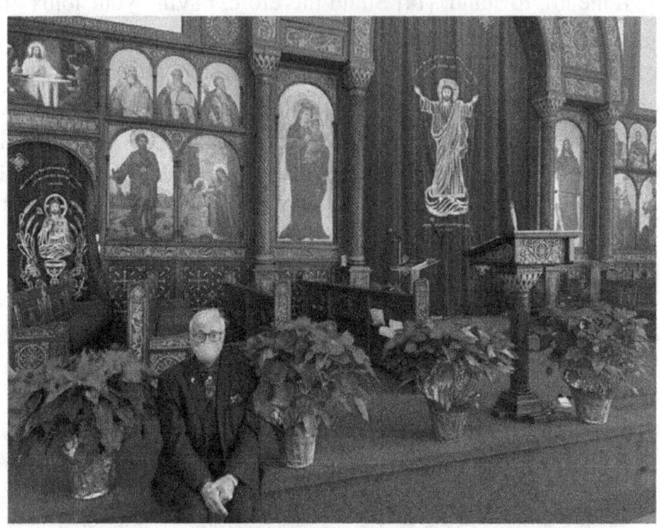

I am in my journey of no return! I am sojourner in a strange land and a foreigner to the land and thy people! Yet I was touched with those the unknowns unrelated to me!!

I am the unknown to thy, yet I was sent somehow to help thy! But don't know why?

I am the unknown to thy and I don't know thy, yet I was directed to be in thy life! But don't know why?

I am the unknown to thy and I was asked to be in thy life! But don't know why?

I am the unknown to thy and I was guided in a mysterious way to support thy! But don't know why?

I am the Unknown to thy and I had intuition to follow thy! But don't know why!

I am the unknown to thy and found myself in thy way and here I am! But don't know why!

I am the unknown to thy and I was called to come to you! But don't know why?

I am the unknown to thy and strange things happened to end in thy court! But don't know why!

+++

Since then, each day passes by, I realize why I am the unknown to thy be in thy life!

It was meant for our path to cross and be on each other life! Indeed, it wasn't a mistake and it had never been an error to get to know thy! It isn't accident to be in my circle and the purpose soon later shall be revealed!

Friend, it had to be from above! God is in control and always working for the best of His children that are calling His Name!

My mother told me one day: "I may not know anyone in the country you going to! I may not have power or money or connection to help you in your lifetime journey! Yet I will always be with you in the spirit, and I won't never stop praying for you!"

And as she wished me the final goodbye, her last words as she kissed me and hugged me tight crying in tears: "O God our Lord, please be with my son wherever he goes, overshadow him with Your wings. You are everywhere. Please dear God, put the good people in my son way and send away those meant to hurt him"

It was the opening prayers that had set in my ears since then in my journey of no return! I am sojourner in a strange land foreigner to the land and thy people! I do believe my mother continue yo pray the same words up high above the clouds!

For all those the Unknowns to me, yet God had sent thy to my life and thy don't know why, yet I know why! I thank thy so much for being in my life! I thank thy for listening to that hidden voice from above! Thy in my life have brought warmth and love to my soul in my sojourning journey! Thank you thy and Thank mom! My endless gratitude and forever appreciations!

Praises to our Lord and Savior, In Jesus our Lord Name, Amen

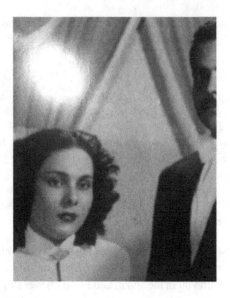

RC, What a lovely Woods!

CG, You have ended your journey and all the people that know you, thank you for who you are and how you have helped heal them. You will continue to heal many more. Bless you!

JT, thank you for being in my life in such a small way but you bring tremendous comfort to me knowing there are truly blessed and kind people left in this small world of ours Ramsis...real friends are one of God's blessings we sometimes never meet in person but feel in our hearts and souls

I was an Earthly Competitor Pursuing My Dream!!

Written by Ramsis Ghaly

I was an Earthly Competitor Pursuing My Endless Dreams!

I was so consumed of gaining power, Money and Richness!!

I Realized Later on It was all Vanity of Vanities!!

"Vanity of vanities, saith the Preacher, vanity of vanities; all is vanity. [3] What profit hath a man of all his labour which he taketh under the sun? [4] One generation passeth away, and another generation cometh: but the earth abideth for ever. [5] The sun also ariseth, and the sun goeth down, and hasteth to his place where he arose. [6] The wind goeth toward the south, and turneth about unto the north; it whirleth about continually, and the wind returneth again according to his circuits. [8] All things are full of labour; man cannot utter it : the eye is not satisfied with seeing, nor the ear filled with hearing. [18] For in much wisdom is much grief: and he that increaseth knowledge increaseth sorrow." Ecclesiastes 1:2-6,8,18 KJV

I was a child pursuing my dreams!

I was walking watching my steps!

I was climbing reaching the top!

I was struggling frightening for the truth!

I was running pursuing my destiny!

I was sweating day and night earning wealth!

I was saving to cumulate a fortune !

I was competing with the powers on earth to be the one!

I took so many adventures to concur the odds with self ego and being eccentric caring less about those around me!

I paid my way and carved my path stepping in so many as long as I stayed ahead climbing quietly!

I achieved all earthy things I have ever dreamed of!

I received much of fame, and I possessed countless savings!

I was sitting guarding my wealth!

I was staring at my gains!

I was totally consumed to be nothing but success and richness!

But I never knew who am I? And why I existed?

I was searching deep unto myself to know who was really me? What was my identity?

I didn't know my purpose and why I was here?

I was lost! While I was surrounded with my goodies and wealth!

I was neither content nor happy but feeling despair, disturbed and unfulfilled!

Only until I heard my Savior words, only then my life has changed! Indeed, as the spoken words of my Lord: "The life is more than meat, and the body is more than raiment! But rather seek ye the kingdom of God"

What did I profit from all these gains and richness, if I lose my own soul as it is written: Matthew 16:26-27 KJV "For what is a man profited, if he shall gain the whole world, and lose his own soul? or what shall a man give in exchange for his soul? [27] For the Son of man shall come in the glory of his Father with his angels; and then he shall reward every man according to his works."

Luke 12:20,22-23,29,31-37 KJV "But God said unto him, Thou fool, this night thy soul shall be required of thee: then whose shall those things be, which thou hast provided? [22] And he said unto his disciples, Therefore I say unto you, Take no thought for your life, what ye shall eat; neither for the body, what ye shall put on. [23] The life is more than meat, and the body is more than raiment. [29] And seek not ye what ye shall eat, or what ye shall drink, neither be ye of doubtful mind. [31] But rather seek ye the kingdom of God; and all these things shall be added unto you. [32] Fear not, little flock; for it is your Father's good pleasure to give you the kingdom. [33] Sell that ye have, and give alms; provide yourselves bags which wax not old, a treasure in the heavens that faileth not, where no thief approacheth, neither moth corrupteth. [34] For where your treasure is, there will your heart be also. [35] Let your loins be girded about, and your lights burning; [36] And ye yourselves like unto men that wait for their lord, when he will return from the wedding; that when he cometh and knocketh, they may open unto him immediately. [37] Blessed are those servants, whom the lord when he cometh shall find watching: verily I say unto you, that he shall gird himself, and make them to sit down to meat, and will come forth and serve them."

Jesus was and is and will forever be my purpose and my life!!

He was within me, and I didn't see Him!

He was inside me and I didn't hear Him!

Jesus was all along watching over ne and I realized not!

Jesus was always walking with me, and I denied Him!

Jesus was living in my being all these years and I didn't acknowledge Him!

I wish I had eyes to see, the ears to hear, the heart to feel and the mind to believe for all the past years!! Yet my heart was hardened, my neck was stiff, and my mind was like a stone!!

But today is the day, O my soul let thy heart harden and thy neck be stiff, and thy mind be as a stone and body was rebellion and rebuked and rejected many eye-opening times!!

Hebrews 3:7-19 ESV "Therefore, as the Holy Spirit says, "Today, if you hear his voice, do not harden your hearts as in the rebellion, on the day of testing in the wilderness, where your fathers put me to the test and saw my works for forty years. Therefore I was provoked with that generation, and said, 'They always go astray in their heart; they have not known my ways.' As I swore in my wrath, 'They shall not enter my rest.'"

Jeremiah 7:23-28 ESV "But this command I gave them: 'Obey my voice, and I will be your God, and you shall be my people. And walk in all the way that I command you, that it may be well with you.' But they did not obey or incline their ear, but walked in their own counsels and the stubbornness of their evil hearts, and went backward and not forward. From the day that your fathers came out of the land of Egypt to this day, I have persistently sent all my servants the prophets to them, day after day. Yet they did not listen to me or incline their ear, but stiffened their neck. They did worse than their fathers. "So you shall speak all these words to them, but they will not listen to you. You shall call to them, but they will not answer you."

Psalm 95:6-8 KJV "O come, let us worship and bow down: let us kneel before the Lord our maker. [7] For he is our God; and we are the people of his pasture, and the sheep of his hand. To day if ye will hear his voice, [8] Harden not your heart, as in the provocation, and as in the day of temptation in the wilderness:"

let us praise our Lord: Psalm 118:19-29 KJV "Open to me the gates of righteousness: I will go into them, and I will praise the Lord : [20] This gate of the Lord, into which the righteous shall enter. [21] I will praise thee: for thou hast heard me, and art become my salvation. [22] The stone which the builders refused is become the head stone of the corner. [23] This is the Lord's doing; it is marvellous in our eyes. [24] This is the day which the Lord hath made; we will rejoice and be glad in it. [25] Save now, I beseech thee, O Lord : O Lord, I beseech thee, send now prosperity. [26] Blessed be he that cometh in the name of the Lord : we have blessed you out of the house of the Lord. [27] God is the Lord, which hath shewed us light: bind the sacrifice with cords, even unto the horns of the altar. [28] Thou art my God, and I will praise thee: thou art my God, I will exalt thee. [29] O give thanks unto the Lord ; for he is good: for his mercy endureth for ever."

Indeed, I was an Earthly Competitor Pursuing My Endless Dreams!

I was so consumed of gaining power, Money and Richness!!

I Realized Later on It was all Vanity of Vanities!!

Amen

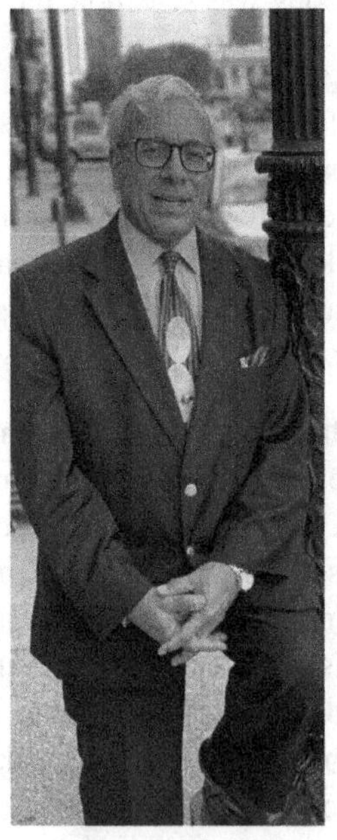

DM, Yes everything without meaning without God

CK, Preach

KH, Amen!

MH, The true richness of your dreams & career comes from the ability that God gave you in helping others to feel well again.

MH, You should take great pride in that. It was a great gift he gave you, in order to help his people to heal & feel good once again. You are a great Dr. And great pride that you are a great servant of the Lord. One of the Best Dr's. Ever!! With a caring &...

CP, So very true. Nice picture.

JD, Bless you!

CK, I wanted to send you this song to you as it goes so well with your post.

JF, Amen and amen!!!

RC, God bless us!

AF, ربنا يحافظ عليك ويبارك حياتك ويفرح قلبك دايما .

CL, God Bless You!

DB, Our lives are better because of what God has done through you, Dr. Ghaly! Thank you, God, and, thank you Dr. Ghaly! Dave & Sue.

Fruit Ripening of a Human Soul and Flowering Plant of a Human Life!

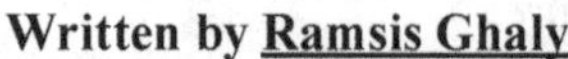

Written by Ramsis Ghaly

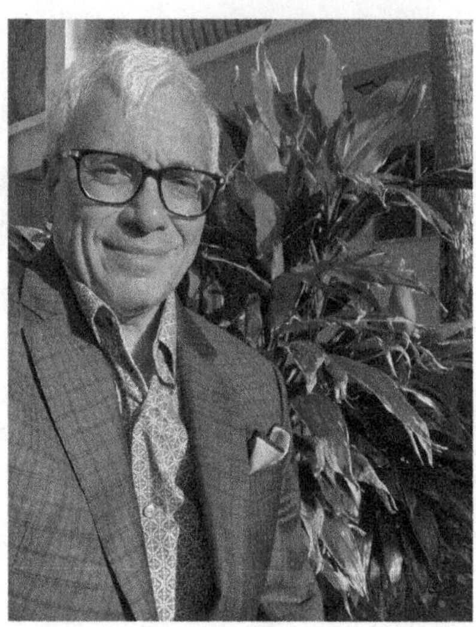

I wonder is it a lifetime of a great song and harmony of a melody is the Fruit Ripening of a Human Soul and Flowering Plant of a Human Life!

It is written that each human soul with a breath of life, a fruit ripen must be asked of her! And every human soul must give rise to a flowering plant ! Since a good human soul gives rise to a fruit ripen, a bad human soul gives no fruit ripen! A good human spirit produces a flowering plant and a bad human soul produces no flowering plant!

A life saved is a Fruit Ripening and a life gained is a Flowering Plant !

The Fruit Ripening of a Human Soul is the resurrection in glory and the Flowering Plant pof a Human Life is a name in the Book of Life!

The Fruit Ripening of a Human Soul is the eternal treasures and the Flowering Plant of a Human Life is entry to the Kingdom of God!

The Fruit Ripening of a Human Soul is dining is the Holy Marriage to the Bridegroom and the Flowering Plant of a Human Life is eternity with the Heavenly Father!

A life that doesn't Ripen is doomed and a life that doesn't Flowering is dead ! A human soul doesn't ripen is casted out and a human soul doesn't flowering be burned with fire!

For the human soul to Ripen, it must abide with the True Vine and for human life to flower must be a living branch in Vine the Savior and shall give rise multitudes of ripen fruits snd flowering plants!!

"Every branch in me that beareth not fruit he taketh away: and every branch that beareth fruit, he purgeth it, that it may bring forth more fruit. [4] Abide in me, and I in you. As the branch cannot bear fruit of itself, except it abide in the vine; no more can ye, except ye abide in me. [5] I am the vine, ye are the branches: He that abideth in me, and I in him, the same bringeth forth much fruit: for without me ye can do nothing. [6] If a man abide not in me, he is cast forth as a branch, and is withered; and men gather them, and cast them into the fire, and they are burned. [7] If ye abide in me, and my words abide in you, ye shall ask what ye will, and it shall be done unto you."John 15:2,4-7 KJV

A human Fruit that doesn't Ripen is unprofitable as that man with one talent! A human plant that doesn't Flower is that man who received one went and digged in the earth, and hid his lord's money and told the Lord, I knew thee that thou art an hard man, reaping where thou hast not sown, and gathering where thou hast not strawed: And I was afraid, and went and hid thy talent in the earth: lo, there thou hast that is thine——

That human soul that does not Ripen, the Lord says Thou wicked and slothful servant, thou knewest that I reap where I sowed not, and gather where I have not strawed: Thou oughtest therefore to have put my money to the exchangers, and then at my coming I should have received mine own with usury. —

That human soul that doesn't flower shall hear the voice of the Master "—Take therefore the talent from him, and give it unto him which hath ten talents. [29] For unto every one that hath shall be given, and he shall have abundance: but from him that hath not shall be taken away even that which he hath. [30] And cast ye the unprofitable servant into outer darkness: there shall be weeping and gnashing of teeth.

"But he that had received one went and digged in the earth, and hid his lord's money. [19] After a long time the lord of those servants cometh, and reckoneth with them. [24] Then he which had received the one talent came and said, Lord, I knew thee that thou art an hard man, reaping where thou hast not sown, and gathering where thou hast not strawed: [25] And I was afraid, and went and hid thy talent in the earth: lo, there thou hast that is thine. [26] His lord answered and said unto him, Thou wicked and slothful servant, thou knewest that I reap where

I sowed not, and gather where I have not strawed: [27] Thou oughtest therefore to have put my money to the exchangers, and then at my coming I should have received mine own with usury. [28] Take therefore the talent from him, and give it unto him which hath ten talents. [29] For unto every one that hath shall be given, and he shall have abundance: but from him that hath not shall be taken away even that which he hath. [30] And cast ye the unprofitable servant into outer darkness: there shall be weeping and gnashing of teeth."Matthew 25:18-19,24-30 KJV

The best times of a life living are at the sunrise and the sunset and in between is just a struggle and so is human life!

As the Fruit Ripening So is a blessed Life! And as the Flowering Plant, So is honorable living!

When that time comes, it shall be best time of the in human lifespan!

At that time is the Pinnacle of beauty and the ultimate maturity!

It is that peak of wisdom and the time when the human soul says "Mission accomplished"!

As the Fruit of the Human Soul is Ripening So is a blessed Life! And as the Flowering of the Human Plant takes place, So is the Honorable Living!

Indeed, the best times of humanity are at the sunrise and the sunset and in between is just a struggle!

Flowering of the human soul is indicative of colorful inward and beauty! Ripening of a human being is a freshness in the soul and health to the body!

The human soul has a time for Flowering and blooming! It that time of spiritual Blossoming!

Through the human soul ripening is joy and happiness and through human soul flowering is peace and state of fulfillment!

The Ripening of the human soul coincides with the reconciled state of the being when the entire person: body, soul and spirit abide firmly with the Divine!

The Flowering of the human soul is the Solidarity of inner Goodness against Evilness, the Light over Darkness, the righteousness over Wickedness and the Holiness over Sinfulness!

Ripening of a human soul before the Lord is when the soul is palatable to the mouth, sweeter to the taste, softer to the teeth, juicy to the stomach and unbitter to the tongue!

So at the Harvest time at the Day of the Lord, be that time coincides with the Ripening of the human soul, the flowering of the human spirit, the sunrise of the saved soul and the sunset toward the past!

https://en.m.wikipedia.org/wiki/Ripening

https://en.m.wikipedia.org/wiki/Flowering_plant

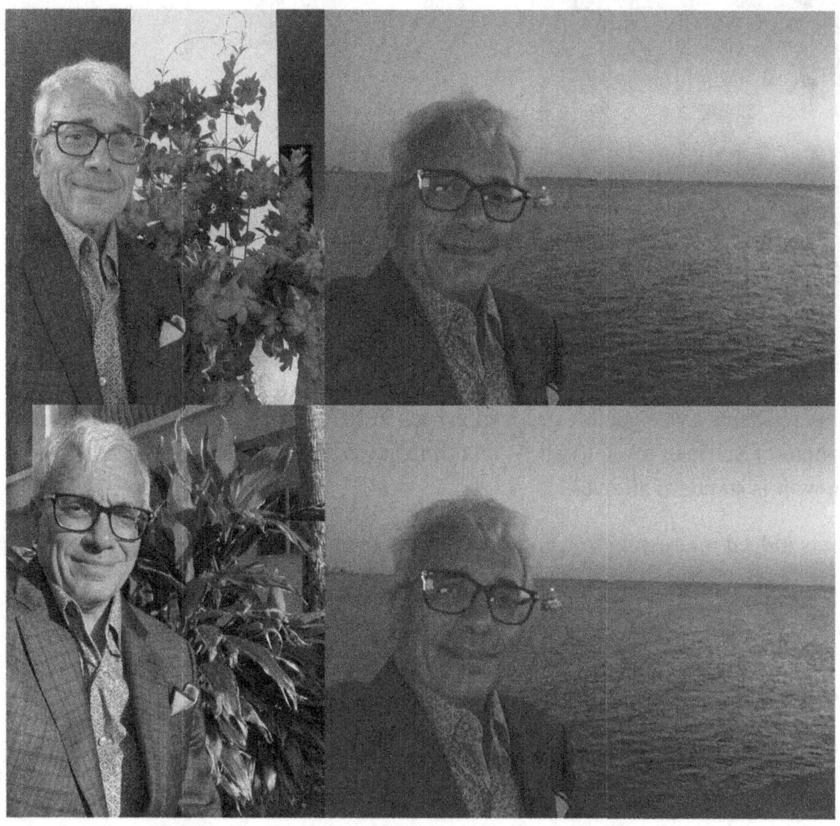

JT, your pen to paper is brilliant

DN, Well said

Selfie of My Selfie: Sharing!!

Written by Ramsis Ghaly

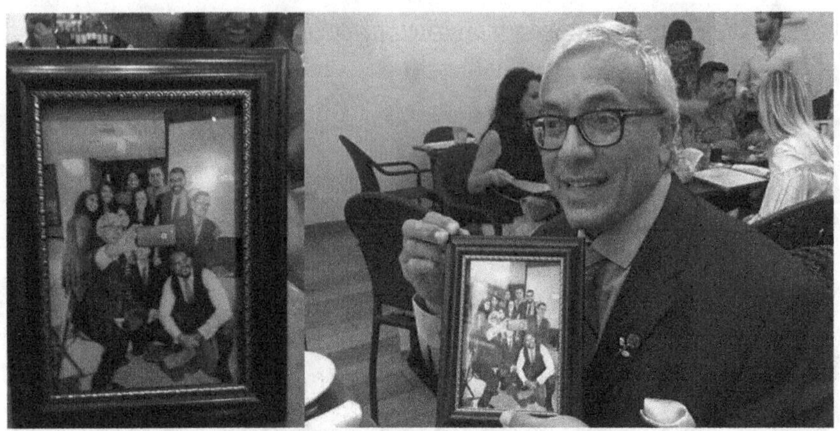

My residents a week before graduation back in 2017 surprised me with this framed photo of Selfie of my selfie!!! At that time, it was still unusual to take selfies and now it is standard all over!!

It is indeed interesting to let others view my own views!

It is called "EMPATHY" as both sides appreciate the views of each other!

The world has never meant to be one sided or just one view but sharing one another! It is called "SHARING"!!

Once both sides views are shared, it is the basis of so called "HARMONY"!!

As more and more views are shared from all sides, it grows unto state of "MERGE" and " UNITY"!

It is the ultimate love that bind human nature together and melting the difference so as all are one in love in God as one sheep to One Shephard as it is written: "As the Father hath loved me, so have I loved you: continue ye in my love. [10] If ye keep my commandments, ye shall abide in my love; even as I have kept my Father's commandments, and abide in his love. [12] This is my commandment, That ye love one another, as I have loved you. [13] Greater love hath no man than this, that a man lay down his life for his friends." John 15:9-10,12-13 KJV And: "I am the good shepherd, and know my sheep, and am known of mine. [15] As the Father knoweth me, even so know I the Father: and I lay down my life for the sheep. [16] And other sheep I have, which are not of this fold: them also I must bring, and they shall hear my voice; and there shall be one fold, and one shepherd. [27] My sheep hear my voice, and I know them, and they follow me: [28] And I give unto them eternal life; and they shall never perish, neither shall any man pluck them out of my hand." John 10:14-16,27-28 KJV

On the other hand, the opposite of selfie of my own only is named "SELF-CENTERED" and my world is my own-self"! It isn't a life worth living! It isn't the world created! It isn't the eternity yo come in the Kingdom our Heavenly Father!

Biblical Verses of "Sharing":

2 Corinthians 9:13 Because of the proof given by this ministry, they will glorify God for your obedience to your confession of the gospel of Christ and for the liberality of your contribution to them and to all,

1 Thessalonians 2:8 Having so fond an affection for you, we were well-pleased to impart to you not only the gospel of God but also our own lives, because you had become very dear to us.

Acts 4:32 And the congregation of those who believed were of one heart and soul; and not one of them claimed that anything belonging to him was his own, but all things were common property to them.

1 Timothy 6:18 Instruct them to do good, to be rich in good works, to be generous and ready to share,

Colossians 1:12 giving thanks to the Father, who has qualified us to share in the inheritance of the saints in Light.

Romans 5:2 through whom also we have obtained our introduction by faith into this grace in which we stand; and we exult in hope of the glory of God.

John 13:18 I do not speak of all of you. I know the ones I have chosen; but it is that the Scripture may be fulfilled, 'He who eats My bread has lifted up his heel against Me.'

1 Corinthians 10:16 Is not the cup of blessing which we bless a sharing in the blood of Christ? Is not the bread which we break a sharing in the body of Christ?

Romans 6:5 For if we have become united with Him in the likeness of His death, certainly we shall also be in the likeness of His resurrection,

Philemon 1:6 and I pray that the fellowship of your faith may become effective through the knowledge of every good thing which is in you for Christ's sake.

For he was counted among us and received his share in this ministry."

Philippians 2:2 make my joy complete by being of the same mind, maintaining the same love, united in spirit, intent on one purpose.

Proverbs 5:17 Let them be yours alone

And not for strangers with you.

Micah 7:5 Do not trust in a neighbor;

Do not have confidence in a friend.

From her who lies in your bosom

Guard your lips.

Philippians 2:1 Therefore if there is any encouragement in Christ, if there is any consolation of love, if there is any fellowship of the Spirit, if any affection and compassion,

Philippians 1:5 in view of your participation in the gospel from the first day until now.

Acts 2:46 Day by day continuing with one mind in the temple, and breaking bread from house to house, they were taking their meals together with gladness and sincerity of heart,

Psalm 41:9 Even my close friend in whom I trusted,

Who ate my bread,

Has lifted up his heel against me.

Psalm 55:14 We who had sweet fellowship together

Walked in the house of God in the throng.

2 Corinthians 8:4 begging us with much urging for the favor of participation in the support of the saints,

Acts 2:42 They were continually devoting themselves to the apostles' teaching and to fellowship, to the breaking of bread and to prayer.

2 Thessalonians 2:14 It was for this He called you through our gospel, that you may gain the glory of our Lord Jesus Christ.

Hebrews 6:4 For in the case of those who have once been enlightened and have tasted of the heavenly gift and have been made partakers of the Holy Spirit,

Philippians 3:10 that I may know Him and the power of His resurrection and the fellowship of His sufferings, being conformed to His death;

Philippians 1:15 Some, to be sure, are preaching Christ even from envy and strife, but some also from good will;

1 Corinthians 10:17 Since there is one bread, we who are many are one body; for we all partake of the one bread.

Job 31:16 "If I have kept the poor from their desire,

Or have caused the eyes of the widow to fail,

John 17:5 Now, Father, glorify Me together with Yourself, with the glory which I had with You before the world was.

Philippians 4:14 Nevertheless, you have done well to share with me in my affliction.

Acts 4:37 and who owned a tract of land, sold it and brought the money and laid it at the apostles' feet.

Philippians 4:15 You yourselves also know, Philippians, that at the first preaching of the gospel, after I left Macedonia, no church shared with me in the matter of giving and receiving but you alone;

Numbers 31:27 and divide the booty between the warriors who went out to battle and all the congregation.

Colossians 1:27 to whom God willed to make known what is the riches of the glory of this mystery among the Gentiles, which is Christ in you, the hope of glory.

Romans 1:12 that is, that I may be encouraged together with you while among you, each of us by the other's faith, both yours and mine.

Isaiah 42:8 "I am the Lord, that is My name;

I will not give My glory to another,

Nor My praise to graven images.

Luke 1:58 Her neighbors and her relatives heard that the Lord had displayed His great mercy toward her; and they were rejoicing with her.

Acts 4:34 For there was not a needy person among them, for all who were owners of land or houses would sell them and bring the proceeds of the sales

Proverbs 25:24 It is better to live in a corner of the roof

Than in a house shared with a contentious woman.

Romans 15:27 Yes, they were pleased to do so, and they are indebted to them. For if the Gentiles have shared in their spiritual things, they are indebted to minister to them also in material things.

Isaiah 58:7 "Is it not to divide your bread with the hungry

And bring the homeless poor into the house;

When you see the naked, to cover him;

And not to hide yourself from your own flesh?

1 Samuel 30:24 And who will listen to you in this matter? For as his share is who goes down to the battle, so shall his share be who stays by the baggage; they shall share alike."

Hebrews 13:13

So, let us go out to Him outside the camp, bearing His reproach.

Hebrews 3:16

And do not neglect doing good and sharing, for with such sacrifices God is pleased.

Romans 12:13 contributing to the needs of the saints, practicing hospitality.

Acts 2:44 And all those who had believed were together and had all things in common;

Galatians 6:6 The one who is taught the word is to share all good things with the one who teaches him.

Acts 2:45 and they began selling their property and possessions and were sharing them with all, as anyone might have need.

2 Corinthians 9:6-8 "The point is this: whoever sows sparingly will also reap sparingly, and whoever sows bountifully will also reap bountifully. 7 Each one must give as he has decided in his heart, not reluctantly or under compulsion, for God loves a cheerful giver. 8 And God is able to make all grace abound to you, so that having all sufficiency in all things at all times, you may abound in every good work."

2 Corinthians 9:10-11 "He who supplies seed to the sower and bread for food will supply and multiply your seed for sowing and increase the harvest of your

righteousness. 11 You will be enriched in every way to be generous in every way, which through us will produce thanksgiving to God."

Acts 20:35 "In all things I have shown you that by working hard in this way we must help the weak and remember the words of the Lord Jesus, how he himself said, 'It is more blessed to give than to receive.'"

Hebrews 13:16 "Do not neglect to do good and to share what you have, for such sacrifices are pleasing to God."

Luke 6:37-38 "Judge not, and you will not be judged; condemn not, and you will not be condemned; forgive, and you will be forgiven; 38 give, and it will be given to you. Good measure, pressed down, shaken together, running over, will be put into your lap. For with the measure you use it will be measured back to you."

Matthew 19:21 "Jesus said to him, "If you would be perfect, go, sell what you possess and give to the poor, and you will have treasure in heaven; and come, follow me."

Proverbs 11:24-25 "One gives freely, yet grows all the richer; another withholds what he should give, and only suffers want. 25 Whoever brings blessing will be enriched, and one who waters will himself be watered."

Proverbs 19:17 "Whoever is generous to the poor lends to the Lord, and he will repay him for his deed."

Psalm 37:21 "The wicked borrows but does not pay back, but the righteous is generous and gives;"

Psalm 104:28 "When you give it to them, they gather it up; when you open your hand, they are filled with good things.

Deuteronomy 15:7-8 "If among you, one of your brothers should become poor, in any of your towns within your land that the Lord your God is giving you, you shall not harden your heart or shut your hand against your poor brother, 8 but you shall open your hand to him and lend him sufficient for his need, whatever it may be."

Deuteronomy 15:10 "You shall give to him freely, and your heart shall not be grudging when you give to him, because for this the Lord your God will bless you in all your work and in all that you undertake."

Leviticus 25:36-37 "Take no interest from him or profit, but fear your God, that your brother may live beside you. 37 You shall not lend him your money at interest, nor give him your food for profit."

Luke 6:30 "Give to everyone who begs from you, and from one who takes away your goods do not demand them back."

Luke 21:1-4 "Jesus looked up and saw the rich putting their gifts into the offering box, 2 and he saw a poor widow put in two small copper coins. 3 And he said, "Truly, I tell you, this poor widow has put in more than all of them. 4 For they all contributed out of their abundance, but she out of her poverty put in all she had to live on."

Matthew 6:1-4 "Beware of practicing your righteousness before other people in order to be seen by them, for then you will have no reward from your Father who is in heaven. 2 "Thus, when you give to the needy, sound no trumpet before you, as the hypocrites do in the synagogues and in the streets, that they may be praised by others. Truly, I say to you, they have received their reward. 3 But when you give to the needy, do not let your left hand know what your right hand is doing, 4 so that your giving may be in secret. And your Father who sees in secret will reward you."

Matthew 10:8 "Heal the sick, raise the dead, cleanse lepers, cast out demons. You received without paying; give without pay."

Proverbs 3:9 "Honor the Lord with your wealth

and with the firstfruits of all your produce;"

Proverbs 3:27 "Do not withhold good from those to whom it is due, when it is in your power to do it."

Proverbs 31:9 "9 Open your mouth, judge righteously, defend the rights of the poor and needy."

Www.ghalyneurosurgeon.com

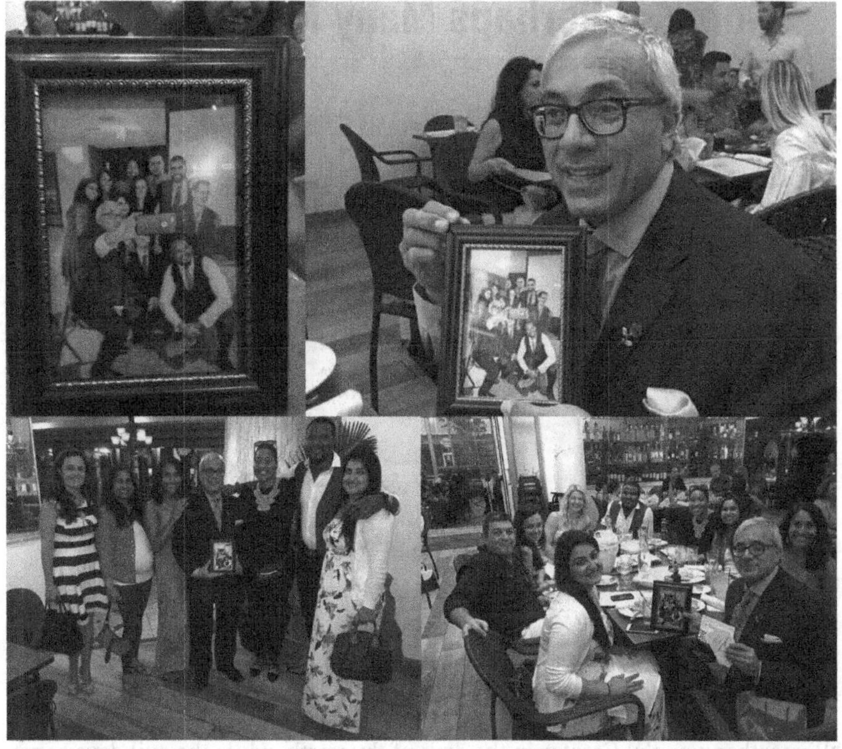

JT, what would you do without your camera Ramsis??

DH, You're too funny

CG, What a great gift for you! I love looking at your self-taken camera photos. It's easier to show something in a picture than to describe it.

AV, Aww, such a great and best group!!

JM, "Fabulous" Groups!!!

Some of Perhaps Many Misnomers!!

Written by Ramsis Ghaly

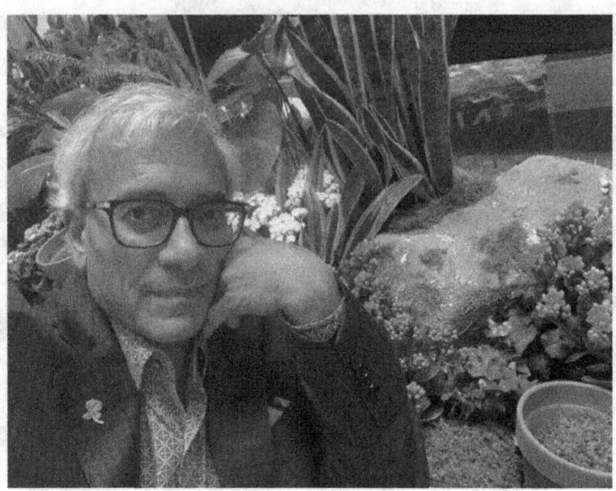

++Church is restricted to elders only!

"Remember now thy Creator in the days of thy youth, while the evil days come not, nor the years draw nigh, when thou shalt say, I have no pleasure in them;" Ecclesiastes 12:1 KJV

- God is only for the sick, poor and incapable!

- It is pessimism when you think or talk or worry about "What is after death" and to believe that there is a Day set for Judgment and giving account to everyone deed before the Savior Jesus the Trye King!

- It is elusion to believe that there is God and Second Coming where it put an end to the world and brand new spiritual life with no end at the kingdom of Gid New Jerusalem where the old earth and universe shall disappear and all things shall be new!

Matthew 24:29-31 KJV "Immediately after the tribulation of those days shall the sun be darkened, and the moon shall not give her light, and the stars shall fall from heaven, and the powers of the heavens shall be shaken: [30] And then shall appear the sign of the Son of man in heaven: and then shall all the tribes of the earth mourn, and they shall see the Son of man coming in the clouds of heaven with power and great glory. [31] And he shall send his angels with a great sound of a trumpet, and they shall gather together his elect from the four winds, from one end of heaven to the other."

Revelation 21:1-8 KJV "And I saw a new heaven and a new earth: for the first heaven and the first earth were passed away; and there was no more sea. [2] And I John saw the holy city, new Jerusalem, coming down from God out of heaven, prepared as a bride adorned for her husband. [3] And I heard a great voice out of heaven saying, Behold, the tabernacle of God is with men, and he will dwell with them, and they shall be his people, and God himself shall be with them, and be their God. [4] And God shall wipe away all tears from their eyes; and there shall be no more death, neither sorrow, nor crying, neither shall there be any more pain: for the former things are passed away. [5] And he that sat upon the throne said, Behold, I make all things new. And he said unto me, Write: for these words are true and faithful. [6] And he said unto me, It is done. I am Alpha and Omega, the beginning and the end. I will give unto him that is athirst of the fountain of the water of life freely. [7] He that overcometh shall inherit all things; and I will be his God, and he shall be my son. [8] But the fearful, and unbelieving, and the abominable, and murderers, and whoremongers, and sorcerers, and idolaters, and all liars, shall have their part in the lake which burneth with fire and brimstone: which is the second death."

- Clergy, Priests, Ministers, Evangelists, Bishops and Popes are all immune from sin anc be trusted blindly!

++Start at a very young age, go out and date as many before you make your mind!

- Have fun and only Play in early years before you get old!

- A good living philosophy is to Live today as if it is you last day and party and drink until you die!

Luke 12:23 KJV "The life is more than meat, and the body is more than raiment." Luke 12:18-22 KJV "And he said, This will I do: I will pull down my barns, and build greater; and there will I bestow all my fruits and my goods. [19] And I will say to my soul, Soul, thou hast much goods laid up for many years; take thine ease, eat, drink, and be merry. [20] But God said unto him, Thou fool, this night thy soul shall be required of thee: then whose shall those things be, which thou hast provided? [21] So is he that layeth up treasure for himself, and is not rich toward God. [22] And he said unto his disciples, Therefore I say unto you, Take no thought for your life, what ye shall eat; neither for the body, what ye shall put on."

++Muscles before minds!

- You win by how much you fight and throw a fit!

- Eye for eye and tooth for tooth goes ways than just let it go!

- Revenge supersede forgiveness!

- You get respected if you show strength!

- Nations respond well by sanctions!

- Economy does well through turfs and punching other countries!

- Dialogues with evildoers and conspirators remark to good politics!

- Professionalism is to be a team player, loose your autonomy and be submissive to the big daddy!!

Matthew 5:38-47 KJV "Ye have heard that it hath been said, An eye for an eye, and a tooth for a tooth: [39] But I say unto you, That ye resist not evil: but whosoever shall smite thee on thy right cheek, turn to him the other also. [40] And if any man will sue thee at the law, and take away thy coat, let him have thy cloke also. [41] And whosoever shall compel thee to go a mile, go with him twain. [42] Give to him that asketh thee, and from him that would borrow of thee turn not thou away. [43] Ye have heard that it hath been said, Thou shalt love thy neighbour, and hate thine enemy. [44] But I say unto you, Love your enemies, bless them that curse you, do good to them that hate you, and pray for them which despitefully use you, and persecute you; [45] That ye may be the children of your Father which is in heaven: for he maketh his sun to rise on the evil and on the good, and sendeth rain on the just and on the unjust. [46] For if ye love them which love you, what reward have ye? do not even the publicans the same? [47] And if ye salute your brethren only, what do ye more than others ? do not even the publicans so?"

++A value of a man is how much he possesses!

Luke 12:15 KJV "And he said unto them, Take heed, and beware of covetousness: for a man's life consisteth not in the abundance of the things which he possesseth."

- Money and richness bring happiness!

- Money is everything in life and to earn more us the good fight!

1 Timothy 6:9-10 KJV But they that will be rich fall into temptation and a snare, and into many foolish and hurtful lusts, which drown men in destruction and perdition. [10] For the love of money is the root of all evil: which while some coveted after, they have erred from the faith, and pierced themselves through with many sorrows."

- Smart household are those who fool the government!

- You are a winner if you find away not to pay taxes!

- Get as much free things from the government as you can and it is okay to lie! It us called white lie!!

Proverbs 10:4 Poor is he who works with a negligent hand,

But the hand of the diligent makes rich.

Proverbs 12:11 He who tills his land will have plenty of bread, But he who pursues worthless things lacks sense.

Ecclesiastes 9:10 Whatever your hand finds to do, do it with all your might; for there is no activity or planning or knowledge or wisdom in Sheol where you are going.

Proverbs 14:23 In all labor there is profit,

But mere talk leads only to poverty.

Proverbs 12:24 The hand of the diligent will rule,

But the slack hand will be put to forced labor.

1 Thessalonians 4:11 and to make it your ambition to lead a quiet life and attend to your own business and work with your hands, just as we commanded you,

Psalm 104:23 Man goes forth to his work

And to his labor until evening.

Psalm 90:10 As for the days of our life, they contain seventy years, Or if due to strength, eighty years,

Yet their pride is but labor and sorrow;

For soon it is gone and we fly away.

2 Thessalonians 3:10 For even when we were with you, we used to give you this order: if anyone is not willing to work, then he is not to eat, either.

++The most intelligent individuals are those achieved high scores in examinations and ranked out of reputable nationwide schools!

Spoil a child, do not chastise, let him do what he wants to do, he is just a kid" is the best strategy to bring up wisdom and learn from his own mistakes!

Children learn better by coercion!

Hebrews 12:5-8 KJV “And ye have forgotten the exhortation which speaketh unto you as unto children, My son, despise not thou the chastening of the Lord, nor faint when thou art rebuked of him: [6] For whom the Lord loveth he chasteneth, and scourgeth every son whom he receiveth. [7] If ye endure chastening, God dealeth with you as with sons; for what son is he whom the father chasteneth not? [8] But if ye be without chastisement, whereof all are partakers, then are ye bastards, and not sons.”

++Face-mask provides the best protection when it doesn’t cover the nose and mouth!

- Vaccines are the only remedy to viruses !

- Health insurance grantee receiving the best treatment!

- The Top 100 hospitals means actual rank out of 100 hospitals!

- Trust your doctors and healthcare blindly and don’t question them, they always gave your best interest!

- A healthy baby is by how much he or she weights! A fatter, smarter he or she!

- If you eat animal brains your memory get better!!

- Drink natural water electrolytes, eat Organic food and daily Vitamins keeps you away from doctors and hospitals!

-If you eat animal brains your memory get better!!

- Peopke who are kind to you are always have no self motivation for evil!

++A good job is that one where you work less and make more!

The new graduates should make decisions primarily based on financial gains?

++The Elevator will arrive faster if you keep pushing the button repeatedly

- You will get things done by yelling and screaming!

- Those are sitting in front will arrive sooner than those are sitting in the back seats!

++ No one does something for nothing!

- It is about money and behind anything there is a “catch”

- Patience, kindness, humility, compassion and gentleness are all signs of weakness and defeat!!

- People are there to get you!

Verses

Whoever is patient has great understanding, but one who is quick-tempered displays folly.

Proverbs 14:29

Love is patient, love is kind. It does not envy, it does not boast, it is not proud. It does not dishonor others, it is not self-seeking, it is not easily angered, it keeps no record of wrongs. 1 Corinthians 13:4-5

Be joyful in hope, patient in affliction, faithful in prayer. Romans 12:12

Be completely humble and gentle; be patient, bearing with one another in love. Ephesians 4:2

But if we hope for what we do not yet have, we wait for it patiently. Romans 8:25

Let us not become weary in doing good, for at the proper time we will reap a harvest if we do not give up. Galatians 6:9

Better a patient person than a warrior, one with self-control than one who takes a city.

Proverbs 16:32

Be still before the Lord and wait patiently for him; do not fret when people succeed in their ways, when they carry out their wicked schemes.

Psalm 37:7

Wait for the Lord; be strong and take heart and wait for the Lord. Psalm 27:14

The Lord will fight for you; you need only to be still.

Exodus 14:14

The Lord is not slow in keeping his promise, as some understand slowness. Instead he is patient with you, not wanting anyone to perish, but everyone to come to repentance. 2 Peter 3:9

Therefore, as God's chosen people, holy and dearly loved, clothe yourselves with compassion, kindness, humility, gentleness and patience.

Colossians 3:12

May the God who gives endurance and encouragement give you the same attitude of mind toward each other that Christ Jesus had.

Romans 15:5

communityencouragementcomforter

For his anger lasts only a moment, but his favor lasts a lifetime; weeping may stay for the night, but rejoicing comes in the morning.

Psalm 30:5

In the morning, Lord, you hear my voice; in the morning I lay my requests before you and wait expectantly.

Psalm 5:3

Yet the Lord longs to be gracious to you; therefore he will rise up to show you compassion. For the Lord is a God of justice. Blessed are all who wait for him! Isaiah 30:18

The Lord is compassionate and gracious, slow to anger, abounding in love. Psalm 103:8

But for that very reason I was shown mercy so that in me, the worst of sinners, Christ Jesus might display his immense patience as an example for those who would believe in him and receive eternal life. 1 Timothy 1:16

But do not forget this one thing, dear friends: With the Lord a day is like a thousand years, and a thousand years are like a day. 2 Peter 3:8

Therefore keep watch, because you do not know on what day your Lord will come.

Matthew 24:42

But the one who stands firm to the end will be saved. Matthew 24:13

Preach the word; be prepared in season and out of season; correct, rebuke and encourage—with great patience and careful instruction. 2 Timothy 4:2

I am coming soon. Hold on to what you have, so that no one will take your crown. Revelation 3:11

Rend your heart and not your garments. Return to the Lord your God, for he is gracious and compassionate, slow to anger and abounding in love, and he relents from sending calamity. Joel 2:13

The prospect of the righteous is joy, but the hopes of the wicked come to nothing. Proverbs 10:28

JT, your wisdom and words keep me believing Ramsis...

JK, We are suffering Enough here...

We need drastically immediate change in Our Government, otherwise America will disappeared...

What a tragedy..

We need Our Loving God Back inside the White House, and come back of President Donald Trump, Prayers to saved our lives and Our Country we love

Jt. your wisdom and words keep me believing Ramsis...

cg, Very interesting as usual.

Mh, Only the Lord can save us now. We are definitely living in the end of day's.

My Identity is No Longer with People But With You O My Lord!

Written by Ramsis Ghaly

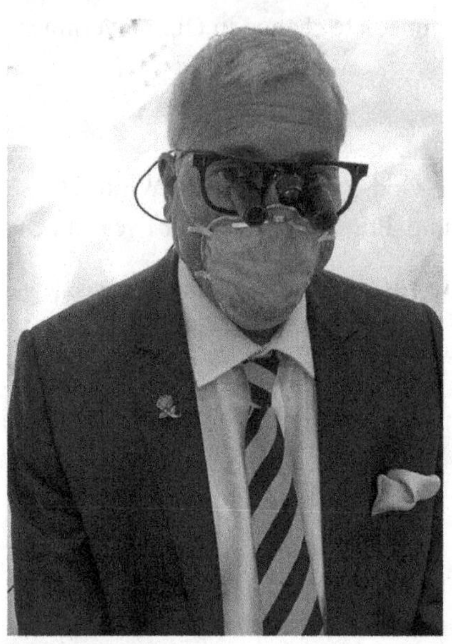

One day, I believed that my identity is only with my parents! And I felt my love is only for my parents! In fact, I thought my identity is my passport and my citizenship and many times I thought who I am but a Driver license ID! I was so proud to be a citizen of the land!

But yet, my true identity, it wasn't just complete in my heritage as my existence it wasn't just justified through my parents! It has never fulfilled my heart deep inside my brain!

So, I have lived my early years in doubt and questioning my true identity and to whom I belong and why I am existed?? Those questions continue to bothersome through my growing up"

My life had been so incomplete even with my parents and my friends as I was growing up! I began to reach out and pray to the God the Lord of heaven and earth !

I said to myself, there was no way I was just formed in my mom womb with the will of my parents to continue their legacy in earth and to represent them after their death!! Human life is much more valuable than this material legacy! In fact, I don't want to live a life that has an end under the ground and no life afterward with an eternal Father that never die!

That time was an eye opening when I looked up to heaven and I prayer to the Creator kneeling in humility: "Please our Heavenly Father let me know more about You! I know You exist and I believe You have created me eternal and in thy Inage! But Yet I don't know You the way I should!!"

After that night, I began to have spiritual visions and began to understand the word of God in the Holy Bible! My ears began to listen and my eyes to see the unseen! In fact, my mind was much more attentive to unseen and spiritual much more than the seen and material!

I looked around and beyond the surface and realized I was surrounded by opportunistic had no true love in me or cared deeply about my future! I saw many took advantage of me and my belongings! I was trapped numerous times with wickedness and victimized in innumerable human traffickers! In my misery and abandonment, Yet I felt Some One is truly love me and care much about me and who am I! But I didn't know Who was that One! It must be a One that actually formed me and doesn't want me to vanish and never took advantage of me! Indeed, That One was already in my temple and found my soul among the list sheep of Israel!

I witnessed my mind was gradually being transformed from Carnal mind to spiritual mind! Even my parts from the flesh and lusts to the wholeness and holiness!

Indeed, I began to find my identity not in my biologic parents but rather in my Heavenly Father and my existence is in my Lord Jesus and not in the legacy of my heritage through flesh and blood but through the Holy Spirit of God the Lord!!

My life forever changed as I began to do that I would not, it is no more I that do it, but sin that dwelleth in me. I find then a law, that, when I would do good, evil is present with me. I find then a law, that, when I would do good, evil is present with me. For I delight in the law of God after t the inward man: …as it is written!!

Years later, my parents were gone, and I felt my identity was gone and I had no existence! At that time, I was so sad and sorrowful if the kids but confident in my Lord Jesus that I shall see them again and they are alive with Him since the true life is at His kingdom! Therefore, my tears were converted to peace and comfort knowing they are alive and not dead in a much better place"

At that night of kissing my parents, I heard while asleep, a soft whispering voice came to my ears at the middle of the night, "You are my son, and I am Your Heavenly Father since you were born!"

For the first time, I woke up from my dreams, joyful and at peace! I kept wandering and my mind drifted to so many thoughts and yes indeed, my identity began with Jesus Baby the Newborn Son of God!

Since then I was confirmed that my identity is neither in a driver license nor in a passport not in a citizenship of the physical land but in heaven with Jesus my Savior and Beloved as it is written: "For our citizenship is in heaven, from which we also eagerly wait for the Savior, the Lord Jesus Christ, 21who will transform our lowly body that it may be conformed to His glorious body, according to the working by which He is able even to subdue all things to Himself." (Philippians 3: 20-21)

O my God Lord Jesus who died for me and kept me safe and protected through the darkness of the world and the harshness of the heat during the day and the freezing cold at night!! Thanksgiving to my Lord Who never gave up in my soul and has always been attentive to my being! My Savior cared for my Salvation and paid my dues so that my soul is no longer condemned unto death!

Since then, I grow unto little christ following His steps and listening to His commandments. I no longer get interested to the flesh but to the Spirit! I no longer inspired by the world existence but the life in Christ! Furthermore, I No longer looking in living in the world but life after death! My inspiration is my name to be written in the Book of life and Not in the Library of the Congress!

My identity is his and my existence is for Him Lord Jesus and my eternal love in Him Jesus my Savior and my purpose is Only Him Jesus my Lord. As it is written; "I am crucified with Christ: nevertheless I live; yet not I, but Christ liveth in me: and the life which I now live in the flesh I live by the faith of the Son of God, who loved me, and gave himself for me." Galatians 2:20 KJV

Yes, my Lord and Savior, You are my identity and I am the little Christ unto Thy!! My Identity is No Longer with People But With You O My Lord!

Pertinent Biblical Verses

"But ye are not in the flesh, but in the Spirit, if so be that the Spirit of God dwell in you. Now if any man have not the Spirit of Christ, he is none of his. [10] And if Christ be in you, the body is dead because of sin; but the Spirit is life because of righteousness. [37] Nay, in all these things we are more than conquerors through him that loved us. [38] For I am persuaded, that neither death, nor life, nor angels, nor principalities, nor powers, nor things present, nor things to come, [39] Nor height, nor depth, nor any other creature, shall be able to separate us from the love of God, which is in Christ Jesus our Lord." Romans 8:9-10,37-39 KJV

"But by the grace of God I am what I am: and his grace which was bestowed upon me was not in vain; but I laboured more abundantly than they all: yet not I, but the grace of God which was with me."1 Corinthians 15:10 KJV

"For we preach not ourselves, but Christ Jesus the Lord; and ourselves your servants for Jesus' sake. [6] For God, who commanded the light to shine out of darkness, hath shined in our hearts, to give the light of the knowledge of the glory of God in the face of Jesus Christ. [8] We are troubled on every side, yet not distressed; we are perplexed, but not in despair; [9] Persecuted, but not forsaken; cast down, but not destroyed; [10] Always bearing about in the body the dying of the Lord Jesus, that the life also of Jesus might be made manifest in our body. [11] For we which live are alway delivered unto death for Jesus' sake, that the life also of Jesus might be made manifest in our mortal flesh. [12] So then death worketh in us, but life in you. [13] We having the same spirit of faith, according as it is written, I believed, and therefore have I spoken; we also believe, and therefore speak; [14] Knowing that he which raised up the Lord Jesus shall raise up us also by Jesus, and shall present us with you. [15] For all things are for your sakes, that the abundant grace might through the thanksgiving of many redound to the glory of God. [16] For which cause we faint not; but though our outward man perish, yet the inward man is renewed day by day. [17] For our light affliction, which is but for a moment, worketh for us a far more exceeding and eternal weight of glory; [18] While we look not at the things which are seen, but at the things which are not seen: for the things which are seen are temporal; but the things which are not seen are eternal."2 Corinthians 4:5-6,8-18 KJV

For they that are after the flesh do mind the things of the flesh; but they that are after the Spirit the things of the Spirit. [6] For to be carnally minded is death; but to be spiritually minded is life and peace. [7] Because the carnal mind is enmity against God: for it is not subject to the law of God, neither indeed can be. [8] So then they that are in the flesh cannot please God. [9] But ye are not in the flesh, but in the Spirit, if so be that the Spirit of God dwell in you. Now if any man have not the Spirit of Christ, he is none of his. [10] And if Christ be in you, the body is dead because of sin; but the Spirit is life because of righteousness. [12] Therefore, brethren, we are debtors, not to the flesh, to live after the flesh. [13] For if ye live after the flesh, ye shall die: but if ye through the Spirit do mortify the deeds of the body, ye shall live." Romans 8:5-10,12-13 KJV

"Was then that which is good made death unto me? God forbid. But sin, that it might appear sin, working death in me by that which is good; that sin by the commandment might become exceeding sinful. [14] For we know that the law is spiritual: but I am carnal, sold under sin. [15] For that which I do I allow not: for what I would, that do I not; but what I hate, that do I. [16] If then I do that which I would not, I consent unto the law that it is good. [17] Now then it is no more I that do it, but sin that dwelleth in me. [18] For I know that in me (that is, in my flesh,) dwelleth no good thing: for to will is present with me; but how to perform that which is good I find not. [19] For the good that I would I do not: but the evil which I would not, that I do. [20] Now if I do that I would not, it is no more I that do it, but sin that dwelleth in me. [21] I find then a law, that, when I would do good, evil is present with me. [22] For I delight in the law of God after the inward man: [23] But I see another law in my members, warring against the law of my mind, and bringing me into captivity to the law of sin which is in my members. [24] O wretched man that I am! who shall deliver me from the body of this death? [25] I thank God through Jesus Christ our Lord. So then with the mind I myself serve the law of God; but with the flesh the law of sin." Romans 7:13-25 KJV

"Therefore if any man be in Christ, he is a new creature: old things are passed away; behold, all things are become new. [18] And all things are of God, who hath reconciled us to himself by Jesus Christ, and hath given to us the ministry of reconciliation; [19] To wit, that God was in Christ, reconciling the world unto himself, not imputing their trespasses unto them; and hath committed unto us the word of reconciliation. [20] Now then we are ambassadors for Christ, as though God did beseech you by us: we pray you in Christ's stead, be ye reconciled to God. [21] For he hath made him to be sin for us, who knew no sin; that we might be made the righteousness of God in him."2 Corinthians 5:17-21 KJV

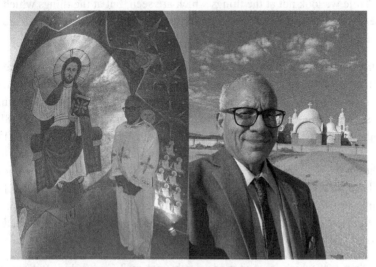

Ms, That was a long thing to read, but I couldn't stop. It was so good.

Fear Not

"You aren't alone"

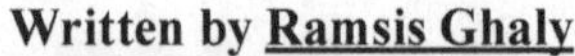

Written by Ramsis Ghaly

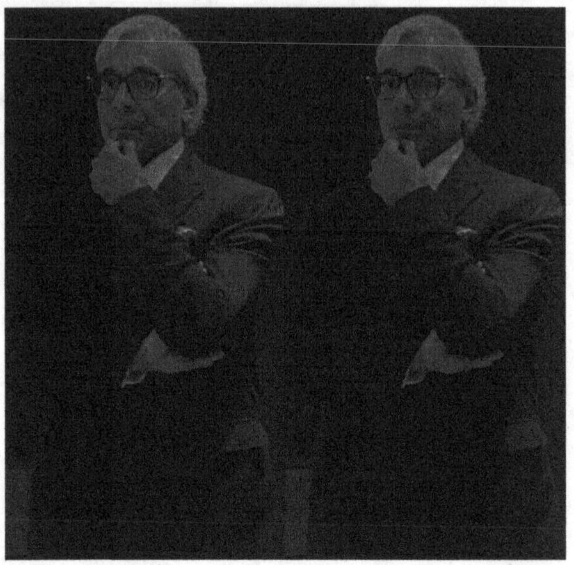

"You aren't alone"

Written by Ramsis Ghaly

It was a moment where I said loudly: "You aren't alone" "You should know that by now"

I was feeling fearful in a deep thought where all of a sudden involuntary my mouth opened, and my tongue spoke up with these words!

It was a moment of doubt and the times were so hard and my Savior spoke in my lips and encouraged my soul: "You aren't alone" "You should know that by now"

"Strange" I said to myself! Where those words came from? I didn't mean to even say a word! I was just shivering in my sorrows of the overwhelming thoughts of what were about to come! And perhaps what was about to be revealed"

I was feeling shaky and feeble laying down in the sick bed as those with no hope!!! And those words descended from heaven: "You aren't alone" "You should know that by now"

I remembers Our Lord Promise: "-and, lo, I am with you alway, even unto the end of the world. Amen." Matthew 28:20 KJV

I said to myself how many fellowmen and women are passing through what I gave experienced feeling hopeless and with no help and all alone???

How many times a man goes through hardship and feels so alone!! Or how many times a man go through various situations in life and believe he is the only one and nobody else has passed through!

As a sojourner in our earthly journey, the message from above: "You aren't alone" "You should know that by now"

As thy soul goes unto hardship, remember thy aren't alone and utter the words to thy soul: "You aren't alone" "You should know that by now"

When thy soul suffers from loneliness, recall the words to thyself: "You aren't alone" "You should know that by now"

When it gets tough and it appears impossible, repeat the words to thy soul: "You aren't alone" "You should know that by now"

At the times of discrimination and persecution—At the times of false accusation—-at the times of hunger and famine—-at the times of loss and sadness—-At the time of sorrows and broken heart—-At the time of affliction —-At the times of the giant waves and quakes—-At the times of freezing rains and heavy tornadoes — At the times of pains and aches— At the times of being downs and failing strength——At the times of under the water and being under—-At the time of wars and unrest——At the time of tribulation——At the time upon the Cross—-At the time of defeat—-At the time of falling—-At the time of failing———At the gloomy times and grim chances—- At whatever the times might be, remember those spoken words and the Promise of our Lord Jesus: Words: "-and, lo, I am with you alway, even unto the end of the world. Amen." Matthew 28:20 KJV

Indeed "You aren't alone" "You should know that by now"

At the moment of death, at the time of sickness, at the depth of darkness, at the time of extreme hardship as the soul is at the end of its rope, at the time of last breath, as the human heart is slowing down to be still and at whatever it might be, the human soul feels trapped in Satan cage with no hope, no relief, no Promise to be filled, and all what is written and hoped for are false as no more life eternity! Thy human soul stand up and utter those words: "You aren't alone" "You should know that by now"

It reminded my soul with St Paul words to the Thessalonians and too I was comforted: "But I would not have you to be ignorant, brethren, concerning them which are asleep, that ye sorrow not, even as others which have no hope. [14] For if we believe that Jesus died and rose again, even so them also which sleep in Jesus will God bring with him. [15] For this we say unto you by the word of the Lord, that we which are alive and remain unto the coming of the Lord shall not prevent them which are asleep. [16] For the Lord himself shall descend from heaven with a shout, with the voice of the archangel, and with the trump of God: and the dead in Christ shall rise first: [17] Then we which are alive and remain shall be caught up together with them in the clouds, to meet the Lord in the air: and so shall we ever be with the Lord. [18] Wherefore comfort one another with these words."1 Thessalonians 4:13-18 KJV

Even if many increased that trouble me! many are they that rise up against me. Many there be which say of my soul, There is no help for him in God, But thou, O Lord, art a shield for me; my glory, and the lifter up of mine head! "You aren't alone" "You should know that by now"

As the multitudes against me and the rise of my enemies, I laid me down and slept; I awaked; for the Lord sustained me!

Psalm 3 "Lord, how are they increased that trouble me! many are they that rise up against me. [2] Many there be which say of my soul, There is no help for him in God. Selah. [3] But thou, O Lord, art a shield for me; my glory, and the lifter up of mine head. [4] I cried unto the Lord with my voice, and he heard me out of his holy hill. Selah. [5] I laid me down and slept; I awaked; for the Lord sustained me. [6] I will not be afraid of ten thousands of people, that have set themselves against me round about. [7] Arise, O Lord ; save me, O my God: for thou hast smitten all mine enemies upon the cheek bone; thou hast broken the teeth of the ungodly. [8] Salvation belongeth unto the Lord : thy blessing is upon thy people. Selah.

In those times of darkness and feelings of "no way out" it is impossible — in those times of doubts or fears when Satan is tempting to take the human mind unto his darkness of the lost land, remembers Our Lord Words: "-and, lo, I am with you alway, even unto the end of the world. Amen." Matthew 28:20 KJV Indeed "You aren't alone" "You should know that by now"

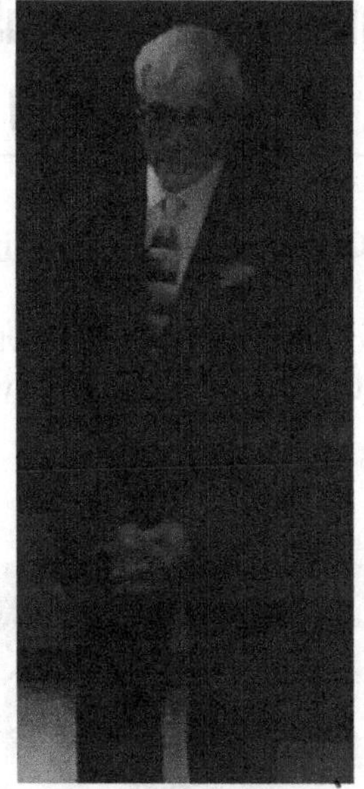

HH, Amen.!!

JT, amen...

NC, Thank you

KG, Amen and Thank you!

You are never alone.

Blessings and God Bless you always.

CG, Thank you for this beautifully written article.

I wish all people knew they are never alone.

JP, I dearly loved this doctor and will share with those I know who are " walking in the valley " feeling alone with no way out. Thank you

SC, **Joan McGrath Pocius** as all of his patienties do

DS, You must have known I needed these wonderful words. Thank-You.

JP, I recommend you carve out a quiet peace-filled moment and read this . We are never really alone

Thou art careful and troubled about many things But one thing is needful!!

Written ON 08/14/2022 by Ramsis Ghaly

"The Lord is near to all who call upon Him, to all who call upon Him in truth. He will fulfill the desire of those who fear Him; He will also hear their cry and will save them."

Psalm 145:18-19

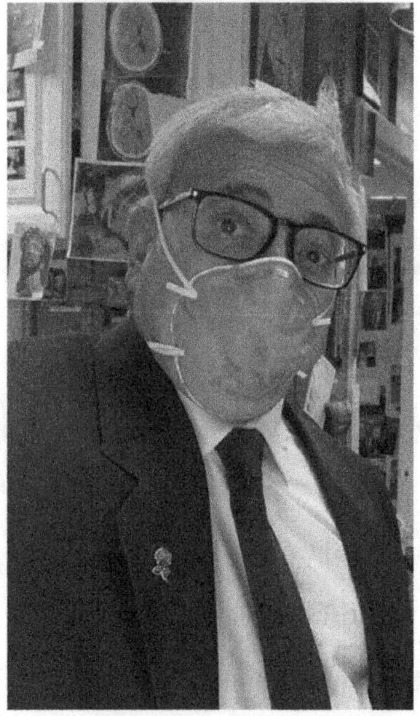

What a timely message:——

"For we are His workmanship, created in Christ Jesus for good works, which God prepared beforehand that we should walk in them" (Ephesians 2:10) "Be diligent to present yourself approved to God as a workman who does not need to be ashamed, accurately handling the word of truth." 2 Timothy 2:15

We are living in a very difficult times and the world is seeing the most horrific days, months and tears and each of us suffering much living minute but minute and doesn't know what to come!!!

And what else since the list doesn't want to end?? But remember that among all those fears and experiences: "One thing is needful!!

Indeed the world is full of wars and worries, violence and crimes, hate and attacks, turmoil and unsettlements, immoralities and inequities, sickness and nightmares, sadness and tears, screams and cries, aches and pains, broken hearts and broken bones, betrayals and deceiving, slavery and abuse, opportunistic and users, cheaters and stabbers, destruction and desolation, quakes and tornadoes, breakdowns and fractures, disobedience and disrespect, untrustworthy and liars, thieves and hijackers, rapes and molestation, trafficking and stealing, ———etc.

And what else since the list doesn't want to end?? But one thing is needful!!

"And Jesus answered and said unto her, Martha, Martha, thou art careful and troubled about many things: [42] But one thing is needful: and Mary hath chosen that good part, which shall not be taken away from her." Luke 10:41-42 KJV

"For we are His workmanship, created in Christ Jesus for good works, which God prepared beforehand that we should walk in them" (Ephesians 2:10)

Matthew 6:34 "Therefore do not be anxious about tomorrow, for tomorrow will be anxious for itself. Sufficient for the day is its own trouble"

Matthew 16:26 "For what will it profit a man if he gains the whole world and forfeits his soul? Or what shall a man give in return for his soul?"

James 4:13-17 KJV "Go to now, ye that say, To day or to morrow we will go into such a city, and continue there a year, and buy and sell, and get gain: [14] Whereas ye know not what shall be on the morrow. For what is your life? It is even a vapour, that appeareth for a little time, and then vanisheth away. [15] For that ye ought to say, If the Lord will, we shall live, and do this, or that. [16] But now ye rejoice in your boastings: all such rejoicing is evil. [17] Therefore to him that knoweth to do good, and doeth it not, to him it is sin."

Colossians 3:12-14 "Put on then, as God's chosen ones, holy and beloved, compassionate hearts, kindness, humility, meekness, and patience, 13 bearing with one another and, if one has a complaint against another, forgiving each other; as the Lord has forgiven you, so you also must forgive. 14 And above all these put on love, which binds everything together in perfect harmony."

Ephesians 4:31-32 "Let all bitterness and wrath and anger and clamor and slander be put away from you, along with all malice. 32 Be kind to one another, tenderhearted, forgiving one another, as God in Christ forgave you."

Hebrews 4:12 "For the word of God is living and active, sharper than any two-edged sword, piercing to the division of soul and of spirit, of joints and of marrow, and discerning the thoughts and intentions of the heart"

Philippians 2:2-8 "complete my joy by being of the same mind, having the same love, being in full accord and of one mind. 3 Do nothing from selfish ambition or conceit, but in humility count others more significant than yourselves. 4 Let each of you look not only to his own interests, but also to the interests of others. 5 Have this mind among yourselves, which is yours in Christ Jesus, 6 who, though he was in the form of God, did not count equality with God a thing to be grasped, 7 but emptied himself, by taking the form of a servant, being born in the likeness of men. 8 And being found in human form, he humbled himself by becoming obedient to the point of death, even death on a cross."

Romans 12:17-21 "Repay no one evil for evil, but give thought to do what is honorable in the sight of all. 18 If possible, so far as it depends on you, live peaceably with all. 19 Beloved, never avenge yourselves, but leave it to the wrath of God, for it is written, "Vengeance is mine, I will repay, says the Lord." 20 To the contrary, "if your enemy is hungry, feed him; if he is thirsty, give him something to drink; for by so doing you will heap burning coals on his head." 21 Do not be overcome by evil, but overcome evil with good"

Revelation 22:12-14 "Behold, I am coming soon, bringing my recompense with me, to repay each one for what he has done. 13 I am the Alpha and the Omega, the first and the last, the beginning and the end. Blessed are those who wash their robes, so that they may have the right to the tree of life and that they may enter the city by the gates"

Matthew 6:9-13 KJV "After this manner therefore pray ye: Our Father which art in heaven, Hallowed be thy name. [10] Thy kingdom come. Thy will be done in earth, as it is in heaven. [11] Give us this day our daily bread. [12] And forgive us our debts, as we forgive our debtors. [13] And lead us not into temptation, but deliver us from evil: For thine is the kingdom, and the power, and the glory, for ever. Amen."

SA, Thank you, Good Doctor, for always sharing inspirational scriptures that speak to my spirit and remind that God is indeed on the throne. Every knee will bow.

CG, Thank you for another of your spiritual lessons. Indeed the one thing that is needful in our lives is our faith .

ED, Thank you so much for sharing Doctor. I can't tell you how much I needed this today. God bless you and keep you safe

Dm, Not only a neurosurgeon but a faithful servant of God.

Do Not Be Down on Thyself But be Down To Earth!

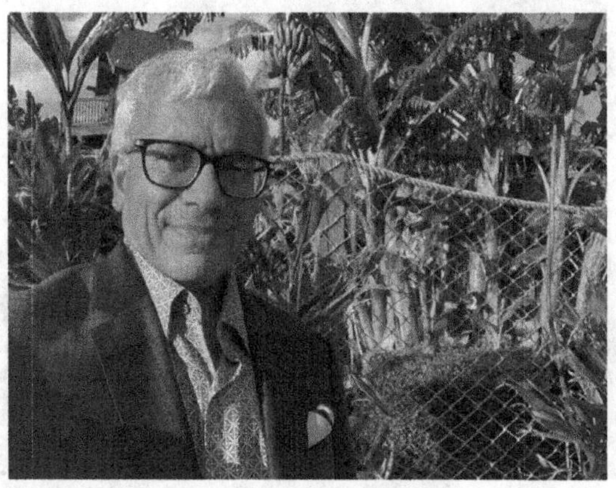

"Don't Be Down On Thyself But Be Down to Earth"

As the world is coming together and globalization is settling in, the people of the world are realizing that so many things are the same and sharing so much over thousands of years!

Thanks to the technology and modern science as a result of Hod increases our knowledge that the entire world indeed one people from one parent Adam and Eve and share similar values!

It is also indeed proof of one God, One Christ, One Savior, one Bible, one people, one flesh, one human body, one human anatomy, one heart, one brain, one blood, one reproductive system, one air, one water, One history, one ground, one roof, one earth planet and one universe.

Looking Up scale is fake, misleading and full of smoke!

Up high is good to visit and be inspired but not a state of living and a life to share if thyself is looking to be above the earth!

Above the earth fur now isn't conks to keep with peaceful living and if thyself can, only for short time!

Don't be hard on thyself all the time but be down to earth and listen to the wide and your loved ones!

Be down to earth and admit your shortcoming at the time of being down in thyself!

It is good to mix with common and gather with all others! And fake science and so called robots and artificial intelligence taking over the world! How many time people walk barefooted down to earth rather than put on their expensive high heal shoes?

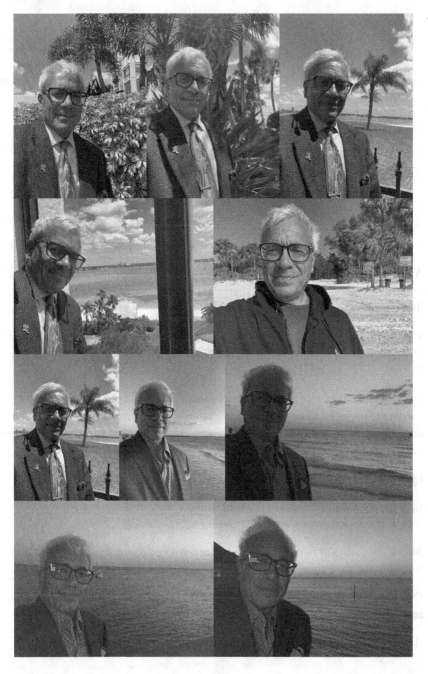

Because of God Grace He Left Not Himself Without Witness in Each Generation!

Written by Ramsis Ghaly

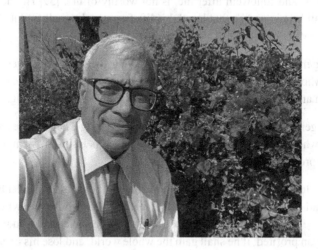

As Lord God was with us so He shall be with our children! Many of us are concern about the future of our children, be of Good cheer and have faith in Jesus!

-No fear for the generations to come since God the Lord shall sail with them as He sailed with our fathers!!

"Nevertheless he left not himself without witness, in that he did good, and gave us rain from heaven, and fruitful seasons, filling our hearts with food and gladness." Acts 14:17 KJV

+In every generation there are un-followers of Christ and there are followers of Christ as those who keep Jesus Cross high and the Nobel statues up protecting humanity from falling!

+In every generation there are haters and destroyers and there are lovers and builders as those who keep Jesus Cross high and the Nobel statues up protecting humanity from falling!

+In every generation there are losers and cowards and there are heroes and patriotists as those who keep Jesus Cross high and the Nobel statues up protecting humanity from falling!

+In every generation there are selfish people and there are those who sacrifice their lives for righteousness and as those who keep Jesus Cross high and the Nobel statues up protecting humanity from falling!

"He that loveth father or mother more than me is not worthy of me: and he that loveth son or daughter more than me is not worthy of me. [38] And he that taketh not his cross, and followeth after me, is not worthy of me. [39] He that findeth his life shall lose it: and he that loseth his life for my sake shall find it."Matthew 10:37-39 KJV

+In every generation there are those who save their lives for themselves and there are those who loose their lives for the sak of righteousness as those who keep Jesus Cross high and the Nobel statues up protecting humanity from falling!

+In every generation there are those who deny carrying Their crosses and there are those who carry their crosses as those who keep Jesus Cross high and the statues up protecting humanity from falling!

"Then said Jesus unto his disciples, If any man will come after me, let him deny himself, and take up his cross, and follow me. [25] For whosoever will save his life shall lose it: and whosoever will lose his life for my sake shall find it. [26] For what is a man profited, if he shall gain the whole world, and lose his own soul? or what shall a man give in exchange for his soul?" Matthew 16:24-26 KJV

+In every generation there are those who follow darkness and there are those who follow the True Light as those who follow the True Light who keep Jesus Cross high and the Nobel statues up protecting humanity from falling!

"Then spake Jesus again unto them, saying, I am the light of the world: he that followeth me shall not walk in darkness, but shall have the light of life."John 8:12 KJV "Then Jesus said unto them, Yet a little while is the light with you. Walk while ye have the light, lest darkness come upon you: for he that walketh in darkness knoweth not whither he goeth." John 12:35 KJV

+In every generation there are those who follow mammons and there are those who follow God as those who keep Jesus Cross high and the Nobel statues up protecting humanity from falling!

"No man can serve two masters: for either he will hate the one, and love the other; or else he will hold to the one, and despise the other. Ye cannot serve God and mammon." Matthew 6:24 KJV

+In every generation there are those who follow Beelzebubs and there are those who follow Jesus as those stewarts who keep Jesus Cross high and the Nobel statues up protecting humanity from falling!

"And Jesus knew their thoughts, and said unto them, Every kingdom divided against itself is brought to desolation; and every city or house divided against itself shall not stand: [26] And if Satan cast out Satan, he is divided against himself; how shall then his kingdom stand? [27] And if I by Beelzebub cast out devils, by whom do your children cast them out? therefore they shall be your judges. [28] But if I cast out devils by the Spirit of God, then the kingdom of God is come unto you." Matthew 12:25-28 KJV

+In every generation there are submissive people and there are the true Believers of the Word as those believers who keep Jesus Cross high and the Nobel statues up protecting humanity from falling!

+In every generation there are the regular people and there are the Good Samaritans extra-mile helper as those believers who keep Jesus Cross high and the Nobel statues up protecting humanity from falling

"And Jesus answering said, A certain man went down from Jerusalem to Jericho, and fell among thieves, which stripped him of his raiment, and wounded him, and departed, leaving him half dead. [31] And by chance there came down a certain priest that way: and when he saw him, he passed by on the other side. [32] And likewise a Levite, when he was at the place, came and looked on him, and passed by on the other side. [33] But a certain Samaritan, as he journeyed, came where he was: and when he saw him, he had compassion on him, [34] And went to him, and bound up his wounds, pouring in oil and wine, and set him on his own beast, and brought him to an inn, and took care of him. [35] And on the morrow when he departed, he took out two pence, and gave them to the host, and said unto him, Take care of him; and whatsoever thou spendest more, when I come again, I will repay thee. [36] Which now of these three, thinkest thou, was neighbour unto him that fell among the thieves? [37] And he said, He that shewed mercy on him. Then said Jesus unto him, Go, and do thou likewise." Luke 10:30-37 KJV

+In every generation there are the materialistic and there are the spiritual as those spiritual who keep Jesus Cross high and the Nobel statues up protecting humanity from falling!

+In every generation there are the trouble makers and violent individuals and there are the meek and peace seeking individuals as those spiritual who keep Jesus Cross high and the Nobel statues up protecting humanity from falling!

+In every generation there are the men servants and maidens and there are the faithful servants as those spiritual who keep Jesus Cross high and the Nobel statues up protecting humanity from falling!

+In every generation there are those aren't watching for that day and those watching for that day as those watching for that day who keep Jesus Cross high and the Nobel statues up protecting humanity from falling!

"Blessed are those servants, whom the lord when he cometh shall find watching: verily I say unto you, that he shall gird himself, and make them to sit down to meat, and will come forth and serve them. [38] And if he shall come in the second watch, or come in the third watch, and find them so, blessed are those servants. [39] And this know, that if the goodman of the house had known what hour the thief would come, he would have watched, and not have suffered his house to be broken through." Luke 12:37-39 KJV

+In every generation there are follower of seen temporary treasure and there are followers of unseen eternal treasures as those who keep Jesus Cross high and the Nobel statues up protecting humanity from falling!

+In every generation there are the corrupted people and there are honest I cooperated people as those who keep Jesus Cross high and the Nobel statues up protecting humanity from falling!

+In every generation there are the follower of mortal things in the present world and there are followers of immortal things in heaven according to the promise as those who keep Jesus Cross high and the Nobel statues up protecting humanity from falling!

1 Corinthians 15:32-34 KJV "If after the manner of men I have fought with beasts at Ephesus, what advantageth it me, if the dead rise not? let us eat and drink; for to morrow we die. [33] Be not deceived: evil communications corrupt good manners. [34] Awake to righteousness, and sin not; for some have not the knowledge of God: I speak this to your shame."

"But have renounced the hidden things of dishonesty, not walking in craftiness, nor handling the word of God deceitfully; but by manifestation of the truth commending ourselves to every man's conscience in the sight of God. [3] But if our gospel be hid, it is hid to them that are lost: [4] In whom the god of this world hath blinded the minds of them which believe not, lest the light of the glorious gospel of Christ, who is the image of God, should shine unto them. [5] For we preach not ourselves, but Christ Jesus the Lord; and ourselves your servants for Jesus' sake. [6] For God, who commanded the light to shine out of darkness, hath shined in our hearts, to give the light of the knowledge of the glory of God in the face of Jesus Christ. [7] But we have this treasure in earthen vessels, that the excellency of the power may be of God, and not of us. [18] While we look not at the things which are seen, but at the things which are not seen: for the things which are seen are temporal; but the things which are not seen are eternal."2 Corinthians 4:2-7,18 KJV

+In every generation there are the followers and there are the leaders as those leaders who keep Jesus Cross high and the Nobel statues up protecting humanity from falling!

+In every generation there are the majority and there are the minority as the minority who keep Jesus Cross high and the Nobel statues up protecting humanity from falling!

+In every generation there are the foolish, naïve views and less intelligent and there are the wise, experienced and intelligent as those spiritual who keep Jesus Cross high and the Nobel statues up protecting humanity from falling!

+In every generation there are the common and there are the uncommon as the uncommon who keep Jesus Cross high and the statues up protecting humanity from falling!

+In every generation there are the passivists and there are the fighters as those fighters who keep Jesus Cross high and the Nobel statues up protecting humanity from falling!

Therefore as Because of Love, Jesus Redeemed His people, Heavenly Father because of His Love< He never forsaken us and let His People be consumed as He left Himself with no Witness as well!

"It is of the LORD's mercies that we are not consumed, because his compassions fail not." Lamentation 3:22 And "For God so loved the world, that he gave his only begotten Son, that whosoever believeth in him should not perish, but have everlasting life. 17 For God sent not his Son into the world to condemn the world; but that the world through him might be saved.18 He that believeth on him is not condemned: but he that believeth not is condemned already, because he hath not believed in the name of the only begotten Son of God." John3:16-18

"Nevertheless he left not himself without witness, in that he did good, and gave us rain from heaven, and fruitful seasons, filling our hearts with food and gladness." Acts 14:17 KJV

DH, Thank you Dr. Ghaly

JT, amen...bless you Ramsis for sharing this with us

CP, Very nice.

ED, Bless you good and wise Doctor.

RC, God is perfect! God bless you!

VW, Thank you, Dr. Ghaly!

JN, Very nice & thank you. Have a blessed Easter.

MH, God Bless you Have a Happy Easter

DN, Thank you god

CG, Your writings always help us understand the words of God.

Thank you and God Bless!I

CL, Amen

SJ, Happiest of Easter, Dr. Ghaly. May this rebirth bring out the goodness of the human heart and our connection to God

God is Gracious to Man!

Written by Ramsis Ghaly

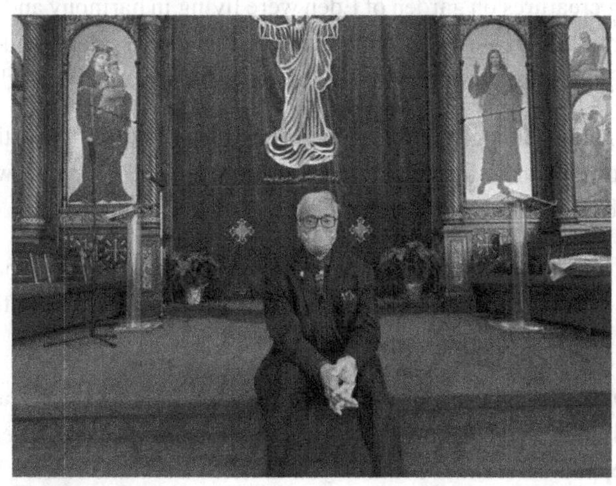

God is Gracious to Man!

Written by Ramsis Ghaly

Joel 2:7 "They run like mighty men,

They climb the wall like soldiers;

And they each march in line,

Nor do they deviate from their paths."

I found myself surrounded by non human living creatures! I start to reflect at each of them!

I shivered when I saw the lion holding the neck of a huge cow 🐄 attempt to suffocate her and murder her to the ground and then group of lions are already began to eat the flesh and the cow 🐄 was still alive!

Joel 1:6 "For a nation has invaded my land,

Mighty and without number;

Its teeth are the teeth of a lion,

And it has the fangs of a lioness."

I couldn't believe it and asked my Lord: "How could an animal created by God becomes so evil when the animals joined Adam and Eve thrown down to earth because of their disobedience to God commandments!!

Adam and Eve never ever hunted animals and murdered them or dare to kill them. All are living creatures on garden of Eden were living in harmony and Adam was dominating over all creatures and conversing with them. Garden of Eden was full of Love and good and there was nothing of darkness or bad or wrong!

While I was in deep thoughts a flying bird came to me saying: "I saw the lion and evil it had done! I am so thankful to our God that He had given me wings and I am a flying bird the lion can't reach me!"

I said to the flying bird : "Well said o my wise bird and I am too very thankful that God created me as a man in His image and always protect me from the horrific teeth of that lion and He grange me away to overcome it"

The flying bird sang a beautiful song and flew away! While I was staring at the bird which already made to the clouds, An animal was so tall fast runner with very long legs stopped before me. I said : "you must be Zarafa Giraffe." The Zarafa replied saying: "Yes I am and I saw with you from far what that dangerous lion did to the cow. The lion is an animal runs around and call itself the king of the zoo so proud of itself and kills as many domestic animals as it could! The lion always hungry and if us also do fast. But I am so grateful to God that He created me as Zarafa with long legs and very fast runner you escape the lion teeth!" I said to Zarafa: "You look gorgeous and I am so grateful to God that He had given you speedy legs to escape. I am also grateful to God that He created me with mind to be able to make steel engines and drive me as fast anywhere even to the space. I can rid s train with speed more than 500 miles an hour, a car more than 100 miles an hour, a ship more than 50 miles an hour, an airplane more than 500 miles an hour and submarine under the oceans. I am also so protected inside. God is indeed gracious to me and you otherwise we would have been victims to dangerous killers such as lions!!"

All of a sudden, the Zarafa ran so fast that it totally disappeared! While I was looking with telescope to locate the Zarafa, a fish came out of the water and said to me: "I am grateful to God that created me as a fish swims under the waters and the lion can never reach me or try to come close! That lion that was killing the cow it will drown in seconds if tries to hunt me. I am all deep under the waters and moons could see me"

I replied to the beautiful fish : "I am so happy for you being so gorgeous and swimming all the time under the water. I am happy for you to be h dear the waters away from the reach of the creeping animals. I am also grateful that God created me to be able to walk on the land and swim under the waters without being attacked from either those on the land or under the land or under the waters"

I got up and head back to my closet praising God. Indeed I learned so much today as it is written in the holy book of Hod Jesus Christ:

Daniel 2:38 "and wherever the sons of men dwell, or the beasts of the field, or the birds of the sky, He has given them into your hand and has caused you to rule over them all. You are the head of gold.

1 Kings 4:33 "He spoke of trees, from the cedar that is in Lebanon even to the hyssop that grows on the wall; he spoke also of animals and birds and creeping things and fish."

Job 12:7 But now ask the beasts and let them teach you; And the birds of the heavens and let them tell you.

Psalm 145:8 "The Lord is gracious and merciful;

Slow to anger and great in lovingkindness."

Psalm 116:5 "Gracious is the Lord, and righteous;

Yes, our God is compassionate."

Isaiah 30:18 "Therefore the Lord longs to be gracious to you,

And therefore He waits on high to have compassion on you. For the Lord is a God of justice;

How blessed are all those who long for Him."

For the Lord your God is gracious and compassionate. He will not turn his face from you if you return to him. 2 Chronicles 30:9

"But in your great mercy you did not put an end to them or abandon them, for you are a gracious and merciful God." Nehemiah 9:31

Genesis 9:2 "The fear of you and the terror of you will be on every beast of the earth and on every bird of the sky; with everything that creeps on the ground, and all the fish of the sea, into your hand they are given."

Genesis 1:26 "Then God said, "Let Us make man in Our image, according to Our likeness; and let them rule over the fish of the sea and over the birds of the sky and over the cattle and over all the earth, and over every creeping thing that creeps on the earth."

Psalm 8:7-8

All sheep and oxen,

And also the beasts of the field,

The birds of the heavens and the fish of the sea,

Whatever passes through the paths of the seas.

Genesis 2:20 “The man gave names to all the cattle, and to the birds of the sky, and to every beast of the field, but for Adam there was not found a helper suitable for him.”

My Heavenly Father Bless thy Holy Name Forever and Ever More!!

Written by Ramsis Ghaly

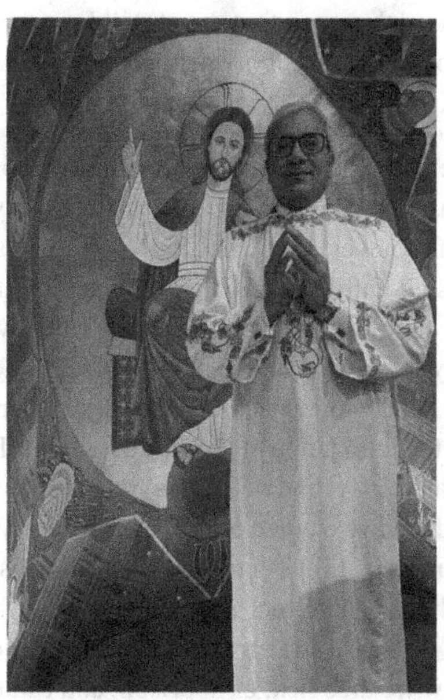

When it comes down to, Not even my father or my mother but it is our Heavenly Father which art in heaven, Hallowed be thy name. [10] Thy kingdom come. Thy will be done in earth, as it is in heaven. [11] Give us this day our daily bread. [12] And forgive us our debts, as we forgive our debtors. [13] And lead us not into temptation, but deliver us from evil: For thine is the kingdom, and the power, and the glory, for ever. Amen." Matthew 6:9-13 KJV

When it comes down to, Not even my father or my mother but it is the Heavenly Father that matters! Let me tell you all about my Heavenly Father God of the earth and Heaven the Lord of seen and unseen, the Creator of all things! You will love my Father and He is waiting for you, too. Let me tell you all about my Heavenly Father God of the earth and Heaven the Lord of seen and unseen, the Creator of all things! He said: "Behold, I stand at the door, and knock: if any man hear my voice, and open the door, I will come in to him, and will sup with him, and he with me. 21To him that overcometh will I grant to sit with me in my throne, even as I also overcame, and am set down with my Father in his throne. 22He that hath an ear, let him hear what the Spirit saith unto the churches." Revelations 3: 20-22

My Heavenly Father is Love full of Love and He is all about Love ! He adopted me before I was born and had watched over me since then all the way to the end! He overshadows my soul throughout my years of living! He has no end He never get upset from me! He is with me and live with me, living in my heart and soul day and night! He is always at my side and many times He carries me to the shore!

"Can a woman forget her sucking child, that she should not have compassion on the son of her womb? yea, they may forget, yet will I not forget thee. [16] Behold, I have graven thee upon the palms of my hands; thy walls are continually before me." Isaiah 49:15-16 KJV

When I die, my Heavenly Father will come and take me home! He is my forever Love and destiny! He us the Lord of my soul! I live fir tgst day when I see Him face to face and be with Him forever! I pray He shall accept my soul saying: Matthew 25:23 KJV "His lord said unto him, Well done, good and faithful servant; thou hast been faithful over a few things, I will make thee ruler over many things: enter thou into the joy of thy lord." Matthew 25:34-40 KJV "Then shall the King say unto them on his right hand, Come, ye blessed of my Father, inherit the kingdom prepared for you from the foundation of the world: [35] For I was an hungred, and ye gave me meat: I was thirsty, and ye gave me drink: I was a stranger, and ye took me in: [36] Naked, and ye clothed me: I was sick, and ye visited me: I was in prison, and ye came unto me. [37] Then shall the righteous answer him, saying, Lord, when saw we thee an hungred, and fed thee ? or thirsty, and gave thee drink? [38] When saw we thee a stranger, and took thee in? or naked, and clothed thee ? [39] Or when saw we thee sick, or in prison, and came unto thee? [40] And the King shall answer and say unto them, Verily I say unto you, Inasmuch as ye have done it unto one of the least of these my brethren, ye have done it unto me."

My Heavenly Father never forgets me and never forsaken my soul! He wipes my tears and forgive my sins! He is my refuge, my fortes and my Rock! He is the Life, The Way, The Truth and The Resurrection! I love Him so much and He loves me more! There is no true Love outside Him and all the Hope and love are in Him! He is what every human soul wants, needs, hunger for and thirst for!!!

John 14:6 KJV "Jesus saith unto him, I am the way, the truth, and the life: no man cometh unto the Father, but by me." John 11:25 KJV "Jesus said unto her, I am the resurrection, and the life: he that believeth in me, though he were dead, yet shall he live:"

My Heavenly Father gives me everything and more than I ever dream! My Father gives me Love ! My Father gives me hope! My Father gives me Life! My Father gives me heavenly peace! My Father gives me bread! My Father gives me Salvation! My Father gives me from what His and feed me from His Own and of that bread that I will never hunger and Waters that I will never thirst! Around Him, there isn't need to worry or to fear or to feel uncomfortable! My Father is always have special place for me, never ever reject me or turn his back or turned His face away from me! He thinks highly of me and never ever ashamed of me! Never once He let me down! His promises never fails! He is the same yesterday, today and tomorrow never change! Living with my Heavenly Father is all what I want! He loved me first and no charge for any service. It is pure love and giving! I appreciate my Heavenly Father so much and my gratitude to Him is always up high. He is a living God and I talk to all the time! I share so much with him all the time! I always hear back from Him and He never busy for me! I am in His fast track and speed dial day and night no matter how early and how late! He comes to me flying over the clouds leaping over the mountains crossing over the valleys in the speed faster than light! He goes through the close the doors, the crashed traffics, in the fires, wars, flooding, earthquakes nothing stops Him and He always reach me!! My Father believes in me! My Father gives me the True freedom and the True liberty! My Heavenly Father never runs out of supplies or resources! My Heavenly Father always gives and never ever take! He is the Heavenly Warrior and has never ever been defeated! He is the Unconquered King and always wins! My Father treats me as His favorite son, always encourages me, supports me and help me to succeed!

He took me many places. At the Dawn my Father picked me up with James and John high in mountain and transfigured as in those days, His face was like the sun and Raymond was white as the light—Matthew 17:1-3 KJV "And after six days Jesus taketh Peter, James, and John his brother, and bringeth them up into an high mountain apart, [2] And was transfigured before them: and his face did shine as the sun, and his raiment was white as the light. [3] And, behold, there appeared unto them Moses and Elias talking with him."

My Heavenly Father has the keys to everlasting life to His Kingdom! He shuts n one can open and open and no one can shut! He is the true Father of the entire human race! My Father is Just and never forgets the little and the least! He is caring for all my people! I pray to Him for them all the time! I always ask for His guidance and Blessing! Seven times a day I pray and praise His Name all day and night! The first word at the dawn and the last word at night I call His Name! My heart and tongue utters Thanksgiving!

My Heavenly Father taught me what is right and what is wrong, how to Love, how to forgive, how to be perfect, how to be holy, how to pray, how to fast, how to do good, how to be Good Samaritan, how to give, how to be truthful, how to be righteous, how to be a man, how to be a christ, how to grow in His faith, how to know Him, how to abide in Him, how to reject darkness, how not to be part of evildoing, give how to do good, how to be cheer giver —-and how to grow in Hid image in the likeness of Him and in the fullness of His glory! My Heavenly Father has given Himself for the world and died for all to provide the eternal sacrifice where mercy and just have met it's the Cross!

I always think about my Heavenly Father, I talk to Him and I pray to Him day and night! He is my Only Love in the world! He is Most Approachable! With Him there is no barrier. He stops what He is doing and listen to me the least! Never once there was a recorded message or waiting on line and He never send His servant or maid but Always Him come at the door and open for me! When I am sick, He runs to kiss me, hugs me and heals me! I always wait for His goodnight kiss and with His hands He touches me and put His arms around me! I tell Him a story and He tell me a night story! Then I go over what is in my mind and day event! My Heavenly Father will always tap on my shoulder and tells me: "I know all about your day, your thoughts and what events had transpired and what is going in your mind for days to come. No worries all good and I am taking care of them for you:!All of them known to you and not unknown!! No worries!

My Heavenly Father is waiting for my soul at the day to say goodbye! He never ask for anything other than to be a good son, a good man and good servant following his commandments and believe in Him! I have given Him my soul, my life, my heart and my mind!! My God Lord is He the Savior of the world and the Heavenly Father for whoever believe in him!

I pray with tears to my Father to protect me from evil and give my soul strength yo overcome! I always dream to live with Him at His Kingdom at the New Jerusalem as My Father will be at its midst: Revelation 21:1-7 KJV "And I saw a new heaven and a new earth: for the first heaven and the first earth were passed away; and there was no more sea. [2] And I John saw the holy city, new Jerusalem, coming down from God out of heaven, prepared as a bride adorned for her husband. [3] And I heard a great voice out of heaven saying, Behold, the tabernacle of God is with men, and he will dwell with them, and they shall be his people, and God himself shall be with them, and be their God. [4] And God shall wipe away all tears from their eyes; and there shall be no more death, neither sorrow, nor crying, neither shall there be any more pain: for the former things are passed away. [5] And he that sat upon the throne said, Behold, I make all things new. And he said unto me, Write: for these words are true and faithful. [6] And he said unto me, It is done. I am Alpha and Omega, the beginning and the end. I will give unto him that is athirst of the fountain of the water of life freely. [7] He that overcometh shall inherit all things; and I will be his God, and he shall be my son."

My Heavenly Father is mine and I am His! He is the Father for all His children and my brethren! Not just the wholly but the sick, the sinful, the poor, the hunger, the thirst, the naked, the homeless, the orphans, the unknown, the rejected, the sentenced, the illiterate, the minorities, the underprivileged, the colored and uncolored, the rich, and all those regardless of whom they are! My Heavenly Father is for Equity, inclusion and no partiality and His judgment is true!

My Heavenly Father has many mansion and He is preparing one for me! He had to go to prepare a house for me: John 14:1-3 KJV "Let not your heart be troubled: ye believe in God, believe also in me. [2] In my Father's house are many mansions: if it were not so, I would have told you. I go to prepare a place for you. [3] And if I go and prepare a place for you, I will come again, and receive you unto myself; that where I am, there ye may be also."

I am at my My Father flock! He asked me to fear not! He had given me gifts as He has done to do many! By His grace, I live day to day and labor at His fields to pile treasures for days to come and follow my heart to be with Him! Luke 12:32-40 KJV "Fear not, little flock; for it is your Father's good pleasure to give you the kingdom. [33] Sell that ye have, and give alms; provide yourselves bags which wax not old, a treasure in the heavens that faileth not, where no thief approacheth, neither moth corrupteth. [34] For where your treasure is, there will your heart be also. [35] Let your loins be girded about, and your lights burning; [36] And ye yourselves like unto men that wait for their lord, when he will return from the wedding; that when he cometh and knocketh, they may open unto him immediately. [37] Blessed are those servants, whom the lord when he cometh shall find watching: verily I say unto you, that he shall gird himself, and make them to sit down to meat, and will come forth and serve them. [38] And if he shall come in the second watch, or come in the third watch, and find them so, blessed are those servants. [39] And this know, that if the goodman of the house had known what hour the thief would come, he would have watched, and not have suffered his house to be broken through. [40] Be ye therefore ready also: for the Son of man cometh at an hour when ye think not."

My Father is my Shepherd. He let me be green pasture by still waters He restore the my soul and lead me in the path of righteousness thy Rod and thy staff comfort my soul —-Psalm 23:1-6 KJV "The Lord is my shepherd; I shall not want. [2] He maketh me to lie down in green pastures: he leadeth me beside the still waters. [3] He restoreth my soul: he leadeth me in the paths of righteousness for his name's sake. [4] Yea, though I walk through the valley of the shadow of death, I will fear no evil: for thou art with me; thy rod and thy staff they comfort me. [5] Thou preparest a table before me in the presence of mine enemies: thou anointest my head with oil; my cup runneth over. [6] Surely goodness and mercy shall follow me all the days of my life: and I will dwell in the house of the Lord for ever."

Revelations 19:15 "And out of his mouth goeth a sharp sword, that with it he should smite the nations: and he shall rule them with a rod of iron: and he treadeth the winepress of the fierceness and wrath of Almighty God" Psalm 2:9-11 KJV "Thou shalt break them with a rod of iron; thou shalt dash them in pieces like a potter's vessel. [10] Be wise now therefore, O ye kings: be instructed, ye judges of the earth. [11] Serve the Lord with fear, and rejoice with trembling." Psalms 23:4

"Yea, though I walk through the valley of the shadow of death, I will fear no evil: for thou [art] with me; thy rod and thy staff they comfort me."

He kiss me with kisses! He adores me and find comfort on me! My Heavenly Father always lift me up, a bruised reed he shall not break and smoking flax he shall never quench! He is so quiet and always smile, never ever scream at me or belittle me or mock me or raise His voice! My Heavenly Father is my forever Father Eternal snd the Most Perfect Father: "Behold my servant, whom I uphold; mine elect, in whom my soul delighteth; I have put my spirit upon him: he shall bring forth judgment to the Gentiles. [2] He shall not cry, nor lift up, nor cause his voice to be heard in the street. [3] A bruised reed shall he not break, and the smoking flax shall he not quench: he shall bring forth judgment unto truth. [4] He shall not fail nor be discouraged, till he have set judgment in the earth: and the isles shall wait for his law." Isaiah 42:1-4 KJV

My Heavenly Father never dies or get sick! He is Most Powerful, Most Genius, Most Wise, Most Holy and Most Perfect! He is the Holy Bread of Life, the source of the Living waters, the Word of God full of light Indescribable, unchangeable and Eternal has no beginning and no End, the Alpha and Omega was dead and alive again one essence!

"And Jesus said unto them, I am the bread of life: he that cometh to me shall never hunger; and he that believeth on me shall never thirst. [37] All that the Father giveth me shall come to me; and him that cometh to me I will in no wise cast out. [51] I am the living bread which came down from heaven: if any man eat of this bread, he shall live for ever: and the bread that I will give is my flesh, which I will give for the life of the world." John 6:35,37,51 KJV

"And in the midst of the seven candlesticks one like unto the Son of man, clothed with a garment down to the foot, and girt about the paps with a golden girdle. [14] His head and his hairs were white like wool, as white as snow; and his eyes were as a flame of fire; [15] And his feet like unto fine brass, as if they burned in a furnace; and his voice as the sound of many waters. [16] And he had in his right hand seven stars: and out of his mouth went a sharp twoedged sword: and his countenance was as the sun shineth in his strength. [18] I am he that liveth, and was dead; and, behold, I am alive for evermore, Amen; and have the keys of hell and of death."Revelation 1:13-16,18 KJV

My Heavenly Father is Most Merciful, Most Gracious and Most Patience never ever give up upon me and His forgiveness has no limit!

He saved my soul and He died for me! The Heavenly Father is watching over me never sleep and never take His eyes from my soul no matter even and where!

My Heavenly Father always heař my prayer listen to my cry and answer my request knows all things before I ask!

My Heavenly Father formed me, made me and engraved me in His palm and one can snatch my soul from His Hand!

My Heavenly Father is my God and Lord who created the entire world, the universe heaven earth seen and unseen and called me His own son! What anyone could ask for!

He Heard my voice! He knows my foot steps! He runs to hug when He sees me from fare! He worries about me more than I worry about myself!

My Heavenly Father feeds me, nourishes my soul and buying all kind of the Most clothing to dress my soul with chains and rare precious stones! He let me eat at His table sitting in the King's table! He wrote my name in His Book of Life and has invited me smears for the Holy wedding of Lamb!

My Heavenly Father loves me so much and one day He came to me and wrote His Holy Name in my forehead! He said this how the world shall identify as my Own good Son!

I always call upon His Name! He manifested Himself to me! I called Him the King of kings and the Lord of lords, the Most High! He ask me to call Him "My Father". My Father is full of Love no One like Him in the entire universe and beyond! He is so humble and meek!

One day, I called Him My God and Lord; "How are You! I know many do not ask how are You!" He said: "Just wait for Me! I am coming" I waited and waited kept looking for a king with so many servants. I saw clouds and He wasn't! I heard thunders and He again wasn't! Then I heard a smooth breeze and I kept looking for my King with a Crown above His head siting upon His Throne with principals and authorities and high ranks worshipping Him! Yet I saw the Most Holy, Innocent Gorgeous, Sweet and Compassionate the True Lamb of God with the mark of the Spear at His Side and the that of the nail at His Palms with Blood stained! I cried and my eyes teared like Rivers and I ran to Him and climbed upon His Shoulder! I cried and kissed Him saying fearfully: "Who dared to that to You my God" My Father replied: "For You as ransom, no One could save you but Me. You and all human descended condemned to death and to bring you back to my Holy Father to gain you back to Me, I descended down and the transgressors done that and worse murdering Me and rejected Me I am the Father!! "Hear, O heavens, and give ear, O earth: for the Lord hath spoken, I have nourished and brought up children, and they have rebelled against me. [3] The ox knoweth his owner, and the ass his master's crib: but Israel doth not know, my people doth not consider." Isaiah 1:2-3 KJV "I am sought of them that asked not for me ; I am found of them that sought me not: I said, Behold me, behold me, unto a nation that was not called by my name. [2] I have spread out my hands all the day unto a rebellious people, which walketh in a way that was not good, after their own thoughts;" Isaiah 65:1-2 KJV

Greater love hath no man than this, that a man lay down his life for his friends. [14] Ye are my friends, if ye do whatsoever I command you. [15] Henceforth I call you not servants; for the servant knoweth not what his lord doeth: but I have called you friends; for all things that I have heard of my Father I have made known unto you: "If ye keep my commandments, ye shall abide in my love; even as I have kept my Father's commandments, and abide in his love. [11] These things have I spoken unto you, that my joy might remain in you, and that your joy might be full. [12] This is my commandment, That ye love one another, as I have loved you. [13] Greater love hath no man than this, that a man lay down his life for his friends. [14] Ye are my friends, if ye do whatsoever I command you. [15] Henceforth I call you not servants; for the servant knoweth not what his lord doeth: but I have called you friends; for all things that I have heard of my Father I have made known unto you. [16] Ye have not chosen me, but I have chosen you, and ordained you, that ye should go and bring forth fruit, and that your fruit should remain: that whatsoever ye shall ask of the Father in my name, he may give it you. [17] These things I command you, that ye love one another." John 15:10-17 KJV

I am the Good shepherd, and know my sheep, and am known of mine. [15] As the Father knoweth me, even so know I the Father: and I lay down my life for the sheep.: "Verily, verily, I say unto you, He that entereth not by the door into the sheepfold, but climbeth up some other way, the same is a thief and a robber. [2] But he that entereth in by the door is the shepherd of the sheep. [3] To him the porter openeth; and the sheep hear his voice: and he calleth his own sheep by name, and leadeth them out. [4] And when he putteth forth his own sheep, he goeth before them, and the sheep follow him: for they know his voice. [5] And a stranger will they not follow, but will flee from him: for they know not the voice of strangers. [7] Then said Jesus unto them again, Verily, verily, I say unto you, I am the door of the sheep. [8] All that ever came before me are thieves and robbers: but the sheep did not hear them. [9] I am the door: by me if any man enter in, he shall be saved, and shall go in and out, and find pasture. [10] The thief cometh not, but for to steal, and to kill, and to destroy: I am come that they might have life, and that they might have it more abundantly. [11] I am the good shepherd: the good shepherd giveth his life for the sheep. [12] But he that is an hireling, and not the shepherd, whose own the sheep are not, seeth the wolf coming, and leaveth the sheep, and fleeth: and the wolf catcheth them, and scattereth the sheep. [13] The hireling fleeth, because he is an hireling, and careth not for the sheep. [14] I am the good shepherd, and know my sheep, and am known of mine. [15] As the Father knoweth me, even so know I the Father: and I lay down my life for the sheep. [16] And other sheep I have, which are not of this fold: them also I must bring, and they shall hear my voice; and there shall be one fold, and one shepherd. [17] Therefore doth my Father love me, because I lay down my life, that I might take it again. [18] No man taketh it from me, but I lay it down of myself. I have power to lay it down, and I have power to take it again. This commandment have I received of my Father."John 10:1-5,7-18 KJV

Let him kiss me with the kisses of his mouth: for thy love is better than wine. [3] Because of the savour of thy good ointments thy name is as ointment poured forth, therefore do the virgins love thee. Song of Songs 1:2-3 KJV "Let him kiss me with the kisses of his mouth: for thy love is better than wine. [3] Because of the savour of thy good ointments thy name is as ointment poured forth, therefore do the virgins love thee." Song of Songs 2:8-10, 14,16-17 KJV "The voice of my beloved! behold, he cometh leaping upon the mountains, skipping upon the hills. [9] My beloved is like a roe or a young hart: behold, he standeth behind our wall, he looketh forth at the windows, shewing himself through the lattice. [10] My beloved spake, and said unto me, Rise up, my love, my fair one, and come away. [14] O my dove, that art in the clefts of the rock, in the secret places of the stairs, let me see thy countenance, let me hear thy voice; for sweet is thy voice, and thy countenance is comely. [16] My beloved is mine, and I am his: he feedeth among the lilies. [17] Until the day break, and the shadows flee away, turn, my beloved, and be thou like a roe or a young hart upon the mountains of Bether." Song of Songs 4:1-4,10-11,16 KJV "Behold, thou art fair, my love; behold, thou art fair; thou hast doves' eyes within thy locks: thy hair is as a flock of goats, that appear from mount Gilead. [2] Thy teeth are like a flock of sheep that are even shorn, which came up from the washing; whereof every one bear twins, and none is barren among them. [3] Thy lips are like a thread of scarlet, and thy speech is comely: thy temples are like a piece of a pomegranate within thy locks. [4] Thy neck is like the tower of David builded for an armoury, whereon there hang a thousand bucklers, all shields of mighty men. [10] How fair is thy love, my sister, my spouse! how much better is thy love than wine! and the smell of thine ointments than all spices! [11] Thy lips, O my spouse, drop as the honeycomb: honey and milk are under thy tongue; and the smell of thy garments is like the smell of Lebanon. [16] Awake, O north wind; and come, thou south; blow upon my garden, that the spices thereof may flow out. Let my beloved come into his garden, and eat his pleasant fruits." Song of Songs 5:10-16 KJV "My beloved is white and ruddy, the chiefest among ten thousand.

[11] His head is as the most fine gold, his locks are bushy, and black as a raven. [12] His eyes are as the eyes of doves by the rivers of waters, washed with milk, and fitly set. [13] His cheeks are as a bed of spices, as sweet flowers: his lips like lilies, dropping sweet smelling myrrh. [14] His hands are as gold rings set with the beryl: his belly is as bright ivory overlaid with sapphires. [15] His legs are as pillars of marble, set upon sockets of fine gold: his countenance is as Lebanon, excellent as the cedars. [16] His mouth is most sweet: yea, he is altogether lovely. This is my beloved, and this is my friend, O daughters of Jerusalem."

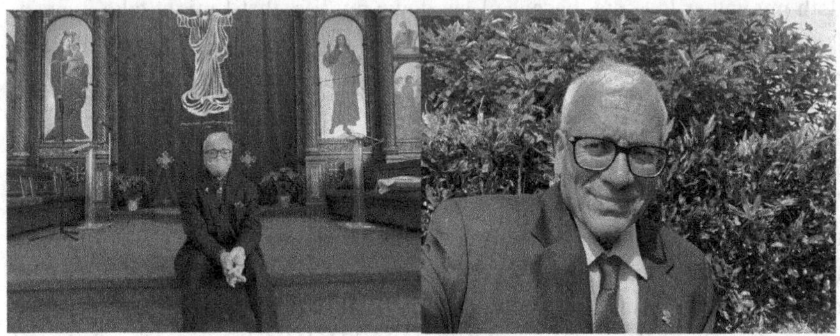

CR, These words were like apples of gold on a silver platter. They brought tears to my eyes and nourishment to my soul.

KG, Your words make me cry and touch my heart. I thank God daily for all his Blessings and even the ones he did not allow. Thank God for you Dr Ghaly. You are a.true inspiration to the world..the gifted healer. Thank God for you. Blessings from Egypt

CG, This is beautifully written. This touches my soul and nourishes it

Always a learned lesson from your writings . Blessings

RC, Touching beuty words

JT, amen

The Story of the Son and the Father!!

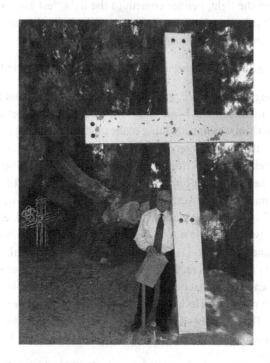

He Always Spoke about His Father!

No one has seen His Father but they had seen His mother!

He had a mother in the flesh but a Father in the Spirit

He had a human mother but a Divine Father!

He had a visible mother but invisible Most Holy Father!

He was the Only One that could see His Father, talk with Him and live with Him inseparable yet He was also in the flesh see all the people!

The world could see the Father because He was from Him from above and everyone else around Him was from below and from the earth! The world hated Him but He loved the world and came to save the world; "For God so loved the world, that he gave his only begotten Son, that whosoever believeth in him should not perish, but have everlasting life. [17] For God sent not his Son into the world to condemn the world; but that the world through him might be saved. [18] He that believeth on him is not condemned: but he that believeth not is condemned already, because he hath not believed in the name of the only begotten Son of God.

[19] And this is the condemnation, that light is come into the world, and men loved darkness rather than light, because their deeds were evil. [20] For every one that doeth evil hateth the light, neither cometh to the light, lest his deeds should be reproved. [21] But he that doeth truth cometh to the light, that his deeds may be made manifest, that they are wrought in God."John 3:16-21 KJV

They can only see His Father through Him for whoever believe in Him!

"In the beginning was the Word, and the Word was with God, and the Word was God. [2] The same was in the beginning with God. [3] All things were made by him; and without him was not any thing made that was made. [4] In him was life; and the life was the light of men. [5] And the light shineth in darkness; and the darkness comprehended it not. [6] There was a man sent from God, whose name was John. [7] The same came for a witness, to bear witness of the Light, that all men through him might believe. [8] He was not that Light, but was sent to bear witness of that Light. [9] That was the true Light, which lighteth every man that cometh into the world. [10] He was in the world, and the world was made by him, and the world knew him not. [11] He came unto his own, and his own received him not. [12] But as many as received him, to them gave he power to become the sons of God, even to them that believe on his name: [13] Which were born, not of blood, nor of the will of the flesh, nor of the will of man, but of God. [14] And the Word was made flesh, and dwelt among us, (and we beheld his glory, the glory as of the only begotten of the Father,) full of grace and truth."John 1

A mystery and no one could figure it out or begin to understand or believe but through the Hoky Spirit!

It confused everyone living in flesh or in spirit that wasn't from Him! Even Satan and all his demons!!'

He wasn't suppose to come down but out of His unconditional Love descended and degraded Himself to a man!

He always called Himself and was called since the Old Testament: The Son of Man!

He was the Mediator to bring the human race back you the heavenly hosts! The earthly fragmented people living in the dark to bring them and join the heavenly kingdom of Him!

Yet those in the world living in darkness, had betrayed Him, mocked Him, called Him liar with all kind of evil words and ultimately became false witness against Him, they rejected Him and refused Him and finally murdered Him and crucified Him!

Yet for that reason He came and made the earthly journey to save the elect those that believe in Him and His Father!

He gave power and glory and taught His earthly children ways to salvations to follow Him!

He became their Father, He adopted them that astray in the world and gave them His blood and flesh to redeem their sins and became sanctified again to be worthy to join His Holy Wedfing and to enter New Jerusalem!

He then resurrected by His own Power as Incarnated Son of God and now is preparing mansions and holy new Eden Garden by the Living Tree the fountain of spring waters as a Good Shepherd and Savior of the world !

At that Day, they will see Him and His Father as eternal celebration begin and He comes in His glory to judge the world and bring the sheep to Him and goats will be sent away, those in the right will be saved and those in the left will be condemned!

In His last long prayers before He departed the world, He prayed to His Father and explained it all!!

"These words spake Jesus, and lifted up his eyes to heaven, and said, Father, the hour is come; glorify thy Son, that thy Son also may glorify thee: [2] As thou hast given him power over all flesh, that he should give eternal life to as many as thou hast given him. [3] And this is life eternal, that they might know thee the only true God, and Jesus Christ, whom thou hast sent. [4] I have glorified thee on the earth: I have finished the work which thou gavest me to do. [5] And now, O Father, glorify thou me with thine own self with the glory which I had with thee before the world was. [6] I have manifested thy name unto the men which thou gavest me out of the world: thine they were, and thou gavest them me; and they have kept thy word. [7] Now they have known that all things whatsoever thou hast given me are of thee. [8] For I have given unto them the words which thou gavest me; and they have received them, and have known surely that I came out from thee, and they have believed that thou didst send me. [9] I pray for them: I pray not for the world, but for them which thou hast given me; for they are thine. [10] And all mine are thine, and thine are mine; and I am glorified in them. [11] And now I am no more in the world, but these are in the world, and I come to thee. Holy Father, keep through thine own name those whom thou hast given me, that they may be one, as we are. [12] While I was with them in the world, I kept them in thy name: those that thou gavest me I have kept, and none of them is lost, but the son of perdition; that the scripture might be fulfilled. [13] And now come I to thee; and these things I speak in the world, that they might have my joy fulfilled in themselves. [14] I have given them thy word; and the world hath hated them, because they are not of the world, even as I am not of the world. [15] I pray not that thou shouldest take them out of the world, but that thou shouldest keep them from the evil. [16] They are not of the world, even as I am not of the world. [17] Sanctify them through thy truth: thy word is truth. [18] As thou hast sent me into the world, even so have I also sent them into the world. [19] And for their sakes I sanctify myself, that they also might be sanctified through the truth. [20] Neither pray I for these alone, but for them also which shall believe on me through their word; [21] That they all may be one; as thou, Father, art in me, and I in thee, that they also may be one in us: that the world may believe that thou hast sent me. [22] And the glory which thou gavest me I have given them; that they may be one, even as we are one: [23] I in them, and thou in me, that they may be made perfect in one; and that the world may know that thou hast sent me, and hast loved them, as thou hast loved me. [24] Father, I will that they also, whom thou hast given me, be with me where I am; that they may behold my glory, which thou hast given me: for thou lovedst me before the foundation of the world. [25] O righteous Father, the world hath not known thee: but I have known thee, and these have known that thou hast sent me. [26] And I have declared unto them thy name, and will declare it : that the love wherewith thou hast loved me may be in them, and I in them."John 17

My Beloved!

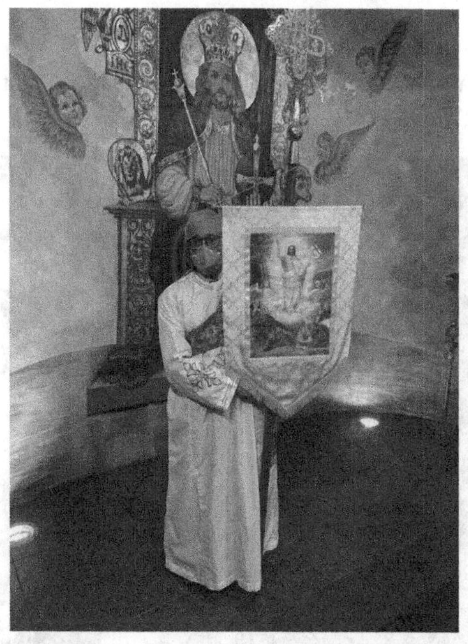

My love and Beloved to Him the Power, the Glory and Dominion fur ever and ever Amen

"Who is this that cometh up from the wilderness, leaning upon her beloved? I raised thee up under the apple tree: there thy mother brought thee forth: there she brought thee forth that bare thee. [7] Many waters cannot quench love, neither can the floods drown it: if a man would give all the substance of his house for love, it would utterly be contemned."Song of Songs 8:5,7 KJV "Let him kiss me with the kisses of his mouth: for thy love is better than wine. [3] Because of the savour of thy good ointments thy name is as ointment poured forth, therefore do the virgins love thee. [4] Draw me, we will run after thee: the king hath brought me into his chambers: we will be glad and rejoice in thee, we will remember thy love more than wine: the upright love thee."Song of Songs 8:5,7 KJV

Ramsis Ghaly

Dl, Amen.

Jm, Magnificent Amen

Ms, Time for Our Lord too. Yes.

To Be With Him!

Written by Ramsis Ghaly

"The glory which You have given Me I have given to them, that they may be one, just as We are one;" John 17:22

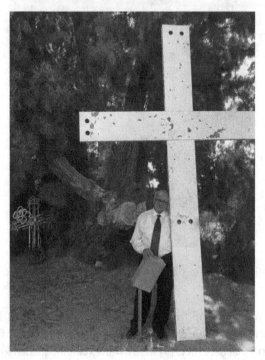

To Follow His Footsteps!

To be solitude with Him!

To be So Close to Him!

To be His Son!

To Join Him!

To Bind in Him!

To be Called by Him!

To Abide in Him!

To Love Him!

To be in Him!

To be in His Kingdom!

To know His Purpose!

To Dwell in Him!

To be in Peace in Him!

To Reconcile with Him!

To be Absorbed in Him!

To be Absent in Him!

To be Perfect in Him!

To be Holy in Him!

To be anointed by Him!

To Search for Him!

To Draw to Him!

To Fly Uphigh to Him!

To Reach Him!

To be in His Court!

To be in His Home!

To Lift Up my soul!

To Subject my Flesh!

To Silence my Needs!

To Kill my Lusts!

To Follow my Destiny to eternity!

To be Destined with Him!

To be Together!

To Hear Him!

To Listen to Him!

To Understand Him!

To Worship Him!

To Praise Him!

To Sing ♫to Him!

To See Him!

To Find Him!

To Know Him!

To Meet Him!

To See Him!

To be with Him Day and Night!

To Walk with Him!

To Eat the Bread of Life!

To Drink His Waters!

To Dine with Him!

To Talk with Him!

To Discuss with Him!

To Be Transformed!

To Be Transfigured!

To Rejuvenate!

To Be Cleansed!

To Be New!

To Run Away from Distraction!

To be one-to-One with Him!

To Live with Him!

To be crucified with Him!

To Die with Him!

To resurrect with Him!

To be Glorified with Him!

To be one in Him!

To be one with Him!

To be one for Him!

Biblical Verses

John 14:23 "Jesus answered and said to him, "If anyone loves Me, he will keep My word; and My Father will love him, and We will come to him and make Our home with him"

John 14:20-21 "At that day you will know that I am in My Father, and you in Me, and I in you. He who has My commandments and keeps them, it is he who loves Me. And he who loves Me will be loved by My Father, and I will love him and manifest Myself to him."

1 John 3:24 "Now he who keeps His commandments abides in Him, and He in him. And by this we know that He abides in us, by the Spirit whom He has given us" John 15:5

"I am the vine, you are the branches. He who abides in Me, and I in him, bears much fruit; for without Me you can do nothing"

Romans 6:5 "For if we have been united together in the likeness of His death, certainly we also shall be in the likeness of His resurrection,"

1 Corinthians 6:17 "But he who is joined to the Lord is one spirit with Him."2 Corinthians 3:18 "But we all, with unveiled face, beholding as in a mirror the glory of the Lord, are being transformed into the same image from glory to glory, just as by the Spirit of the Lord."

Romans 8:10-15 "And if Christ is in you, the body is dead because of sin, but the Spirit is life because of righteousness. But if the Spirit of Him who raised Jesus from the dead dwells in you, He who raised Christ from the dead will also give life to your mortal bodies through His Spirit who dwells in you. Therefore, brethren, we are debtors—not to the flesh, to live according to the flesh. For if you live according to the flesh you will die; but if by the Spirit you put to death the deeds of the body, you will live. For as many as are led by the Spirit of God, these are sons of God. For you did not receive the spirit of bondage again to fear, but you received the Spirit of adoption by whom we cry out, "Abba, Father."

Ephesians 2:18-20 “For through Him we both have access by one Spirit to the Father. Now, therefore, you are no longer strangers and foreigners, but fellow citizens with the saints and members of the household of God, having been built on the foundation of the apostles and prophets, Jesus Christ Himself being the chief cornerstone,”

Philippians 2:5-6 “Let this mind be in you which was also in Christ Jesus, who, being in the form of God, did not consider it robbery to be equal with God,”

1 Corinthians 12:13 “For by one Spirit we were all baptized into one body—whether Jews or Greeks, whether slaves or free—and have all been made to drink into one Spirit.”

2 Corinthians 5:17 “Therefore, if anyone is in Christ, he is a new creation; old things have passed away; behold, all things have become new”

Galatians 3:27-28 “For as many of you as were baptized into Christ have put on Christ. There is neither Jew nor Greek, there is neither slave nor free, there is neither male nor female; for you are all one in Christ Jesus”

Ephesians 1:11 “In Him also we have obtained an inheritance, being predestined according to the purpose of Him who works all things according to the counsel of His will,”

2 Chronicles 15:2 “And he went out to meet Asa, and said to him: “Hear me, Asa, and all Judah and Benjamin. The LORD is with you while you are with Him. If you seek Him, He will be found by you; but if you forsake Him, He will forsake you.”

Philippians 1:27 “Only let your conduct be worthy of the gospel of Christ, so that whether I come and see you or am absent, I may hear of your affairs, that you stand fast in one spirit, with one mind striving together for the faith of the gospel,”

Colossians 1:19-20 “For it pleased the Father that in Him all the fullness should dwell, and by Him to reconcile all things to Himself, by Him, whether things on earth or things in heaven, having made peace through the blood of His cross.”

Colossians 1:27 “To them God willed to make known what are the riches of the glory of this mystery among the Gentiles: which is Christ in you, the hope of glory.”

Colossians 2:13 “And you, being dead in your trespasses and the uncircumcision of your flesh, He has made alive together with Him, having forgiven you all trespasses,

Hebrews 8:10 "For this is the covenant that I will make with the house of Israel after those days, says the LORD: I will put My laws in their mind and write them on their hearts; and I will be their God, and they shall be My people."

James 4:10 "Humble yourselves in the sight of the Lord, and He will lift you up."

1 Peter 1:15 "but as He who called you is holy, you also be holy in all your conduct,"

1 Peter 4:1 "Therefore, since Christ suffered for us in the flesh, arm yourselves also with the same mind, for he who has suffered in the flesh has ceased from sin,"

1 John 2:5 "But whoever keeps His word, truly the love of God is perfected in him. By this we know that we are in Him."

1 John 2:27-28 "But the anointing which you have received from Him abides in you, and you do not need that anyone teach you; but as the same anointing teaches you concerning all things, and is true, and is not a lie, and just as it has taught you, you will abide in Him. And now, little children, abide in Him, that when He appears, we may have confidence and not be ashamed before Him at His coming."

1 John 3:2 "Beloved, now we are children of God; and it has not yet been revealed what we shall be, but we know that when He is revealed, we shall be like Him, for we shall see Him as He is."

1 John 3:6 "Whoever abides in Him does not sin. Whoever sins has neither seen Him nor known Him."

1 John 3:9 "Whoever has been born of God does not sin, for His seed remains in him; and he cannot sin, because he has been born of God."

1 John 4:12-13 "No one has seen God at any time. If we love one another, God abides in us, and His love has been perfected in us. By this we know that we abide in Him, and He in us, because He has given us of His Spirit."

1 John 4:15-16 "Whoever confesses that Jesus is the Son of God, God abides in him, and he in God. And we have known and believed the love that God has for us. God is love, and he who abides in love abides in God, and God in him."

1 John 5:20 "And we know that the Son of God has come and has given us an understanding, that we may know Him who is true; and we are in Him who is true, in His Son Jesus Christ. This is the true God and eternal life."

Revelation 20:4 "And I saw thrones, and they sat on them, and judgment was committed to them. Then I saw the souls of those who had been beheaded for their witness to Jesus and for the word of God, who had not worshiped the beast or his image, and had not received his mark on their foreheads or on their hands. And they lived and reigned with Christ for a thousand years."

Revelation 20:6 "Blessed and holy is he who has part in the first resurrection. Over such the second death has no power, but they shall be priests of God and of Christ, and shall reign with Him a thousand years."

JM, "Beautiful" Amen

JC, Beautiful

KG, Beautiful! God Bless you, Dr **Ramsis Ghaly**

BCD, Very moving words. Thank you Sir

CG, This is truly wonderful! Great picture, compliments your writing.

CL, Love this!

IW, Amen

God Bless you.

RR, Powerfully moving! Thank you for sharing.

John 14:6, I am the way, the truth and the life. No one comes to the Father, but by Me.

CL, Amen thank you

CR, Beautiful reminders

God is my Great Rock The Splendor Majesty!

Written by Ramsis Ghaly

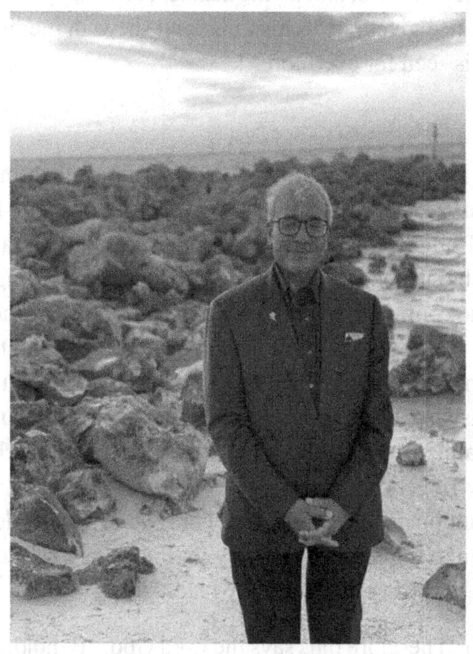

Rock and stone are known of being indestructible strength!

Rocks are standing strong before the unrelenting recurrent day and night hits by the strong waves and giant storms at the seas!

Rock is thy faith is so powerful and solid as it is standing upon the Rock!

Thy Savior is a The Great Rock and Rock of thy salvation!

Thy love is sitting upon a Rock pure and sturdy!

Thy character is refined before the rock of thy faith and love!

Thy protection is that Rock and thy Deliverance!

Thy foundation is established in that Rock the Splendor Majesty!

Thy resurrection is that Most Holy Lamb of God thy Rock!

Matthew 16:18 "18 And I tell you that you are Peter,and on this rock I will build my church, and the gates of Hadeswill not overcome it." Samuel-2 22:2 "And he said, The LORD [is] my rock, and my fortress, and my deliverer;" Psalm 18:1-2,49-50 KJV "I will love thee, O Lord, my strength. [2] The Lord is my rock, and my fortress, and my deliverer; my God, my strength, in whom I will trust; my buckler, and the horn of my salvation, and my high tower. [49] Therefore will I give thanks unto thee, O Lord, among the heathen, and sing praises unto thy name. [50] Great deliverance giveth he to his king; and sheweth mercy to his anointed, to David, and to his seed for evermore."!

Biblical Verses

Psalms 89:26 "26 He will call out to me, 'You are my Father, my God, the Rock my Savior.'" Psalms 18:46 "46 The LORD lives! Praise be to my Rock! Exalted be God my Savior!" Psalms 62:6 "6 Truly he is my rock and my salvation; he is my fortress, I will not be shaken." Psalms 71:3 "3 Be my rock of refuge, to which I can always go; give the command to save me, for you are my rock and my fortress." Psalms 28:1 "1 To you, LORD, I call; you are my Rock, do not turn a deaf ear to me. For if you remain silent, I will be like those who go down to the pit." Psalm 95 "1 Come, let us sing for joy to the LORD; let us shout aloud to the Rock of our salvation." Psalms 144:1 "1 Praise be to the LORD my Rock, who trains my hands for war, my fingers for battle." Psalm 28:1-2 "To you, LORD, I call; you are my Rock, do not turn a deaf ear to me. For if you remain silent, I will be like those who go down to the pit. Hear my cry for mercy as I call to you for help, as I lift up my hands toward your Most Holy Place.".

Isaiah 28:16 (ESV) "Therefore thus says the Lord God, "Behold, I am the one who has laid as a foundation in Zion, a stone, a tested stone, a precious cornerstone, of a sure foundation: 'Whoever believes will not be in haste." Isaiah 51:1 1 "Listen to me, you who pursue righteousness and who seek the LORD: Look to the rock from which you were cut and to the quarry from which you were hewn;" Isaiah 32:2 "Each one will be like a shelter from the wind and a refuge from the storm, like streams of water in the desert and the shadow of a great rock in a thirsty land."

Samuel-2 22:3 "The God of my rock; in him will I trust: [he is] my shield, and the horn of my salvation, my high tower, and my refuge, my saviour; thou savest me from violence." Samuel-2 22:32 "For who [is] God, save the LORD? and who [is] a rock, save our God?" Samuel-2 22:47 "The LORD liveth; and blessed [be] my rock; and exalted be the God of the rock of my salvation." Samuel-2 23:3 "The God of Israel said, the Rock of Israel spake to me, He that ruleth over men [must be] just, ruling in the fear of God." Samuel-1 2:2 "There is] none holy as the LORD: for [there is] none beside thee: neither [is there] any rock like our God." Isaiah

2:10 "10 Go into the rocks, hide in the ground from the fearful presence of the LORDand the splendor of his majesty."

Numbers 20:8 "Take the rod, and gather thou the assembly together, thou, and Aaron thy brother, and speak ye unto the rock before their eyes; and it shall give forth his water, and thou shalt bring forth to them water out of the rock: so thou shalt give the congregation and their beasts drink." Deuteronomy 32:4 "He is] the Rock, his work [is] perfect: for all his ways [are] judgment: a God of truth and without iniquity, just and right [is] he." Deuteronomy 32:13 "He made him ride on the high places of the earth, that he might eat the increase of the fields; and he made him to suck honey out of the rock, and oil out of the flinty rock;" Judges 6:26 "And build an altar unto the LORD thy God upon the top of this rock, in the ordered place, and take the second bullock, and offer a burnt sacrifice with the wood of the grove which thou shalt cut down."

Luke 6:48 "48 They are like a man building a house, who dug down deep and laid the foundation on rock. When a flood came, the torrent struck that house but could not shake it, because it was well built." 1 Corinthians 10:4 "4 and drank the same spiritual drink; for they drank from the spiritual rock that accompanied them, and that rock was Christ."

Romans 9:32 "Why not? Because they were trying to get right with God by keeping the law instead of by trusting in him. They stumbled over the great rock in their path." 1 Peter 2:4 "4 As you come to him, the living Stone—rejected by humans but chosen by God and precious to him—"

Revelation 21:11 "11 It shone with the glory of God, and its brilliance was like that of a very precious jewel, like a jasper, clear as crystal."

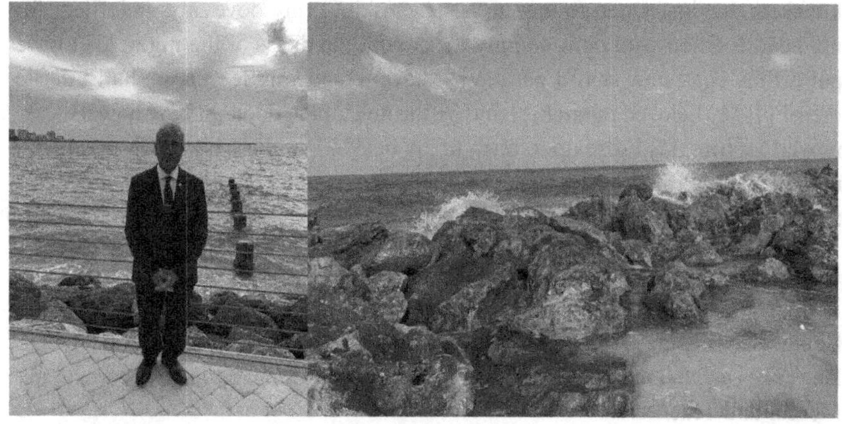

SY, Christ is my firm foundation. The rock on which I stand! Amen Dr. Ghaly!

He is my True Hero He is my True Being!

Written by Ramsis Ghaly

Jesus is my True Hero! Jesus is my True Being! Jesus is my Living! Jesus is my life! Jesus is my True Hero!! "For in him we live, and move, and have our being; as certain also of your own poets have said, For we are also his offspring." Acts 17:28 KJV

He is my Hero! I wish the entire world knows He is my Hero! Come and meet my Hero!! He is my Lord! I live unto the Lord, and I am for the lord's! He is my True Hero! "For whether we live, we live unto the Lord; and whether we die, we die unto the Lord: whether we live therefore, or die, we are the Lord's." Romans 14:8 KJV

I went to sleep, I put Jesus' picture by my side! I hugged Him all night long and dreamed about Him the entire night long! He is my Lord and God! He is my True Hero!!!

He is my True Hero!!!

I went to sleep but I woke up by the voice of my love—- I put off my coat! I washed my feet! I defiled Not my bed—I am so ready to be with my Love!! I wonder every night, if He will knock my door and be with me!! I always have the door open for Him! I told Him where I put the keys and what is the password of my inner home!! I bought an extra/ garage parking for His car and I always have to Cara plate at my dining table!! I wish He comes and come soon!! He is my Hero! He is my refuge and my fortress!! "I sleep, but my heart waketh: it is the voice of my beloved that knocketh, saying, Open to me, my sister, my love, my dove, my undefiled: for my head is filled with dew, and my locks with the drops of the night. [3] I have put off my coat; how shall I put it on? I have washed my feet; how shall I defile them? [4] My beloved put in his hand by the hole of the door, and my bowels were moved for him. [5] I rose up to open to my beloved; and my hands dropped with myrrh, and my fingers with sweet smelling myrrh, upon the handles of the lock." Song of Songs 5:2-5 KJV

He is everywhere in my life! He is my True Hero! He is everywhere in my home, in my soul, and in my heart ! I love Him much and He loves me more! He is my Being!! He is Mine! He is my Beginning and my End my Alpha and my Omega! He is my Day and my Night! He is my Sun and my Moon! He is my Star and my Mentor and Teacher!

He washes me and cleanse me so shall be white like the snow—Purge me with hyssop, and I shall be clean: wash me, and I shall be whiter than snow. [8] Make me to hear joy and gladness; that the bones which thou hast broken may rejoice." Psalm 51:7-8 KJV

He is my True shelter! My True Refuge! He is my True Fortess:,He that dwelleth in the secret place of the most High shall abide under the shadow of the Almighty. [2] I will say of the Lord, He is my refuge and my fortress: my God; in him will I trust. [3] Surely he shall deliver thee from the snare of the fowler, and from the noisome pestilence. [4] He shall cover thee with his feathers, and under his wings shalt thou trust: his truth shall be thy shield and buckler. [5] Thou shalt not be afraid for the terror by night; nor for the arrow that flieth by day; [6] Nor for the pestilence that walketh in darkness; nor for the destruction that wasteth at noonday. [7] A thousand shall fall at thy side, and ten thousand at thy right hand; but it shall not come nigh thee."Psalm 91:1-7 KJV

He restores my soul and bring me joy—"Restore unto me the joy of thy salvation; and uphold me with thy free spirit." Psalm 51:12 KJV

In my distress I cried to my Love, and He heard me! He us my Being and my True Hero! "In my distress I cried unto the Lord, and he heard me. [2] Deliver my soul, O Lord, from lying lips, and from a deceitful tongue." Psalm 120:1-2 KJV

I stood behind Him at His feet weeping and began to wash His feet with tears and did wipe them with the hairs of her head, and kissed his feet, and anointed them with the ointment—He wrapped His arms around me and hold my Hand! He spoke to me the heavenly words full of life saying "Thy sins are forgiven.Thy faith hath saved thee; go in peace."''And stood at his feet behind him weeping, and began to wash his feet with tears, and did wipe them with the hairs of her head, and kissed his feet, and anointed them with the ointment. [48] And he said unto her, Thy sins are forgiven. [50] And he said to the woman, Thy faith hath saved thee; go in peace."Luke 7:38,48,50 KJV

As the night get darker and the time is late, I take Him in my arms and say: "Lord, now lettest thou thy servant depart in peace, according to thy word: For mine eyes have seen thy salvation"

"Then took he him up in his arms, and blessed God, and said, [29] Lord, now lettest thou thy servant depart in peace, according to thy word: [30] For mine eyes have seen thy salvation," Luke 2:28-30 KJV

And as I take the last breath of the day before I drift in my dreams, I utter His words at the Cross: "Father, into thy hands I commend my spirit" "And when Jesus had cried with a loud voice, he said, Father, into thy hands I commend my spirit: and having said thus, he gave up the ghost."Luke 23:46 KJV

He is my True Hero!!!

If my Love comes, He will like my office and my practice! There is a gorgeous garden and His pictures all over! His name is sky high and His cross is my glory!!! He is my Bridegroom! He is in my heart, in mind, my soul, my strength and my thoughts!! And my love to Him exceeds the love of all!! He is my True Hero!!! "Jesus said unto him, Thou shalt love the Lord thy God with all thy heart, and with all thy soul, and with all thy mind. [38] This is the first and great commandment. [39] And the second is like unto it, Thou shalt love thy neighbour as thyself. [40] On these two commandments hang all the law and the prophets." Matthew 22:37-40 KJV

He is my True Hero!!!

Nowadays I go to bed early and with prayers and incense I kneel to my Beloved and I wait for Him every night! I have a huge space for Him dressed in precious linen and aroma. I dream about Him every night! I pray to Him minute by minute! He is with me day and night!! He is my True Hero!!!

He is my True Hero!!!

I wonder how He did He look like when He was in the flesh?? What His disciples saw in Him?? And how soon those fell in love with my Lord! I can tell you a secret: He open the eyes to those who love Him and indeed they see heaven of heavens, springs of waters running by the green pasture and uphigh in the mountains! He is my True Hero!!!

He is my True Hero!!!

Before the night over, I begin to praise Him, my True Hero! My true Being saying: "Praise ye the Lord. Praise God in his sanctuary: praise him in the firmament of his power. [2] Praise him for his mighty acts: praise him according to his excellent greatness. [3] Praise him with the sound of the trumpet: praise him with the psaltery and harp. [4] Praise him with the timbrel and dance: praise him with stringed instruments and organs. [5] Praise him upon the loud cymbals: praise him upon the high sounding cymbals. [6] Let every thing that hath breath praise the Lord. Praise ye the Lord." Psalm 150

I saw Him many years ago when He handed me my path and this time I asked Him when is He coming back! "For to me, to live is Christ, and to die is gain. Philippians 1:21

There is nothing worth loving and be with but Him! I love my Savior and I don't what to do without Him! I wish the world knows Who is my True Hero!

He is my Being! He is my Beloved! He is my Savior! I live not me but Christ livery in me!! "I am crucified with Christ: nevertheless I live; yet not I, but Christ liveth in me: and the life which I now live in the flesh I live by the faith of the Son of God, who loved me, and gave himself for me." Galatians 2:20 KJV

It isn't me and it isn't them, but He is the One! How much I wish the entire world knows Whi is my Hero?? And how much I pray that He will be their Hero, Too!!!!

He is mine and I am His! He spoke to me last night and when I woke up, I saw His picture framed and hanged in every room of my house! As I was walking in the hallway, I found Him! And when I ride my car, He was with me! And when I went to work He was with me! And when I was operating He was by my side!!! My Hero is with my all the time day snd night!! I don't even have to call Him any longer He livery within my soul!! "My beloved is mine, and I am his: he feedeth among the lilies. [17] Until the day break, and the shadows flee away, turn, my beloved, and be thou like a roe or a young hart upon the mountains of Bether." Song of Songs 2:16-17 KJV

Ephesians 3:17—"That Christ may make His home in your hearts through faith, that you, being rooted and grounded in love."

Colossians 1:27 "To whom God willed to make known what are the riches of the glory of this mystery among the Gentiles, which is Christ in you, the hope of glory."

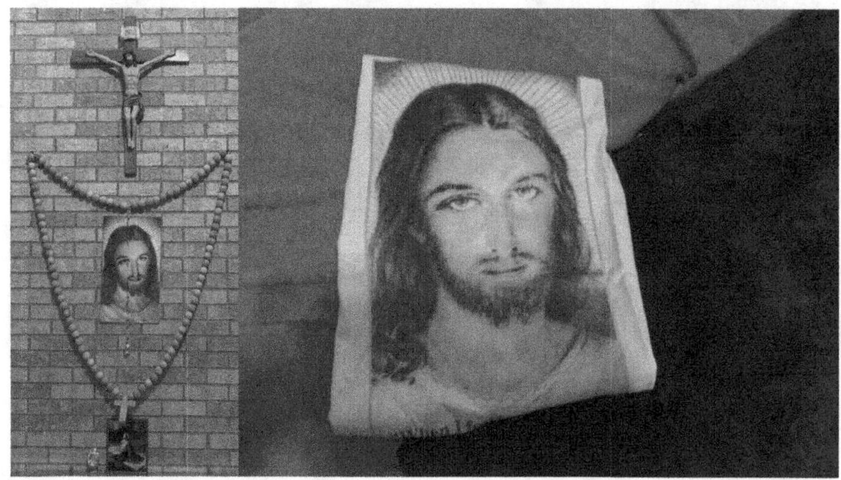

NC, Mine too

SY, Mine too! He loves you so much too

JK, This is one of favor picture of Jesus...

I TRUST IN YOU.

DN, Amen

KH, Amen

MH, Amen

JT, amen...

SA, Amen

GM, He is my hero too! Amén

CR, The most beautiful tribute to Jesus as your Lord and savior that I have ever read. My prayer is that I would experience Him in the same way.

MP, Beautiful words written, he is my Hero too. I wish for him to live within me. I know the Lord is with you all the time day and night, Ramsis. It's special what you do and how well you do it, and he guides you.

JM, "Glorious" Text Dr. Ghaly AMEN To These Gorgeous Visuals

AV, Such beautiful words & thoughts! May our Heavenly Father continue to bless u Dr Ghaly!!

The Sun!!

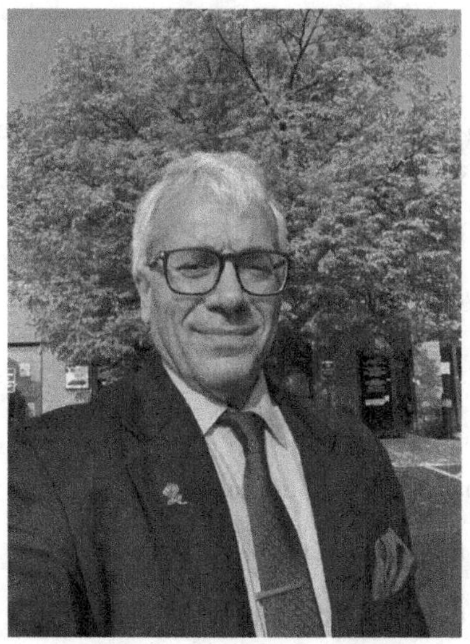

The Sun! The Light! The Warms! The Mighty! The glory of the Almighty! The Truth! The Sight! The Revealing! The Manifestation! The Praises to the Creator!

Who won't feel the same about the sun?

Biblical Verses!!

Psalm 113:3

Verse Concepts

From the rising of the sun to its setting

The name of the Lord is to be praised.

Genesis 1:16

Verse Concepts

God made the two great lights, the greater light to govern the day, and the lesser light to govern the night; He made the stars also.

Deuteronomy 17:3

Verse Concepts

and has gone and served other gods and worshiped them, or the sun or the moon or any of the heavenly host, which I have not commanded,

Joshua 10:12

Verse Concepts

Then Joshua spoke to the Lord in the day when the Lord delivered up the Amorites before the sons of Israel, and he said in the sight of Israel,

“O sun, stand still at Gibeon,

And O moon in the valley of Aijalon.”

Psalm 19:4

Verse Concepts

Their line has gone out through all the earth,

And their utterances to the end of the world.

In them He has placed a tent for the sun,

Psalm 121:6

Verse Concepts

The sun will not smite you by day,

Nor the moon by night.

Ecclesiastes 1:5

Verse Concepts

Also, the sun rises and the sun sets;

And hastening to its place it rises there again.

Isaiah 38:8

Verse Concepts

Behold, I will cause the shadow on the stairway, which has gone down with the sun on the stairway of Ahaz, to go back ten steps.” So the sun’s shadow went back ten steps on the stairway on which it had gone down.

Joel 2:31

Verse Concepts

"The sun will be turned into darkness

And the moon into blood

Before the great and awesome day of the Lord comes.

Acts 26:13

Verse Concepts

at midday, O King, I saw on the way a light from heaven, brighter than the sun, shining all around me and those who were journeying with me.

Judges 9:33

Verse Concepts

In the morning, as soon as the sun is up, you shall rise early and rush upon the city; and behold, when he and the people who are with him come out against you, you shall do to them whatever you can."

Isaiah 60:19

Verse Concepts

"No longer will you have the sun for light by day,

Nor for brightness will the moon give you light;

But you will have the Lord for an everlasting light,

And your God for your glory.

Genesis 19:23-24

The sun had risen over the earth when Lot came to Zoar. Then the Lord rained on Sodom and Gomorrah brimstone and fire from the Lord out of heaven,

Amos 8:9

Verse Concepts

"It will come about in that day," declares the Lord God,

"That I will make the sun go down at noon

And make the earth dark in broad daylight.

Malachi 4:2

Verse Concepts

“But for you who fear My name, the sun of righteousness will rise with healing in its wings; and you will go forth and skip about like calves from the stall.

Job 30:28

Verse Concepts

“I go about mourning without comfort;

I stand up in the assembly and cry out for help.

Deuteronomy 33:14

Verse Concepts

And with the choice yield of the sun,

And with the choice produce of the months.

Exodus 16:21

Verse Concepts

They gathered it morning by morning, every man as much as he should eat; but when the sun grew hot, it would melt.

Mark 4:6

Verse Concepts

And after the sun had risen, it was scorched; and because it had no root, it withered away.

James 1:11

Verse Concepts

For the sun rises with a scorching wind and withers the grass; and its flower falls off and the beauty of its appearance is destroyed; so too the rich man in the midst of his pursuits will fade away.

Genesis 28:11

Verse Concepts

He came to a certain place and spent the night there, because the sun had set; and he took one of the stones of the place and put it under his head, and lay down in that place.

Deuteronomy 24:13

Verse Concepts

When the sun goes down you shall surely return the pledge to him, that he may sleep in his cloak and bless you; and it will be righteousness for you before the Lord your God.

Mark 1:32

Verse Concepts

When evening came, after the sun had set, they began bringing to Him all who were ill and those who were demon-possessed.

Numbers 21:11

Verse Concepts

They journeyed from Oboth and camped at Iye-abarim, in the wilderness which is opposite Moab, to the east.

Deuteronomy 4:41

Verse Concepts

Then Moses set apart three cities across the Jordan to the east,

Deuteronomy 4:47

Verse Concepts

They took possession of his land and the land of Og king of Bashan, the two kings of the Amorites, who were across the Jordan to the east,

Joshua 12:1

Verse Concepts

Now these are the kings of the land whom the sons of Israel defeated, and whose land they possessed beyond the Jordan toward the sunrise, from the valley of the Arnon as far as Mount Hermon, and all the Arabah to the east:

Joshua 1:4

Verse Concepts

From the wilderness and this Lebanon, even as far as the great river, the river Euphrates, all the land of the Hittites, and as far as the Great Sea toward the setting of the sun will be your territory.

Psalm 50:1

Verse Concepts

A Psalm of Asaph.

The Mighty One, God, the Lord, has spoken,

And summoned the earth from the rising of the sun to its setting.

Isaiah 45:6

Verse Concepts

That men may know from the rising to the setting of the sun

That there is no one besides Me.

I am the Lord, and there is no other,

Deuteronomy 4:19

Verse Concepts

And beware not to lift up your eyes to heaven and see the sun and the moon and the stars, all the host of heaven, and be drawn away and worship them and serve them, those which the Lord your God has allotted to all the peoples under the whole heaven.

Genesis 1:16-18

God made the two great lights, the greater light to govern the day, and the lesser light to govern the night; He made the stars also. God placed them in the expanse of the heavens to give light on the earth, and to govern the day and the night, and to separate the light from the darkness; and God saw that it was good.

Psalm 136:7

To Him who made the great lights,

For His lovingkindness is everlasting:

The sun to rule by day,

For His lovingkindness is everlasting,

Genesis 1:14

Verse Concepts

Then God said, "Let there be lights in the expanse of the heavens to separate the day from the night, and let them be for signs and for seasons and for days and years;

Genesis 29:7

Verse Concepts

He said, "Behold, it is still high day; it is not time for the livestock to be gathered. Water the sheep, and go, pasture them."

Exodus 22:26

Verse Concepts

If you ever take your neighbor's cloak as a pledge, you are to return it to him before the sun sets,

1 Samuel 11:9

Verse Concepts

They said to the messengers who had come, "Thus you shall say to the men of Jabesh-gilead, 'Tomorrow, by the time the sun is hot, you will have deliverance.'" So the messengers went and told the men of Jabesh; and they were glad.

Exodus 27:13

The width of the court on the east side shall be fifty cubits.

Deuteronomy 11:30

Verse Concepts

Are they not across the Jordan, west of the way toward the sunset, in the land of the Canaanites who live in the Arabah, opposite Gilgal, beside the oaks of Moreh?

Joshua 19:12

Verse Concepts

Then it turned from Sarid to the east toward the sunrise as far as the border of Chisloth-tabor, and it proceeded to Daberath and up to Japhia.

Deuteronomy 33:13-14

Of Joseph he said,

"Blessed of the Lord be his land,

With the choice things of heaven, with the dew,

And from the deep lying beneath,

And with the choice yield of the sun,

And with the choice produce of the months.

Job 8:16

Verse Concepts

"He thrives before the sun,

And his shoots spread out over his garden.

Matthew 5:45

Verse Concepts

so that you may be sons of your Father who is in heaven; for He causes His sun to rise on the evil and the good, and sends rain on the righteous and the unrighteous.

Jonah 4:8

Verse Concepts

When the sun came up God appointed a scorching east wind, and the sun beat down on Jonah's head so that he became faint and begged with all his soul to die, saying, "Death is better to me than life."

Isaiah 49:10

Verse Concepts

"They will not hunger or thirst,

Nor will the scorching heat or sun strike them down;

For He who has compassion on them will lead them

And will guide them to springs of water.

Matthew 13:6

Verse Concepts

But when the sun had risen, they were scorched; and because they had no root, they withered away.

Revelation 7:16

Verse Concepts

They will hunger no longer, nor thirst anymore; nor will the sun beat down on them, nor any heat;

Deuteronomy 17:2-5

"If there is found in your midst, in any of your towns, which the Lord your God is giving you, a man or a woman who does what is evil in the sight of the Lord your God, by transgressing His covenant, and has gone and served other gods and worshiped them, or the sun or the moon or any of the heavenly host, which I have not commanded, and if it is told you and you have heard of it, then you shall inquire thoroughly. Behold, if it is true and the thing certain that this detestable thing has been done in Israel,read more.

Job 31:26-28

If I have looked at the sun when it shone

Or the moon going in splendor,

And my heart became secretly enticed,

And my hand threw a kiss from my mouth,

That too would have been an iniquity calling for judgment,

For I would have denied God above.

Ezekiel 8:16

Verse Concepts

Then He brought me into the inner court of the Lord's house. And behold, at the entrance to the temple of the Lord, between the porch and the altar, were about twenty-five men with their backs to the temple of the Lord and their faces toward the east; and they were prostrating themselves eastward toward the sun.

2 Kings 23:5-11

He did away with the idolatrous priests whom the kings of Judah had appointed to burn incense in the high places in the cities of Judah and in the surrounding area of Jerusalem, also those who burned incense to Baal, to the sun and to the moon and to the constellations and to all the host of heaven. He brought out the Asherah from the house of the Lord outside Jerusalem to the brook Kidron, and burned it at the brook Kidron, and ground it to dust, and threw its dust on the graves of the common people. He also broke down the houses of the male cult prostitutes which were in the house of the Lord, where the women were weaving hangings for the Asherah.read more.

Jeremiah 8:1-2

“At that time,” declares the Lord, “they will bring out the bones of the kings of Judah and the bones of its princes, and the bones of the priests and the bones of the prophets, and the bones of the inhabitants of Jerusalem from their graves. They will spread them out to the sun, the moon and to all the host of heaven, which they have loved and which they have served, and which they have gone after and which they have sought, and which they have worshiped. They will not be gathered or buried; they will be as dung on the face of the ground.

Jeremiah 43:13

Verse Concepts

He will also shatter the obelisks of Heliopolis, which is in the land of Egypt; and the temples of the gods of Egypt he will burn with fire.”””

Matthew 24:29-30

“But immediately after the tribulation of those days the sun will be darkened, and the moon will not give its light, and the stars will fall from the sky, and the powers of the heavens will be shaken. And then the sign of the Son of Man will appear in the sky, and then all the tribes of the earth will mourn, and they will see the Son of Man coming on the clouds of the sky with power and great glory.

Mark 13:24

Verse Concepts

“But in those days, after that tribulation, the sun will be darkened and the moon will not give its light,

Luke 21:25-26

“There will be signs in sun and moon and stars, and on the earth dismay among nations, in perplexity at the roaring of the sea and the waves, men fainting from fear and the expectation of the things which are coming upon the world; for the powers of the heavens will be shaken.

Exodus 10:21-23

Then the Lord said to Moses, "Stretch out your hand toward the sky, that there may be darkness over the land of Egypt, even a darkness which may be felt." So Moses stretched out his hand toward the sky, and there was thick darkness in all the land of Egypt for three days. They did not see one another, nor did anyone rise from his place for three days, but all the sons of Israel had light in their dwellings.

Isaiah 13:9-10

Behold, the day of the Lord is coming,

Cruel, with fury and burning anger,

To make the land a desolation;

And He will exterminate its sinners from it.

For the stars of heaven and their constellations

Will not flash forth their light;

The sun will be dark when it rises

And the moon will not shed its light.

Jeremiah 4:28

Verse Concepts

"For this the earth shall mourn

And the heavens above be dark,

Because I have spoken, I have purposed,

And I will not change My mind, nor will I turn from it."

Ezekiel 32:7-8

"And when I extinguish you,

I will cover the heavens and darken their stars;

I will cover the sun with a cloud

And the moon will not give its light.

"All the shining lights in the heavens

I will darken over you

And will set darkness on your land,"

Declares the Lord God.

Joel 3:14-15

Multitudes, multitudes in the valley of decision!

For the day of the Lord is near in the valley of decision.

The sun and moon grow dark

And the stars lose their brightness.

Amos 5:20

Verse Concepts

Will not the day of the Lord be darkness instead of light,

Even gloom with no brightness in it?

Matthew 27:45

Verse Concepts

Now from the sixth hour darkness fell upon all the land until the ninth hour.

Mark 15:33

Verse Concepts

When the sixth hour came, darkness fell over the whole land until the ninth hour.

Luke 23:44

Verse Concepts

It was now about the sixth hour, and darkness fell over the whole land until the ninth hour,

Acts 2:20

Verse Concepts

'The sun will be turned into darkness

And the moon into blood,

Before the great and glorious day of the Lord shall come.

Revelation 6:12-17

I looked when He broke the sixth seal, and there was a great earthquake; and the sun became black as sackcloth made of hair, and the whole moon became like blood; and the stars of the sky fell to the earth, as a fig tree casts its unripe figs when shaken by a great wind. The sky was split apart like a scroll when it is rolled up, and every mountain and island were moved out of their places.read more.

Job 9:7

Verse Concepts

Who commands the sun not to shine,

And sets a seal upon the stars;

Psalm 74:16

Verse Concepts

Yours is the day, Yours also is the night;

You have prepared the light and the sun.

Joshua 10:12-13

Then Joshua spoke to the Lord in the day when the Lord delivered up the Amorites before the sons of Israel, and he said in the sight of Israel,

"O sun, stand still at Gibeon,

And O moon in the valley of Aijalon."

So the sun stood still, and the moon stopped,

Until the nation avenged themselves of their enemies.

Is it not written in the book of Jashar? And the sun stopped in the middle of the sky and did not hasten to go down for about a whole day.

2 Kings 20:8-11

Now Hezekiah said to Isaiah, "What will be the sign that the Lord will heal me, and that I shall go up to the house of the Lord the third day?" Isaiah said, "This shall be the sign to you from the Lord, that the Lord will do the thing that He has spoken: shall the shadow go forward ten steps or go back ten steps?" So Hezekiah answered, "It is easy for the shadow to decline ten steps; no, but let the shadow turn backward ten steps."read more.

Psalm 19:1-6

For the choir director. A Psalm of David.

The heavens are telling of the glory of God;

And their expanse is declaring the work of His hands.

Day to day pours forth speech,

And night to night reveals knowledge.

There is no speech, nor are there words;

Their voice is not heard.

read more.

Psalm 148:3-5

Praise Him, sun and moon;

Praise Him, all stars of light!

Praise Him, highest heavens,

And the waters that are above the heavens!

Let them praise the name of the Lord,

For He commanded and they were created.

Jeremiah 31:35-36

Thus says the Lord,

Who gives the sun for light by day

And the fixed order of the moon and the stars for light by night,

Who stirs up the sea so that its waves roar;

The Lord of hosts is His name:

"If this fixed order departs

From before Me," declares the Lord,

"Then the offspring of Israel also will cease

From being a nation before Me forever."

Habakkuk 3:11

Verse Concepts

Sun and moon stood in their places;

They went away at the light of Your arrows,

At the radiance of Your gleaming spear.

Luke 1:78-79

Because of the tender mercy of our God,

With which the Sunrise from on high will visit us,

To shine upon those who sit in darkness and the shadow of death,

To guide our feet into the way of peace."

Psalm 84:11

Verse Concepts

For the Lord God is a sun and shield;

The Lord gives grace and glory;

No good thing does He withhold from those who walk uprightly.

Isaiah 9:2

Verse Concepts

The people who walk in darkness

Will see a great light;

Those who live in a dark land,

The light will shine on them.

Habakkuk 3:4

Verse Concepts

His radiance is like the sunlight;

He has rays flashing from His hand,

And there is the hiding of His power.

Matthew 17:2

Verse Concepts

And He was transfigured before them; and His face shone like the sun, and His garments became as white as light.

2 Corinthians 4:6

Verse Concepts

For God, who said, "Light shall shine out of darkness," is the One who has shone in our hearts to give the Light of the knowledge of the glory of God in the face of Christ.

Revelation 1:16

Verse Concepts

In His right hand He held seven stars, and out of His mouth came a sharp two-edged sword; and His face was like the sun shining in its strength.

Revelation 21:23

Verse Concepts

And the city has no need of the sun or of the moon to shine on it, for the glory of God has illumined it, and its lamp is the Lamb.

Isaiah 24:23

Verse Concepts

Then the moon will be abashed and the sun ashamed,

For the Lord of hosts will reign on Mount Zion and in Jerusalem,

And His glory will be before His elders.

Isaiah 60:19-20

"No longer will you have the sun for light by day,

Nor for brightness will the moon give you light;

But you will have the Lord for an everlasting light,

And your God for your glory.

"Your sun will no longer set,

Nor will your moon wane;

For you will have the Lord for an everlasting light,

And the days of your mourning will be over.

Revelation 22:5

Verse Concepts

And there will no longer be any night; and they will not have need of the light of a lamp nor the light of the sun, because the Lord God will illumine them; and they will reign forever and ever.

Psalm 37:6

Verse Concepts

He will bring forth your righteousness as the light

And your judgment as the noonday.

Matthew 13:43

Verse Concepts

Then the righteous will shine forth as the sun in the kingdom of their Father. He who has ears, let him hear.

2 Samuel 23:3-4

"The God of Israel said,

The Rock of Israel spoke to me,

'He who rules over men righteously,

Who rules in the fear of God,

Is as the light of the morning when the sun rises,

A morning without clouds,

When the tender grass springs out of the earth,

Through sunshine after rain.'

Proverbs 4:18

Verse Concepts

But the path of the righteous is like the light of dawn,

That shines brighter and brighter until the full day.

Isaiah 58:8-10

“Then your light will break out like the dawn,

And your recovery will speedily spring forth;

And your righteousness will go before you;

The glory of the Lord will be your rear guard.

“Then you will call, and the Lord will answer;

You will cry, and He will say, ‘Here I am.’

If you remove the yoke from your midst,

The pointing of the finger and speaking wickedness,

And if you give yourself to the hungry

And satisfy the desire of the afflicted,

Then your light will rise in darkness

And your gloom will become like midday.

Isaiah 62:1

Verse Concepts

For Zion’s sake I will not keep silent,

And for Jerusalem’s sake I will not keep quiet,

Until her righteousness goes forth like brightness,

And her salvation like a torch that is burning.

Daniel 12:3

Verse Concepts

Those who have insight will shine brightly like the brightness of the expanse of heaven, and those who lead the many to righteousness, like the stars forever and ever.

Hosea 6:3

Verse Concepts

"So let us know, let us press on to know the Lord.

His going forth is as certain as the dawn;

And He will come to us like the rain,

Like the spring rain watering the earth."

Psalm 72:5-17

Let them fear You while the sun endures,

And as long as the moon, throughout all generations.

May he come down like rain upon the mown grass,

Like showers that water the earth.

In his days may the righteous flourish,

And abundance of peace till the moon is no more.

read more.

Psalm 89:36

Verse Concepts

"His descendants shall endure forever

And his throne as the sun before Me.

Jeremiah 15:9

Verse Concepts

"She who bore seven sons pines away;

Her breathing is labored.

Her sun has set while it was yet day;

She has been shamed and humiliated.

So I will give over their survivors to the sword

Before their enemies," declares the Lord.

Micah 3:6

Verse Concepts

Therefore it will be night for you—without vision,

And darkness for you—without divination.

The sun will go down on the prophets,

And the day will become dark over them.

Ramsis Ghaly

The True Spring of My life!

The Spring and Flowers in Photos!!! A Journey to Search for thy Spring!
Written on 3/26/2022 by Ramsis Ghaly

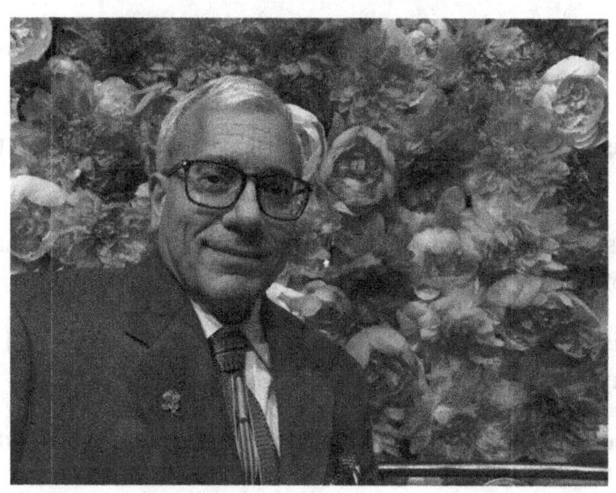

Each human soul is a rising Spring in its own!

That Spring is always full in its eyes and kind in its heart!

That Spring brings peace and comfort!

That Spring rejuvenates thy soul and renew thy energy from day to day!

The Spring in thy gives nourishment to the soul and water to thy thirst!

That Spring of thy life is always shines inward and keep thy going!

That Spring gives that smooth breeze to the turbulent mind!

That Spring is my Life Living and Dreams to my soul!

That Spring overwhelms my soul and overshadow me!

That Spring is the Armour of God and the Breastplate of righteousness !

That Spring is the Loin girt of Truth and Shield of my Faith!

That Spring is the Helmet of Salivation and the flying Eagle of my life!

That Spring is my Pride and Champion at the end of thy day!

That Spring is my Defense in the wars and my Advocate among the multitudes!

That Spring is the that riding on the White horse he that sat upon him was called Faithful and True, and in righteousness he doth judge and make war. [12] His eyes were as a flame of fire, and on his head were many crowns; and he had a name written, that no man knew, but he himself. [13] And he was clothed with a vesture dipped in blood: and his name is called The Word of God." Revelation 19:11-13 KJV

At the end of day, that Spring within thy shepherd quiescence and satisfaction to thy soul!

That Spring is the Garden of my Eden the Heaven of my Life and the Paradise of my Land!

That Spring is the Only Fountain in my life, the True Living Tree and the Owner of the Book of Life!

That Spring is what I always search for, my Purpose, my Goal and my Destiny throughout my lifetime!

I searched deeply and the Spring of my life revealed to my soul and manifested its love to me!

The Spring is that who is saying to my soul living deep in my heart: I am the rose of Sharon, and the lily of the valleys!

That is my Spring: the lily among thorns, so is my love among the daughters!

The Spring is that written: the apple tree among the trees of the wood, so is my beloved among the sons. I sat down under his shadow with great delight, and his fruit was sweet to my taste!

The Spring is that written: the flowers appear on the earth; the time of the singing of birds is come, and the voice of the turtle is heard in our land!

The Spring is that written: The fig tree putteth forth her green figs, and the vines with the tender grape give a good smell. Arise, my love, my fair one, and come away!

The Spring is that written: O my dove, that art in the clefts of the rock, in the secret places of the stairs, let me see thy countenance, let me hear thy voice; for sweet is thy voice, and thy countenance is comely!

My Spring the True Resurrection of my Soul!

Indeed I finally realized there is a spring of its own at each day living in a human soul!

As there is a Rose in each day living of a human soul!

I wonder if each human soul is aware of that Spring and that Rose at each day living!!!!

Perhaps if I just make announcement to the world of turmoil to look each day of living for that Spring and that Rose !

It is that hope that keeps thy going each day of living until thy enters to the Everlasting Spring and to Rose of Sharon!!

Indeed, now I know that spring is my Beloved the Almighty Rose of Sharon!!

My Spring is my Love! My beloved is mine, and I am his: he feedeth among the lilies!!

"I am the rose of Sharon, and the lily of the valleys. [2] As the lily among thorns, so is my love among the daughters. [3] As the apple tree among the trees of the wood, so is my beloved among the sons. I sat down under his shadow with great delight, and his fruit was sweet to my taste. [8] The voice of my beloved! behold, he cometh leaping upon the mountains, skipping upon the hills. [9] My beloved is like a roe or a young hart: behold, he standeth behind our wall, he looketh forth at the windows, shewing himself through the lattice. [10] My beloved spake, and said unto me, Rise up, my love, my fair one, and come away. [12] The flowers appear on the earth; the time of the singing of birds is come, and the voice of the turtle is heard in our land; [13] The fig tree putteth forth her green figs, and the vines with the tender grape give a good smell. Arise, my love, my fair one, and come away. [14] O my dove, that art in the clefts of the rock, in the secret places of the stairs, let me see thy countenance, let me hear thy voice; for sweet is thy voice, and thy countenance is comely. [16] My beloved is mine, and I am his: he feedeth among the lilies." Song of Songs 2:1-3,8-10,12-14,16 KJV

"Finally, my brethren, be strong in the Lord, and in the power of his might. [11] Put on the whole armour of God, that ye may be able to stand against the wiles of the devil. [12] For we wrestle not against flesh and blood, but against principalities, against powers, against the rulers of the darkness of this world, against spiritual wickedness in high places. [13] Wherefore take unto you the whole armour of God, that ye may be able to withstand in the evil day, and having done all, to stand. [14] Stand therefore, having your loins girt about with truth, and having on the breastplate of righteousness; [15] And your feet shod with the preparation of the gospel of peace; [16] Above all, taking the shield of faith, wherewith ye shall be able to quench all the fiery darts of the wicked. [17] And take the helmet of salvation, and the sword of the Spirit, which is the word of God: [18] Praying always with all prayer and supplication in the Spirit, and watching thereunto with all perseverance and supplication for all saints;"Ephesians 6:10-18 KJV

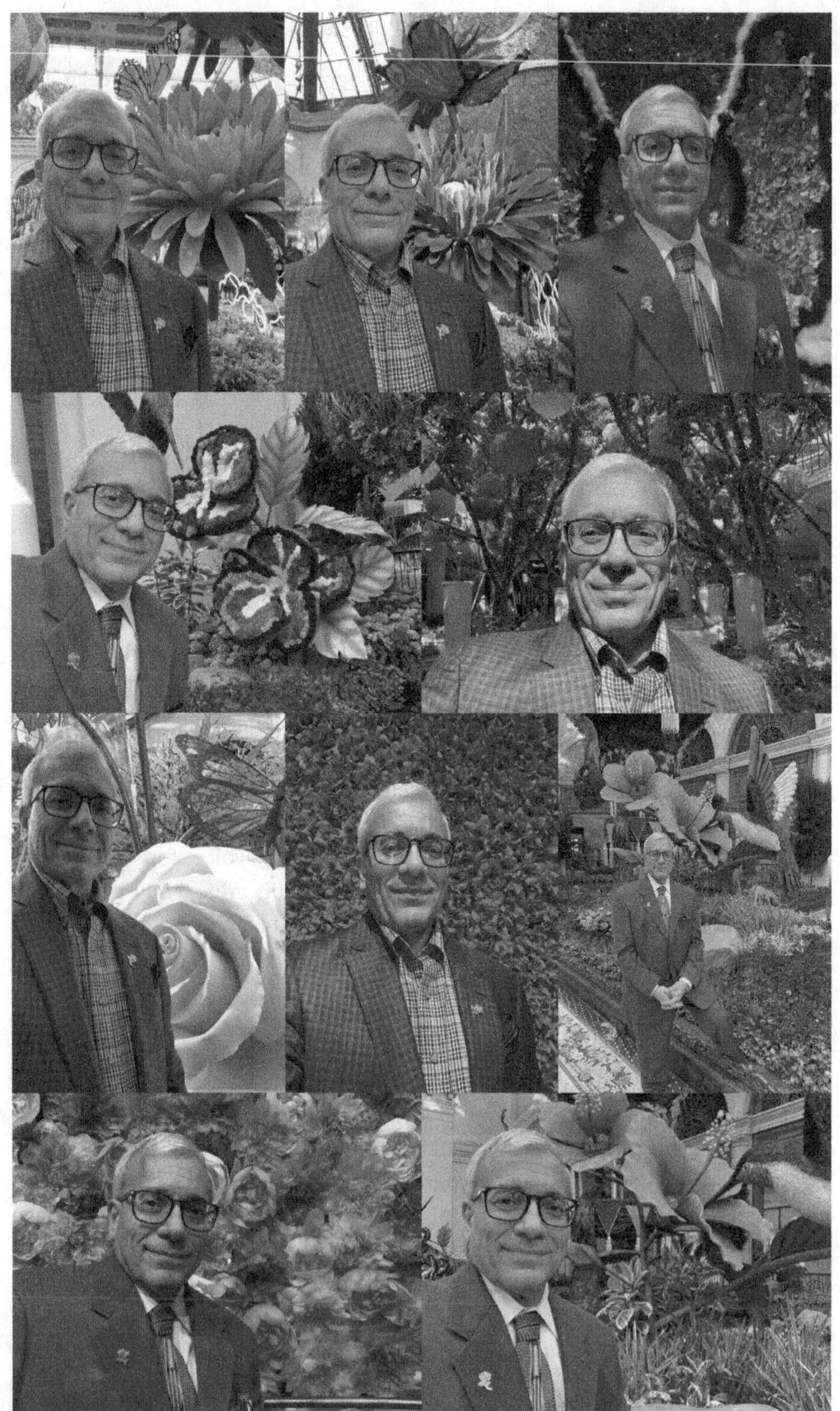

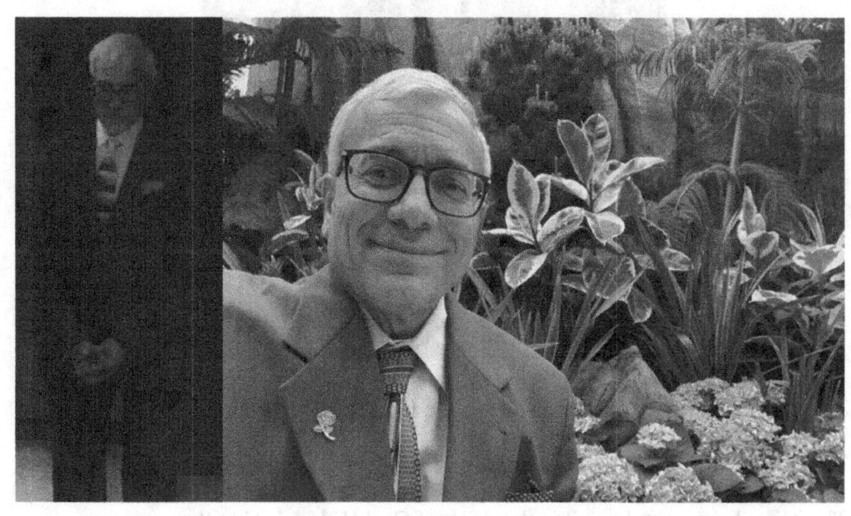

God Hidden's Hand! And so His Child!

Ramsis Ghaly

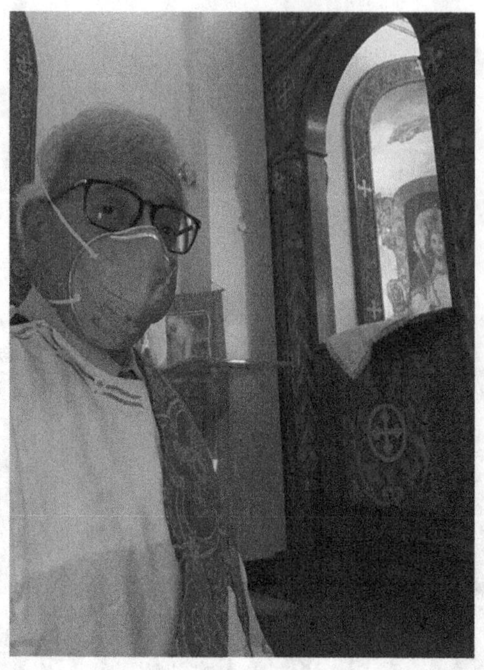

The goodness a man does, it is due to the God Hidden's Hand!

The good work a man does, it is a result of the God's Hidden Hand!

The miracles a man does, it is the work of God Hidden's Hand!

The magic supernatural service, a man does, it is from the God Hidden's Hand!

The Light shining from a man, it is due to the God Hidden's Hand!

The righteousness oddly a man, it is due to the God Hidden's Hand!

The glory of a man, it is due to the God Hidden's Hand!

The life eternity of a man, it is due to the God Hidden's Hand!

The Healing of a man, it is due to the God Hidden's Hand!

And so a righteous man does goodness in silence and hidden from the world eyes!!

A Christian man while he is doing, he is uttering His Lord words: "unprofitable servants: we have done that which was our duty to do" Ax if us written: "So likewise ye, when ye shall have done all those things which are commanded you, say, We are unprofitable servants: we have done that which was our duty to do. "Luke 17:10 KJV

The true servant of the Lord is too silent and hidden, his deeds is buried with him unto the grave but follow him to be revealed at That Day!

"Take heed that ye do not your alms before men, to be seen of them: otherwise ye have no reward of your Father which is in heaven. [2] Therefore when thou doest thine alms, do not sound a trumpet before thee, as the hypocrites do in the synagogues and in the streets, that they may have glory of men. Verily I say unto you, They have their reward. [3] But when thou doest alms, let not thy left hand know what thy right hand doeth: [4] That thine alms may be in secret: and thy Father which seeth in secret himself shall reward thee openly. [5] And when thou prayest, thou shalt not be as the hypocrites are : for they love to pray standing in the synagogues and in the corners of the streets, that they may be seen of men. Verily I say unto you, They have their reward. [6] But thou, when thou prayest, enter into thy closet, and when thou hast shut thy door, pray to thy Father which is in secret; and thy Father which seeth in secret shall reward thee openly. [16] Moreover when ye fast, be not, as the hypocrites, of a sad countenance: for they disfigure their faces, that they may appear unto men to fast. Verily I say unto you, They have their reward. [17] But thou, when thou fastest, anoint thine head, and wash thy face; [18] That thou appear not unto men to fast, but unto thy Father which is in secret: and thy Father, which seeth in secret, shall reward thee openly."Matthew 6:1-6,16-18 KJV

At That Time, nothing shall be secret but all things shall be revealed snd manifest as it is written; "For nothing is secret, that shall not be made manifest; neither any thing hid, that shall not be known and come abroad." Luke 8:17 KJV

Biblical Verses:

Psalm 90:16

Let Your work appear to Your servants

And Your majesty to their children." 2 Peter 1:3 ESV

"His divine power has granted to us all things that pertain to life and godliness, through the knowledge of him who called us to his own glory and excellence," Psalm 107:1-43 ESV

"Oh give thanks to the Lord, for he is good, for his steadfast love endures forever! Let the redeemed of the Lord say so, whom he has redeemed from trouble and gathered in from the lands, from the east and from the west, from the north and from the south. Some wandered in desert wastes, finding no way to a city to dwell in; hungry and thirsty, their soul fainted within them. ..." John 14:13 ESV

"Whatever you ask in my name, this I will do, that the Father may be glorified in the Son." Romans 11:36 ESV

2 Corinthians 10:17-18 KJV "But he that glorieth, let him glory in the Lord. [18] For not he that commendeth himself is approved, but whom the Lord commendeth."

"Every good gift and every perfect gift is from above, and cometh down from the Father of lights, with whom is no variableness, neither shadow of turning." James 1:17, KJV

"Therefore let no man glory in men. For all things are yours;" 1 Corinthians 3:21, KJV

"For from him and through him and to him are all things. To him be glory forever. Amen.

DN, Amen

JT, amen...God has blessed your hands!

RC, Good is a manifestation of well done things like you do

AV, Amen & God continue to Bless your hands!

CG, Amen! Gods hands hold our problems and let's feel at peace.

JM, AMEN

Life Back to Normal Without Mask! Transitioning Slowly But Surely!

Written on 10/16/2022 by Ramsis Ghaly

Life Back to Normal Without Mask! Transitioning Slowly But Surely!

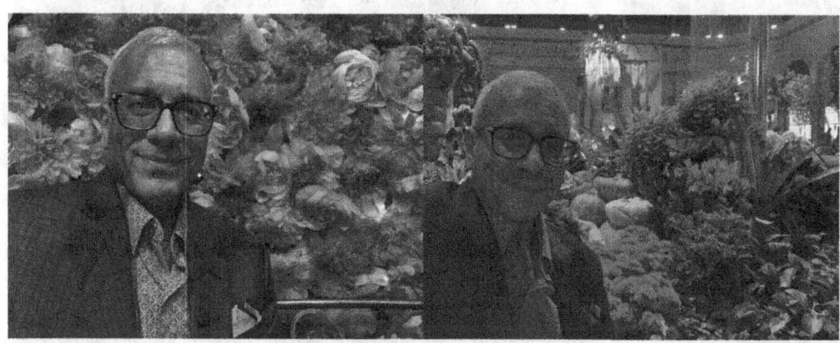

It isn't an easy decision to remove the facemask. There are still many doubts that COVID is truly gone. But I started slowly to take mask off id no much of crowd or sickness around, keep good ventilation and watch the surrounding!!

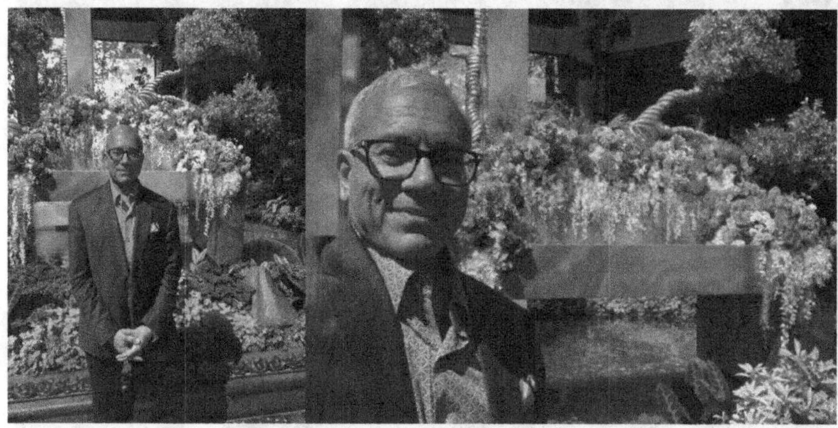

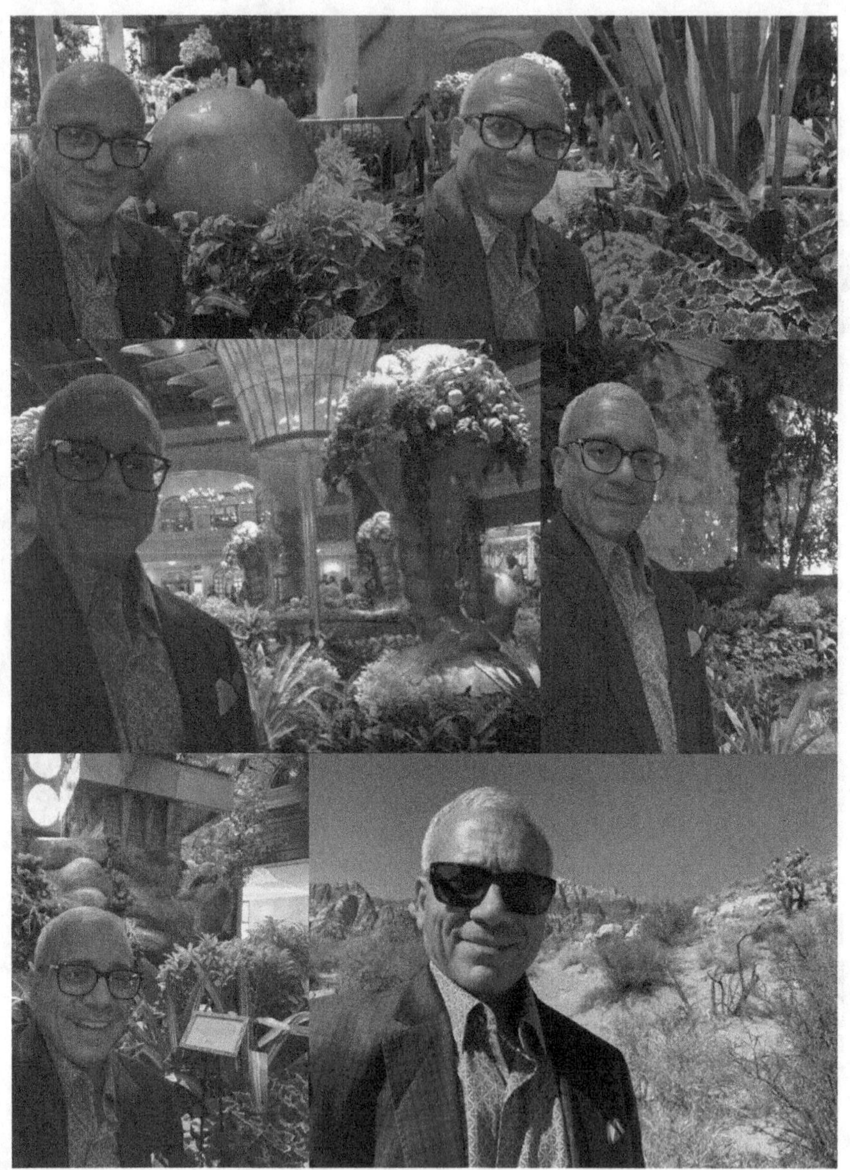

What a Nobility Other than to give while in dire need!!

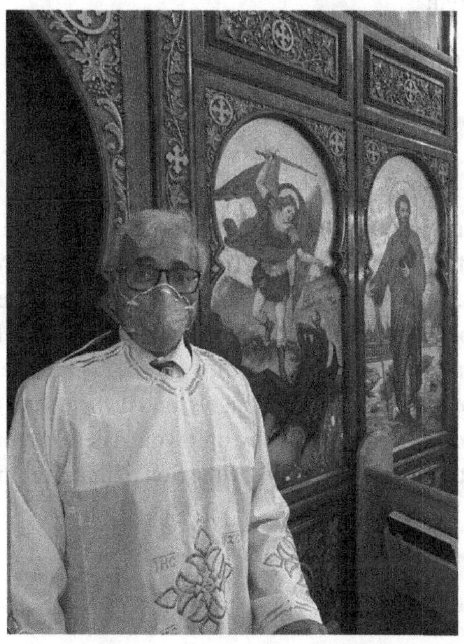

What a Nobility Other than to give while in dire need!! Or even to be perfect to give all what you have to the poor and follow the Savior as it is written: "Jesus said unto him, If thou wilt be perfect, go and sell that thou hast, and give to the poor, and thou shalt have treasure in heaven: and come and follow me."

What a Nobility other than to give while in dire need!!

It is when someone is in dire need, yet he gives from his own!

To help while in need of help!

To give while in need! As the biblical lady that gave all what she had: "And he called unto him his disciples, and saith unto them, Verily I say unto you, That this poor widow hath cast more in, than all they which have cast into the treasury: [44] For all they did cast in of their abundance; but she of her want did cast in all that she had, even all her living." Mark 12:43-44 KJV

To forgive while hanged on the Cross! As our Savior: "Then said Jesus, Father, forgive them; for they know not what they do. And they parted his raiment, and cast lots."

To restore life while dying! As our God and Savior: "And Jesus said unto him, Verily I say unto thee, To day shalt thou be with me in paradise." Luke 23:43 KJV

To heal while sick!

To do while impaired!

To comfort while in pain!

To deny while

Matthew 16:24-28 KJV

[24] Then said Jesus unto his disciples, If any man will come after me, let him deny himself, and take up his cross, and follow me. [25] For whosoever will save his life shall lose it: and whosoever will lose his life for my sake shall find it. [26] For what is a man profited, if he shall gain the whole world, and lose his own soul? or what shall a man give in exchange for his soul? [27] For the Son of man shall come in the glory of his Father with his angels; and then he shall reward every man according to his works. [28] Verily I say unto you, There be some standing here, which shall not taste of death, till they see the Son of man coming in his kingdom.

My Lord and Father

Long ago There were three crucified One was risen and two others didn't!

Dedicated to Our Savior in the Memory of His Passion Week and Resurrection!!
Written by Ramsis Ghaly

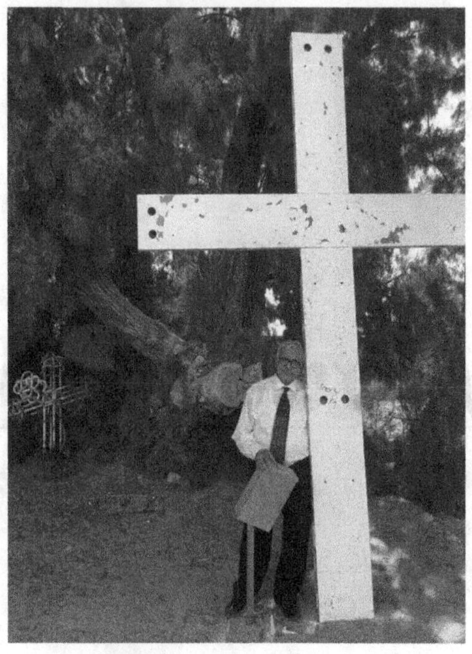

At the dawn of Sunday morning before the sun rise while so many were asleep, I visited that site

I stood in fear and trembling, yet my mind was drifted to the events occurred long ago!!

I kissed the cross and tears ran out of my eyes like rivers! I worshiped to the One hanged in the cross and bowed on my knees praying! I hugged the Cross and the memories raced unto my head as my soul began to meditate as follows:

+ Long ago, There were three Crosses, One gives life eternity and the two others bring death and damnation!

+ Long ago, There were three Crosses, One gives life eternity and the two others bring death and damnation! Centuries later, No one could find the crosses but

Queen Helena. A long Journey she took and her people. The Cross that raised the dead was the One. That One Cross was the one that heals all people and sabe all lives. That One is Holy and Divine and the Son of Good was crucified upon it. Because of that One. The entire world was redeemed and the heavens were open again. Through that One the earth was reconciled with the heaven where Justice and mercy were met at that One in that Moment!!

+ Long ago, There were three Crosses, One had the Promise of the Heavenly Father as follows: Fear not, little flock; for it is your Father's good pleasure to give you the kingdom. [33] Sell that ye have, and give alms; provide yourselves bags which wax not old, a treasure in the heavens that faileth not, where no thief approacheth, neither moth corrupteth. [34] For where your treasure is, there will your heart be also. [35] Let your loins be girded about, and your lights burning;" while the other two have none! Luke 12:32-35 KJV

+ Long ago, There were three hanged upon the cross that Friday very long ago, One performed all kind of miracles and raised the dead and the two others didn't!

+ Long ago, There were three hanged upon the cross that Friday very long ago, One died because of Love and the other two didn't!

+ Long ago, There were Three crucified outside the city before all people humiliated and murdered, One volunteered as a result of His unconditional Love and the two others hanged because of their crimes!

+ Long ago, There were three hanged upon the cross Friday's very long ago, One Lay down His Life to save the world from their sins and other two didn't!

+ Long ago, There were three hanged upon the cross that Friday very long ago, One give Himself to rescue His people from the everlasting death and other two didn't!

"For God so loved the world, that he gave his only begotten Son, that whosoever believeth in him should not perish, but have everlasting life." John 3:16 KJV

+ Long ago, There were three hanged upon the cross that Friday very long ago, One died for others and other two didn't!

+ Long ago, There were three hanged upon the cross that Friday very long ago, One died as Ransom for many and other two didn't!

+ Long ago, There were three hanged upon the cross that Friday very long ago, One redeemed His people and the other right benefitted from Him and other left died in his sin!

+ Long ago, There were three hanged upon the cross that Friday very long ago, One Lay down His Life by His own power for the world and other two didn't!

"Therefore doth my Father love me, because I lay down my life, that I might take it again. [18] No man taketh it from me, but I lay it down of myself. I have power to lay it down, and I have power to take it again. This commandment have I received of my Father." John 10:17-18 KJV

+ Long ago, There were three hanged upon the cross Friday very long ago, One died to pay the dues of the sins of the world and other two didn't!

+ Long ago, There were three hanged upon the cross that Friday very long ago and died, One was risen and was and is snd is to come Jesus saith unto him, I am the way, the truth, and the life: no man cometh unto the Father, but by me. [7] If ye had known me, ye should have known my Father also: and from henceforth ye know him, and have seen him." And the two others were dead! John 14:6-7 KJV

+ Long ago, There were Three ordered to be crucified, One was innocent and two were guilt of their sins!

+ Long ago, There were Three ordered to be crucified, One every soul on earth and heaven worship, the other one we adore and the third we ignore!

+ Long ago, There were Three ordered to be crucified, One forgive all sins, the other one intercede for us and the third is no longer remembered!

+ Long ago, There were Three ordered to be crucified, One taught us Love and He loved us first, the second taught us to repent even at the cross sentence and the third taught us what not to be!

+ Long ago, There were Three ordered to be crucified, One invited us to His Father heavenly Kingdom and the two others didn't!

+ Long ago, There were Three indicted with serious crimes and put to death, One for no cause and no wrongdoing and two for their crimes!

+ Long ago, There were Three were accused with sins and weren't acquitted, One falsely and two others deserved sentence!

+ Long ago, There were Three crucified, One was tortured severely and entire city was shaken by His glory in suffering and the other two were quietly sentenced for their deeds!

+ Long ago, There were Three crucified Friday morning, One was dragged in the streets of Jerusalem spit upon and beaten up with 41 except one stripes and the other two didn't!

+ Long ago, There were Three sentenced to death is the famous city of the Lord, One was sentenced wrongly by His Own and the other two sentenced by their court!

+ Long ago, There were Three charged of death by crucifix, One received a throne of spikes pierced His head in pains and blood and two others weren't!

"The governor answered and said unto them, Whether of the twain will ye that I release unto you? They said, Barabbas. [22] Pilate saith unto them, What shall I do then with Jesus which is called Christ? They all say unto him, Let him be crucified. [23] And the governor said, Why, what evil hath he done? But they cried out the more, saying, Let him be crucified. [25] Then answered all the people, and said, His blood be on us, and on our children. [26] Then released he Barabbas unto them: and when he had scourged Jesus, he delivered him to be crucified. [27] Then the soldiers of the governor took Jesus into the common hall, and gathered unto him the whole band of soldiers. [28] And they stripped him, and put on him a scarlet robe. [29] And when they had platted a crown of thorns, they put it upon his head, and a reed in his right hand: and they bowed the knee before him, and mocked him, saying, Hail, King of the Jews! [30] And they spit upon him, and took the reed, and smote him on the head. [31] And after that they had mocked him, they took the robe off from him, and put his own raiment on him, and led him away to crucify him. [35] And they crucified him, and parted his garments, casting lots: that it might be fulfilled which was spoken by the prophet, They parted my garments among them, and upon my vesture did they cast lots. [36] And sitting down they watched him there; [37] And set up over his head his accusation written, THIS IS JESUS THE KING OF THE JEWS. [38] Then were there two thieves crucified with him, one on the right hand, and another on the left. [39] And they that passed by reviled him, wagging their heads, [40] And saying, Thou that destroyest the temple, and buildest it in three days, save thyself. If thou be the Son of God, come down from the cross. [41] Likewise also the chief priests mocking him, with the scribes and elders, said, [42] He saved others; himself he cannot save. If he be the King of Israel, let him now come down from the cross, and we will believe him. [43] He trusted in God; let him deliver him now, if he will have him: for he said, I am the Son of God. [44] The thieves also, which were crucified with him, cast the same in his teeth. [45] Now from the sixth hour there was darkness over all the land unto the ninth hour. [46] And about the ninth hour Jesus cried with a loud voice, saying, Eli, Eli, lama sabachthani? that is to say, My God, my God, why hast thou forsaken me? [47] Some of them that stood there, when they heard that, said, This man calleth for Elias. [48] And straightway one of them ran, and took a spunge, and filled it with vinegar, and put it on a reed, and gave him to drink. [49] The rest said, Let be, let us see whether Elias will come to save him. [50] Jesus, when he had cried again with a loud voice, yielded up the ghost. [51] And, behold, the veil of the temple was rent in twain from the top to the bottom; and the earth did quake, and the rocks rent; [52] And the graves were opened; and many bodies of the saints which slept arose, [53] And came out of the graves after his resurrection, and went into the holy city, and appeared unto many."Matthew 27:21-23,25-31,35-53 KJV

+ Long ago, There were Three charged of death by crucifix, One was a tender plant, and the transgressors tortured Him as a root out of a dry ground: He hath no form nor comeliness; and when we shall see him, there is no beauty that we should desire him and the other two weren't!

+ Long ago, There were Three charged of death by crucifix, One was despised and rejected of men; a man of sorrows, and acquainted with grief: and we hid as it were our faces from him; he was despised, and we esteemed him not and the other two weren't!

+ Long ago, There were Three charged of death by crucifix, One was Surely he hath borne our griefs, and carried our sorrows: yet we did esteem him stricken, smitten of God, and afflicted and the other two weren't!

+ Long ago, There were Three charged of death by crucifix, One was wounded for our transgressions, he was bruised for our iniquities: the chastisement of our peace was upon him; and with his stripes we are healed and the other two weren't!

+ Long ago, There were Three charged of death by crucifix, One where the Lord hath laid on him the iniquity of us all and the other two among all like sheep have gone astray; we have turned every one to his own way!!

+ Long ago, There were Three charged of death by crucifix, One was oppressed, and he was afflicted, yet he opened not his mouth: he is brought as a lamb to the slaughter, and as a sheep before her shearers is dumb, so he openeth not his mouth and the other two weren't!

+ Long ago, There were Three charged of death by crucifix, One was taken from prison and from judgment: and who shall declare his generation? for he was cut off out of the land of the living: for the transgression of my people was he stricken and the other two weren't!

+ Long ago, There were Three charged of death by crucifix, One made his grave with the wicked, and with the rich in his death; because he had done no violence, neither was any deceit in his mouth and the other two weren't!

+ Long ago, There were Three charged of death by crucifix, One Yet it pleased the Lord to bruise him; he hath put him to grief: when thou shalt make his soul an offering for sin, he shall see his seed, he shall prolong his days, and the pleasure of the Lord shall prosper in his hand and the two others weren't!

+ Long ago, There were Three charged of death by crucifix, One saw of the travail of his soul, and shall be satisfied: by his knowledge shall my righteous servant justify many; for he shall bear their iniquities and the other two weren't!

+ Long ago, There were Three charged of death by crucifix, One poured out his soul unto death: and he was numbered with the transgressors; and he bare the sin of many, and made intercession for the transgressors and others weren't!

Isaiah 53:2 "For he shall grow up before him as a tender plant, and as a root out of a dry ground: he hath no form nor comeliness; and when we shall see him, there is no beauty that we should desire him. [3] He is despised and rejected of men; a man of sorrows, and acquainted with grief: and we hid as it were our faces from him; he was despised, and we esteemed him not. [4] Surely he hath borne our griefs, and carried our sorrows: yet we did esteem him stricken, smitten of God, and afflicted. [5] But he was wounded for our transgressions, he was bruised for our iniquities: the chastisement of our peace was upon him; and with his stripes we are healed. [6] All we like sheep have gone astray; we have turned every one to his own way; and the Lord hath laid on him the iniquity of us all. [7] He was oppressed, and he was afflicted, yet he opened not his mouth: he is brought as a lamb to the slaughter, and as a sheep before her shearers is dumb, so he openeth not his mouth. [8] He was taken from prison and from judgment: and who shall declare his generation? for he was cut off out of the land of the living: for the transgression of my people was he stricken. [9] And he made his grave with the wicked, and with the rich in his death; because he had done no violence, neither was any deceit in his mouth. [10] Yet it pleased the Lord to bruise him; he hath put him to grief: when thou shalt make his soul an offering for sin, he shall see his seed, he shall prolong his days, and the pleasure of the Lord shall prosper in his hand. [11] He shall see of the travail of his soul, and shall be satisfied: by his knowledge shall my righteous servant justify many; for he shall bear their iniquities. [12] Therefore will I divide him a portion with the great, and he shall divide the spoil with the strong; because he hath poured out his soul unto death: and he was numbered with the transgressors; and he bare the sin of many, and made intercession for the transgressors."

+ Long ago, There were Three hanged on the cross, One a sign was written "The King of the Jews" and the other two didn't!

+ Long ago, There were Three hanged in the tree, One the sun hidden it's face from Him, the Moon shut it's light, the clouds covert the face of the universe and the earth shacked it's foundation and the other two didn't! earth!

+ Long ago, There were Three crucified, One in the middle of the two others, one in the right repented and was saved and the other mocked Him and died forever!

"And when they were come to the place, which is called Calvary, there they crucified him, and the malefactors, one on the right hand, and the other on the left. [35] And the people stood beholding. And the rulers also with them derided him, saying, He saved others; let him save himself, if he be Christ, the chosen of God. [36] And the soldiers also mocked him, coming to him, and offering him vinegar, [37] And saying, If thou be the king of the Jews, save thyself. [38] And a superscription also was written over him in letters of Greek, and Latin, and Hebrew, THIS IS THE KING OF THE JEWS. [44] And it was about the sixth hour, and there was a darkness over all the earth until the ninth hour. [45] And the sun was darkened, and the veil of the temple was rent in the midst."Luke 23:33,35-38,44-45 KJV

+ Long ago, There were three hanged upon a tree, One they didn't break His legs and the other two they did so!

+ Long ago, There were Three sentenced together in one Friday, one was a sacrifice for the world and the two others were thieves deserved death one confessed with sins and believed in the true God before he died and the other didn't!

"And one of the malefactors which were hanged railed on him, saying, If thou be Christ, save thyself and us. [40] But the other answering rebuked him, saying, Dost not thou fear God, seeing thou art in the same condemnation? [41] And we indeed justly; for we receive the due reward of our deeds: but this man hath done nothing amiss. [42] And he said unto Jesus, Lord, remember me when thou comest into thy kingdom. [43] And Jesus said unto him, Verily I say unto thee, To day shalt thou be with me in paradise."Luke 23:39-43 KJV

+ Long ago, There were Three crucified together, One the Holy One comment His soul unto thy Hand of His Father and the other two didn't!

"And when Jesus had cried with a loud voice, he said, Father, into thy hands I commend my spirit: and having said thus, he gave up the ghost."Luke 23:46 KJV

+ Long ago, There were Three crucified together, One died first and the two others followed before the evening according to the Jewish tradition!

+ Long ago, There were Three crucified in that day called Good Friday, One died early and at His death … the veil of the temple was rent y in twain from the top to the bottom; and the earth did quake, and the rocks rent; And the graves were opened; and many bodies of the saints which slept arose, And came out of the graves after his resurrection, and went into the holy city, and appeared unto many. Matthew 27:51-53 KJV

+ Long ago, There were Three crucified, One after His death, the centurion feared Him believed in Him and not of the other two!

"Now when the centurion, and they that were with him, watching Jesus, saw the earthquake, and those things that were done, they feared greatly, saying, Truly this was the Son of God." Matthew 27:54 KJV

+ Long ago, There were three hanged upon the cross that Friday very long ago, One was awaken by His own in the third day and two others couldn't and their bodies remained buried!

"And the angel answered and said unto the women, Fear not ye: for I know that ye seek Jesus, which was crucified. [6] He is not here: for he is risen, as he said. Come, see the place where the Lord lay. [7] And go quickly, and tell his disciples that he is risen from the dead; and, behold, he goeth before you into Galilee; there shall ye see him: lo, I have told you."Matthew 28:5-7 KJV

+ Long ago, There were Three sentenced together and crucified in one Friday and died, one was The Son of God and the two others were his creation!

+ Long ago, There were Three sentenced together and crucified in one Friday and died, one was the Creator and His Own didn't know Him and the other two were forever condemned to the second death!

+ Long ago, There were Three sentenced together and crucified in one Friday and died, one was The King of Glory and the other two weren't!

+ Long ago, There were Three sentenced together and crucified in one Friday and died, one was The Lord strong and mighty, the Lord mighty in battle, and the other two weren't!

+ Long ago, There were Three sentenced together and crucified in one Friday and died, One was The Lord of hosts, he is the King of glory. Selah and others two weren't!

"Lift up your heads, O ye gates; and be ye lift up, ye everlasting doors; and the King of glory shall come in. [8] Who is this King of glory? The Lord strong and mighty, the Lord mighty in battle. [9] Lift up your heads, O ye gates; even lift them up, ye everlasting doors; and the King of glory shall come in. [10] Who is this King of glory? The Lord of hosts, he is the King of glory. Selah." Psalm 24:7-10 KJV

+ Long ago, There were Three sentenced together and crucified in one Friday and died, One was risen and no longer here and when they entered seculchre, "they saw a young man sitting on the right side, clothed in a long white garment; b and they were affrighted. c And he saith unto them, Be not affrighted: Ye seek Jesus of

Nazareth, which was crucified: he is risen; he is not here: behold the place where they laid him. But go your way, tell his disciples and Peter that he goeth before you into Galilee: there shall ye see him, as he said unto you. …" and the other two were dead! Mark 16:5-7 KJV

+ Long ago, There were Three sentenced together and crucified in one Friday and died, One was risen and as His disciples went inside His sculpture fearful, the angels -"said unto them, Why seek ye the living among the dead? [6] He is not here, but is risen: remember how he spake unto you when he was yet in Galilee, [7] Saying, The Son of man must be delivered into the hands of sinful men, and be crucified, and the third day rise again." and the other two were dead! Luke 24:5-7 KJV

+ Long ago, There were Three sentenced together and crucified in one Friday and died, One His burial was empty as He was risen in His glory and appeared to His disciple Mary Magdalene "Jesus saith unto her, Woman, why weepest thou? whom seekest thou? She, supposing him to be the gardener, saith unto him, Sir, if thou have borne him hence, tell me where thou hast laid him, and I will take him away. [16] Jesus saith unto her, Mary. She turned herself, and saith unto him, Rabboni; which is to say, Master. [17] Jesus saith unto her, Touch me not; for I am not yet ascended to my Father: but go to my brethren, and say unto them, I ascend unto my Father, and your Father; and to my God, and your God." and other two died! John 20:15-17 KJV

+ Long ago, There were Three sentenced together and crucified in one Friday and died, One rose from the dead and showed His Disciple Thomas His marks "And after eight days again his disciples were within, and Thomas with them: then came Jesus, the doors being shut, and stood in the midst, and said, Peace be unto you. [27] Then saith he to Thomas, Reach hither thy finger, and behold my hands; and reach hither thy hand, and thrust it into my side: and be not faithless, but believing. [28] And Thomas answered and said unto him, My Lord and my God. [29] Jesus saith unto him, Thomas, because thou hast seen me, thou hast believed: blessed are they that have not seen, and yet have believed." And two others died! John 20:26-29 KJV

+ Long ago, There were Three sentenced together and crucified in one Friday and died, One was risen and appeared to His children And as they thus spake, Jesus himself stood in the midst of them, and saith unto them, Peace be unto you. -Why are ye troubled? and why do thoughts n arise in your hearts? [39] Behold my hands and my feet, that it is I myself: handle me, and see; for a spirit hath not flesh and bones, as ye see me have." and the other two were dead! Luke 24: 36, 38-39 KJV

+ Long ago, There were Three sentenced together and crucified in one Friday and died, One conquered the sting of death and became the firstfruit and appeared before His disciples ate with them and taught them all what was written and the promises "And while they yet believed not for joy, and wondered, he said unto them, Have ye here any meat? [42] And they gave him a piece of a broiled fish, and of an honeycomb. [43] And he took it, and did eat before them. [44] And he said unto them, These are the words which I spake unto you, while I was yet with you, that all things must be fulfilled, which were written in the law of Moses, and in the prophets, and in the psalms, concerning me. [46] And said unto them, Thus it is written, and thus it behoved Christ to suffer, and to rise from the dead the third day: [47] And that repentance and remission of sins should be preached in his name among all nations, beginning at Jerusalem. [48] And ye are witnesses of these things. [49] And, behold, I send the promise of my Father upon you: but tarry ye in the city of Jerusalem, until ye be endued with power from on high." and the other two were dead! Luke 24:41-44,46-49 KJV

+ Long ago, There were Three sentenced together and crucified in one Friday and died, One resurrected from death on the third day and spent time with His children and blessed them and "And he led them out as far as to Bethany, and he lifted up his hands, and blessed them. [51] And it came to pass, while he blessed them, he was parted from them, and carried up into heaven. [52] And they worshipped him, and returned to Jerusalem with great joy: [53] And were continually in the temple, praising and blessing God. Amen." and the other two were dead! Luke 24:50-53 KJV

+ Long ago, There were three hanged upon the cross that Friday very long ago and died, One rose and appeared to His disciples saying "Be not afraid: go tell my brethren that they go into Galilee, and there shall they see me." And the other two were dead! Matthew 28:10 KJV

+ Long ago, There were three hanged upon the cross that Friday very long ago, One was Jesus Christ the Savior of the world and was dead but alive again came while the doors were closed and spake unto them, saying, All power is given unto me in heaven and in earth. [19] Go ye therefore, and teach all nations, baptizing them in the name of the Father, and of the Son, and of the Holy Ghost: [20] Teaching them to observe all things whatsoever I have commanded you: and, lo, I am with you alway, even unto the end of the world. Amen. And the other two were dead! Matthew 28:18-20 KJV

+ Long ago, There were Three sentenced together and crucified in one Friday and died, One was Jesus the Christ and after His death rose on the third day "And many other signs truly did Jesus in the presence of his disciples, which are not written in this book: [31] But these are written, that ye might believe that Jesus is the Christ, the Son of God; and that believing ye might have life through his name." and other two were dead and remained dead! John 20:30-31 KJV

+ Long ago, There were three hanged upon the cross that Friday very long ago and died, One was Jesus Christ the Savior of the world and was dead but alive again came while the doors were closed and spake unto them, saying, "Go ye into all the world, and preach the gospel to every creature. [16] He that believeth and is baptized shall be saved; but he that believeth not shall be damned. [17] And these signs shall follow them that believe; In my name shall they cast out devils; they shall speak with new tongues; [18] They shall take up serpents; and if they drink any deadly thing, it shall not hurt them; they shall lay hands on the sick, and they shall recover." And the other two were dead! Mark 16:15-18 KJV

Long ago, There were three hanged upon the cross that Friday very long ago and died, One is risen to his Father and fulfilling the promise "In my Father's house are many mansions: if it were not so, I would have told you. I go to prepare a place for you. [3] And if I go and prepare a place for you, I will come again, and receive you unto myself; that where I am, there ye may be also. [4] And whither I go ye know, and the way ye know." And the two others were dead! John 14:2-4 KJV

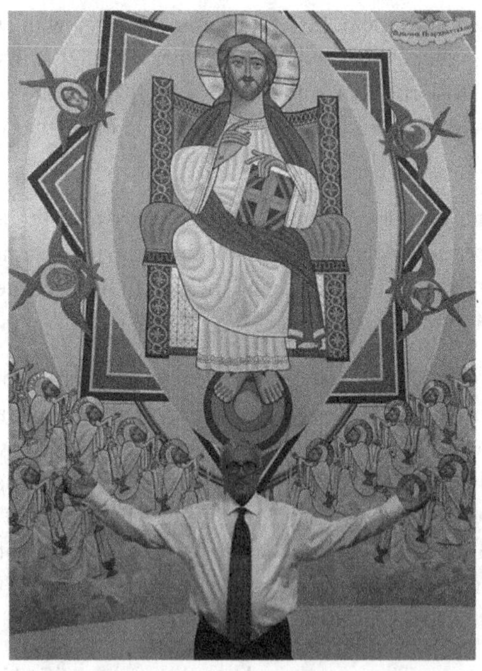

For I have suffered many things this day in a dream because of Him!!

Written On 8/7/2022 by Ramsis Ghaly

At that time, the wife was the only voice whispering the truth and no one listen including the headman at that time and so is in our time!! As an innocent voice calling for the salvation of the world and was murdered by them, so is what the current world doing for that innocent voice calling for their own goodness!

A gorgeous lady the prettiest in her town married to the most powerful man in that city lived at a luxury king's house with so many maids and servants always dressed in the best exuberant dresses putting on the fragrant perfumes and precious stones!!

Everyone envied her for her wealthiness and prettiness, and no one dared to come close to her but only the governor her husband Pontius Pilate!! They worshipped her feet steps and adored her at that time!

At the dawn of that day, she wasn't the same! A highly disturbed soul trembling in fears running away for her life searching by all means in her husband! She saw Lord Jesus in a dream as an innocent angel who stood before the aggressors and accused Him wrongly and was killed by them!! But in the same dream she also saw Him in His second coming as the Son of the Most High and the hell planned for the unrepented aggressors!! She has seen early in her dream the glory of heaven and angelic innocents. However, the dream had ended by the unceasing fires where the lake of brimstone and torture to those liars and all followers Satan!!

An early morning, she ran to her husband who already had departed the house to attend early the court hall! She looked for him so worried and fearful, but he wasn't around! She asked her servants to take her to his office and he was about to start his day!

It turns out that when the morning had come, Pontius Pilate's arose from a horrific dream!!

What the Pontius Pilate's wife had seen all night??

What things she had suffered from that night??

Why had she demanded from her husband, the governor, to Have nothing to do with that just man??

Why she said so as Pontius Pilate the governor sat by the Judgment Seat in the Great Hall to hear the case against the Son of God??

How she was able to let the governor say to the accusers: "Why, what evil hath he done? But they cried out the more, saying, Let him be crucified." Matthew 27:23 KJV

It had to be an unimaginable night an extremely painful experience! A night was full of true terrors and overwhelming nightmares! It must have been an agonizing restless night!

She must have slept so irritable alone in her own bed that was sweaty soaked with blood!

It must be night full of fears and dreams of punishments to injustice! The dream was an honest holy man went through horrific injustice and was murdered! And the entire display of hell and second death in the lake of fire and eternal damnation of Daniel revealed to the Pontius Pilate's wife at that night before her husband sat at the Judgment seat early that morning!!

She arrived at the Judgment Hall dressed in the darkest cloth appeared to her husband with the angriest face with extreme trembling and apprehension gasping her breath sweating profusely with droplets of blood!! And that governor didn't sense and

And yet Pontius Pilate didn't listen and gave in to the accusers fearing his job and statue!!!

Pirate's wife was the last warning toward justice and No One cared to consider!

"When he was set down on the judgment seat, his wife sent unto him, saying, have thou nothing to do with that just man: for I have suffered many things this day in a dream because of him." Matthew 27:19 KJV

The world loved darkness than light as it is written: "And the light shineth in darkness; and the darkness comprehended it not. [10] He was in the world, and the world was made by him, and the world knew him not. [11] He came unto his own, and his own received him not." John 1:5,10-11 KJV

In in fact the world doesn't know the Truth because it's deeds are evil and like the darkness. As st that time, the world didn't receive the truth and so is now!! "And this is the condemnation, that light is come into the world, and men loved darkness rather than light, because their deeds were evil. [20] For every one that doeth evil hateth the light, neither cometh to the light, lest his deeds should be reproved. [21] But he that doeth truth cometh to the light, that his deeds may be made manifest, that they are wrought in God." John 3:19-21 KJV

MR, I appreciate your writing because what you said is the truth and made feel good what you have written and I hope continue success in your professional writing God bless you doctor you are the best friend in Facebook I ever I had because the way you put the words together make feel good

ED, Amen Doctor. Thank you for sharing. The words have deep meaning. God please protect us from the evil in this world

kg, Amen,Dr Ghaly and God Bless you always. You move me to tears with the truth of your words.

God be with you always

Blessings from Egypt

LA, "Then the disciples came to Jesus and asked,, "Why do You speak to the people in parables?"

He replied, "The knowledge of the mysteries of the kingdom of heaven has been given to you, but not to them. Whoever has will be given more, and he will have an abundance. Whoever does not have, even what he has will be taken away from him. This is why I speak to them in parables:

'Though seeing, they do not see; though hearing, they do not hear or understand.' In them the prophecy of Isaiah is fulfilled:

'You will be ever hearing but never understanding; you will be ever seeing but never perceiving. For this people's heart has grown callous; they hardly hear with their ears, and they have closed their eyes. Otherwise they might see with their eyes, hear with their ears, understand with their hearts, and turn, and I would heal them.'"- Matthew 13: 10-15

Some will come to truth desiring,

Some, I'm told, would rather not.

Some will find in Him fulfillment,

Some will simply come to nought.

Some will find this precious treasure

That lay hidden in the field.

Some will find the pearl of wisdom

And will know the Truth revealed.

Some will turn away with Pilate,

Shrug then simply wash their hands.

Some will see true Truth unfolding

In the light of God's Commands*.

Some will see the Cross of Calv'ry

And see nothing really there.

They will take the desert broad way…

Into endless dark despair.

Some will bow before the Maker,

Some will trust in make believe.

Some will find the Grace-Gift given,

Some will choose not to receive.

---

* Before this faith came, we were held in custody under the law, locked up until faith should be revealed.. So the law became our guardian to lead us to Christ, that we might be justified by faith.." - Galatians 3:23

Eloi Eloi lama sabachthani!

"And at the ninth hour Jesus cried with a loud voice, saying, Eloi, Eloi, lama sabachthani? which is, being interpreted, My God, my God, why hast thou forsaken me?" Mark 15:34 KJV

If my Master felt abandoned at the most critical breath of His life saying to His Father, Eloi, Eloi, lama sabachthani? as His own brutally wounded Him unfairly, who am I to complain!

If my Savior cried at the ninth hour while the aggressors mocking Him in public disfigured His body and nailed Him to the cross with no cause spitting at His face cried to His Father saying, Eloi, Eloi, lama sabachthani?, I am nothing and unworthy but to burry my face in the sands!

As I hear those words from my Savior, my soul cries profusely with Him saying, Eloi, Eloi, lama sabachthani?

But who am I but a sinful soul deserve to be cursed and live all my life in sorrows, pains; thorns, thistles, sweats, aches and suffering till I return unto the ground; for out of it wast taken: for dust art, and unto dust shalt return as it is written: "Unto the woman he said, I will greatly multiply thy sorrow and thy conception; in sorrow thou shalt bring forth children; and thy desire shall be to thy husband, and he shall rule over thee. [17] And unto Adam he said, Because thou hast hearkened unto the voice of thy wife, and hast eaten of the tree, of which I commanded thee, saying, Thou shalt not eat of it: cursed is the ground for thy sake; in sorrow shalt thou eat of it all the days of thy life; [18] Thorns also and thistles shall it bring forth to thee; and thou shalt eat the herb of the field; [19] In the sweat of thy face shalt thou eat bread, till thou return unto the ground; for out of it wast thou taken: for dust thou art, and unto dust shalt thou return." Genesis 3:16-19 KJV

The life living wasn't meant to be all joy, murry and laugh! Indeed, I often mediate as the first sound of a newborn is a sudden loud cry while the mother screaming from pains and pushing her soul out of her womb!

In the midst of darkness I looked up to heaven screaming 😱 to my heavenly Father saying, Eloi, Eloi, lama sabachthani

At times of gloominess I can't help it but bow down crying appealing to the Lord of hosts: saying, Eloi, Eloi, lama sabachthani

To the victimized souls and those accused of wrong-doing, look up to Heaven raising you arms and hearts crying to the Lord of hosts: saying, Eloi, Eloi, lama sabachthani

A man's journey is full of hardships, betrayals, injustice and sweating

It isn't far to view a human life on earth as a curse sojourning

A man does to his fellow man evil destruction, the innocent man has no help but to scream to the Lord of mercy saying, Eloi, Eloi, lama sabachthani

A life where injustice is overwhelming and the innocent voices are buried and the malicious stronger among them eat the vulnerable souls alive as multitudes of crying sheep day and night screaming in one voice to their Heavenly Father saying, Eloi, Eloi, lama sabachthani

The children of Bethlehem land of Judas are slaughtered two years old and younger by the swords of the coward Herods of the world and those innocent little angels have no one to go to but their Heavenly Father saying, Eloi, Eloi, lama sabachthani As it is written: "Then Herod, when he saw that he was mocked of the wise men, was exceeding wroth, and sent forth, and slew all the children that were in Bethlehem, and in all the coasts thereof, from two years old and under, according to the time which he had diligently enquired of the wise men. [17] Then was fulfilled that which was spoken by Jeremy the prophet, saying, [18] In Rama was there a voice heard, lamentation, and weeping, and great mourning, Rachel weeping for her children, and would not be comforted, because they are not." Matthew 2:16-18 KJV

Indeed the lamentations of the victims ascending up from all the corners of the earth up to the Heavenly Father screaming with loud voice day and night since the foundation of the world till its end saying the words of Jermiah the prophet: "there a voice heard, lamentation, and weeping, and great mourning, Rachel weeping for her children, and would not be comforted, because they are not"

My Heavenly Father descended to my soul comforting my heart holding my hand saying with a soft voice to those innocent souls crying to Him saying, Eloi, Eloi, lama sabachthani, O My Love daughter of Jerusalem I am sick of love ♡ come to Me: "I charge you, O daughters of Jerusalem, if ye find my beloved, that ye tell him, that I am sick of love." Song of Songs 5:8 KJV "I am my beloved's, and his desire is toward me. [11] Come, my beloved, let us go forth into the field; let us lodge in the villages. [12] Let us get up early to the vineyards; let us see if the vine flourish, whether the tender grape appear, and the pomegranates bud forth: there will I give thee my loves."Song of Songs 7:10-12 KJV

To every crying soul of injustice and false witness crying to the Lord saying, Eloi, Eloi, lama sabachthani, a day soon is coming to hear the Heavenly Father and His hosts; "Gracious is the Lord, and righteous; yea, our God is merciful. [6] The Lord preserveth the simple: I was brought low, and he helped me. [7] Return unto thy rest, O my soul; for the Lord hath dealt bountifully with thee. [8] For thou hast delivered my soul from death, mine eyes from tears, and my feet from falling. [9] I will walk before the Lord in the land of the living. [10] I believed, therefore have I spoken: I was greatly afflicted:" Psalm 116:5-10 KJV

To the crying souls saying, Eloi, Eloi, lama sabachthani, whether living or dying, they are unto the Lord:"For none of us liveth to himself, and no man dieth to himself. [8] For whether we live, we live unto the Lord; and whether we die, we die unto the Lord: whether we live therefore, or die, we are the Lord's. [9] For to this end Christ both died, and rose, and revived, that he might be Lord both of the dead and living." Romans 14:7-9 KJV

As the crying souls at the cross patiently to the end saying, Eloi, Eloi, lama sabachthani, a crown of life is waiting for the; "For I am now ready to be offered, and the time of my departure is at hand. [7] I have fought a good fight, I have finished my course, I have kept the faith: [8] Henceforth there is laid up for me a crown of righteousness, which the Lord, the righteous judge, shall give me at that day: and not to me only, but unto all them also that love his appearing." 2 Timothy 4:6-8 KJV

To the crying souls at the cross saying, Eloi, Eloi, lama sabachthani, let not be troubled "Let not your heart be troubled: ye believe in God, believe also in me. [2] In my Father's house are many mansions: if it were not so, I would have told you. I go to prepare a place for you. [3] And if I go and prepare a place for you, I will come again, and receive you unto myself; that where I am, there ye may be also." John 14:1-3 KJV

To each crying soul appealing to the Heavenly Father saying saying, Eloi, Eloi, lama sabachthani, the Lord is thee Shephard coming to lead thee to the green pasture beside the still waters comfort anoint thee head with oil and thee shall dwell in the House of the Lord for ever: "The Lord is my shepherd; I shall not want. [2] He maketh me to lie down in green pastures: he leadeth me beside the still waters. [3] He restoreth my soul: he leadeth me in the paths of righteousness for his name's sake. [4] Yea, though I walk through the valley of the shadow of death, I will fear no evil: for thou art with me; thy rod and thy staff they comfort me. [5] Thou preparest a table before me in the presence of mine enemies: thou anointest my head with oil; my cup runneth over. [6] Surely goodness and mercy shall follow me all the days of my life: and I will dwell in the house of the Lord for ever." Psalm 23:1-6 KJV

To those crying at the cross screaming saying, Eloi, Eloi, lama sabachthani, Jesus our Savior is coming leaping upon the mountains skipping upon the hills: "The voice of my beloved! behold, he cometh leaping upon the mountains, skipping upon the hills. [14] O my dove, that art in the clefts of the rock, in the secret places of the stairs, let me see thy countenance, let me hear thy voice; for sweet is thy voice, and thy countenance is comely. [16] My beloved is mine, and I am his: he feedeth among the lilies. [17] Until the day break, and the shadows flee away, turn, my beloved, and be thou like a roe or a young hart upon the mountains of Bether." Song of Songs 2:8,14,16-17 KJV

To those shedding tears at the ninth hour with our Savior at Cross saying, Eloi, Eloi, lama sabachthani, He is coming in His glory the Lamb is the Eternal light to receive thee: "And I saw no temple therein: for the Lord God Almighty and the Lamb are the temple of it. [23] And the city had no need of the sun, neither of the moon, to shine in it: for the glory of God did lighten it, and the Lamb is the light thereof." Revelation 21:22-23 KJV

Indeed, O My human Soul:
After Labor Pains and Screams, there is a joy with a Newborn Baby!
After Eloi, Eloi, lama sabachthan, Heavenly rest for the soul!
After the Cross there is Glory!
After Death there is Eternal Life!
After Loss of life there is Gain of the soul!
After Defeat, there is heavenly Triumph!
After the Good Fight, there is a Crown of Righteousness from the Righteous Judge!
After Injustice, there is heavenly Justice!
To every Herod, there is Almighty God!
To every Goliath, there is blessed David!
To every Sheep, there is a Good Shepherd!
To every fruitful Branch; there is a Vine and a Vinedresser!

"And God shall wipe away all tears from their eyes; and there shall be no more death, neither sorrow, nor crying, neither shall there be any more pain: for the former things are passed away. [6] And he said unto me, It is done. I am Alpha and Omega, the beginning and the end. I will give unto him that is athirst of the fountain of the water of life freely. [7] He that overcometh shall inherit all things; and I will be his God, and he shall be my son." Revelation 21:4,6-7 KJV

"Behold, I come quickly: blessed is he that keepeth the sayings of the prophecy of this book. [12] And, behold, I come quickly; and my reward is with me, to give every man according as his work shall be. [13] I am Alpha and Omega, the beginning and the end, the first and the last. [14] Blessed are they that do his commandments, that they may have right to the tree of life, and may enter in through the gates into the city. [20] He which testifieth these things saith, Surely I come quickly. Amen. Even so, come, Lord Jesus." Revelation 22:7,12-14,20 KJV

Amen Jesus Come

The Lance of Longinus The Holy Spear of Destiny!

Reflection Written by Ramsis Ghaly

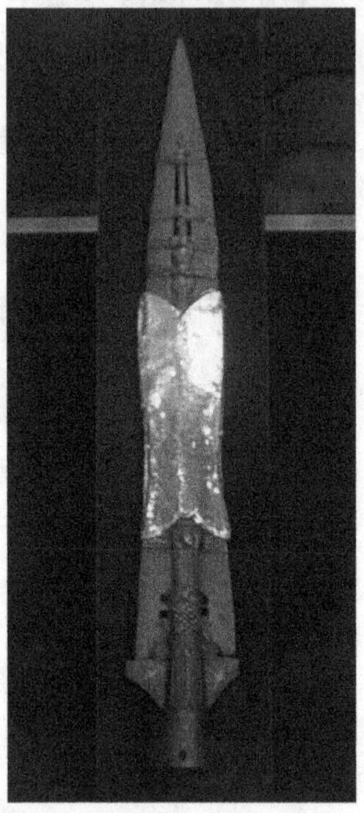

Whoever Find That Lance of Glory, shall Conquer in faith and Nothing stand before thee. The Spear caused pouring of the Most precious Blood and Waters from God Almighty the Lord of Life renal the source of Life in the final the moments of Jesus Christ in the Flesh!

"One of the soldiers pierced his side with a lance (λόγχη), and immediately there came out blood and water." John 29:34

The Spear of Longinus is Dark but Lovely Black but comely! It was so dark and brutal and meant to kill my Lord, yet it was lovely and comely as it was stopped by the Love of God: "I am black, but comely, O ye daughters of Jerusalem, as the tents of Kedar, as the curtains of Solomon." Song of Songs 1:5 KJV I am dark, but lovely, O daughters of Jerusalem, Like the tents of Kedar, Like the curtains of Solomon."

It is the love and mercy of my Beloved! He is mine and I am His: "I am my beloved's, and my beloved is mine: he feedeth among the lilies. [4] Thou art beautiful, O my love, as Tirzah, comely as Jerusalem, terrible as an army with banners. [5] Turn away thine eyes from me, for they have overcome me: thy hair is as a flock of goats that appear from Gilead." Song of Songs 6:3-5 KJV

Draw me and we will run after thee: the King has brought me unto His chamber: "Draw me, we will run after thee: the king hath brought me into his chambers: we will be glad and rejoice in thee, we will remember thy love more than wine: the upright love thee." Song of Songs 1:4 KJV

"For God so loved the world, that he gave his only begotten Son, that whosoever believeth in him should not perish, but have everlasting life. [17] For God sent not his Son into the world to condemn the world; but that the world through him might be saved. [18] He that believeth on him is not condemned: but he that believeth not is condemned already, because he hath not believed in the name of the only begotten Son of God." John 3:16-18 KJV

With the Lance at His side pouring Blood and waters, His Love overcome me! It is the Love of my Beloved to me: "I am my beloved's, and my beloved is mine: he feedeth among the lilies. [4] Thou art beautiful, O my love, as Tirzah, comely as Jerusalem, terrible as an army with banners. [5] Turn away thine eyes from me, for they have overcome me: thy hair is as a flock of goats that appear from Gilead." Song of Songs 6:3-5 KJV

From the hand of a strong Roman soldier, it flew so high to target the core of God of Love ! That spear lodged unto the side of Life, the Living Tree, the Fountain of spring waters, the Shore of Peace, the Good Ground of Righteousness, the Core of humility, the Center of Reconciliation, the Intersection between Just and Mercy, the Side of Forgiveness, the True God of Salvation and the Destiny to Life Eternity!!

That Spear made by evil man to kill, Yet the Divine Love made it the Spear of Salvation, the Core of Divine Love, the Mystery of Incarnation!

Whenever the Sharpe Lance touches Love, it brings up Life and gives out waters and blood !

The Spear of Destiny is a Testimonial of The Two-in-One: The Divinity and Humanity and The Two Natures in One: The Divine Nature and the Human Nature! While Jesus was bleeding to death and nailed to the Cross, The Everlasting Divinity never ever departed His Humanity made Him an Eternal Sacrifice before the Heavenly Father in the behalf of all people as the Everlasting Redemption of sins!

The Spear of Destiny is the certain mark of reconciliation where it took away the human aggression and transformed it Sacrifice of Love !

The Spear of Destiny is the Sure Sign of complete acceptance of the Heavenly Justice to the new man and to the First Fruit of the New Testament through the Holy Lamb of God!

As the Spear flew to pierce the side of the Savior of the World, Our God and Lord, Jesus Christ, it poured Love from the Son of Man, living waters from the True God in the Flesh! A Divine Love out of Love poured Blood and forever the last Sign in the Cross of the Everlasting Love !

Although the Spear was meant to kill and it was coming out of extreme hate, yet once it was intercepted by the Divine Love, It grinded the gate and melted away the aggression of human race and sanctified to Love and Forgiveness!

Even to the last breath, the aggressors didn't stop torturing our Lord and as it penetrates painfully to shatter the organs of the Savior of the world, and it met with absolute mercy and Love from the Holy Lamb of God!

It is the spear that the Roman soldier pierced with Jesus side and came blood and water after Jesus gave up the ghost in the cross for the world as it is written: "But when they came to Jesus, and saw that he was dead already, they brake not his legs: [34] But one of the soldiers with a spear pierced his side, and forthwith came there out blood and water." John 19:33-34 KJV

The Holy Lance, also known as the Lance of Longinus, (named after Saint Longinus), the Spear of Destiny, or the Holy Spear, is the lance that pierced the side of Jesus as he hung on the cross during his crucifixion! The name of the soldier who pierced Christ's side with a lonchē is identified as a centurion and called Longinus (making the spear's Latin name Lancea Longini)

Jesus Wounds

+ Crown of Thorns: "They stripped him and put a scarlet robe on him, and twisting together a crown of thorns, they put it on his head and put a reed in his right hand. And kneeling before him, they mocked him, saying, "Hail, King of the Jews!" And they spit on him and took the reed and struck him on the head. (Matt 27:28-30, ESV)

+ Stripes and smites to the face and the entire flesh: "Then did they spit in his face and buffeted him; and others smote him with the palms of their hands," Matthew 26:67 KJV "And they stripped him, and put on him a scarlet robe. [30] And they spit upon him, and took the reed, and smote him on the head. [31] And after that they had mocked him, they took the robe off from him, and put his own raiment on him, and led him away to crucify him." Matthew 27:28,30-31 KJV

+ Nails in His Hands and Feet: "And when they came to the place that is called The Skull, there they crucified him, and the criminals, one on his right and one on his left." (Luke 23:33, ESV)

+ Pierced Side: "But when they came to Jesus and saw that he was already dead, they did not break his legs. But one of the soldiers pierced his side with a spear, and at once there came out blood and water." (John 19:33-34, ESV)

+ Pierced Heart and sadness: "And about the ninth hour, Jesus cried out with a loud voice, saying, "Eli, Eli, lema sabachthani?" that is, "My God, my God, why have you forsaken me?" (Matt 27:46, ESV)

Those piercing wounds in the Holy Lamb of God the crown of thorns in the head, the smites, the scourging, the nails in each hand and wrist and each foot and the last The Spear pierced His side, poured out His Soul unto death as He was numbered among transgressors to bare the sin of many and made intercession fur the transgressors as it is written: "He is despised and rejected of men; a man of sorrows, and acquainted with grief: and we hid as it were our faces from him; he was despised, and we esteemed him not. [4] Surely he hath borne our griefs and carried our sorrows: yet we did esteem him stricken, smitten of God, and afflicted. But he was wounded for our transgressions, he was bruised for our iniquities: the chastisement of our peace was upon him; and with his stripes we are healed. [6] All we like sheep have gone astray; we have turned every one to his own way; and the Lord hath laid on him the iniquity of us all. [7] He was oppressed, and he was afflicted, yet he opened not his mouth: he is brought as a lamb to the slaughter, and as a sheep before her shearers is dumb, so he openeth not his mouth. [10] Yet it pleased the Lord to bruise him; he hath put him to grief: when thou shalt make his soul an offering for sin, he shall see his seed, he shall prolong his days, and the pleasure of the Lord shall prosper in his hand. [12] Therefore will I divide him a portion with the great, and he shall divide the spoil with the strong; because he hath poured out his soul unto death: and he was numbered with the transgressors; and he bare the sin of many, and made intercession for the transgressors."Isaiah 53:3-7,10,12 KJV

Jesus wounds are forever the unimaginable Price of Salvation, the True Divine Love and the scars of what man had done to the Son of God!

"But Thomas, one of the twelve, called Didymus, was not with them when Jesus came. [27] Then saith he to Thomas, Reach hither thy finger, and behold my hands; and reach hither thy hand, and thrust it into my side: and be not faithless, but believing. [28] And Thomas answered and said unto him, My Lord and my God. [29] Jesus saith unto him, Thomas, because thou hast seen me, thou hast believed: blessed are they that have not seen, and yet have believed." John 20:24,27-29 KJV

As the nails at the hands of our Savior hands and wrists sign forever so is the spear entry at side of God shall be forever signs of salvation and condemnation! "Ought not Christ to have suffered these things, and to enter into his glory? [38] And he said unto them, Why are ye troubled? and why do thoughts arise in your hearts? [39] Behold my hands and my feet, that it is I myself: handle me, and see; for a spirit hath not flesh and bones, as ye see me have." Luke 24:26,38-39 KJV

Jesus wounds aren't forgotten even at the second Coming in His Glory where He shall Judge the world! "Behold, he cometh with clouds; and every eye shall see him, and they also which pierced him: and all kindreds of the earth shall wail because of him. Even so, Amen. [18] I am he that liveth, and was dead; and, behold, I am alive for evermore, Amen; and have the keys of hell and of death."Revelation 1:7,18 KJV

Colossians 1:20 "and through Him to reconcile all things to Himself, whether things on earth or things in heaven have made peace through the blood of His cross." Later in Colossians 2:14, Paul states, "having canceled the certificate of debt consisting of decrees against us, which was hostile to us; and He has taken it out of the way, having nailed it to the cross."4. Philippians 2:5-8 "In your relationships with one another, have the same mindset as Christ Jesus: 6 Who, being in very nature God, did not consider equality with God something to be used to his own advantage; 7 rather, he made himself nothing by taking the very nature of a servant, being made in human likeness. 8 And being found in appearance as a man, he humbled himself by becoming obedient to death—even death on a cross!"7. 1 Peter 2:24 "He himself bore our sins" in his body on the cross, so that we might die to sins and live for righteousness; "by his wounds you have been healed."22. Romans 5:21 "so that, just as sin reigned in death, so also grace might reign through righteousness to bring eternal life through Jesus Christ our Lord." Romans 4:25 "He was delivered over to death for our sins and was raised to life for our justification." Galatians 6:17 "From now on let no one cause trouble for me, for I bear on my body the brand-marks of Jesus."

"He healeth the broken in heart, and bindeth up their wounds. [5] Great is our Lord, and of great power: his understanding is infinite. [7] Sing unto the Lord with thanksgiving; sing praise upon the harp unto our God: [12] Praise the Lord, O Jerusalem; praise thy God, O Zion."Psalm 147:3,5,7,12 KJV

Historic Remarks about the Lance of Longinus:

Divine Mercy

Divine Compassion

The Blood of Salvation

Baptismal Waters

The emanating Blood and water after death is a miracle as in the First Council of Nicaea, that "Jesus Christ was both true God and true man." The blood symbolizes his humanity, the water his divinity. Saint Faustina Kowalska, a Polish nun whose advocacy and writings led to the establishment of the Divine Mercy devotion, also acknowledged the miraculous nature of the blood and water, explaining that the blood is a symbol of the divine mercy of Christ, while the water is a symbol of His divine compassion and of baptismal waters.

It is done so that they may believe the He is the Savior of the world: John 19:35-37 KJV "And he that saw it bare record, and his record is true: and he knoweth that he saith true, that ye might believe.

For these things were done, that the scripture should be fulfilled, A bone of him shall not be broken. And again, another scripture saith, They shall look on him whom they pierced."

It is the Blood and waters for eternal life —-And this is the record, that God hath given to us eternal life, and this life is in his Son. [12] He that hath the Son hath life; and he that hath not the Son of God hath not life. [13] These things have I written unto you that believe on the name of the Son of God; that ye may know that ye have eternal life,—-

1 John 5:1,4-13,20-21 KJV "Whosoever believeth that Jesus is the Christ is born of God: and everyone that loveth him that begat loveth him also that is begotten of him. [4] For whatsoever is born of God overcometh the world: and this is the victory that overcometh the world, even our faith. [5] Who is he that overcometh the world, but he that believeth that Jesus is the Son of God? [6] This is he that came by water and blood, even Jesus Christ; not by water only, but by water and blood. And it is the Spirit that beareth witness, because the Spirit is truth. [7] For there are three that bear record in heaven, the Father, the Word, and the Holy Ghost: and these three are one. [8] And there are three that bear witness in earth, the Spirit, and the water, and the blood: and these three agree in one. [9] If we receive the witness of men, the witness of God is greater: for this is the witness of God which he hath testified of his Son. [10] He that believeth on the Son of God hath the witness in himself: he that believeth not God hath made him a liar;

because he believeth not the record that God gave of his Son. [11] And this is the record, that God hath given to us eternal life, and this life is in his Son. [12] He that hath the Son hath life; and he that hath not the Son of God hath not life. [13] These things have I written unto you that believe on the name of the Son of God; that ye may know that ye have eternal life, and that ye may believe on the name of the Son of God. [20] And we know that the Son of God is come, and hath given us an understanding, that we may know him that is true, and we are in him that is true, even in his Son Jesus Christ. This is the true God, and eternal life. [21] Little children, keep yourselves from idols. Amen."

The Journey of The Holy Spear of Destiny?

No one knows where is it now??

Vienna, Germany, Rome, —-?

Summary

Holy Lance in Rome beneath the dome of Saint Peter's Basilica,

the Church of the Holy Sepulchre. The alleged presence in Jerusalem

to Constantinople and deposited it in the church of Hagia Sophia, and later to the Church of the Virgin of the Pharos.

The Latin Emperor Baldwin II of Constantinople, who later sold it to Louis IX of France. The point of the lance was then enshrined with the crown of thorns in the Sainte Chapelle in Paris.

During the French Revolution these relics were removed to the Bibliothèque Nationale but the point subsequently disappeared,

Nuremberg Holy Lance in Vienna, in the Imperial Treasury or Weltliche Schatzkammer (lit. Worldly Treasure Room) at the Hofburg Palace in Vienna,

In the tenth century, the Holy Roman Emperors came into possession of the lance, In 1000, Otto III gave Bolesław I of Poland a replica of the Holy Lance at the Congress of Gniezno. In 1084, Henry IV had a silver band with the inscription "Nail of Our Lord" added to it. Around 1350, Charles IV had a golden sleeve put over the silver one, inscribed Lancea et clavus Domini (Lance and nail of the Lord). In 1424, Sigismund had a collection of relics, including the lance, moved from his capital in Prague to his birthplace, Nuremberg, and decreed them to be kept there forever. This collection was called the Imperial Regalia. When the French Revolutionary army approached Nuremberg in the spring of 1796, the city councilors decided to remove the Reichskleinodien to Vienna for safe keeping. The collection was entrusted to a Baron von Hügel, who promised to return the objects once the threat was resolved. However, the Holy Roman Empire was disbanded in 1806 and in the confusion, he sold the collection to the Habsburgs.The city councillors asked for the return of the collection after the defeat of Napoleon's army at the Battle of Waterloo, but the Austrian authorities refused. During the Anschluss, when Austria was annexed to Germany, the Nazis brought the Reichskleinodien to Nuremberg, where they displayed them during the September 1938 Party Congress. They then transferred them to the Historischer Kunstbunker, a bunker.

On August 7, 1945 Horn and a U.S. army captain escorted Fries and Schmeiszner to the entrance of the Panier Platz Bunker, where they located the treasures hidden behind a wall of masonry in a small room off of a subterranean corridor, roughly eighty feet below ground.The Regalia were first brought back to Nuremberg castle to be reunited with the rest of the Reichskleinodien, and then transferred with the entire collection to Austrian officials the following January. researchers at the Interdisciplinary Research Institute for Archeology in Vienna used X-ray and other technology to examine a range of lances, and determined that the Vienna lance dates from around the 8th to the beginning of the 9th century, with the nail apparently being of the same metal, and ruled out the possibility of it dating back to the 1st century AD.

Relics

A relic described as the Holy Lance in Rome is preserved beneath the dome of Saint Peter's Basilica, although the Catholic Church makes no claim as to its authenticity. The first historical reference to a lance was made in AD 570 by an unknown pilgrim from Piacenza (often erroneously identified with St. Antoninus of Piacenza)

A lance is mentioned in the so-called Breviarius at the Church of the Holy Sepulchre. n 615, Jerusalem was captured by the Persian forces of King Khosrau II (Chosroes II). According to the Chronicon Paschale, the point of the lance, which had been broken off, was given in the same year to Nicetas, who took it to Constantinople and deposited it in the church of Hagia Sophia, and later to the Church of the Virgin of the Pharos. This point of the lance, which was now set in an icon, was acquired by the Latin Emperor Baldwin II of Constantinople, who later sold it to Louis IX of France. The point of the lance was then enshrined with the crown of thorns in the Sainte Chapelle in Paris. During the French Revolution these relics were removed to the Bibliothèque Nationale but the point subsequently disappeared.

John Mandeville declared in 1357 that he had seen the blade of the Holy Lance both at Paris and at Constantinople, and that the latter was a much larger relic than the former; it is worth adding that Mandeville is not generally regarded as one of the Middle Ages' most reliable witnesses, and his supposed travels are usually treated as an eclectic amalgam of myths, legends and other fictions. "The lance which pierced Our Lord's side" was among the relics at Constantinople shown in the 1430s to Pedro Tafur, who added "God grant that in the overthrow of the Greeks they have not fallen into the hands of the enemies of the Faith, for they will have been ill-treated and handled with little reverence."

Whatever the Constantinople relic was, it did fall into the hands of the Turks, and in 1492, under circumstances minutely described in Pastor's History of the Popes, the Sultan Bayezid II sent it to Pope Innocent VIII to encourage the pope to continue to keep his brother and rival Zizim (Cem Sultan) prisoner. At this time great doubts as to its authenticity were felt at Rome, as Johann Burchard records,[9] because of the presence of other rival lances in Paris (the point that had been separated from the lance), Nuremberg (see Holy Lance in Vienna below), and Armenia (see Holy Lance in Echmiadzin below). In the mid-18th century Pope Benedict XIV states that he obtained from Paris an exact drawing of the point of the lance, and that in comparing it with the larger relic in St. Peter's he was satisfied that the two had originally formed one blade. This relic has never since left Rome, and its resting place is at Saint Peter's.

The Holy Lance in Vienna is displayed in the Imperial Treasury or Weltliche Schatzkammer (lit. Worldly Treasure Room) at the Hofburg Palace in Vienna, Austria. It is a typical winged lance of the Carolingian dynasty. At different times, it was said to be the lance of Saint Maurice or that of Constantine the Great. In the tenth century, the Holy Roman Emperors came into possession of the lance, according to sources from the time of Otto I (912–973). In 1000, Otto III gave Bolesław I of Poland a replica of the Holy Lance at the Congress of Gniezno. In 1084, Henry IV had a silver band with the inscription "Nail of Our Lord" added to it. This was based on the belief that the nail embedded in the spear-tip was one that had been used for the Crucifixion of Jesus. It was only in the thirteenth century that the Lance became identified with that of Longinus, which had been used to pierce Christ's side and had been drenched in water and the blood of Christ.

In 1273, the Holy Lance was first used in a coronation ceremony. Around 1350, Charles IV had a golden sleeve put over the silver one, inscribed Lancea et clavus Domini (Lance and nail of the Lord). In 1424, Sigismund had a collection of relics, including the lance, moved from his capital in Prague to his birthplace, Nuremberg, and decreed them to be kept there forever. This collection was called the Imperial Regalia (Reichskleinodien).

When the French Revolutionary army approached Nuremberg in the spring of 1796, the city councilors decided to remove the Reichskleinodien to Vienna for safe keeping. The collection was entrusted to a Baron von Hügel, who promised to return the objects once the threat was resolved. However, the Holy Roman Empire was disbanded in 1806 and in the confusion, he sold the collection to the Habsburgs.The city councillors asked for the return of the collection after the defeat of Napoleon's army at the Battle of Waterloo, but the Austrian authorities refused.

n Mein Kampf, Hitler wrote that the Imperial Insignia "were still preserved in Vienna and appeared to act as magical relics rather than as the visible guarantee of an everlasting bond of union. When the Habsburg State crumbled to pieces in 1918, the Austrian Germans instinctively raised an outcry for union with their German fatherland". During the Anschluss, when Austria was annexed to Germany, the Nazis brought the Reichskleinodien to Nuremberg, where they displayed them during the September 1938 Party Congress. They then transferred them to the Historischer Kunstbunker, a bunker that had been built into some of the medieval cellars of old houses underneath Nuremberg Castle to protect historic art from air raids.

Most of the Regalia were recovered by the Allies at the end of the war, but the Nazis had hidden the five most important pieces in hopes of using them as political symbols to help them rally for a return to power, possibly at the command of Nazi Commander Heinrich Himmler. Walter Horn — a Medieval studies scholar who had fled Nazi Germany and served in the Third Army under General George S. Patton — became a special investigator in the Monuments, Fine Arts, and Archives program after the end of the war, and was tasked with tracking the missing pieces down. After a series of interrogations and false rumors, Nuremberg city councilor Stadtrat Fries confessed that he, fellow-councilman Stadtrat Schmeiszner, and an SS official had hidden the Imperial Regalia on March 31, 1945, and he agreed to bring Horn's team to the site. On August 7, Horn and a U.S. army captain escorted Fries and Schmeiszner to the entrance of the Panier Platz Bunker, where they located the treasures hidden behind a wall of masonry in a small room off of a subterranean corridor, roughly eighty feet below ground. The Regalia were first brought back to Nuremberg castle to be reunited with the rest of the Reichskleinodien, and then transferred with the entire collection to Austrian officials the following January.

A Holy Lance is conserved in Vagharshapat (previously known as Echmiadzin), the religious capital of Armenia. It was previously held in the monastery of Geghard. The first source that mentions it is a text Holy Relics of Our Lord Jesus Christ, in a thirteenth-century Armenian manuscript. According to this text, the spear which pierced Jesus was to have been brought to Armenia by the Apostle

Thaddeus. The manuscript does not specify precisely where it was kept, but the Holy Lance gives a description that exactly matches the lance, the monastery gate, since the thirteenth century precisely, the name of Geghardavank (Monastery of the Holy Lance).

In 1655, the French traveler Jean-Baptiste Tavernier was the first Westerner to see this relic in Armenia. In 1805, the Russians captured the monastery and the relic was moved to Tchitchanov Geghard, Tbilisi, Georgia. It was later returned to Armenia, and is still on display at the Manoogian museum in Vagharshapat, enshrined in a 17th-century reliquary.

During the June 1098 Siege of Antioch, a monk named Peter Bartholomew reported that he had a vision in which St. Andrew told him that the Holy Lance was buried in the Church of St. Peter in Antioch. After much digging in the cathedral, Bartholomew allegedly discovered a lance. Despite the doubts of many, including the papal legate Adhemar of Le Puy, the discovery of the Holy Lance of Antioch inspired the starving Crusaders to break the siege and secure the city.

In the 18th century, Roman cardinal Prospero Lambertini claimed the Antiochian lance was a fake.

Another lance has been preserved at Kraków, Poland, since at least the 13th century

A mitred Adhémar de Monteil carrying one of the instances of the Holy Lance in one of the battles of the First Crusade. And 1898 there is a drawing of the Holy Lance In Rome

Holy Lance displayed in the Imperial Treasury at the Hofburg Palace in Vienna, Austria

Size of this preview: 274 × 599 pixels. Other resolutions: 110 × 240 pixels | 219 × 480 pixels | 351 × 768 pixels | 1,161 × 2,536 pixels.

Original file (1,161 × 2,536 pixels, file size: 2.17 MB, MIME type: image/jpeg).

Deutsch: Die Heilige Lanze

Karolingisch, 8. Jahrhundert Stahl, Eisen, Messing, Silber, Gold, Leder 50,7 cm lang

SK Inv.-Nr. XIII 19

English: The Holy Lance

Carolingian, 8th century Steel, iron, brass, silver, gold, leather 50.7 cm long

https://en.m.wikipedia.org/wiki/Imperial_Treasury,_Vienna

Holy_Lance_Detail.jpg (800 × 533 pixels, file size: 62 KB, MIME type: image/jpeg)

Armenia Holy Lance in Echmiadzin

Psalm 22 "My God, my God, why hast thou forsaken me? why art thou so far from helping me, and from the words of my roaring? b [2] O my God, I cry in the daytime, but thou hearest not; and in the night season, and am not silent. [3] But thou art holy, O thou that inhabitest the praises of Israel. [4] Our fathers trusted in thee: they trusted, and thou didst deliver them. [5] They cried unto thee, and were delivered: they trusted in thee, and were not confounded. [6] But I am a worm, and no man; a reproach of men, and despised of the people. [7] All they that see me laugh me to scorn: they shoot out the lip, they shake the head, saying, [8] He trusted on the Lord that he would deliver him: let him deliver him, seeing he delighted in him. [9] But thou art he that took me out of the womb: thou didst make me hope when I was upon my mother's breasts. [10] I was cast upon thee from the womb: thou art my God from my mother's belly. [11] Be not far from me; for trouble is near; for there is none to help. [12] Many bulls have compassed me: strong bulls of Bashan have beset me round. [13] They gaped upon me with their mouths, as a ravening and a roaring lion. [14] I am poured out like water, and all my bones are out of joint: my heart is like wax; it is melted in the midst of my bowels. [15] My strength is dried up like a potsherd; and my tongue cleaveth to my jaws; and thou hast brought me into the dust of death. [16] For dogs have compassed me: the assembly of the wicked have inclosed me: they pierced my hands and my feet. [17] I may tell all my bones: they look and stare upon me. [18] They part my garments among them, and cast lots upon my vesture. [19] But be not thou far from me, O Lord : O my strength, haste thee to help me. [20] Deliver my soul from the sword; my darling from the power of the dog. [21] Save me from the lion's mouth: for thou hast heard me from the horns of the unicorns. [22] I will declare thy name unto my brethren: in the midst of the congregation will I praise thee. [23] Ye that fear the Lord, praise him; all ye the seed of Jacob, glorify him; and fear him, all ye the seed of Israel. [24] For he hath not despised nor abhorred the affliction of the afflicted; neither hath he hid his face from him; but when he cried unto him, he heard. [25] My praise shall be of thee in the great congregation: I will pay my vows before them that fear him. [26] The meek shall eat and be satisfied: they shall praise the Lord that seek him: your heart shall live for ever. [27] All the ends of the world shall remember and turn unto the Lord : and all the kindreds of the nations shall worship before thee. [28] For the kingdom is the Lord's : and he is the governor among the nations. [29] All they that be fat upon earth shall eat and worship: all they that go down to the dust shall bow before him: and none can keep alive his own soul. [30] A seed shall serve him; it shall be accounted to the Lord for a generation. [31] They shall come, and shall declare his righteousness unto a people that shall be born, that he hath done this …"

https://en.m.wikipedia.org/wiki/Holy_Lance....

https://en.m.wikipedia.org/wiki/Five_Holy_Wounds

Review of the Historic Fathers!

Written by Ramsis Ghaly

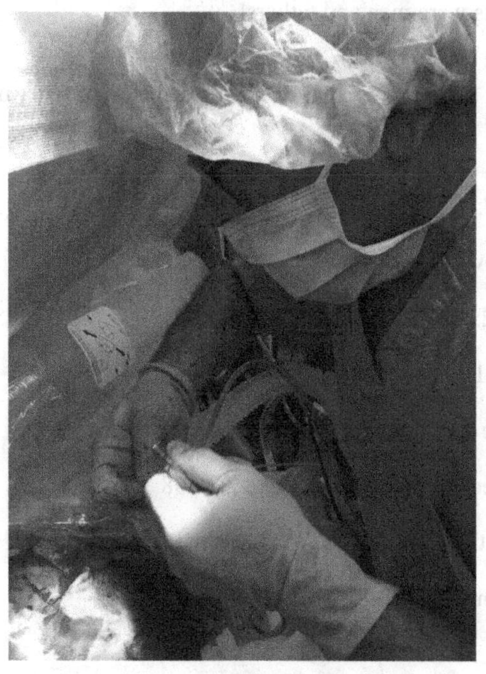

The very first human creation was a man named Adam!

The father of all men and women dependents until the end of the world was a man named Adam!

The first husband was a man named Adam!

The first biologic father was a man named Adam!

The very first criminal was a man and a father named Cain!

The very first patriot was a man and father named Noah!

The very first patriarch was a man and a father!

The very first head of household was a man and a father!

The very first prophet was a man and a father!

The very first human biblical teacher and Leader was a man and a father Moses!

The very first clergyman was a man and a father!

The very first king was a man and a father named Saul!

The very first psalmist was a man and father Psalmist David!

The first prophets were men and fathers!

List o Christian prophets were men with exception of few women as follows:

A

Aaron (Exodus 7:1)

Abraham (Hebrews 11:8)

Adam (Genesis 2:7–8)

Ahijah (1 Kings 11:29)

Amos (one of the 12 Minor Prophets)

Anna (Luke - Dedication of Jesus) Luke 2:36-38

Agabus (Acts of the Apostles 11:27–28)

Azariah (2 Chronicles 15:1–8)

D

Daniel (Matthew 24:15)

David (Hebrews 11:32)

Deborah (Judges 4:4)

E

Elijah (1 Kings 18:36)

Eber (Genesis 16:16–17)

Elisha (2 Kings 9:1)

Enoch (Jude 1:14)

Ezekiel (Ezekiel 1:3)

Ezra (Ezra 7:1)

G

Gad (1 Samuel 22:5)

Gideon (Judges 6 through

H

Habakkuk (Habakkuk 1:1)

Haggai (Haggai 1:1)

Hanani (2 Chronicles 16:7)

Hosea (Hosea 1:1)

Huldah (2 Kings 22:14)

I

Iddo (2 Chronicles 13:22)

Isaac (Genesis 26:2–7)

Isaiah (2 Kings 19:2)

Ishmael (Genesis 16:11–16)

Jacob (Genesis 28:11–16)

Jehu (1 Kings 16:7)

Jeremiah (Jeremiah 20:2)

Jethro (Exodus 2:18)

Joel (Acts 2:16)

John the Baptist (Luke 7:28)

John of Patmos (Revelation 1:1–3)

Jonah (2 Kings 14:25)

Joshua (Joshua 1:1)

Judas Barsabbas (Acts 15:32)

Job (Job 1:1)

L

Lamech (father of Noah) (Genesis 5:28–29)

Lucius of Cyrene (Acts 13:1)

Lot (Genesis 11:27)

M

Malachi (Malachi 1:1)

Manahen (Acts 13:1)

Melchizedek (Genesis 14:18–24)

Micah (Micah 1:1)

Micaiah (1 Kings 22:9)

Moses (Deuteronomy 34:10)

N

Nahum (Nahum 1:1)

Nathan (2 Samuel 7:2)

Noah (Genesis 7:1)

O

Obadiah (Obadiah 1:1)

Oded (2 Chronicles 15:8) Father of Azariah the prophet

Oded (2 Chronicles 28:9)

P

Philip the Evangelist (Acts 8:26) Note: His four daughters also prophesied (Acts 21:8, 9)

Paul the Apostle (Acts of the Apostles 9:20)

S

Samuel (1 Samuel 3:20)

Shemaiah (1 Kings 12:22)

Silas (Acts 15:32)

Simeon Niger (Acts 13:1)

T

Two Witnesses (Revelation 11:3)

U

Uriah (Jeremiah 26:20)

Z

Zechariah, son of Berechiah (Zechariah 1:1)

Zechariah, son of Jehoiada (2 Chronicles 24:20)

Zephaniah (Zephaniah 1:1)

https://en.m.wikipedia.org/wiki/Prophets_of_Christianity

The very first known Baptist is a man and father to his children in the spirit named John the Baptist!

The first apostles of Jesus were man and fathers!

The first known Betrayer was a man and a father Judas Iscariot!

The very first individual brought death was a man and a father named Adam and the First Man brought forgiveness, salvation, life and resurrection to mankind is a Man and Heavenly Father Jesus Christ the Son of God the Most High!

The very First Savior was a Man and Heavenly Father, God is Jesus Christ the Lord!

The Very First and the Only Owner of the Holy Teaching, beatitudes and all the Heavenly Commandments is a man and Heavenly Father, Jesus the Lord!

The Very First-fruit of Resurrection is A Man and God, Jesus the Lord!

The very First and Only One in the Second Coming is A Man and God, Jesus Christ the Lord!

The very First Heavenly Judge to judge the entire world including Adam and Eve and all the descendants is a Man and God, Jesus the Lord!

The very First Heavenly Kingdom and the Owner of New Jerusalem is a Man and God, Jesus Christ the King!

1 Corinthians 15:20-23 KJV "But now is Christ risen from the dead, and become the firstfruits of them that slept. [21] For since by man came death, by man came also the resurrection of the dead. [22] For as in Adam all die, even so in Christ shall all be made alive. [23] But every man in his own order: Christ the firstfruits; afterward they that are Christ's at his coming."

The Very First Two Fathers and The Human Cycle!

Adam, our father, was born from God and not from a mother! Adam never followed the standard human cycle from a womb to an adult but was a mature adult from the start!

Eve, our mother, was born from a Adam rib and flesh and not from a mother! Eve never followed the standard human cycle from a womb to an adult but was a mature adult from the start!

But both followed the life of parenthood and the blessing of laboring and sweating and raising children all the way to age of 930 years old!

The very first father that followed the classic human cycle was Cain since Abel was killed by Cain. And the very first war made by a man as Cain was the first bloody murder where a human blood soaked the ground of earth!

Since the time of Adam and Eve (both were Off human Cycle), their descendants followed religiously the traditional in-human cycle for a man and a woman creation!

An embryo

A newborn

An infant

A child

An adolescent

A student

A dult

A senior

A thinker

A labor

A servant

A partner

A parent

A granda

Biblical Verses to Adam and Descendents

Genesis 1:26-28 KJV "And God said, Let us make man in our image, after our likeness: and let them have dominion over the fish of the sea, and over the fowl of the air, and over the cattle, and over all the earth, and over every creeping thing that creepeth upon the earth. [27] So God created man in his own image, in the image of God created he him; male and female created he them. [28] And God blessed them, and God said unto them, Be fruitful, and multiply, and replenish the earth, and subdue it: and have dominion over the fish of the sea, and over the fowl of the air, and over every living thing that moveth upon the earth."

Genesis 2:7-8,15-23 KJV "And the Lord God formed man of the dust of the ground, and breathed into his nostrils the breath of life; and man became a living soul. [8] And the Lord God planted a garden eastward in Eden; and there he put the man whom he had formed. [15] And the Lord God took the man, and put him into the garden of Eden to dress it and to keep it. [16] And the Lord God commanded the man, saying, Of every tree of the garden thou mayest freely eat: [17] But of the tree of the knowledge of good and evil, thou shalt not eat of it: for in the day that thou eatest thereof thou shalt surely die. [18] And the Lord God said, It is not good that the man should be alone; I will make him an help meet for him. [19] And out of the ground the Lord God formed every beast of the field, and every fowl of the air; and brought them unto Adam to see what he would call them: and whatsoever Adam called every living creature, that was the name thereof. [20] And Adam gave names to all cattle, and to the fowl of the air, and to every beast of the field; but for Adam there was not found an help meet for him. [21] And the Lord God caused a deep sleep to fall upon Adam, and he slept: and he took one of his ribs, and closed up the flesh instead thereof; [22] And the rib, which the Lord God had taken from man, made he a woman, and brought her unto the man. [23] And Adam said, This is now bone of my bones, and flesh of my flesh: she shall be called Woman, because she was taken out of Man."

Genesis 3:16-21,24 KJV "Unto the woman he said, I will greatly multiply thy sorrow and thy conception; in sorrow thou shalt bring forth children; and thy desire shall be to thy husband, and he shall rule over thee. [17] And unto Adam he said, Because thou hast hearkened unto the voice of thy wife, and hast eaten of the tree, of which I commanded thee, saying, Thou shalt not eat of it: cursed is the ground for thy sake; in sorrow shalt thou eat of it all the days of thy life; [18] Thorns also and thistles shall it bring forth to thee; and thou shalt eat the herb of the field; [19] In the sweat of thy face shalt thou eat bread, till thou return unto the ground; for out of it wast thou taken: for dust thou art, and unto dust shalt thou return. [20] And Adam called his wife's name Eve; because she was the mother of all living. [21] Unto Adam also and to his wife did the Lord God make coats of skins, and clothed them. [24] So he drove out the man; and he placed at the east of the garden of Eden Cherubims, and a flaming sword which turned every way, to keep the way of the tree of life."

Genesis 4:1-2,17-23,25-26 KJV "And Adam knew Eve his wife; and she conceived, and bare Cain, and said, I have gotten a man from the Lord. [2] And she again bare his brother Abel. And Abel was a keeper of sheep, but Cain was a tiller of the ground. [17] And Cain knew his wife; and she conceived, and bare Enoch: and he builded a city, and called the name of the city, after the name of his son, Enoch. [18] And unto Enoch was born Irad: and Irad begat Mehujael: and Mehujael begat Methusael: and Methusael begat Lamech. [19] And Lamech took unto him two wives: the name of the one was Adah, and the name of the other Zillah. [20] And Adah bare Jabal: he was the father of such as dwell in tents, and of such as have cattle. [21] And his brother's name was Jubal: he was the father of all such as handle the harp and organ. [22] And Zillah, she also bare Tubal-cain, an instructer of every artificer in brass and iron: and the sister of Tubal-cain was Naamah. [23] And Lamech said unto his wives, Adah and Zillah, Hear my voice; ye wives of Lamech, hearken unto my speech: for I have slain a man to my wounding, and a young man to my hurt. [25] And Adam knew his wife again; and she bare a son, and called his name Seth: For God, said she, hath appointed me another seed instead of Abel, whom Cain slew. [26] And to Seth, to him also there was born a son; and he called his name Enos: then began men to call upon the name of the Lord."

Genesis 5:1-32 KJV "This is the book of the generations of Adam. In the day that God created man, in the likeness of God made he him; [2] Male and female created he them; and blessed them, and called their name Adam, in the day when they were created. [3] And Adam lived an hundred and thirty years, and begat a son in his own likeness, after his image; and called his name Seth: [4] And the days of Adam after he had begotten Seth were eight hundred years: and he begat sons and daughters: [5] And all the days that Adam lived were nine hundred and thirty years: and he died. [6] And Seth lived an hundred and five years, and begat Enos: [7] And Seth lived after he begat Enos eight hundred and seven years, and begat sons and daughters: [8] And all the days of Seth were nine hundred and twelve years: and he died. [9] And Enos lived ninety years, and begat Cainan: [10] And

Enos lived after he begat Cainan eight hundred and fifteen years, and begat sons and daughters: [11] And all the days of Enos were nine hundred and five years: and he died. [12] And Cainan lived seventy years, and begat Mahalaleel: [13] And Cainan lived after he begat Mahalaleel eight hundred and forty years, and begat sons and daughters: [14] And all the days of Cainan were nine hundred and ten years: and he died. [15] And Mahalaleel lived sixty and five years, and begat Jared: [16] And Mahalaleel lived after he begat Jared eight hundred and thirty years, and begat sons and daughters: [17] And all the days of Mahalaleel were eight hundred ninety and five years: and he died. [18] And Jared lived an hundred sixty and two years, and he begat Enoch: [19] And Jared lived after he begat Enoch eight hundred years, and begat sons and daughters: [20] And all the days of Jared were nine hundred sixty and two years: and he died. [21] And Enoch lived sixty and five years, and begat Methuselah: [22] And Enoch walked with God after he begat Methuselah three hundred years, and begat sons and daughters: [23] And all the days of Enoch were three hundred sixty and five years: [24] And Enoch walked with God: and he was not; for God took him. [25] And Methuselah lived an hundred eighty and seven years, and begat Lamech: [26] And Methuselah lived after he begat Lamech seven hundred eighty and two years, and begat sons and daughters: [27] And all the days of Methuselah were nine hundred sixty and nine years: and he died. [28] And Lamech lived an hundred eighty and two years, and begat a son: [29] And he called his name Noah, saying, This same shall comfort us concerning our work and toil of our hands, because of the ground which the Lord hath cursed. [30] And Lamech lived after he begat Noah five hundred ninety and five years, and begat sons and daughters: [31] And all the days of Lamech were seven hundred seventy and seven years: and he died. [32] And Noah was five hundred years old: and Noah begat Shem, Ham, and Japheth."

Biblical Verses about Human Man the Father

Ephesians 5:22-24 ESV Wives, submit to your own husbands, as to the Lord. For the husband is the head of the wife even as Christ is the head of the church, his body, and is himself its Savior. Now as the church submits to Christ, so also wives should submit in everything to their husbands.

1 Corinthians 11:3 ESV But I want you to understand that the head of every man is Christ, the head of a wife is her husband, and the head of Christ is God.

1 Peter 3:7 ESV Likewise, husbands, live with your wives in an understanding way, showing honor to the woman as the weaker vessel, since they are heirs with you of the grace of life, so that your prayers may not be hindered.

1 Timothy 2:11-15 ESV Let a woman learn quietly with all submissiveness. I do not permit a woman to teach or to exercise authority over a man; rather, she is to remain quiet. For Adam was formed first, then Eve; and Adam was not deceived, but the woman was deceived and became a transgressor. Yet she will be saved through childbearing—if they continue in faith and love and holiness, with self-control.

Ephesians 5:23 ESV For the husband is the head of the wife even as Christ is the head of the church, his body, and is himself its Savior.

Genesis 3:16 ESV To the woman he said, "I will surely multiply your pain in childbearing; in pain you shall bring forth children. Your desire shall be for your husband, and he shall rule over you."

Genesis 2:18 ESV Then the Lord God said, "It is not good that the man should be alone; I will make him a helper fit for him."

Ephesians 6:4 ESV Fathers, do not provoke your children to anger, but bring them up in the discipline and instruction of the Lord.

Ephesians 5:25 ESV Husbands, love your wives, as Christ loved the church and gave himself up for her,

1 Corinthians 7:1-40 ESV Now concerning the matters about which you wrote: "It is good for a man not to have sexual relations with a woman." But because of the temptation to sexual immorality, each man should have his own wife and each woman her own husband. The husband should give to his wife her conjugal rights, and likewise the wife to her husband. For the wife does not have authority over her own body, but the husband does. Likewise the husband does not have authority over his own body, but the wife does. Do not deprive one another, except perhaps by agreement for a limited time, that you may devote yourselves to prayer; but then come together again, so that Satan may not tempt you because of your lack of self-control. ...

1 Timothy 5:8 ESV But if anyone does not provide for his relatives, and especially for members of his household, he has denied the faith and is worse than an unbeliever.

Ephesians 5:33 ESV However, let each one of you love his wife as himself, and let the wife see that she respects her husband.

Ephesians 5:22 ESV Wives, submit to your own husbands, as to the Lord.

Colossians 3:19 ESV Husbands, love your wives, and do not be harsh with them.

Proverbs 31:1-31 ESV The words of King Lemuel. An oracle that his mother taught him: What are you doing, my son? What are you doing, son of my womb? What are you doing, son of my vows? Do not give your strength to women, your ways to those who destroy kings. It is not for kings, O Lemuel, it is not for kings to drink wine, or for rulers to take strong drink, lest they drink and forget what has been decreed and pervert the rights of all the afflicted. ...

Matthew 19:5-6 ESV And said, 'Therefore a man shall leave his father and his mother and hold fast to his wife, and the two shall become one flesh'? So they are no longer two but one flesh. What therefore God has joined together, let not man separate."

Galatians 3:28 ESV There is neither Jew nor Greek, there is neither slave nor free, there is no male and female, for you are all one in Christ Jesus.

1 Timothy 2:12 ESV I do not permit a woman to teach or to exercise authority over a man; rather, she is to remain quiet.

Colossians 3:21 ESV Fathers, do not provoke your children, lest they become discouraged.

Ephesians 5:28 ESV In the same way husbands should love their wives as their own bodies. He who loves his wife loves himself.

Colossians 3:18 ESV Wives, submit to your husbands, as is fitting in the Lord.

1 Peter 3:1 ESV Likewise, wives, be subject to your own husbands, so that even if some do not obey the word, they may be won without a word by the conduct of their wives,

Ephesians 5:1-33 ESV Therefore be imitators of God, as beloved children. And walk in love, as Christ loved us and gave himself up for us, a fragrant offering and sacrifice to God. But sexual immorality and all impurity or covetousness must not even be named among you, as is proper among saints. Let there be no filthiness nor foolish talk nor crude joking, which are out of place, but instead let there be thanksgiving. For you may be sure of this, that everyone who is sexually immoral or impure, or who is covetous (that is, an idolater), has no inheritance in the kingdom of Christ and God. ...

Colossians 1:18 ESV And he is the head of the body, the church. He is the beginning, the firstborn from the dead, that in everything he might be preeminent.

1 Peter 3:1-2 ESV Likewise, wives, be subject to your own husbands, so that even if some do not obey the word, they may be won without a word by the conduct of their wives, when they see your respectful and pure conduct.

Ephesians 1:22 ESV And he put all things under his feet and gave him as head over all things to the church,

1 Timothy 2:11-14 ESV Let a woman learn quietly with all submissiveness. I do not permit a woman to teach or to exercise authority over a man; rather, she is to remain quiet. For Adam was formed first, then Eve; and Adam was not deceived, but the woman was deceived and became a transgressor.

Titus 2:5 ESV To be self-controlled, pure, working at home, kind, and submissive to their own husbands, that the word of God may not be reviled.

Colossians 3:20 ESV Children, obey your parents in everything, for this pleases the Lord.

John 3:16 ESV "For God so loved the world, that he gave his only Son, that whoever believes in him should not perish but have eternal life.

1 Timothy 3:12 ESV Let deacons each be the husband of one wife, managing their children and their own households well.

Ephesians 5:24 ESV Now as the church submits to Christ, so also wives should submit in everything to their husbands.

Ephesians 4:15 ESV Rather, speaking the truth in love, we are to grow up in every way into him who is the head, into Christ,

1 Corinthians 11:1-34 ESV Be imitators of me, as I am of Christ. Now I commend you because you remember me in everything and maintain the traditions even as I delivered them to you. But I want you to understand that the head of every man is Christ, the head of a wife is her husband, and the head of Christ is God. Every man who prays or prophesies with his head covered dishonors his head, but every wife who prays or prophesies with her head uncovered dishonors her head, since it is the same as if her head were shaven. ...

Genesis 3:1-24 ESV Now the serpent was more crafty than any other beast of the field that the Lord God had made. He said to the woman, "Did God actually say, 'You shall not eat of any tree in the garden'?" And the woman said to the serpent, "We may eat of the fruit of the trees in the garden, but God said, 'You shall not eat of the fruit of the tree that is in the midst of the garden, neither shall you touch it, lest you die.'" But the serpent said to the woman, "You will not surely die. For God knows that when you eat of it your eyes will be opened, and you will be like God, knowing good and evil." ...

Genesis 2:24 ESV / 33 helpful votes

Therefore a man shall leave his father and his mother and hold fast to his wife, and they shall become one flesh.

1 Timothy 5:14 ESV So I would have younger widows marry, bear children, manage their households, and give the adversary no occasion for slander.

2 Timothy 1:5 ESV I am reminded of your sincere faith, a faith that dwelt first in your grandmother Lois and your mother Eunice and now, I am sure, dwells in you as well.

1 Timothy 3:1-16 ESV The saying is trustworthy: If anyone aspires to the office of overseer, he desires a noble task. Therefore an overseer must be above reproach, the husband of one wife, sober-minded, self-controlled, respectable, hospitable, able to teach, not a drunkard, not violent but gentle, not quarrelsome, not a lover of money. He must manage his own household well, with all dignity keeping his children submissive, for if someone does not know how to manage his own household, how will he care for God's church? ...

Titus 2:3-5 ESV Older women likewise are to be reverent in behavior, not slanderers or slaves to much wine. They are to teach what is good, and so train the young women to love their husbands and children, to be self-controlled, pure, working at home, kind, and submissive to their own husbands, that the word of God may not be reviled.

Proverbs 22:6 ESV Train up a child in the way he should go; even when he is old he will not depart from it.

Joshua 24:15 ESV And if it is evil in your eyes to serve the Lord, choose this day whom you will serve, whether the gods your fathers served in the region beyond the River, or the gods of the Amorites in whose land you dwell. But as for me and my house, we will serve the Lord."

1 Peter 3:1-6 ESV Likewise, wives, be subject to your own husbands, so that even if some do not obey the word, they may be won without a word by the conduct of their wives, when they see your respectful and pure conduct. Do not let your adorning be external—the braiding of hair and the putting on of gold jewelry, or the clothing you wear— but let your adorning be the hidden person of the heart with the imperishable beauty of a gentle and quiet spirit, which in God's sight is very precious. For this is how the holy women who hoped in God used to adorn themselves, by submitting to their own husbands, ...

1 Corinthians 14:34 ESV The women should keep silent in the churches. For they are not permitted to speak, but should be in submission, as the Law also says.

1 Peter 3:5-6 ESV For this is how the holy women who hoped in God used to adorn themselves, by submitting to their own husbands, as Sarah obeyed Abraham, calling him lord. And you are her children, if you do good and do not fear anything that is frightening.

1 Timothy 3:2 ESV Therefore an overseer must be above reproach, the husband of one wife, sober-minded, self-controlled, respectable, hospitable, able to teach,

1 Timothy 2:1-15 ESV First of all, then, I urge that supplications, prayers, intercessions, and thanksgivings be made for all people, for kings and all who are in high positions, that we may lead a peaceful and quiet life, godly and dignified in every way. This is good, and it is pleasing in the sight of God our Savior, who desires all people to be saved and to come to the knowledge of the truth. For there is one God, and there is one mediator between God and men, the man Christ Jesus, ...

Colossians 3:18-19 ESV Wives, submit to your husbands, as is fitting in the Lord. Husbands, love your wives, and do not be harsh with them.

Romans 5:8 ESV But God shows his love for us in that while we were still sinners, Christ died for us.

Ephesians 6:1-3 ESV Children, obey your parents in the Lord, for this is right. “Honor your father and mother” (this is the first commandment with a promise), “that it may go well with you and that you may live long in the land.”

Ephesians 6:1 ESV Children, obey your parents in the Lord, for this is right.

Ephesians 5:25-26 ESV Husbands, love your wives, as Christ loved the church and gave himself up for her, that he might sanctify her, having cleansed her by the washing of water with the word,

Ephesians 1:22-23 ESV And he put all things under his feet and gave him as head over all things to the church, which is his body, the fullness of him who fills all in all.

Acts 5:29 ESV But Peter and the apostles answered, “We must obey God rather than men.

Romans 16:3 ESV Greet Prisca and Aquila, my fellow workers in Christ Jesus,

Genesis 2:1-25 ESV Thus the heavens and the earth were finished, and all the host of them. And on the seventh day God finished his work that he had done, and he rested on the seventh day from all his work that he had done. So God blessed the seventh day and made it holy, because on it God rested from all his work that he had done in creation. These are the generations of the heavens and the earth when they were created, in the day that the Lord God made the earth and the heavens. When no bush of the field was yet in the land and no small plant of the field had yet sprung up—for the Lord God had not caused it to rain on the land, and there was no man to work the ground, ...

1 Timothy 2:11-12 ESV Let a woman learn quietly with all submissiveness. I do not permit a woman to teach or to exercise authority over a man; rather, she is to remain quiet.

Acts 20:28 ESV Pay careful attention to yourselves and to all the flock, in which the Holy Spirit has made you overseers, to care for the church of God, which he obtained with his own blood.

1 John 4:19 ESV We love because he first loved us.

Titus 1:5-9 ESV This is why I left you in Crete, so that you might put what remained into order, and appoint elders in every town as I directed you— if anyone is above reproach, the husband of one wife, and his children are believers and not open to the charge of debauchery or insubordination. For an overseer, as God's steward, must be above reproach. He must not be arrogant or quick-tempered or a drunkard or violent or greedy for gain, but hospitable, a lover of good, self-controlled, upright, holy, and disciplined. He must hold firm to the trustworthy word as taught, so that he may be able to give instruction in sound doctrine and also to rebuke those who contradict it.

1 Timothy 3:15 ESV If I delay, you may know how one ought to behave in the household of God, which is the church of the living God, a pillar and buttress of the truth.

1 Timothy 3:4 ESV He must manage his own household well, with all dignity keeping his children submissive,

1 Timothy 2:9-15 ESV Likewise also that women should adorn themselves in respectable apparel, with modesty and self-control, not with braided hair and gold or pearls or costly attire, but with what is proper for women who profess godliness—with good works. Let a woman learn quietly with all submissiveness. I do not permit a woman to teach or to exercise authority over a man; rather, she is to remain quiet. For Adam was formed first, then Eve; ...

Ephesians 5:22-33 ESV Wives, submit to your own husbands, as to the Lord. For the husband is the head of the wife even as Christ is the head of the church, his body, and is himself its Savior. Now as the church submits to Christ, so also wives should submit in everything to their husbands. Husbands, love your wives, as Christ loved the church and gave himself up for her, that he might sanctify her, having cleansed her by the washing of water with the word, ...

Ephesians 5:21-24 ESV Submitting to one another out of reverence for Christ. Wives, submit to your own husbands, as to the Lord. For the husband is the head of the wife even as Christ is the head of the church, his body, and is himself its Savior. Now as the church submits to Christ, so also wives should submit in everything to their husbands.

1 Corinthians 11:8-10 ESV For man was not made from woman, but woman from man. Neither was man created for woman, but woman for man. That is why a wife ought to have a symbol of authority on her head, because of the angels.

Romans 2:4 ESV Or do you presume on the riches of his kindness and forbearance and patience, not knowing that God's kindness is meant to lead you to repentance?

Romans 16:1-2 ESV I commend to you our sister Phoebe, a servant of the church at Cenchreae, that you may welcome her in the Lord in a way worthy of the saints, and help her in whatever she may need from you, for she has been a patron of many and of myself as well.

Colossians 2:10 And you have been filled in him, who is the head of all rule and authority.

1 Corinthians 14:37 ESV If anyone thinks that he is a prophet, or spiritual, he should acknowledge that the things I am writing to you are a command of the Lord.

1 Corinthians 11:3-10 ESV But I want you to understand that the head of every man is Christ, the head of a wife is her husband, and the head of Christ is God. Every man who prays or prophesies with his head covered dishonors his head, but every wife who prays or prophesies with her head uncovered dishonors her head, since it is the same as if her head were shaven. For if a wife will not cover her head, then she should cut her hair short. But since it is disgraceful for a wife to cut off her hair or shave her head, let her cover her head. For a man ought not to cover his head, since he is the image and glory of God, but woman is the glory of man. ...

Acts 16:31 ESV And they said, "Believe in the Lord Jesus, and you will be saved, you and your household."

Matthew 21:42 ESV Jesus said to them, "Have you never read in the Scriptures: "'The stone that the builders rejected has become the cornerstone; this was the Lord's doing, and it is marvelous in our eyes'?

1 Timothy 2:14 ESV And Adam was not deceived, but the woman was deceived and became a transgressor.

Titus 1:6 ESV If anyone is above reproach, the husband of one wife, and his children are believers and not open to the charge of debauchery or insubordination.

1 Timothy 5:4 ESV But if a widow has children or grandchildren, let them first learn to show godliness to their own household and to make some return to their parents, for this is pleasing in the sight of God.

2 Thessalonians 3:10 ESV For even when we were with you, we would give you this command: If anyone is not willing to work, let him not eat.

Ephesians 5:26-27 ESV That he might sanctify her, having cleansed her by the washing of water with the word, so that he might present the church to himself in splendor, without spot or wrinkle or any such thing, that she might be holy and without blemish.

Acts 10:1-48 ESV At Caesarea there was a man named Cornelius, a centurion of what was known as the Italian Cohort, a devout man who feared God with all his household, gave alms generously to the people, and prayed continually to God. About the ninth hour of the day he saw clearly in a vision an angel of God come in and say to him, "Cornelius." And he stared at him in terror and said, "What is it, Lord?" And he said to him, "Your prayers and your alms have ascended as a memorial before God. And now send men to Joppa and bring one Simon who is called Peter. ...

1 Timothy 3:4-5 ESV He must manage his own household well, with all dignity keeping his children submissive, for if someone does not know how to manage his own household, how will he care for God's church?

1 Timothy 2:15 ESV Yet she will be saved through childbearing—if they continue in faith and love and holiness, with self-control.

Ephesians 5:28-29 ESV In the same way husbands should love their wives as their own bodies. He who loves his wife loves himself. For no one ever hated his own flesh, but nourishes and cherishes it, just as Christ does the church,

Proverbs 31:28-31 ESV Her children rise up and call her blessed; her husband also, and he praises her: "Many women have done excellently, but you surpass them all." Charm is deceitful, and beauty is vain, but a woman who fears the Lord is to be praised. Give her of the fruit of her hands, and let her works praise her in the gates.

1 Timothy 2:13 ESV For Adam was formed first, then Eve;

Malachi 2:14 ESV But you say, "Why does he not?" Because the Lord was witness between you and the wife of your youth, to whom you have been faithless, though she is your companion and your wife by covenant.

Hebrews 13:17 ESV Obey your leaders and submit to them, for they are keeping watch over your souls, as those who will have to give an account. Let them do this with joy and not with groaning, for that would be of no advantage to you.

1 Timothy 3:11 ESV Their wives likewise must be dignified, not slanderers, but sober-minded, faithful in all things.

1 Timothy 3:2-4 ESV Therefore an overseer must be above reproach, the husband of one wife, sober-minded, self-controlled, respectable, hospitable, able to teach, not a drunkard, not violent but gentle, not quarrelsome, not a lover of money. He must manage his own household well, with all dignity keeping his children submissive,

Colossians 3:1-25 ESV If then you have been raised with Christ, seek the things that are above, where Christ is, seated at the right hand of God. Set your minds on things that are above, not on things that are on earth. For you have died, and your life is hidden with Christ in God. When Christ who is your life appears, then you also will appear with him in glory. Put to death therefore what is earthly in you: sexual immorality, impurity, passion, evil desire, and covetousness, which is idolatry. ...

1 Corinthians 14:34-35 ESV The women should keep silent in the churches. For they are not permitted to speak, but should be in submission, as the Law also says. If there is anything they desire to learn, let them ask their husbands at home. For it is shameful for a woman to speak in church.

1 Corinthians 11:4-10 ESV Every man who prays or prophesies with his head covered dishonors his head, but every wife who prays or prophesies with her head uncovered dishonors her head, since it is the same as if her head were shaven. For if a wife will not cover her head, then she should cut her hair short. But since it is disgraceful for a wife to cut off her hair or shave her head, let her cover her head. For a man ought not to cover his head, since he is the image and glory of God, but woman is the glory of man. For man was not made from woman, but woman from man. ...

1 Corinthians 11:1-16 ESV Be imitators of me, as I am of Christ. Now I commend you because you remember me in everything and maintain the traditions even as I delivered them to you. But I want you to understand that the head of every man is Christ, the head of a wife is her husband, and the head of Christ is God. Every man who prays or prophesies with his head covered dishonors his head, but every

wife who prays or prophesies with her head uncovered dishonors her head, since it is the same as if her head were shaven. ...

Revelation 1:6 ESV And made us a kingdom, priests to his God and Father, to him be glory and dominion forever and ever. Amen.

Revelation 1:1 ESV The revelation of Jesus Christ, which God gave him to show to his servants the things that must soon take place. He made it known by sending his angel to his servant John,

1 Corinthians 14:1-40 ESV Pursue love, and earnestly desire the spiritual gifts, especially that you may prophesy. For one who speaks in a tongue speaks not to men but to God; for no one understands him, but he utters mysteries in the Spirit. On the other hand, the one who prophesies speaks to people for their upbuilding and encouragement and consolation. The one who speaks in a tongue builds up himself, but the one who prophesies builds up the church. Now I want you all to speak in tongues, but even more to prophesy. The one who prophesies is greater than the one who speaks in tongues, unless someone interprets, so that the church may be built up. ...

Ecclesiastes 3:11 ESV He has made everything beautiful in its time. Also, he has put eternity into man's heart, yet so that he cannot find out what God has done from the beginning to the end.

Genesis 18:19 ESV For I have chosen him, that he may command his children and his household after him to keep the way of the Lord by doing righteousness and justice, so that the Lord may bring to Abraham what he has promised him."

Revelation 1:1-20 ESV The revelation of Jesus Christ, which God gave him to show to his servants the things that must soon take place. He made it known by sending his angel to his servant John, who bore witness to the word of God and to the testimony of Jesus Christ, even to all that he saw. Blessed is the one who reads aloud the words of this prophecy, and blessed are those who hear, and who keep what is written in it, for the time is near. John to the seven churches that are in Asia: Grace to you and peace from him who is and who was and who is to come, and from the seven spirits who are before his throne, and from Jesus Christ the faithful witness, the firstborn of the dead, and the ruler of kings on earth. To him who loves us and has freed us from our sins by his blood ...

Titus 2:4-5 ESV And so train the young women to love their husbands and children, to be self-controlled, pure, working at home, kind, and submissive to their own husbands, that the word of God may not be reviled.

1 Corinthians 11:4 ESV Every man who prays or prophesies with his head covered dishonors his head,

Many times I look around and say to myself: "Thanks to God that there is a God"

Written by Ramsis Ghaly

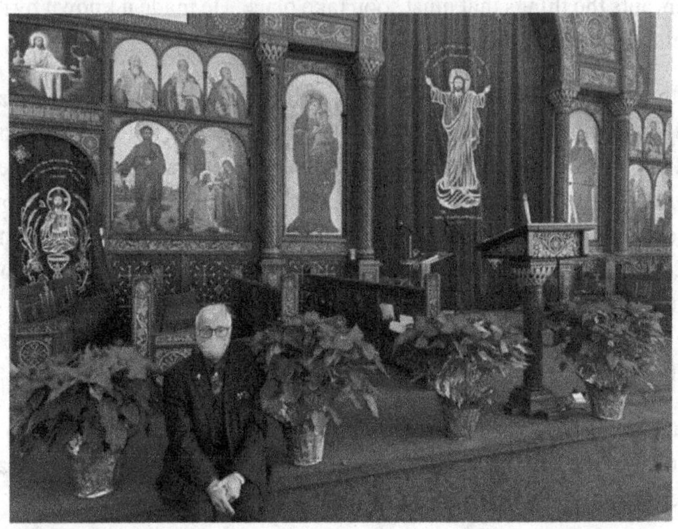

+ When I am not loved without a cause except by God the Lord, I kneel before my God saying: "Thanks to God that there is a God"

"Beloved, let us love one another: for love is of God; and every one that loveth is born of God, and knoweth God. [8] He that loveth not knoweth not God; for God is love. [9] In this was manifested the love of God toward us, because that God sent his only begotten Son into the world, that we might live through him. [10] Herein is love, not that we loved God, but that he loved us, and sent his Son to be the propitiation for our sins."1 John 4:7-10 KJV

+ When I am not adopted son except by God the Lord, I worship my Hod the Lord saying: "Thanks to God that there is a God"

"Henceforth I call you not servants; for the servant knoweth not what his lord doeth: but I have called you friends; for all things that I have heard of my Father I have made known unto you. [16] Ye have not chosen me, but I have chosen you, and ordained you, that ye should go and bring forth fruit, and that your fruit should remain: that whatsoever ye shall ask of the Father in my name, he may give it you." John 15:15-16 KJV

+ I might be forgotten by many! I might be at the bottom list! I might be that homeless person! I might be that very poor soul! I might be the failed individual at my class! I might be the one who is being mocked and bullied! I might be the sick laying at the bed of death! I might be the helpless soul living with no hope! I might be that person dying in my sins saying: "No salvation to my soul"!! Whatever it might be, I look at heaven to my Savior that saved my life, redeemed me and paid my dues and became ransom to many saying: "Thanks to God that there is a God"

"For by grace are ye saved through faith; and that not of yourselves: it is the gift of God: [9] Not of works, lest any man should boast. [10] For we are his workmanship, created in Christ Jesus unto good works, which God hath before ordained that we should walk in them. [13] But now in Christ Jesus ye who sometimes were far off are made nigh by the blood of Christ. [16] And that he might reconcile both unto God in one body by the cross, having slain the enmity thereby: [17] And came and preached peace to you which were afar off, and to them that were nigh. [18] For through him we both have access by one Spirit unto the Father. [19] Now therefore ye are no more strangers and foreigners, but fellowcitizens with the saints, and of the household of God; [20] And are built upon the foundation of the apostles and prophets, Jesus Christ himself being the chief corner stone ; [21] In whom all the building fitly framed together groweth unto an holy temple in the Lord: [22] In whom ye also are builded together for an habitation of God through the Spirit."Ephesians 2:8-10,13,16-22 KJV

+ When I am saddened broken hearted filled with sorrows, grieves and loses and I turn see God running toward me with open arms speaking to me: "Come unto me, all ye that labour and are heavy laden, and I will give you rest. [29] Take my yoke upon you, and learn of me; for I am meek and lowly in heart: and ye shall find rest unto your souls. [30] For my yoke is easy, and my burden is light." Matthew 11:28-30 KJV, I kneel down before God the Lord saying: "Thanks to God that there is a God"

+ When I know that Only One God that never ever lose hope in me or turn His back or his Face from me regardless and moreover, "He shall not cry, nor lift up, nor cause his voice to be heard in the street. [3] A bruised reed shall he not break, and the smoking flax shall he not quench: he shall bring forth judgment unto truth. [4] He shall not fail nor be discouraged, till he have set judgment in the earth: and the isles shall wait for his law." Isaiah 42:2-4 KJV, I cry in tears loving and believing in God the Lord saying: "Thanks to God that there is a God"

+ When the flowers weathers away, the vapors fade away and existence becomes not existed but God the Lord remains the Lord of living forever and ever more, I sing the praises to my Heavrnlh Father saying: "Thanks to God that there is a God"

+ When man gives up and so is the world and my destiny is doomed forever and my only Hope is in God the Lord, I cry saying: "Thanks to God that there is a God"

+ When death of the flesh is inevitable and the end of the world is a matter of when and the crumbling of the universe at the Second Coming of our Lord Jesus and the beginning of the New earth and New Heaven the New Jerusalem at life eternity, I call upon the Lord The Holy Lamb of God saying: "Thanks to God that there is a God"

+ When I know I am hated by all but loved sincerely by One God the Lord, I shed tears in Love saying: "Thanks to God that there is a God"

+ When I am lowly, poor and underprivileged and no one to lift me up, wipe my tears, wash me from all my sins and let me sit in the kings table, I kneel down to that One God the Lord saying: "Thanks to God that there is a God"

+ When I am surrounded by untruth and nothing but fake and game but Only One God the Truth, I stand up in courage believing and saying: "Thanks to God that there is a God"

+ When I am treated badly by all and blamed wrongly by all but One God the Lord, I raise my arms to heaven saying: "Thanks to God that there is a God"

+ When I know I am dead but alive again by God the Almighty, I cry in joy saying: "Thanks to God that there is a God"

+ When I take the last breath and give up the ghost knowing that my spirit shall commit in thy Hand my Heavenly Father, I look up to Heaven saying: "Thanks to God that there is a God"

+ When I see the animosity of men, the atrocities of nations, the wars and news of wars, my heart bleeds and eyes tears looking up to heaven saying: "Thanks to God that there is a God"

+ When I hear of famine, earthquakes, flooding and epidemics of illnesses, I look up to my Savior crying in tears believing and saying: "Thanks to God that there is a God"

+ When I learn that Adam and Eve and their descendants have been condemned to death for ever and Lord Jesus, the Son of God was the Only Essence to save the entire race, I kneeled down worshipped His Name saying: "Thanks to God that there is a God"

+ When I am blind since birth and no one could let me see but the Son of God, I praised my Savior saying: "Thanks to God that there is a God"

+ When I am unable to walk because of my infirmity snd no one could heal my infirmity except my Lord God of Heaven and Earth, I believed in thy Name praying thankfully saying: "Thanks to God that there is a God"

+ When I am sick dying of my illness and No True Healer but Him, the God the Lord, I put my body under His feet saying: "Thanks to God that there is a God"

+ When science has no answer and men have no remedy but only God the Lord incarnated in the flesh has all the remedies and answers, I kneel to that Savior of mankind saying: "Thanks to God that there is a God"

+ When I am having day and night seizures and my entire body convulse and no one else permanently cure my body from those evil seizures by God the Crestor of all things seen and unseen, I cried to God saying: "Thanks to God that there is a God"

+ When I got obsessed with demons and ruled over my life and threw me unto the Camentary with the dead and no One else could cast them out of my body but the Savior of the world who died for me, I threw myself under His feet by the Cross where He shed Hid blood for me and Sayed by loud voice: "Thanks to God that there is a God"

+ When men deny my rights and line up to be false witness accusing me with all kinds of evil and no One else can stand to say the truth and defend ne but God the Lord, I shed my tears before my Savior saying: "Thanks to God that there is a God"

+ When I am being persecuted and jailed for no reason but for righteousness and no One else to bring me hope and open His doors to His kingdom but God the Lord, I lift up my eyes and raise my arms up to heaven saying: "Thanks to God that there is a God"

+ When I am vanishing away from this mortal world and evil world, I look up to heaven admire the King of Heaven appreciative to His eternal sacrifice saying: "Thanks to God that there is a God"

+ When I am hated by all people living in the world full of inequities and injustice and care about itself only going after lusts and power and control, I stand strong rejecting to be part of that world and choosing to follow the True Light of the World saying: "Thanks to God that there is a God"

+ When I am hungry and thirsty and never fulfilled from the world food and drinks, I look up to the True Bread of Life and the True Drink of Salvation that I will no longer be hungry or thirst ever again saying: "Thanks to God that there is a God"

If heroism is forgotten by men, never ever by God!

"Thanks to God that there is a God"

John 3:16-19 KJV "For God so loved the world, that he gave his only begotten Son, that whosoever believeth in him should not perish, but have everlasting life. [17] For God sent not his Son into the world to condemn the world; but that the world through him might be saved. [18] He that believeth on him is not condemned: but he that believeth not is condemned already, because he hath not believed in the name of the only begotten Son of God. [19] And this is the condemnation, that light is come into the world, and men loved darkness rather than light, because their deeds were evil."

John 14:1-4,6,18-21,23,27-29 KJV "Let not your heart be troubled: ye believe in God, believe also in me. [2] In my Father's house are many mansions: if it were not so, I would have told you. I go to prepare a place for you. [3] And if I go and prepare a place for you, I will come again, and receive you unto myself; that where I am, there ye may be also. [4] And whither I go ye know, and the way ye know. [6] Jesus saith unto him, I am the way, the truth, and the life: no man cometh unto the Father, but by me. [18] I will not leave you comfortless: I will come to you. [19] Yet a little while, and the world seeth me no more; but ye see me: because I live, ye shall live also. [20] At that day ye shall know that I am in my Father, and ye in me, and I in you. [21] He that hath my commandments, and keepeth them, he it is that loveth me: and he that loveth me shall be loved of my Father, and I will love him, and will manifest myself to him. [23] Jesus answered and said unto him, If a man love me, he will keep my words: and my Father will love him, and we will come unto him, and make our abode with him. [27] Peace I leave with you, my peace I give unto you: not as the world giveth, give I unto you. Let not your heart be troubled, neither let it be afraid. [28] Ye have heard how I said unto you, I go away, and come again unto you. If ye loved me, ye would rejoice, because I said, I go unto the Father: for my Father is greater than I. [29] And now I have told you before it come to pass, that, when it is come to pass, ye might believe."

Av, Amen

Cg, Every article you write is just a unique experience of your faith in and your devotion to God. Thank you for sharing with us.

Jm, AGREE

Sc, Amen my friend

mh, Amen thanks for sending this. I really did need to hear this. God is good & loves us so much.

Dh, Amen

Sj, Amen

Jk, Beautifully done..

I Wonder Who Nowadays Shall Be That One??

Written by Ramsis Ghaly

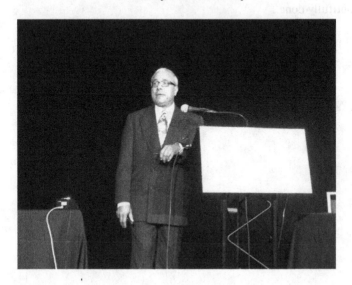

"The Lord is near to the brokenhearted and saves those who are crushed in spirit. Many are the afflictions of the righteous, but the Lord delivers him out of them all."

Psalm 34:18-19

Who stand for injustice whatever the cost?

Who sacrifice for others for the sake of righteousness?

"Greater love hath no man than this, that a man lay down his life for his friends. [17] These things I command you, that ye love one another." John 15:13,17 KJV

No matter what shall it cost or threat it shall create or risk to thy life, Who shall be the voice of the voiceless, the rescuer to the victim, the advocate to the innocent, the supporter to the underprivileged, the cheer giver to the needy, the Shephard to astray sheep, the councilor to the disturbed, the healer to sick, thr shield to the fallen, the shoulder to the feeble, the father to the fatherless, the mother to the motherless, the brother to the brotherless, the sister to the sisterless, the friend to the stranger, and the mentor to mentee??

Who? Who? Who? "Thus saith the Lord ; Execute ye judgment and righteousness, and deliver the spoiled out of the hand of the oppressor: and do no wrong, do no violence to the stranger, the fatherless, nor the widow, neither shed innocent blood in this place. [4] For if ye do this thing indeed, then shall there enter in by the gates of this house kings sitting upon the throne of David, riding in chariots and on horses, he, and his servants, and his people. [29] O earth, earth, earth, hear the word of the Lord." Jeremiah 22:3-4,29 KJV

"Is not this the fast that I have chosen? to lose the bands of wickedness, to undo the heavy burdens, and to let the oppressed go free, and that ye break every yoke? [7] Is it not to deal thy bread to the hungry, and that thou bring the poor that are cast out to thy house? when thou seest the naked, that thou cover him; and that thou hide not thyself from thine own flesh? [8] Then shall thy light break forth as the morning, and thine health shall spring forth speedily: and thy righteousness shall go before thee; the glory of the Lord shall be thy rereward. [9] Then shalt thou call, and the Lord shall answer; thou shalt cry, and he shall say, Here I am. If thou take away from the midst of thee the yoke, the putting forth of the finger, and speaking vanity; [10] And if thou draw out thy soul to the hungry, and satisfy the afflicted soul; then shall thy light rise in obscurity, and thy darkness be as the noonday: [11] And the Lord shall guide thee continually, and satisfy thy soul in drought, and make fat thy bones: and thou shalt be like a watered garden, and like a spring of water, whose waters fail not. [12] And they that shall be of thee shall build the old waste places: thou shalt raise up the foundations of many generations; and thou shalt be called, The repairer of the breach, The restorer of paths to dwell in."saiah 58:6-12 KJV

Proverbs 31:9 KJV

[9] Open thy mouth, judge righteously, and plead the cause of the poor and needy.

"How amiable are thy tabernacles, O Lord of hosts! [2] My soul longeth, yea, even fainteth for the courts of the Lord : my heart and my flesh crieth out for the living God. [3] Yea, the sparrow hath found an house, and the swallow a nest for herself, where she may lay her young, even thine altars, O Lord of hosts, my King, and my God. [4] Blessed are they that dwell in thy house: they will be still praising thee. Selah. [5] Blessed is the man whose strength is in thee; in whose heart are the ways of them. [6] Who passing through the valley of Baca make it a well; the rain also filleth the pools. [7] They go from strength to strength, every one of them in Zion appeareth before God. [8] O Lord God of hosts, hear my prayer: give ear, O God of Jacob. Selah. [9] Behold, O God our shield, and look upon the face of thine anointed. [10] For a day in thy courts is better than a thousand. I had rather be a doorkeeper in the house of my God, than to dwell in the tents of wickedness. [11] For the Lord God is a sun and shield: the Lord will give grace and glory: no good thing will he withhold from them that walk uprightly. [12] O Lord of hosts, blessed is the man that trusteth in thee." Psalm 84

Psalm 10:14 "But you, God, see the trouble of the afflicted; you consider their grief and take it in hand. The victims commit themselves to you; you are the helper of the fatherless.

Hebrews 10:22-25 KJV "Let us draw near with a true heart in full assurance of faith, having our hearts sprinkled from an evil conscience, and our bodies washed with pure water. [23] Let us hold fast the profession of our faith without wavering; (for he is faithful that promised;) [24] And let us consider one another to provoke unto love and to good works: [25] Not forsaking the assembling of ourselves together, as the manner of some is ; but exhorting one another : and so much the more, as ye see the day approaching."

Ramsis Ghaly

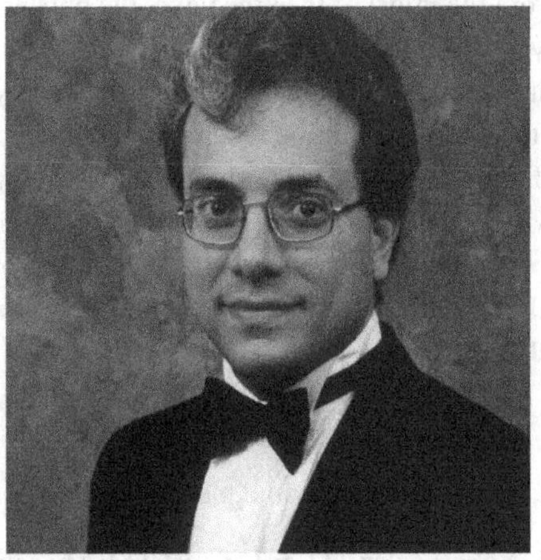

CG, A righteous man is the only one who will stand against injustice. Martin Luther King was righteous.

My angel is My Guardian Partner For Life!

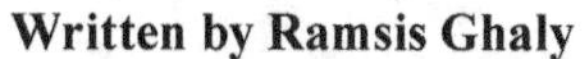

Written by Ramsis Ghaly

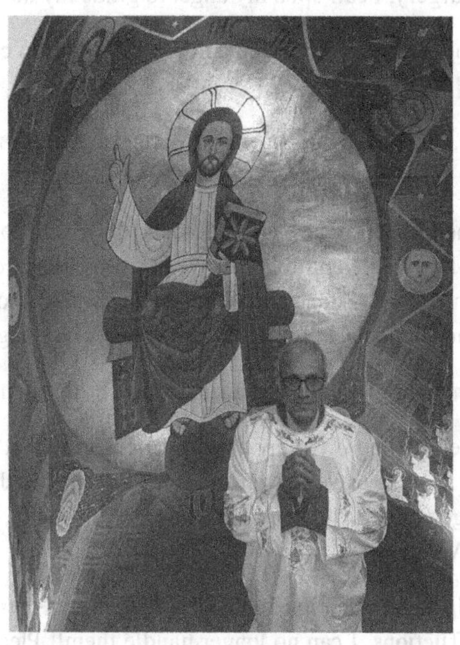

Searching for my Angel O Daughter's of Jerusalem! Have You Seen my Angel?? My angel is My Guardian Partner For Life! By my angel I am safe and not alone! My angel is always by my side even before I call!

My heavenly angel sent from God is all around me and is unseen yet my angel never leaves me!! I am God's child and the day He formed me inside the womb of my mom, He introduced me to my angel and angels of life bless my angel and bless them all!

Many times I feel mankind doesn't thank the guardian angels send from our Heavenly Father from heaven to earth and earth to heaven back and forth since He opened the Heaven again by His salvation! Let man acknowledge, recognize, bless and give thanksgiving yo the angels!

Sometimes I find myself looking for an angel ! Indeed, many times, I pray to my Savior to send me an angel !

Through my tough times, all I hope is for an angel to come down and be by my troubled soul!

Laying down in my sickness, I call upon my angel to come and be by my side!

As I touch my patients, I call upon my angel to let me know and guide my soul to heal!

When I perform surgery, I call upon my angel to guide my hands to rescue me!

When I walk in the darkness, I look up and ask my angel to come down and to walk with me!

In my dining table, there always a plate for my angel as I know my angel is eating with me!

My best time is when I sleep and my angel descend down and go through the walls and appear as a white Eagle and together we start to debrief of the neither day events and what should I had done and didn't do and what I should think about it and reflect unto the abundance of my Heavenly Father blessing!

Even, In my deep thoughts, I ask for my angel to guide me through decision-making!

Lately, I find myself calling often my angel to the degree that one time I felt so sorry to bother my angel to leave heaven and come be with me! Just before I ended my words, my angel smiled: "O son of God thy never bother, we all serve One Lord and Savior, Amen"

I screamed for help and I cried in tears: "O Angel of my Heavenly Father don't leave me in my afflictions, I can no longer handle them!! Please I beseech thee come down and be with me!!"

Every day, as I close my eyes and before I drift to sleep,I call upon my angel and hear a voice: "Here am I: I have you in my arms O child of the Most High"

And in times, I open my eyes and I get so surprised as I see Whom my soul Love with my angel !! I cry with loud voice: My Savior and my Lord: "It was but a little that I passed from them, but I found him whom my soul loveth: I held him, and would not let him go, until I had brought him into my mother's house, and into the chamber of her that conceived me.." Song of Songs 3:4 KJV

Innumerable times, I called upon my Savior and my angel ! I couldn't count how many times!! But I can't live without them!! O my soul why thy continue to stir up and disturb whom my soul Loveth and my angel?? I charged daughters of Jerusalem not to stir them up: "I charge you, O ye daughters of Jerusalem, by the roes, and by the hinds of the field, that ye stir not up, nor awake my love, till he please."Song of Songs 3:5 KJV

One episode I called upon my Beloved and He withdrew Himself from me! I was like a dead man with no single heartbeat and my face was as yellow as it could be: “I opened to my beloved; but my beloved had withdrawn himself and was gone: my soul failed when he spake: I sought him, but I could not find him; I called him, but he gave me no answer. [7] The watchmen that went about the city found me, they smote me, they wounded me; the keepers of the walls took away my veil from me.” Song of Songs 5:6-7 KJV

I ran in the streets looking for my Beloved and my angel crying to the daughters of Jerusalem: “The watchmen that went about the city found me, they smote me, they wounded me; the keepers of the walls took away my veil from me. [8] I charge you, O daughters of Jerusalem, if ye find my beloved, that ye tell him, that I am sick of love. [9] What is thy beloved more than another beloved, O thou fairest among women? what is thy beloved more than another beloved, that thou dost so charge us? [10] My beloved is white and ruddy, the chiefest among ten thousand. [16] His mouth is most sweet: yea, he is altogether lovely. This is my beloved, and this is my friend, O daughters of Jerusalem.”Song of Songs 5:7-10,16 KJV

I called upon His Name Day and night: “Return, Return, Return O my Dove the most beauty and pure unfixed white—; “Whither is thy beloved gone, O thou fairest among women? whither is thy beloved turned aside? that we may seek him with thee. [3] I am my beloved’s, and my beloved is mine: he feedeth among the lilies. [4] Thou art beautiful, O my love, as Tirzah, comely as Jerusalem, terrible as an army with banners. [9] My dove, my undefiled is but one; she is the only one of her mother, she is the choice one of her that bare her. The daughters saw her, and blessed her; yea, the queens and the concubines, and they praised her. [13] Return, return, O Shulamite; return, return, that we may look upon thee. What will ye see in the Shulamite? As it were the company of two armies.” Song of Songs 6:1,3-4,9,13 KJV

Come! Coe! Come! my Beloved I laid Up for thee—: “I am my beloved’s, and his desire is toward me. [11] Come, my beloved, let us go forth into the field; let us lodge in the villages. [12] Let us get up early to the vineyards; let us see if the vine flourish, whether the tender grape appear, and the pomegranates bud forth: there will I give thee my loves. [13] The mandrakes give a smell, and at our gates are all manner of pleasant fruits, new and old, which I have laid up for thee, O my beloved.” Song of Songs 7:10-13 KJV

My Beloved coming up from the wilderness, seal my soul upon thine heart, Many waters cannot quench love, neither can the floods drown it: “Who is this that cometh up from the wilderness, leaning upon her beloved? I raised thee up under the apple tree: there thy mother brought thee forth: there she brought thee forth that bare thee. [6] Set me as a seal upon thine heart, as a seal upon thine arm: for love is strong as death; jealousy is cruel as the grave: the coals thereof are coals of fire, which hath a most vehement flame. [7] Many waters cannot quench love, neither can the floods drown it: if a man would give all the substance of his house for love, it would utterly be contemned. Song of Songs 8:5-7 KJV

Amen

The Lord's Lovingkindness never cease to His children! Angels of the Lord descend from heaven from God! I am a child of God and from the moment He formed me inside the womb of my mom, my angel and angels are all around me! They never sleep and always there for me! They are unseen yet I do! I don't hear them yet I do!

"The Lord's lovingkindnesses indeed never cease, for His compassions never fail. They are new every morning; great is Your faithfulness."

Lamentations 3:21-23

The angels of God are descending and ascending since that time: "And he saith unto him, Verily, verily, I say unto you, Hereafter ye shall see heaven open, and the angels of God ascending and descending upon the Son of man." John 1:51 KJV

Let man render Thanksgiving to the angel and angels of heaven! Let man welcome the angels of the Lord and cast out the evil spirits! Let man, call upon his angel and angels and work together to fulfill the purpose of the Almighty! Let man, receive them with open arms and let them in? Let man, worship God the Lord and Praise His Name with his angels unceasingly! Let man, provides them with appreciation and appropriate acknowledgment and recognition!

Let the world praise the Lord God and glorify the Lord of hosts with new songs: "And suddenly there was with the angel a multitude of the heavenly host praising God, and saying, [14] Glory to God in the highest, and on earth peace, good will toward men." Luke 2:13-14 KJV

It was a new day when the heavens opened and angels came down when Baby Jesus was born and broke all the barriers: "And, lo, the angel of the Lord came upon them, and the glory of the Lord shone round about them: and they were sore afraid. [10] And the angel said unto them, Fear not: for, behold, I bring you good tidings of great joy, which shall be to all people. [11] For unto you is born this day in the city of David a Saviour, which is Christ the Lord. [12] And this shall be a sign unto you; Ye shall find the babe wrapped in swaddling clothes, lying in a manger." Luke 2:9-12 KJV

Indeed, my soul reaches out to my angel and angels dine and have frequent conversations! My angel shares my existence and accompany me wherever I go and whenever, since I was born until the moment I commit my soul in my Heavenly Father's Hand! My angel of life is mine and I am his! Together my guardian angel leads me to my salvation and bring me to light and closer and closer!

Angels of heaven are the earth co-inhabitants since our Savior descended down, born and lived among us! They are no longer strangers but one creation with us praising God, the Creator of all things seen and unseen!

It was the birth of new day not only to angels but mankind as Jesus message Kingdom of God is at hand: "And saying, The time is fulfilled, and the kingdom of God is at hand: repent ye, and believe the gospel." Mark 1:15 KJV

Biblical Verses

Psalm 103:20 Bless the Lord, you His angels,

Mighty in strength, who perform His word,

Obeying the voice of His word!

Hebrews 1:7 And of the angels He says,

"Who makes His angels winds,

And His ministers a flame of fire."

Psalm 104:4 He makes the winds His messengers,

Flaming fire His ministers.

Daniel 10:13 But the prince of the kingdom of Persia was withstanding me for twenty-one days; then behold, Michael, one of the chief princes, came to help me, for I had been left there with the kings of Persia.

Revelation 12:7 And there was war in heaven, Michael and his angels waging war with the dragon. The dragon and his angels waged war,

Daniel 8:16 And I heard the voice of a man between the banks of Ulai, and he called out and said, "Gabriel, give this man an understanding of the vision."

Luke 1:19 The angel answered and said to him, "I am Gabriel, who stands in the presence of God, and I have been sent to speak to you and to bring you this good news.

Hebrews 1:14 Are they not all ministering spirits, sent out to render service for the sake of those who will inherit salvation?

Exodus 23:23 For My angel will go before you and bring you in to the land of the Amorites, the Hittites, the Perizzites, the Canaanites, the Hivites and the Jebusites; and I will completely destroy them.

Numbers 20:16 But when we cried out to the Lord, He heard our voice and sent an angel and brought us out from Egypt; now behold, we are at Kadesh, a town on the edge of your territory.

Isaiah 63:8-9 For He said, "Surely, they are My people,

Sons who will not deal falsely."

So He became their Savior.

In all their affliction He was afflicted,

And the angel of His presence saved them;

In His love and in His mercy He redeemed them,

And He lifted them and carried them all the days of old.

Isaiah 37:36 Then the angel of the Lord went out and struck 185,000 in the camp of the Assyrians; and when men arose early in the morning, behold, all of these were dead.

Acts 5:19 But during the night an angel of the Lord opened the gates of the prison, and taking them out he said,

Acts 7:53 You who received the law as ordained by angels, and yet did not keep it."

Job 33:22-26

"Then his soul draws near to the pit,

And his life to those who bring death.

"If there is an angel as mediator for him,

One out of a thousand,

To remind a man what is right for him,

Then let him be gracious to him, and say,

'Deliver him from going down to the pit,

I have found a ransom';

Acts 7:38 This is the one who was in the congregation in the wilderness together with the angel who was speaking to him on Mount Sinai, and who was with our fathers; and he received living oracles to pass on to you.

Galatians 3:19 Why the Law then? It was added because of transgressions, having been ordained through angels by the agency of a mediator, until the seed would come to whom the promise had been made.

Hebrews 2:2 For if the word spoken through angels proved unalterable, and every transgression and disobedience received a just penalty,

Zechariah 1:8-10 I saw at night, and behold, a man was riding on a red horse, and he was standing among the myrtle trees which were in the ravine, with red, sorrel and white horses behind him. Then I said, "My lord, what are these?" And the angel who was speaking with me said to me, "I will show you what these are." And the man who was standing among the myrtle trees answered and said, "These are those whom the Lord has sent to patrol the earth."

l 7:15-16 "As for me, Daniel, my spirit was distressed within me, and the visions in my mind kept alarming me. I approached one of those who were standing by and began asking him the exact meaning of all this. So he told me and made known to me the interpretation of these things:

Zechariah 4:11-14 Then I said to him, "What are these two olive trees on the right of the lampstand and on its left?" And I answered the second time and said to him, "What are the two olive branches which are beside the two golden pipes, which empty the golden oil from themselves?" So he answered me, saying, "Do you not know what these are?" And I said, "No, my lord."read more.

Revelation 17:1Then one of the seven angels who had the seven bowls came and spoke with me, saying, "Come here, I will show you the judgment of the great harlot who sits on many waters,

Zechariah 3:4 He spoke and said to those who were standing before him, saying, "Remove the filthy garments from him." Again he said to him, "See, I have taken your iniquity away from you and will clothe you with festal robes."

Numbers 22:21-35 So Balaam arose in the morning, and saddled his donkey and went with the leaders of Moab. But God was angry because he was going, and the angel of the Lord took his stand in the way as an adversary against him. Now he was riding on his donkey and his two servants were with him. When the donkey saw the angel of the Lord standing in the way with his drawn sword in his hand, the donkey turned off from the way and went into the field; but Balaam struck the donkey to turn her back into the way.read more.

Psalms 91:11 - For he shall give his angels charge over thee, to keep thee in all thy ways.

Hebrews 13:2 - Be not forgetful to entertain strangers: for thereby some have entertained angels unawares.

Hebrews 1:14 - Are they not all ministering spirits, sent forth to minister for them who shall be heirs of salvation?

Psalms 103:20 - Bless the LORD, ye his angels, that excel in strength, that do his commandments, hearkening unto the voice of his word.

Psalms 34:7 - The angel of the LORD encampeth round about them that fear him, and delivereth them.

Isaiah 6:2 - Above it stood the seraphims: each one had six wings; with twain he covered his face, and with twain he covered his feet, and with twain he did fly.

Jude 1:6 - And the angels which kept not their first estate, but left their own habitation, he hath reserved in everlasting chains under darkness unto the judgment of the great day.

Revelation 19:10 - And I fell at his feet to worship him. And he said unto me, See thou do it not: I am thy fellowservant, and of thy brethren that have the testimony of Jesus: worship God: for the testimony of Jesus is the spirit of prophecy.

Matthew 24:31 - And he shall send his angels with a great sound of a trumpet, and they shall gather together his elect from the four winds, from one end of heaven to the other.

Matthew 18:10 - Take heed that ye despise not one of these little ones; for I say unto you, That in heaven their angels do always behold the face of my Father which is in heaven.

Searching for my Angel O Daughter's of Jerusalem! Have You Seen my Angel??
My angel is My Guardian Partner for Life! By my angel I am safe and not alone!
My angel is always by my side even before I call!

Searching for my Angel O Daughter's of Jerusalem! Have You Seen my Angel??
My angel is My Guardian Partner for Life! By my angel I am safe and not alone!

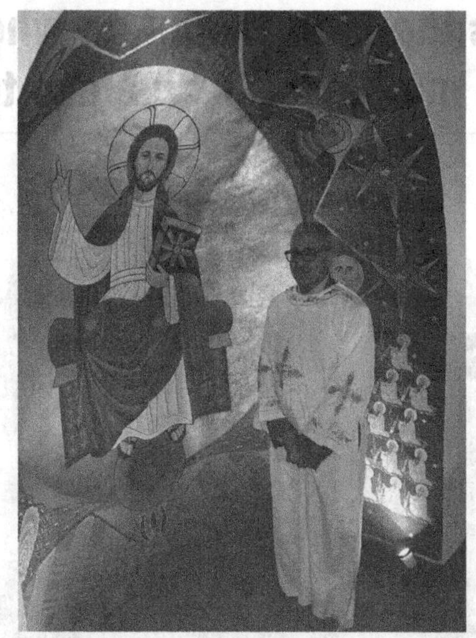

ES, Thank you so much for posting this. There really is no other reason that I should be alive right now if it weren't for Jesus sending down His Angels to protect me. So many times I should have died. When I feel lost, lonely, ugly, not good enough……. I have to ask for the Power of the Holy Spirit to fill me w His truth. I am a daughter of the King most high!!!! I am loved!!!!! I am accepted as I am by the blood of Christ out Savior NOT by anything I can do or earn. Man's opinion of me (should) mean nothing to me. Only God our Creator

What is the First thing I do when I go and see my Savior Jesus face to face?

Written by Ramsis Ghaly

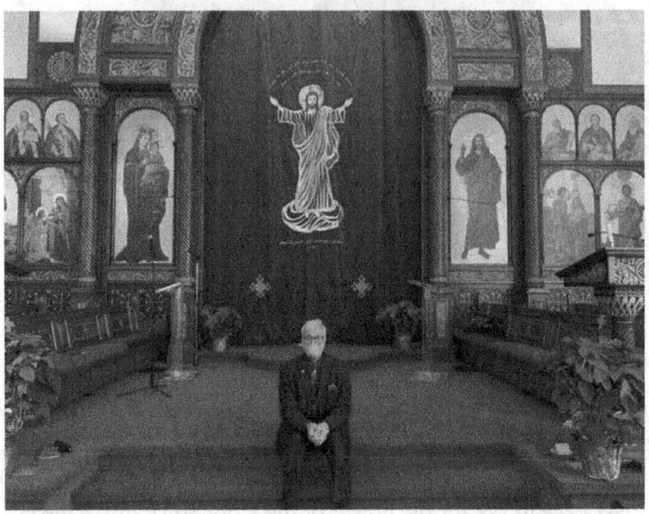

This night, I asked my soul: What is the First thing, I will do when I go and see my Savior Jesus Face -to-face?

The very very first thing I will do, do what the publican did: Worship my Savior, kneel before Him afar off, would not lift up my eyes smite upon my breast, saying: "God be merciful to me a sinner." As it is written: "And the publican, standing afar off, would not lift up so much as his eyes unto heaven, but smote upon his breast, saying, God be merciful to me a sinner." Luke 18:13 KJV

The very second thing I will do is what Simon Peter, son of Jonas said: "Yea, Lord; thou knowest that I love thee. Lord, thou knowest all things; thou knowest that I love thee." As it is written:

"So when they had dined, Jesus saith to Simon Peter, Simon, son of Jonas, lovest thou me more than these? He saith unto him, Yea, Lord; thou knowest that I love thee. He saith unto him, Feed my lambs. [16] He saith to him again the second time, Simon, son of Jonas, lovest thou me? He saith unto him, Yea, Lord; thou knowest that I love thee. He saith unto him, Feed my sheep. [17] He saith unto him the third time, Simon, son of Jonas, lovest thou me? Peter was grieved because he said unto him the third time, Lovest thou me? And he said unto him, Lord, thou knowest all things; thou knowest that I love thee. Jesus saith unto him, Feed my sheep." John 21:15-17 KJV

Then I shall Scream in joy, Cry with tears of happiness, Run and sit at His feet, Kiss Him and sit by His side, Love Him and put my head by His chest!

Once I am in the bosom of whom my soul loveth: I will hold Him, and would not let Him go as it is written: "It was but a little that I passed from them, but I found him whom my soul loveth: I held him, and would not let him go, until I had brought him into my mother's house, and into the chamber of her that conceived me." Song of Songs 3:4 KJV

My Savior Jesus is coming —"And the Spirit and the bride say, Come. And let him that heareth say, Come. And let him that is athirst come. And whosoever will, let him take the water of life freely. [20] He which testifieth these things saith, Surely I come quickly. Amen. Even so, come, Lord Jesus. [21] The grace of our Lord Jesus Christ be with you all. Amen." Revelation 22:17,20-21 KJV

"And, behold, I come quickly; and my reward is with me, to give every man according as his work shall be. [13] I am Alpha and Omega, the beginning and the end, the first and the last. [14] Blessed are they that do his commandments, that they may have right to the tree of life, and may enter in through the gates into the city. [16] I Jesus have sent mine angel to testify unto you these things in the churches. I am the root and the offspring of David, and the bright and morning star." Revelation 22:12-14,16 KJV

Amen

JT, i will kneel and give thanks

AV, Beautiful message! GBYD

CG, Being in His presence will be your greatest present.

Kings and Queens

Jesus The True King of the World and St Mary the Mother of God the True Queen of the World!

Written on 9/12/2022 by Ramsis Ghaly

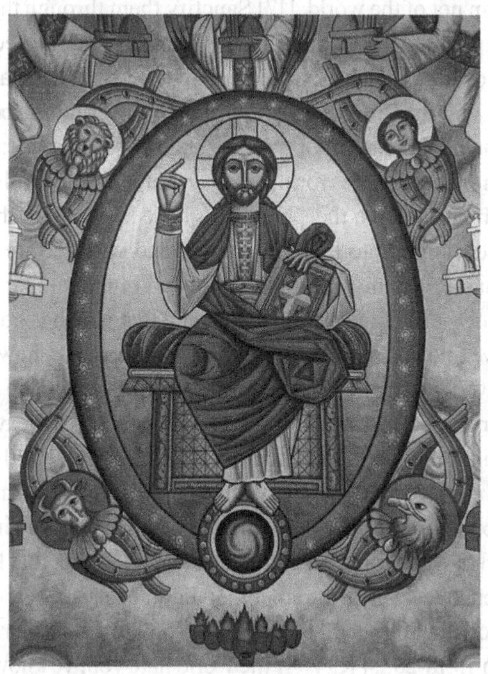

As the World is celebrating the earthly king and British monarchy and Commonwealth realms, Royal Family, House of Windsor 9/8/22, Queen Elizabeth death and king Charles III coronation,, let the world Not forget Jesus is the True King NEVER DIES EVERLASTING!

Revelation 19:16 KJV "And he hath on his vesture and on his thigh a name written, KING OF KINGS, AND LORD OF LORDS."

Jesus Christ the True King

But Jesus kingdom is not from the world! It isn't materialistic and earthly but eternal and of Truth and Righteousness as He spoke to Pilate saying: John 18:36-37 KJV "Jesus answered, My kingdom is not of this world: if my kingdom were of this world, then would my servants fight, that I should not be delivered to the Jews: but now is my kingdom not from hence. [37] Pilate therefore said unto him, Art thou a king then? Jesus answered, Thou sayest that I am a king. To this end was I born, and for this cause came I into the world, that I should bear witness unto the truth. Every one that is of the truth heareth my voice." And John 17:14-17,23-26 KJV "I have given them thy word; and the world hath hated them, because they are not of the world, even as I am not of the world. [15] I pray not that thou shouldest take them out of the world, but that thou shouldest keep them from the evil. [16] They are not of the world, even as I am not of the world. [17] Sanctify them through thy truth: thy word is truth. [23] I in them, and thou in me, that they may be made perfect in one; and that the world may know that thou hast sent me, and hast loved them, as thou hast loved me. [24] Father, I will that they also, whom thou hast given me, be with me where I am; that they may behold my glory, which thou hast given me: for thou lovedst me before the foundation of the world. [25] O righteous Father, the world hath not known thee: but I have known thee, and these have known that thou hast sent me. [26] And I have declared unto them thy name, and will declare it : that the love wherewith thou hast loved me may be in them, and I in them."John 3:6,12-13,17-19 KJV "That which is born of the flesh is flesh; and that which is born of the Spirit is spirit. [12] If I have told you earthly things, and ye believe not, how shall ye believe, if I tell you of heavenly things? [13] And no man hath ascended up to heaven, but he that came down from heaven, even the Son of man which is in heaven. [17] For God sent not his Son into the world to condemn the world; but that the world through him might be saved. [18] He that believeth on him is not condemned: but he that believeth not is condemned already, because he hath not believed in the name of the only begotten Son of God. [19] And this is the condemnation, that light is come into the world, and men loved darkness rather than light, because their deeds were evil." John 4:24 KJV God is a Spirit: and they that worship him must worship him in spirit and in truth."John 15:18-20,24 KJV "If the world hate you, ye know that it hated me before it hated you. [19] If ye were of the world, the world would love his own: but because ye are not of the world, but I have chosen you out of the world, therefore the world hateth you. [20] Remember the word that I said unto you, The servant is not greater than his lord. If they have persecuted me, they will also persecute you; if they have kept my saying, they will keep yours also. [24] If I had not done among them the works which none other man did, they had not had sin: but now have they both seen and hated both me and my Father."

Jesus refused the glory of the world and rejected the desire of people to make Him a material king for material world and went to pray alone: John 6:14-15 KJV "Then those men, when they had seen the miracle that Jesus did, said, This is of a truth that prophet that should come into the world. [15] When Jesus therefore perceived that they would come and take him by force, to make him a king, he departed again into a mountain himself alone."

Jesus is the Way, Truth and Life but The prince of world is evil John 14:6,30-31 KJV "Jesus saith unto him, I am the way, the truth, and the life: no man cometh unto the Father, but by me. [30] Hereafter I will not talk much with you: for the prince of this world cometh, and hath nothing in me. [31] But that the world may know that I love the Father; and as the Father gave me commandment, even so I do. Arise, let us go hence."

Yet Jesus is my True King who descended from His glory to live as a poor man, carried my sins and tolerated my poverty, thirst and hunger and nakedness and ultimately shed His Own blood as God for His people and took nothing from His people but hell, hunger and pains. His people killed Him, yet with no single pay back, He gives the world His own kingdom and saying to His people:

Matthew 11:28-30 KJV "Come unto me, all ye that labour and are heavy laden, and I will give you rest. [29] Take my yoke upon you, and learn of me; for I am meek and lowly in heart: and ye shall find rest unto your souls. [30] For my yoke is easy, and my burden is light."

Jesus the True King and not the earthly king. Jesus loved us first for no reason and not to get anything from us but love back. 1 John 4:8-9,19 KJV "He that loveth not knoweth not God; for God is love. [9] In this was manifested the love of God toward us, because that God sent his only begotten Son into the world, that we might live through him. [19] We love him, because he first loved us."

Jesus is full of True Love to mankind; ***John 3:16-18 KJV "For God so loved the world, that he gave his only begotten Son, that whosoever believeth in him should not perish, but have everlasting life. [17] For God sent not his Son into the world to condemn the world; but that the world through him might be saved. [18] He that believeth on him is not condemned: but he that believeth not is condemned already, because he hath not believed in the name of the only begotten Son of God."***

How much glorious when Our Creator The Savior of the World, The Holy Lamb of God, The True King of Kings, Lord of Lords Jesus Christ, comes in His second coming to judge the world and bring His children to Him at His Kingdom where He shall be their true King and Heavenly Father and they shall be His own. Jesus won't be in Roll Royce luxury car and the crowd be in the street, but Jesus shall be in their midst wiping their tears, shining His Light, nourishing their souls, giving them the true eternal life,—- Jesus the True King shall let His children live with Him in His own Castle in His own kingdom inseparable of Him. They won't wait outside The Buckingham palace or waive for them from the balcony, but He shall walk with them. He shall bring them to sit by His dining table and entering in His

Holy wedding. It shall be no television screen to see Him or radio to hear Him but Jesus shall be One to one with His children.

As it is written ***Revelation 21:3-7 KJV "And I heard a great voice out of heaven saying, Behold, the tabernacle of God is with men, and he will dwell with them, and they shall be his people, and God himself shall be with them, and be their God. [4] And God shall wipe away all tears from their eyes; and there shall be no more death, neither sorrow, nor crying, neither shall there be any more pain: for the former things are passed away. [5] And he that sat upon the throne said, Behold, I make all things new. And he said unto me, Write: for these words are true and faithful. [6] And he said unto me, It is done. I am Alpha and Omega, the beginning and the end. I will give unto him that is athirst of the fountain of the water of life freely. [7] He that overcometh shall inherit all things; and I will be his God, and he shall be my son."***

Jesus shall never take a penny or taxes or anything from His children, but He shall give them true Love and springs of waters full of glory. Jesus the True King shall be with His people by the Tree of Life! Jesus the True King is the only King able to give the True Life and true eternity and cast out death and cast out from His people all the pains, aches, injustice, suffering, darkness and all evil!

Jesus, the Savior of the world died for His people and descended down from His glory to live in person with His people and carried their sins and open the gate for whoever follow Him regardless of his color and form to enter to His own kingdom

Jesus Christ is the True King worth watching, following His footsteps and obey His commandments and waiting for Him all other kings are fake and nothing compared to our Lord Jesus!

Praise our Lord Jesus the True King and never put hope in any earthly king as the psalmist wrote: ***Psalm 146 KJV "Praise ye the Lord. Praise the Lord, O my soul. [2] While I live will I praise the Lord : I will sing praises unto my God while I have any being. [3] Put not your trust in princes, nor in the son of man, in whom there is no help. [4] His breath goeth forth, he returneth to his earth; in that very day his thoughts perish. [5] Happy is he that hath the God of Jacob for his help, whose hope is in the Lord his God: [6] Which made heaven, and earth, the sea, and all that therein is : which keepeth truth for ever: [7] Which executeth judgment for the oppressed: which giveth food to the hungry. The Lord looseth the prisoners: [8] The Lord openeth the eyes of the blind: the Lord raiseth them that are bowed down: the Lord loveth the righteous: [9] The Lord preserveth the strangers; he relieveth the fatherless and widow: but the way of the wicked he turneth upside down. [10] The Lord shall reign for ever, even thy God, O Zion, unto all generations. Praise ye the Lord."***

Jesus is the Lord of Lords King of Kings:

Revelation 17:14 KJV "These shall make war with the Lamb, and the Lamb shall overcome them: for he is Lord of lords, and King of kings: and they that are with him are called, and chosen, and faithful."

God Save the king

O earth thy reminded of biblical citation of "God Save the king" as follows:

Saul the king

"God save the king"

1 Samuel 10:24 KJV "And Samuel said to all the people, See ye him whom the Lord hath chosen, that there is none like him among all the people? And all the people shouted, and said, God save the king."

Solomon the king

"God save the king"

1 Kings 1:39 KJV "And Zadok the priest took an horn of oil out of the tabernacle, and anointed Solomon. And they blew the trumpet; and all the people said, God save king Solomon."

1 Samuel 10:24 "And Samuel said to all the people, See ye him whom the LORD hath chosen, that there is none like him among all the people? And all the people shouted, and said, God save the king."

KJV, 2 Samuel 16:16 "And it came to pass, when Hushai the Archite, David's friend, was come unto Absalom, that Hushai said unto Absalom, God save the king, God save the king."

KJV, 2 Kings 11:12 "And he brought forth the king's son, and put the crown upon him, and gave him the testimony; and they made him king, and anointed him; and they clapped their hands, and said, God save the king."

KJV, 2 Chronicles 23:11 "Then they brought out the king's son, and put upon him the crown, and gave him the testimony, and made him king. And Jehoiada and his sons anointed him, and said, God save the king."

KJV, WBS, MSTC Nehemiah 2:3 "Nevertheless I was sore afraid and said unto the king, "God save the king's life forever, should I not look sadly? The city of my fathers' burial lieth waste and the gates thereof are consumed with fire."

PROPLE chose their king and refused His anointee

We will have our king

1 Samuel 8:19-20 KJV "Nevertheless the people refused to obey the voice of Samuel; and they said, Nay; but we will have a king over us; [20] That we also may be like all the nations; and that our king may judge us, and go out before us, and fight our battles."

God repented

1 Samuel 15:11 KJV "It repenteth me that I have set up Saul to be king: for he is turned back from following me, and hath not performed my commandments. And it grieved Samuel; and he cried unto the Lord all night."

Jesus is the True King

Revelation 19:13, 16

He is clothed in a robe dipped in blood, and the name by which he is called is The Word of God. . . . On his robe and on his thigh he has a name written, King of kings and Lord of lords.

John 18:36

Jesus answered, "My kingdom is not of this world. If my kingdom were of this world, my servants would have been fighting, that I might not be delivered over to the Jews. But my kingdom is not from the world."

Isaiah 9:6–7

For to us a child is born, to us a son is given; and the government shall be upon his shoulder, and his name shall be called Wonderful Counselor, Mighty God, Everlasting Father, Prince of Peace. Of the increase of his government and of peace there will be no end, on the throne of David and over his kingdom, to establish it and to uphold it with justice and with righteousness from this time forth and forevermore. The zeal of the Lord of hosts will do this.

Ephesians 1:20–21

. . . that he worked in Christ when he raised him from the dead and seated him at his right hand in the heavenly places, far above all rule and authority and power and dominion, and above every name that is named, not only in this age but also in the one to come.

Daniel 7:13–14

I saw in the night visions, and behold, with the clouds of heaven there came one like a son of man, and he came to the Ancient of Days and was presented before him. And to him was given dominion and glory and a kingdom, that all peoples, nations, and languages should serve him; his dominion is an everlasting dominion, which shall not pass away, and his kingdom one that shall not be destroyed.

Acts 2:30–32

Being therefore a prophet, and knowing that God had sworn with an oath to him that he would set one of his descendants on his throne, he foresaw and spoke about the resurrection of the Christ, that he was not abandoned to Hades, nor did his flesh see corruption. This Jesus God raised up, and of that we all are witnesses.

Revelation 17:14

They will make war on the Lamb, and the Lamb will conquer them, for he is Lord of lords and King of kings, and those with him are called and chosen and faithful.

1 Timothy 6:13–15

I charge you in the presence of God, who gives life to all things, and of Christ Jesus, who in his testimony before Pontius Pilate made the good confession, to keep the commandment unstained and free from reproach until the appearing of our Lord Jesus Christ, which he will display at the proper time—he who is the blessed and only Sovereign, the King of kings and Lord of lords.

Hebrews 1:3–4

He is the radiance of the glory of God and the exact imprint of his nature, and he upholds the universe by the word of his power. After making purification for sins, he sat down at the right hand of the Majesty on high, having become as much superior to angels as the name he has inherited is more excellent than theirs.

Revelation 1:5–6

. . . and from Jesus Christ the faithful witness, the firstborn of the dead, and the ruler of kings on earth. To him who loves us and has freed us from our sins by his blood and made us a kingdom, priests to his God and Father, to him be glory and dominion forever and ever. Amen.

Who is he, this King of glory? The Lord Almighty— he is the King of glory. Psalm 24:10

I will exalt you, my God the King; I will praise your name for ever and ever. Psalm 145:1

For the Lord is our judge, the Lord is our lawgiver, the Lord is our king; it is he who will save us. Isaiah 33:22

Above his head they placed the written charge against him: this is jesus, the king of the jews.

Matthew 27: 37

Now to the King eternal, immortal, invisible, the only God, be honor and glory for ever and ever. Amen. 1 Timothy 1:17

The Lord will be king over the whole earth. On that day there will be one Lord, and his name the only name. Zechariah 14:9

After Jesus was born in Bethlehem in Judea, during the time of King Herod, Magi from the east came to Jerusalem and asked, "Where is the one who has been born king of the Jews? We saw his star when it rose and have come to worship him."

Matthew 2:1-2

Now I, Nebuchadnezzar, praise and exalt and glorify the King of heaven, because everything he does is right and all his ways are just. And those who walk in pride he is able to humble. Daniel 4:37

Rejoice greatly, Daughter Zion! Shout, Daughter Jerusalem! See, your king comes to you, righteous and victorious, lowly and riding on a donkey, on a colt, the foal of a donkey. Zechariah 9:9

I thank and praise you, God of my ancestors: You have given me wisdom and power, you have made known to me what we asked of you, you have made known to us the dream of the king. Daniel 2:23

Heal the sick who are there and tell them, 'The kingdom of God has come near to you.' Luke 10:9

Do not be afraid, little flock, for your Father has been pleased to give you the kingdom. Luke 12:32

From that time on Jesus began to preach, "Repent, for the kingdom of heaven has come near."

Matthew 4:17

"The time has come," he said. "The kingdom of God has come near. Repent and believe the good news!" Mark 1:15

Jesus replied, "Very truly I tell you, no one can see the kingdom of God unless they are born again."

John3:3

Blessed are those who are persecuted because of righteousness, for theirs is the kingdom of heaven.

Matthew 5:10

But seek first his kingdom and his righteousness, and all these things will be given to you as well.

Matthew 6:33

Therefore anyone who sets aside one of the least of these commands and teaches others accordingly will be called least in the kingdom of heaven, but whoever practices and teaches these commands will be called great in the kingdom of heaven. Matthew 5:19

Jesus answered, "Very truly I tell you, no one can enter the kingdom of God unless they are born of water and the Spirit." John 3:5

Jesus said, "Let the little children come to me, and do not hinder them, for the kingdom of heaven belongs to such as these." Matthew 19:14

Not everyone who says to me, 'Lord, Lord,' will enter the kingdom of heaven, but only the one who does the will of my Father who is in heaven. Matthew 7:21

The Lord will rescue me from every evil attack and will bring me safely to his heavenly kingdom. To him be glory for ever and ever. Amen. 2 Timothy 4:18

Or do you not know that wrongdoers will not inherit the kingdom of God? Do not be deceived: Neither the sexually immoral nor idolaters nor adulterers nor men who have sex with men nor thieves nor the greedy nor drunkards nor slanderers nor swindlers will inherit the kingdom of God. 1 Corinthians 6:9-10

Prayers for the Earthly king

Psalm 72 "Give the king thy judgments, O God, and thy righteousness unto the king's son. [2] He shall judge thy people with righteousness, and thy poor with judgment. [3] The mountains shall bring peace to the people, and the little hills, by righteousness. [4] He shall judge the poor of the people, he shall save the children of the needy, and shall break in pieces the oppressor. [5] They shall fear thee as long as the sun and moon endure, throughout all generations. [6] He shall come down like rain upon the mown grass: as showers that water the earth. [7] In his days shall the righteous flourish; and abundance of peace so long as the moon endureth. [8] He shall have dominion also from sea to sea, and from the river unto the ends of the earth. [9] They that dwell in the wilderness shall bow before him; and his enemies shall lick the dust. [10] The kings of Tarshish and of the isles shall bring presents: the kings of Sheba and Seba shall offer gifts. [11] Yea, all kings shall fall down before him: all nations shall serve him. [12] For he shall deliver the needy when he crieth; the poor also, and him that hath no helper. [13] He shall spare the poor and needy, and shall save the souls of the needy. [14] He shall redeem their soul from deceit and violence: and precious shall their blood be in his sight. [15] And he shall live, and to him shall be given of the gold of Sheba: prayer also shall be made for him continually; and daily shall he be praised. [16] There shall be an handful of corn in the earth upon the top of the mountains; the fruit thereof shall shake like Lebanon: and they of the city shall flourish like grass of the earth. [17] His name shall endure for ever: his name shall be continued as long as the sun: and men shall be blessed in him: all nations shall call him blessed. [18] Blessed be the Lord God, the God of Israel, who only doeth wondrous things. [19] And blessed be his glorious name for ever: and let the whole earth be filled with his glory; Amen, and Amen. [20] The prayers of David the son of Jesse are ended."

THIS IS MY EVERLASTING TRUE KING AND THE WORLD TRUE KING THAT NEVER DIES HAD THE TRUE KEYS TO HEAVEN AND HADES: "*He is despised and rejected of men; a man of sorrows, and acquainted with grief: and we hid as it were our faces from him; he was despised, and we esteemed him not. [4] Surely he hath borne our griefs, and carried our sorrows: yet we did esteem him stricken, smitten of God, and afflicted. [5] But he was wounded for our transgressions, he was bruised for our iniquities: the chastisement of our peace was upon him; and with his stripes we are healed. [6] All we like sheep have gone astray; we have turned every one to his own way; and the Lord hath laid on him the iniquity of us all. [7] He was oppressed, and he was afflicted, yet he opened not his mouth: he is brought as a lamb to the slaughter, and as a sheep before her shearers is dumb, so he openeth not his mouth. [8] He was taken from prison and from judgment: and who shall declare his generation? for he was cut off out of the land of the living: for the transgression of my people was he stricken. [9] And he made his grave with the wicked, and with the rich in his death; because he had done no violence, neither was any deceit in his mouth. [10] Yet it pleased the Lord to bruise him; he hath put him to grief: when thou shalt make his soul an offering for sin, he shall see his seed, he shall prolong his days, and the pleasure of the Lord shall prosper in his hand. [11] He shall see of the travail of his soul, and shall be satisfied: by his knowledge shall my righteous servant justify many; for he shall bear their iniquities. [12] Therefore* *will I divide him a portion with the great, and he shall divide the spoil with the strong; because he hath poured out his soul unto death: and he was numbered with the transgressors; and he bare the sin of many, and made intercession for the transgressors."Isaiah 53*

Queen of Heaven is St Mary!

Written on 9/14/2022 by Ramsis Ghaly
Written by

How many are celebrating Queen Mary, the Theotokos, mother of God Jesus Christ the Savior of the world and the True King of all seen and unseen God the Lord Jesus Christ as the world celebrate Queen Elisabeth and King Charles III of Britain??

It is an eye opening and waking call of nowadays celebrating the Earthly king and queen and how much resources spent and more than 250 million people worldwide watching!!

I wonder if the world celebrates the True King Jesus Christ and Savior of the world all people and Queen Mary the Mother of God with even the same attention as the world currently celebrate the King Charles III and the queen Elizabeth of British Empire!

While celebrating Queen Elizabeth the Mother of the Savior of the world Jesus, let us remember and celebrate the true Queen of Heaven, the mother of God, Virgin St Mary!

Queen of Heaven (Latin: Regina Caeli) is a title given to the Virgin Mary, by Christians mainly of the Catholic Church and, to a lesser extent, in Anglicanism, Lutheranism, and Eastern Orthodoxy.

Queen of Heaven Mary is sitting by the King Jesus Her Son and God!

The queen in gold of Ophir, the king greatly desire thy beauty: for he is thy Lord; and worship thou him, I will make thy name to be remembered in all generations: therefore shall the people praise thee for ever and ever."

Psalm 45:9-17 KJV. "Kings' daughters were among thy honourable women: upon thy right hand did stand the queen in gold of Ophir. [10] Hearken, O daughter, and consider, and incline thine ear; forget also thine own people, and thy father's house; [11] So shall the king greatly desire thy beauty: for he is thy Lord; and worship thou him. [12] And the daughter of Tyre shall be there with a gift; even the rich among the people shall intreat thy favour. [13] The king's daughter is all glorious within: her clothing is of wrought gold. [14] She shall be brought unto the king in raiment of needlework: the virgins her companions that follow her shall be brought unto thee. [15] With gladness and rejoicing shall they be brought: they shall enter into the king's palace. [16] Instead of thy

fathers shall be thy children, whom thou mayest make princes in all the earth. [17] I will make thy name to be remembered in all generations: therefore shall the people praise thee for ever and ever."

Acts 7:49, "Heaven is My throne, and earth is My footstool",

https://en.m.wikipedia.org/wiki/Queen_of_Heaven

"MARY" which means "Royal Incense"

St. Mary the Virgin is the Mother of God; Theotokos. (Lk 1:43). She was the seed of David (Rom 3:1); the bride-to-be of Joseph (Mt 1:18-25); kinswoman of Elizabeth the mother of John the Baptist (Lk 1:36); attended to ceremonial purification (Lk 2:22-38); fled into Egypt with Joseph and Jesus (Mt 2:13-15); lived in Nazareth (Mt 2:19-23); took twelve-year old Jesus to the temple in Jerusalem (Lk 2:41-50); at the wedding in Cana of Galilee (Jn 2:1-11); concerned for Jesus' safety (Mt 12:46, Mk 3:21-31, Lk 8:19-21); at the cross where she was entrusted by Our Lord Jesus Christ to care of John the Evangelist (Jn 19:25-27); in the Upper Room with the disciples where the Holy Spirit came down upon them (Acts 1:14).

St. Mary's parents, Joachim and Anne, were righteous people in front of God. They prayed earnestly asking God to grant them a child. Six years after they were married, they had Mary, and they knew that she was a special gift from God. They gave her the name "MARY" which means "Royal Incense" because she would become a special offering to God. When Mary was three years old, Joachim and Anne took her to the temple and dedicated their child to God. She spent nine years in the temple

https://st-takla.org/.../Saint-Mary-Fast_Virgin-Life...

The 'Theotokos'

This is a Greek word composed of two syllables: 'Theo' meaning 'God', and 'tokos' meaning 'bearer'; that is, 'she who bore God in her womb'.

https://en.m.wikipedia.org/wiki/Queen_of_Heaven

Luke 1:28,31-33,35,37-38 KJV

[28] And the angel came in unto her, and said, Hail, thou that art highly favoured, the Lord is with thee: blessed art thou among women. [31] And, behold, thou shalt conceive in thy womb, and bring forth a son, and shalt call his name JESUS. [32] He shall be great, and shall be called the Son of the Highest: and the Lord God shall give unto him the throne of his father David: [33] And he shall reign over the house of Jacob for ever; and of his kingdom there shall be no end. [35] And the angel answered and said unto her, The Holy

Ghost shall come upon thee, and the power of the Highest shall overshadow thee: therefore also that holy thing which shall be born of thee shall be called the Son of God. [37] For with God nothing shall be impossible. [38] And Mary said, Behold the handmaid of the Lord; be it unto me according to thy word. And the angel departed from her.

Luke 2:10-14,16 KJV "And the angel said unto them, Fear not: for, behold, I bring you good tidings of great joy, which shall be to all people. [11] For unto you is born this day in the city of David a Saviour, which is Christ the Lord. [12] And this shall be a sign unto you; Ye shall find the babe wrapped in swaddling clothes, lying in a manger. [13] And suddenly there was with the angel a multitude of the heavenly host praising God, and saying, [14] Glory to God in the highest, and on earth peace, good will toward men. [16] And they came with haste, and found Mary, and Joseph, and the babe lying in a manger."

Isaiah 7:14 ESV "Therefore the Lord himself will give you a sign. Behold, the virgin shall conceive and bear a son, and shall call his name Immanuel."

St Mary Theotokos, Queen for life earth and heave!

Queen Elizabeth Wueen in earth for 70 years!

St Mary found worthy to be the mother of God!

Queen Elizabeth found worthy to be queen of Britain!

The True Queen of World is St Mary!

The Queen of the British Empire is queen Elizabeth!

The Queen of Heaven is St Mary!

The queen of England and commonwealth is Queen Elizabeth!

The eternal Queen is St Mary!

The seventy-year Queen of Britain is Queen Elizabeth!

The Queen that brought salvation through her Son is St Mary the Theotokos and put an end to death and grant the entire human race life eternity through her Son bloodshed!

Queen Mary of Heaven lived in a manger consecrated her life to the True King and Savior Jesus!

Queen Mary of Heaven brought heaven to earth and earth to heaven and became mankind second gate!

Queen Mary of Heaven free gave and continue to give and appear and perform incredible miracles through her apparitions!!

The world is interceding to St Mary to pray for each before the throne of her Son and Savior Jesus Christ!

DN, So very true

JT, i had to read this a few times to understand...

BN, Amen

cg, Wonderful article!

Our Lord Jesus is indeed the King of Kings.

Kings use force and killing to get their way. With Jesus, none of these is true. Kings are identified with wealth. They have everything they need. Jesus llved a life of poverty. He is indeed our King. Amen

DL, Amén.

KB, So 100 percent Right.

MB, 100%

JT, agreed

CG, Blessed Virgin Mary pray for us.

A Poem Dedicated to Queen Elizabth II and The Era of Elizabethan!

Written on 09/19/2022 by Ramsis Ghaly

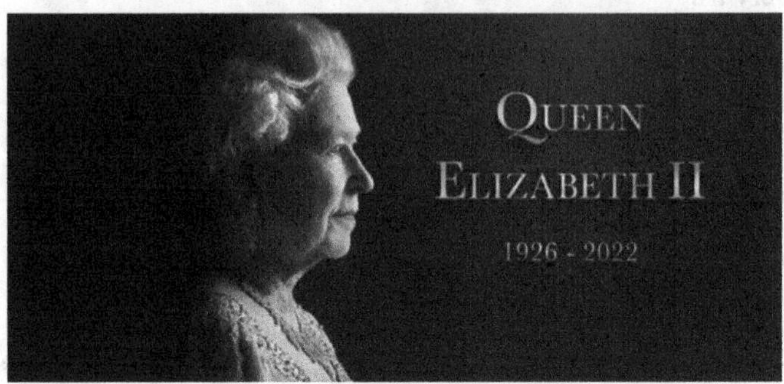

A Life Anointed by the Holy Spirit to a Monarch! A Life to Remember and Footsteps to follow! A Life of Duty and Service!

A Life of Faith and Love!

A Life of a Queen forever admired and Unmatched dignities, today we the world came together to say thank you and final goodbye!

A Life of a Queen ordained as Monarch at age of 25th reigned February 6, 1952 coronated to the British Throne, June, 2, 1953, In the Name of the Father, The Son and The Holy Sprit in the Order of the Most High Gaza, a Defender of the Faith, Sovereign the most High order of Gaza, born April 21, 1926 and departed September 8, 2022, queen regent of 32 sovereign states to fifteen states for little more than 70 years the longest of any British!

A life of Queen serve and endured to the end, deep in faith, Patron followed Christ with silent prayers!

A Life of Queen inspired the entire world during her State funeral showed outpouring of love united tens of thousands of leaders, royalties and dignitaries!

A Life of a Queen from the Nineteenth century to the Twentieth Century, marks an era named under her name the "Elizabethan Era"!

A Life of Crowns and Politics!

A Life of Queen Full of Loyalty and Character!

A Life of a Deeply Christian Queen with roots of royal family transcended from the Divine through thousands of years!

A Life of Broadcasts and Sermons!

A Life Among the Kings and Queens!

A Life Among the World Leaders and Global Prime-ministers!

A Life of Vow Kept and an Imperial Family to Follow!

A Life Began of Very Young Age Twenty-Five Years of Age!

A Life Full of Male's World and Arm Forces!

A Life Faced Repetitive Adversaries and Controversies!

A Life of Freedom and Changes!

A Life of Great Chief and Phenomenal Commander!

A Life of a Class, Down-to-Earth Person and Part of All of Socioeconomic Classes!

A Life Through Tragedies, Atrocities and Wars Including COVID-19!

A Life of a queen at a time of failing in British colonization resulted in Decolonization and liberation with establishment instead of family of commonwealth in love, stability and continuity!

A Life of a Queen under which British Empire was falling yet her monarchy was rising up high exceeded the sky!

A Life of Queen Head of State the longest ran monarchy From a age of steam tarins with black and white TV to digital technology and Transformation to Modern Britain, Commonwealth and world!

A Life of a Queen where liberation took place and multiracial nation!

A Life of a Queen of the Ages took the monarchy up high through the Tribulating world and Frequently changing!

A Life of a Queen United the world when there were divisions and united the world Globally in her presence and her absence and beyond her death!

A Life of Royal Highness and Causal Togetherness's!

A Life Beyond a Queen, a Wife, a Mother, a Servicewoman, Grandma and Beyond!

A Life of Laughs, Smiles and Joy!

A Life breading and Raising Horses and Dogs!

A Life of Public Servant and Privat Family!

A Life of Sense of NO Ego full of Resilience and Dignity!

A Life of Constant Changes and Manages!

A Life of Jubilees Sliver and Diamond Monarchy!

A Life of Mourning and Burden!

A life Dedicated to Service and People!

A life Full of Energy and Prosperity with Extreme Loyalty and Humility!

A Lifelong beyond Ninety Years and Prominence Beyond Seventy Years!

A Life Filled with Unmeasured Accomplishments, wisdom and sense gifted by the Holy Spirit!

A Life Reached to the Four Coroners of Earth !

A Life Began Standing Alone and Ended A Saden Widow Alone!

A Life Where Many of Loved Ones Passed Away and Much of Gains and Loses!

A Life of an Era That is Well-Done, and It Won't Ever Come Again!

A Life to Celebrate and a One Person Represented all ages!

A Life of Strength and Constancy!

A Life of Blessing and a Life to Bless!

A Life of Queen Elizabeth II, cared about people, visited and met those she rolled over and encountered!

A Life dedicated and Pledged to Reign to Serve and a World to Bring Together!

A Life of a Royal Exceeded Hundred Folds Set Before Her and Beyond!

A Life of Iconic Figure, Fame and Ever Recognized!

A Life of Queen of Commonwealth, Queen of All People and Queen of the World!

A Life of Majesty and Daily Full Schedule with Millions of Events!

A Life of Personal Sacrifices, Compassion, Kindness and Heart of Gold!

A Life of Hope, Sharing and Support!

A Life Sympathy, Empathy, Selflessness Quietly, Hard on Herself and Cheer-giver!

A Life of Compassion, Empathy and Serenity!

A life of a Queen full of knowledge, understanding, with perspective of history, uplifting standing up to her values immensely, selfless service!

A Life of a caring Queen full of kindness connected to people unashamed of her God and Savior Jesus the Lord!

A Life of a humble Queen that never raised above the norm, the common and underprivileged kept sense of humor and multitudes of charities!

A Life of Queen maintained the inherited customs and traditions from thousands of years values wondering in communities, walking in streets mixing with ordinary people yet standing by the British parliaments, Buckingham Palace and Castles!

A Life of Stability and Steady with Spirit Never Wavering from Duty or Service!

A Life Throughout the Upheaved Events National and International!

A Life Full of Prayers, Thanksgiving and Inspired Christmas Wishes!

A Life of a Royal Faced Unparalleled Challenges Headed and Ran for So Long Close to a Century!

A Life of Unheard-of Devotions and Held the Constitution to the Heart!

A life of a Leader with Seventy Years of Cumulative Wisdom!

A Life of Faithful Servant and an Example to Modern Shaky leaders to Look Up To!

A Life Lived to Full, grieving to millions of souls and hard to say goodbye!

A Life Reflective of the Queen of people reign over people much loved by people with witnessed outpouring of love and outshining many other kings and queens!

A Life of Queen Began with “God Save the Queen “and Handed to the Son “God Save the King”!

A Life Arrived Naked of the Warm Womb to a Coffin Surrounded with Millions of Loves, Prayers, Pay Respect, Commemorations and Goodbyes for Now!

In Summary.

A Life Walk-In in Unexpected Destiny and Uncertain Future Carried Jesus Cross While Living in Christ and Dying in Christ to be Glorified with Him at That Day!

A Life a Queen Followed the Footsteps of the Good Shephard!

A Life of a Warrior that Never Dies in Jesus Name, the Lord of Resurrection that Eternal Never End!

"His lord said unto him, Well done, thou good and faithful servant: thou hast been faithful over a few things, I will make thee ruler over many things: enter thou into the joy of thy lord." Matthew 25:21 KJV

"I have fought a good fight, I have finished my course, I have kept the faith: [8] Henceforth there is laid up for me a crown of righteousness, which the Lord, the righteous judge, shall give me at that day: and not to me only, but unto all of them also that love his appearing."2 Timothy 4:7-8 KJV

"For to me to live is Christ, and to die is gain." Philippians 1:21 KJV

"I have been crucified with Christ; and it is no longer I who live, but Christ lives in me; and the life which I now live in the flesh I live by faith in the Son of God, who loved me and gave Himself up for me." Galatians 2:20

A Life with Story Incredibly Moving and Now Going to a Resting Place by the Westminster Abby on Earth while returning to God of Heaven by Phillip and George: "Return unto thy rest, O my soul; for the Lord hath dealt bountifully with thee. [8] For thou hast delivered my soul from death, mine eyes from tears, and my feet from falling. [9] I will walk before the Lord in the land of the living. [10] I believed, therefore have I spoken: I was greatly afflicted:" Psalm 116:7-10 KJV

"Lord, now You are letting Your servant depart in peace,

According to Your word; For my eyes have seen Your salvation Which You have prepared before the face of all peoples, A light to *bring* revelation to the Gentiles, And the glory of Your people Israel." (Luke 2:29-32)

Biblical scriptures Read During Queen Elizabeth II Funeral Prayers!

A touchy and holy deeply spiritual Funeral ceremony full of Words of Jesus the Savior of the world and Christian lyrics!! Let me share:

An Era began thousands of years and shall be named in her honor the Elizabethan Era forever!

Grief felt by all and rituals of comfort and hope!

Queen Elizabeth II (born Princess Elizabeth of York), 96, the mother of the United Kingdom's King Charles III, died September 8, 2022 at Balmoral Castle in Aberderdeenshire, Scotland, a residence of the British Royal Family for thousands of Years. The unforgettable funeral Journey in Hierarchy order of Gaza founded more than 600 years ago. In Peace passed by Westminster Abby, Windsor to St Geroge's Castle.

Her televised State Funeral September 19 Westminster Abbey, watched by an estimated 4 billion people, was attended by heads of state and dignitaries from around the world, including US President Joe Biden. She reigned 70 years, the longest of any British monarch and the longest recorded of any female head of state in history in Sovereignty.

A life celebrated in an incredible State Funeral with a huge scale of crowd lined up paying tribute, respect, show appreciation, saying final farewell, to the Queen of people who dedicated her life, devoted herself since teenager for service and duty for more than seventy years, among unheard of a worldwide mourners, statesmen and women, presidents, prime-minsters, royalties and dignitaries in hundreds of thousands all got together to celebrate a Life of Queen that Had given so much to the world!!

A Deeply religious scented in hymns, psalms, scriptures procession for A Life of the longest served queen unashamed of her Christian faith and a spectacular mother figure and grandmother while serving the people of the world touching multitudes following procession of Queen Victoria from 1900!

Westminster Abby of thirteen centuries of history where she was married and coronated as a Queen of great Britain and commonwealth in a splendid deep spiritual ceremony to lay to rest at the Windsor St George's Chapel alongside where her family were buried too, her husband King Phillip, her father, George II, mother Queen Elizabeth, and sister Margret, and monarchs Queen Mary, king George I, queen Victoria, king Charles I, king Henry-- .

As Queen Elizabeth Beloved people say farewell, those who served, her dogs and horses say goodbye, as her Monarch Imperial Precious State Crown, Orb, and Sceptre depart her body to be placed in great Alter separating her body as she is making her final place of rest alone again to the burial committing her soul in the hands of God as profound Christian with unrelenting service flourished so many multitudes of fruits nation and international worldwide, in courage and hope, in a complicated ever changing world, long life in blessing with honorable memories to follow and set an example what a man can do if follow the Savior footsteps and commandments, in faith as her Lord Jesus the Precious Corner Stone, living for ever. The merciful God grant life to whoever fear Him and hold His Children in His Righteousness.

John 11:25-26
Buy your copy of The Faith of Queen Elizabeth: The Poise, Grace and Quiet Strength Behind the Crown in the FaithGateway Store where you'll enjoy low prices every day. Jesus said unto her, I am the resurrection, and the life: he that believeth in me, though he were dead, yet shall he live: and whosoever liveth and believeth in me shall never die.

Job 19:25-27
I know that my redeemer liveth, and that he shall stand at the latter day upon the earth: and though after my skin worms destroy this body, yet in my flesh shall I see God: Whom I shall see for myself, and mine eyes shall behold, and not another.

1 Timothy 6:7
We brought nothing into this world, and it is certain we can carry nothing out.

Revelation 14:13
I heard a voice from heaven, saying unto me, "Write, From henceforth blessed are the dead which die in the Lord: even so saith the Spirit; for they rest from their labours. Amen.

1 Corinthians 15:20–26, 53–58
Now is Christ risen from the dead, and become the firstfruits of them that slept. For since by man came death, by man came also the resurrection of the dead. For as in Adam all die, even so in Christ shall all be made alive. But every man in his own order: Christ the firstfruits; afterward they that are Christ's at his coming. Then cometh the end, when he shall have delivered up the kingdom to God, even the Father; when he shall have put down all rule and all authority and power. For he must reign, till he hath put all enemies under his feet. The last enemy that shall be destroyed is death. For this corruptible must put on incorruption, and this mortal must put on immortality. So when this corruptible shall have put on incorruption, and this mortal shall have put on immortality, then shall be brought to pass the saying that is written, Death is swallowed up in victory. O death, where is thy sting? O grave, where is thy victory? The sting of death is sin; and the strength

of sin is the law. But thanks be to God, which giveth us the victory through our Lord Jesus Christ. Therefore, my beloved brethren, be ye steadfast, unmoveable, always abounding in the work of the Lord, forasmuch as ye know that your labour is not in vain in the Lord.Psalm 42:1–7

Like as the hart desireth the water-brooks
so longeth my soul after thee, O God.
My soul is athirst for God, yea, even for the living God
when shall I come to appear before the presence of God?
My tears have been my meat day and night
while they daily say unto me, Where is now thy God?
Now when I think thereupon, I pour out my heart by myself
for I went with the multitude, and brought them forth into the house of God;
In the voice of praise and thanksgiving
among such as keep holy-day.
Why art thou so full of heaviness, O my soul
and why art thou so disquieted within me?
Put thy trust in God
for I will yet give him thanks for the help of his countenance.

John 14:1–9a

"Let not your heart be troubled: ye believe in God, believe also in me. In my Father's house are many mansions: if it were not so, I would have told you. I go to prepare a place for you. And if I go and prepare a place for you, I will come again, and receive you unto myself; that where I am, there ye may be also. And whither I go ye know, and the way ye know." Thomas saith unto him, "Lord, we know not whither thou goest; and how can we know the way?" Jesus saith unto him, "I am the way, the truth, and the life: no man cometh unto the Father, but by me. If ye had known me, ye should have known my Father also: and from henceforth ye know him, and have seen him." Philip saith unto him, "Lord, shew us the Father, and it sufficeth us." Jesus saith unto him, "Have I been so long time with you, and yet hast thou not known me, Philip? He that hath seen me hath seen the Father."

Psalm 34:8

Taste and see how gracious the LORD is blest is the man that trusteth in him.

Matthew 6:9–13

Our Father which art in heaven, Hallowed be thy name. Thy kingdom come. Thy will be done in earth, as it is in heaven. Give us this day our daily bread. And forgive us our debts, as we forgive our debtors. And lead us not into temptation, but deliver us from evil: For thine is the kingdom, and the power, and the glory, for ever. Amen.

Romans 8:35a, 38b–39
Who shall separate us from the love of Christ? Neither death, nor life, nor angels, nor principalities, nor powers, nor things present, nor things to come, nor height, nor depth, nor any other creature, shall be able to separate us from the love of God, which is in Christ Jesus our Lord. Alleluia! Amen.

[Read the "Order of Service for a Service of Thanksgiving for the Life of Her Majesty The Queen" at St Giles' Cathedral, Edinburgh, Scotland, Monday September 12.]

Following The State Funeral was the Committal Service later in the day at St. George's Chapel, Windsor. The following Bible verses were either alluded to or directly read during the service:

Psalm 121
I will lift up mine eyes unto the hills
from whence cometh my help.
My help cometh even from the LORD
who hath made heaven and earth.
He will not suffer thy foot to be moved
and he that keepeth thee will not sleep.
Behold, he that keepeth Israel: shall neither slumber nor sleep.
The LORD himself is thy keeper
the LORD is thy defence upon thy right hand;
So that the sun shall not burn thee by day
neither the moon by night.
The LORD shall preserve thee from all evil
yea, it is even he that shall keep thy soul.
The LORD shall preserve thy going out, and thy coming in
from this time forth for evermore.

Revelation 21:1–7
I saw a new heaven and a new earth: for the first heaven and the first earth were passed away; and there was no more sea. And I John saw the holy city, new Jerusalem, coming down from God out of heaven, prepared as a bride adorned for her husband. And I heard a great voice out of heaven saying, "Behold, the tabernacle of God is with men, and he will dwell with them, and they shall be his people, and God himself shall be with them, and be their God. And God shall wipe away all tears from their eyes; and there shall be no more death, neither sorrow, nor crying, neither shall there be any more pain: for the former things are passed away." And he that sat upon the throne said, "Behold, I make all things new." And

he said unto me, "Write: for these words are true and faithful." And he said unto me, "It is done. I am Alpha and Omega, the beginning and the end. I will give unto him that is athirst of the fountain of the water of life freely. He that overcometh shall inherit all things; and I will be his God, and he shall be my son."

Psalm 103:13–17
Like as a father pitieth his own children:
even so is the LORD merciful unto them that fear him.
For he knoweth whereof we are made:
he remembereth that we are but dust.
The days of man are but as grass:
for he flourisheth as a flower of the field.
For as soon as the wind goeth over it, it is gone:
and the place thereof shall know it no more.
But the merciful goodness of the LORD endureth for ever and ever upon them that fear him:
and his righteousness upon children's children.

The Lyrics
The Day Thou Gavest, Lord, Is Ended

The Queen chose this hymn to be sung at her funeral.

It was written by John Ellerton in 1870 and is often sung to the tune of St Clement.

The hymn was also played at the celebrations for the Diamond Jubilee of Queen Victoria in 1897.

It is the official evening hymn of the Royal Navy, with the words focusing on the worldwide fellowship of the church.

The lyrics are:

The day you gave us, Lord, is ended,
the darkness falls at your request;
to you our morning hymns ascended,
your praise shall sanctify our rest.

We thank you that your Church, unsleeping
while earth rolls onward into light,
through all the world her watch is keeping
and never rests by day or night.

As over continent and island
each dawn leads to another day,
the voice of prayer is never silent,
nor do the praises die away.

So be it, Lord! Your throne shall never,
like earth's proud empires, pass away;
your kingdom stands and grows forever
until there dawns your glorious day.

The Lord Is My Shepherd

This hymn is actually Psalm 23 and its main theme is the trust one holds in God.

It is a very important psalm in the Church of England, often sung as a response at funerals - and is believed to be a favorite to the queen. Many people will find the words familiar as they are used in the theme tune for popular BBC comedy The Vicar Of Dibley. The tune used for the show was written by composer Howard Goodall, whereas in church it is commonly sung to Crimond, which is generally credited to Jessie Seymour Irvine.

The traditional lyrics are:

The Lord's my shepherd; I'll not want.
He makes me down to lie
in pastures green; he leadeth me
the quiet waters by.

He leadeth me, he leadeth me
the quiet waters by.
My soul he doth restore again
and me to walk doth make
within the paths of righteousness,
e'en for his own name's sake;

within the paths of righteousness,
e'en for his own name's sake.
Yea, though I walk in death's dark vale,
yet will I fear no ill;
for thou art with me, and thy rod
and staff me comfort still;
for thou art with me, and thy rod
and staff me comfort still.

My table thou hast furnished
in presence of my foes;
my head thou dost with oil anoint,
and my cup overflows.
My head thou dost with oil anoint,
and my cup overflows.

Goodness and mercy all my life
shall surely follow me,
and in God's house forevermore
my dwelling place shall be;
and in God's house forevermore
my dwelling place shall be.

Love Divine, All Loves Excelling

The Queen also chose Love Divine, All Loves Excelling for her funeral. This hymn was written by leader of the Methodist movement Charles Wesley in 1747 and it describes Christian perfection.

The tune is Blaenwern by William Penfro Rowlands.

It was sung during the wedding of Prince William and Kate Middleton in 2011.

The lyrics are:

Love divine, all loves excelling,
joy of heav'n, to earth come down,
fix in us thy humble dwelling,
all thy faithful mercies crown.
Jesus, thou art all compassion,
pure, unbounded love thou art.
Visit us with thy salvation;
enter ev'ry trembling heart.

Breathe, O breathe thy loving Spirit
into ev'ry troubled breast.
Let us all in thee inherit,
let us find the promised rest.
Take away the love of sinning;
Alpha and Omega be.
End of faith, as its beginning,
set our hearts at liberty.

Come, Almighty, to deliver,
let us all thy life receive.
Suddenly return, and never,
nevermore they temples leave.
Thee we would be always blessing,
serve thee as thy hosts above,
pray, and praise thee without ceasing,
glory in thy perfect love.

Finish, then, thy new creation;
true and spotless let us be.
Let us see thy great salvation
perfectly restored in thee.
Changed from glory into glory,
till in heav'n we take our place,
till we cast our crowns before thee,
lost in wonder, love and praise.

The Sentences

During the procession of the coffin into the Abbey, the choir will sing verses from the Bible.

These will be:

John 11 verses 25-26: "I am the resurrection and the life, saith the Lord: he that believeth in me, though he were dead, yet shall he live: and whosoever liveth and believeth in me shall never die.

Job 9 verses 25-27: "I know that my Redeemer liveth, and that he shall stand at the latter day upon the earth: and though after my skin worms destroy this body, yet in my flesh shall I see God; whom I shall see for myself, and mine eyes shall behold, and not another."

1 Timothy 6 verse 7 and Job 1 verse 21: "We brought nothing into this world, and it is certain we can carry nothing out. The Lord gave, and the Lord hath taken away; blessed be the name of the Lord."

The Book of Common Prayer: "Thou knowest, Lord, the secrets of our hearts; shut not thy merciful ears unto our prayer; but spare us, Lord most holy, O God most mighty, O holy and most merciful Saviour, thou most worthy Judge eternal, suffer us not, at our last hour, for any pains of death, to fall from thee. Amen."

Revelation 14 verse 13: "I heard a voice from heaven, saying unto me, Write, From henceforth blessed are the dead which die in the Lord: even so saith the Spirit; for they rest from their labours. Amen."

The Bidding

The Bidding will be read by the Dean of Westminster, Dr David Hoyle.

IN grief and also in profound thanksgiving we come to this House of God, to a place of prayer, to a church where remembrance and hope are sacred duties.

Here, where Queen Elizabeth was married and crowned, we gather from across the nation, from the Commonwealth, and from the nations of the world, to mourn our loss, to remember her long life of selfless service, and in sure confidence to commit her to the mercy of

God our maker and redeemer.

With gratitude we remember her unswerving commitment to a high calling over so many years as Queen and Head of the Commonwealth. With admiration we recall her life-long sense of duty and dedication to her people. With thanksgiving we praise God for her constant example of Christian faith and devotion.

With affection we recall her love for her family and her commitment to the causes she held dear. Now, in silence, let us in our hearts and minds recall our many reasons for thanksgiving, pray for all members of her family, and commend Queen Elizabeth to the care and keeping of almighty God.

This is followed by the prayer:

O MERCIFUL God, the Father of our Lord Jesus Christ, who is the resurrection and the life; in whom whosoever believeth shall live, though he die; and whosoever liveth, and believeth in him, shall not die eternally; who hast taught us, by his holy Apostle Saint Paul, not to be sorry, as men without hope, for them that sleep in him:

We meekly beseech thee, O Father, to raise us from the death of sin unto the life of righteousness; that, when we shall depart this life, we may rest in him, as our hope is this our sister doth; and that, at the general Resurrection in the last day, we may be found acceptable in thy sight; and receive that blessing, which thy well-beloved Son

shall then pronounce to all that love and fear thee, saying, Come, ye blessed children of my Father, receive the kingdom prepared for you from the beginning of the world. Grant this, we beseech thee, O merciful Father, through Jesus Christ, our mediator and redeemer. Amen.

The First Lesson

Baroness Scotland will read from 1 Corinthians 15, verses 20-26 and 53 to the end.

Now is Christ risen from the dead, and become the first fruits of them that slept.

For since by man came death, by man came also the resurrection of the dead.

For as in Adam all die, even so in Christ shall all be made alive. But every man in his own order: Christ the firstfruits; afterward they that are Christ's at his coming.

Then cometh the end, when he shall have delivered up the kingdom to God, even the Father; when he shall have put down all rule and all authority and power.

For he must reign, till he hath put all enemies under his feet. The last enemy that shall be destroyed is death.

For this corruptible must put on incorruption, and this mortal must put on immortality. So when this corruptible shall have put on incorruption, and this mortal shall have put on immortality, then shall be brought to pass the saying that is written, Death is swallowed up in victory.

O death, where is thy sting? O grave, where is thy victory? The sting of death is sin; and the strength of sin is the law.

But thanks be to God, which giveth us the victory through our Lord Jesus Christ.

Therefore, my beloved brethren, be ye steadfast, unmoveable, always abounding in the work of the Lord, forasmuch as ye know that your labour is not in vain in the Lord.

The Psalm

The choir will sing Psalm 42 verses 1-7.

It was composed by Judith Weir in 1954.

The words are:

Like as the hart desireth the water-brooks : so longeth my soul after thee, O God.

My soul is athirst for God, yea, even for the living God : when shall I come to appear before the presence of God?
My tears have been my meat day and night : while they daily say unto me, Where is now thy God?
Now when I think thereupon, I pour out my heart by myself : for I went with the multitude, and brought them forth into the house of God;

In the voice of praise and thanksgiving : among such as keep holy-day.
Why art thou so full of heaviness, O my soul : and why art thou so disquieted within me?

Put thy trust in God : for I will yet give him thanks for the help of his countenance.

The Second Lesson

The second lesson read by PM Liz Truss is from John 14 verses 1-9a.

Let not your heart be troubled: ye believe in God, believe also in me.

In my Father's house are many mansions: if it were not so, I would have told you. I go to prepare a place for you.

And if I go and prepare a place for you, I will come again, and receive

you unto myself; that where I am, there ye may be also. And whither I go ye know, and the way ye know.

Thomas saith unto him, Lord, we know not whither thou goest; and

how can we know the way? Jesus saith unto him, I am the way, the truth, and the life: no man cometh unto the Father, but by me.

If ye had known me, ye should have known my Father also: and from henceforth ye know him, and have seen him.

Philip saith unto him, Lord, shew us the Father, and it sufficeth us. Jesus saith unto him, Have I been so long time with you, and yet hast thou not known me, Philip? He that hath seen me hath seen the Father.

The Anthem from Songs of Farewell

The choir will sing The Anthem from Songs of Farewell, which was written by Hubert Parry in the First World War.

It comprises six choral motets, with My Soul, There Is A Country by Henry Vaughan being sung as the anthem at the Queen's funeral.

Songs from the series became the main hymns in services given by the Church of England.

The words are:

My soul, there is a country
Far beyond the stars,
Where stands a winged sentry

All skilful in the wars:

There, above noise and danger
Sweet Peace sits crowned with smiles
And One, born in a manger
Commands the beauteous files.

He is thy gracious friend
And, O my soul, awake!
Did in pure love descend
To die here for thy sake.

If thou canst get but thither,
There grows the flow'r of Peace,
The Rose that cannot wither,
Thy fortress and thy ease.

Leave then thy foolish ranges,
For none can thee secure
But One who never changes,
Thy God, thy life, thy cure.

Prayers

A series of seven prayers will be read giving thanks for the Queen as well as praying for those who are grieving.

Let us give thanks to God for Queen Elizabeth's long life and reign, recalling with gratitude her gifts of wisdom, diligence, and service.

GOD, from whom cometh everything that is upright and true: accept our thanks for the gifts of heart and mind that thou didst bestow upon thy daughter Elizabeth, and which she showed forth among us in her words and deeds; and grant that we may have grace to live our lives in accordance with thy will, to seek the good of others, and to remain faithful servants unto our lives' end; through Jesus Christ our Lord. Amen

Confident in God's love and compassion, let us pray for all those whose hearts are heavy with grief and sorrow.

ALMIGHTY God, Father of all mercies and giver of all comfort: deal graciously, we pray thee, with those who mourn, that casting every care on thee, they may know the consolation of thy love; through Jesus Christ our Lord. Amen.

Let us pray for His Majesty The King and all the Royal Family; that they may know the sustaining power of God's love and the prayerful fellowship of God's people.

ALMIGHTY God, the fountain of all goodness, we humbly beseech thee to bless our most gracious Sovereign Lord King Charles, Camilla The Queen Consort, William Prince of Wales, and all the Royal Family: endue them with thy Holy Spirit, enrich them with thy heavenly grace; prosper them with all happiness; and bring them to thine everlasting kingdom; through Jesus Christ our Lord. Amen.

In recognition of Queen Elizabeth's service to this United Kingdom, let us rejoice in her unstinting devotion to duty, her compassion for her subjects, and her counsel to her ministers; and we pray for the continued health and prosperity of this Nation.

ALMIGHTY God, whose will it is that all thy children should serve thee in serving one another: look with love, we pray thee, on this Nation. Grant to its citizens grace to work together with honest and faithful hearts, each caring for the good of all; that, seeking first thy kingdom and its righteousness, they may possess all things needful for their daily sustenance and the common good; through Jesus Christ our Lord. Amen.

Let us give thanks for Queen Elizabeth's commitment to the Commonwealth throughout her reign, for her service and dedication to its peoples, and for the rich bonds of unity and mutual support she sustained.

ALMIGHTY and everlasting God, hear our prayer for the Commonwealth, and grant it the guidance of thy wisdom. Inspire those in authority, that they may promote justice and the common good; give to all its citizens the spirit of mutual honour and respect; and grant to us all grace to strive for the establishment of righteousness and peace; for the honour of thy name. Amen.

We give thanks to God for Queen Elizabeth's loyalty to the faith she inherited through her baptism and confirmation, and affirmed at her coronation; for her unswerving devotion to the Gospel; and for her steadfast service as Supreme Governor of the Church of England.

LORD, we beseech thee to keep thy household the Church in continual godliness; that through thy protection she may be free from all adversities, and devoutly given to serve thee in all good works, to the glory of thy name; through Jesus Christ our Lord. Amen.

Let us pray that we may be given grace to live as those who believe in the communion of saints, the forgiveness of sins, and the resurrection to eternal life.

BRING us, O Lord God, at our last awakening into the house and gate of heaven, to enter into that gate and dwell in that house, where there shall be no darkness nor dazzling, but one equal light; no noise nor silence, but one equal music; no fears nor hopes, but one equal possession; no ends nor beginnings, but one equal eternity; in the habitation of thy glory and dominion, world without end. Amen.

The choir sings: "O TASTE and see how gracious the Lord is :
blest is the man that trusteth in him."

The Lord's Prayer

Then The Lord's Prayer will be said:

In confidence and hope, let us pray to the Father in the words our Saviour taught us,

OUR Father, who art in heaven, hallowed be thy name; thy kingdom come; thy will be done; on earth as it is in heaven.

Give us this day our daily bread. And forgive us our trespasses, as we forgive those who trespass against us.

And lead us not into temptation; but deliver us from evil. For thine is the kingdom, the power, and the glory, for ever and ever. Amen

The Commendation

The commendation will be read by the Archbishop of Canterbury, Justin Welby.

He will begin: "Let us commend to the mercy of God, our maker and redeemer, the soul of Elizabeth, our late Queen."

This will be followed by two prayers of commendation.

HEAVENLY Father, King of kings, Lord and giver of life, who of thy grace in creation didst form mankind in thine own image, and in thy great love offerest us life eternal in Christ Jesus; claiming the promises of thy most blessed Son, we entrust the soul of Elizabeth, our sister here departed, to thy merciful keeping, in sure and certain hope of the resurrection to eternal life, when Christ shall be all in all; who died and rose again to save us, and now liveth and reigneth with thee and the Holy Spirit, in glory for ever. Amen.

GO forth, O Christian soul, from this world, in the name of God the Father almighty, who created thee; in the name of Jesus Christ, Son of the living God, who suffered for thee; in the name of the Holy Spirit, who was poured out upon thee and anointed thee. In communion with all the blessed saints, and aided by the angels and archangels and all the armies of the heavenly host, may thy portion this day be in peace, and thy dwelling in the heavenly Jerusalem. Amen.

The Anthem

The second anthem was composed by James MacMillan for this service, and will be sung by the choir.

The words are adapted from Romans 8 verses 35a and 38b.

They are: *"Who shall separate us from the love of Christ? Neither death, nor life, nor angels, nor principalities, nor powers, nor things present, nor things to come, nor height, nor depth, nor any other creature, shall be able to separate us from the love of God, which is in Christ Jesus our Lord. Alleluia! Amen."*

The Blessing

The final blessing will be read by the Dean:

GOD grant to the living grace; to the departed rest; to the Church, The King, the Commonwealth, and all people, peace and concord, and to us sinners, life everlasting; and the blessing of God almighty, the Father, the Son, and the Holy Spirit, be among you and remain with you always. Amen.

The final blessing will be read by the Dean:

GOD grant to the living grace; to the departed rest; to the Church, The King, the Commonwealth, and all people, peace and concord, and to us sinners, life everlasting; and the blessing of God almighty, the Father, the Son, and the Holy Spirit, be among you and remain with you always. Amen.

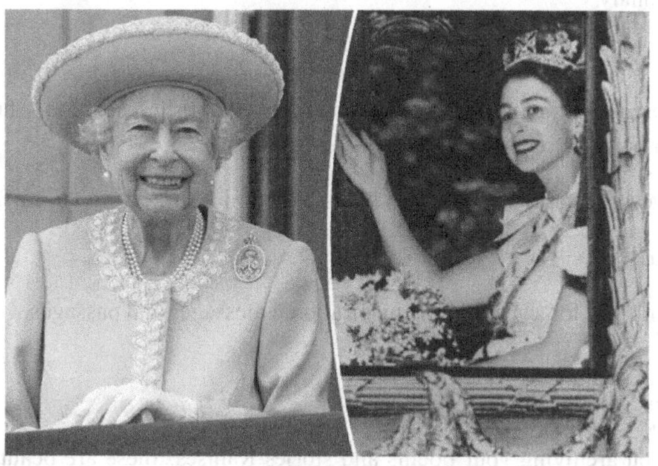

A Life of a Queen strived to be a Faithful Servant to Lord Jesus!

Queen Ellizabeth II, a LIFE Story Incredibly Moving and Now Going to a Resting Place by the Westminster Abby on Earth while returning to God of Heaven by Phillip and George: "Return unto thy rest, O my soul; for the Lord hath dealt bountifully with thee. [8] For thou hast delivered my soul from death, mine eyes from tears, and my feet from falling. [9] I will walk before the Lord in the land of the living. [10] I believed, therefore have I spoken: I was greatly afflicted:" Psalm 116:7-10 KJV

"Lord, now You are letting Your servant depart in peace,

According to Your word; For my eyes have seen Your salvation Which You have prepared before the face of all peoples, A light to bring revelation to the Gentiles, And the glory of Your people Israel." (Luke 2:29-32)

<u>Ramsis Ghaly</u>

LM, Beautiful

CG, What a beautiful tribute to a beautiful lady.

KB, Have a great day well said God bless you for all surgery you do.

JT, are you archiving your poems and stories Ramses...these are beautiful and insightful...they would make amazing publications

LB, This was posted by a wonderful man who loves God and his fellow man, Dr Ramsis Ghaly.

Read this when you have time to absorb and contemplate.

<u>CG,</u> These words are perfect for the final farewell to the Queen. May she finally rest after her long reign.

KB, Have a great day well said God bless you for all surgery you do.

LM, Beautiful

BL, Thank you for sharing these inspirational messages and passages. God bless you.

TF, Thank You for sharing

JT, are you archiving your poems and stories Ramses...these are beautiful and insightful...they would make amazing publications

CG, What a beautiful tribute to a beautiful lady.

I am Not A Royal Yet Good Pity on Me!

Written on 9/23/2022 by Ramsis Ghaly

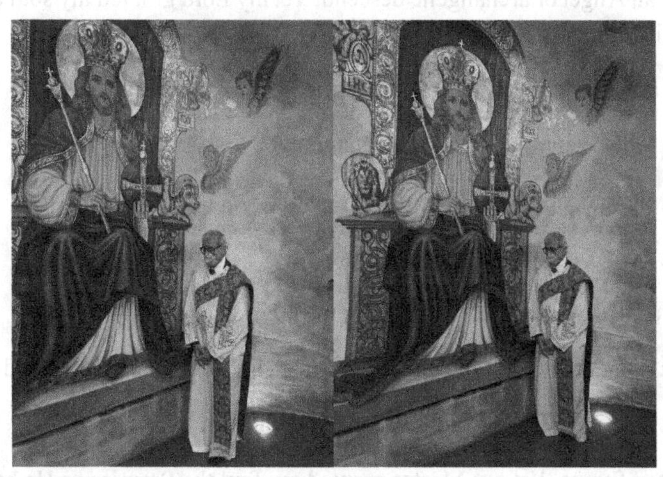

I am Not A Royal Yet Good Pity on Me!

I am Not Royal, Yet God has forgiven me!

I am Not Royal, Yet my Lord let me enter His Court!

I am not Royal, Yet God my Lord Drew me to Him!

I am Not a Royal, yet my Savior Died for me!

I am Not from a Royal Family, Yet my God Redeemed my soul!

I am a Sinner, Yet Jesus my Lord Saved my soul!

I am of No Existence, Yet my Lord God Formed me!

I am from Dust and Ashes, Yet God made me in His Image in His Likeness!

I am Nothing, Yet Rause me from the pit to sit by Him at the King's table!

I am Not invited to His Holy Wedding, Yet the Heavenly Father added my name to the List!

I am Not of any Prominence, Yet Jesus elected me among the tens of thousands of the heavenly hosts!

I am Not a Deacon in His Army, Yet my God let me Praise Him and Sing new songs with His angels!

I am Not Worthy, Yet my Lord paid my Dues!

I am Not an Angel or archangelic descend, Yet my Lord granted my soul eternity in His Kingdom!

I am not a Star, Yet my Heavenly Father Love me!

I am Not Holy, Yet my Redeemer Listen to my Outcry!

I am Not literate, Yet God chose me to Speak!

I am Not rich, Yet my Lord enriched my soul!

I am No a Healer, Yet my Creator made me a Physician!

I am Not of any fame, Yet my Lord Introduced my soul to His saints and hosts!

I sm Not Known, Yet my Lord made me known!

I am Not of Statue, Yet my Master granted my foul the Promise as He had done with Zaccheus!

I am of No Sight for thirty-eight years born in sin, Yet my Lord brought dight to my eyes and Spiritual Vision to my dreams!

I am Not Wholly but sick with infirmity, Yet my Lord made me wholly!

I am with broken bones and can't stand or walk, Yet my Lord lifted me up and granted me the Eagle's wings to fly so high!

I am deemed condemned for ever, Yet my Savior found a way to remove the penalty of death to leave His glory and live in the flesh among the transgressors and shed His blood for me!

I am Hungry and I am dying of no nourishment m, Yet my God became my Bread of Life!

I am Thirsty and I am dying of no waters, Yet God made waters erupt from the rock and became the fountains of living waters!

Biblical Verses

Ecclesiastes 7:20 Indeed, there is not a righteous man on earth who continually does good and who never sins.

Galatians 5:17 For the flesh sets its desire against the Spirit, and the Spirit against the flesh; for these are in opposition to one another, so that you may not do the things that you please.

Genesis 6:5 Then the Lord saw that the wickedness of man was great on the earth, and that every intent of the thoughts of his heart was only evil continually.

Romans 3:9-19 What then? Are we better than they? Not at all; for we have already charged that both Jews and Greeks are all under sin; as it is written, "There is none righteous, not even one; There is none who understands, There is none who seeks for God;

Romans 9:5 whose are the fathers, and from whom is the Christ according to the flesh, who is over all, God blessed forever. Amen.

Jeremiah 17:23 Yet they did not listen or incline their ears, but stiffened their necks in order not to listen or take correction.

2 Peter 2:14 having eyes full of adultery that never cease from sin, enticing unstable souls, having a heart trained in greed, accursed children;

John 3:19 This is the judgment, that the Light has come into the world, and men loved the darkness rather than the Light, for their deeds were evil.

Titus 1:15-16 To the pure, all things are pure; but to those who are defiled and unbelieving, nothing is pure, but both their mind and their conscience are defiled. They profess to know God, but by their deeds they deny Him, being detestable and disobedient and worthless for any good deed.

Romans 3:23 for all have sinned and fall short of the glory of God,

Psalm 51:5 Behold, I was brought forth in iniquity, And in sin my mother conceived me.

Mark 7:21 For from within, out of the heart of men, proceed the evil thoughts, fornications, thefts, murders, adulteries,

Ephesians 5:8 for you were formerly darkness, but now you are Light in the Lord; walk as children of Light

Jeremiah 17:9 "The heart is more deceitful than all else. And is desperately sick;

Who can understand it?

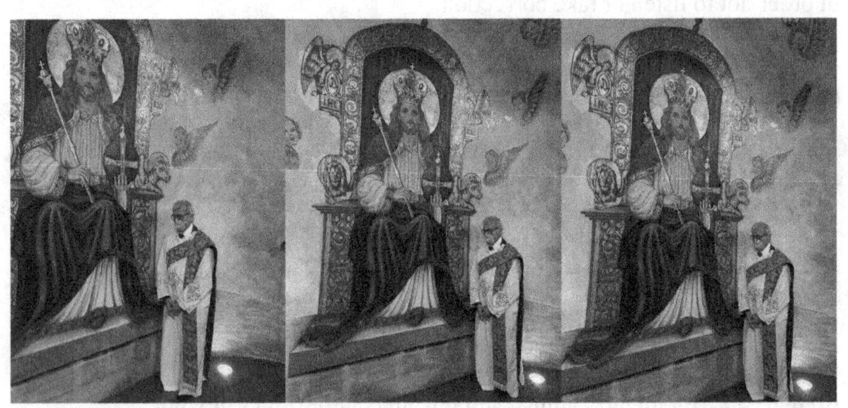

Does Royal Gene Exist??

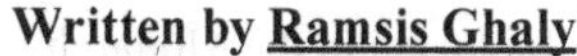

Written by Ramsis Ghaly

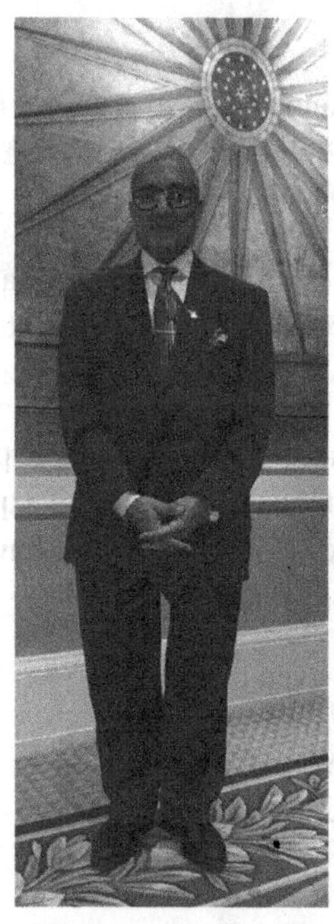

Why the Royal Family and their Descendants mandated to be a king and a queen?? The Sovereign Dynasties, Monarchies and Empires are based sole in blood inheritance! Although, their role has changed recently not to include public affairs, currently in some monarchies, the Crown in society is largely symbolic, remainder of traditions passed down during the monarchy's thousand-year reign.

What is the Importance and Uniqueness in regard to blood inheritance?

I continued to search what is in the blood of Royal Family and Descendants that make them kings and queens and not the public?? Is there a specific blood type for Royalty!

I am trying to find why only the Royal Family and their Descendants can be appointed to be kings and queens forever.

I am looking for what possible reasons why God, Bless His Name, anoint kings and queens by the Holy Spirit based some in the blood inheritance!

It isn't the Blood inheritance or race to justify the man and a king of a queen but deep in the heart within the brain and deeds!! With God No favoritism or partiality! There is no difference!

There is Neither Equity nor Inclusion in the Monarchy system and a race is better than another!

In fact, the words of wisdom stated no one has unique blood and born distinguished from another: Ecclesiastes 7:20 Indeed, there is not a righteous man on earth who continually does good and who never sins."

And the psalmist also indicates no one is a king or a queen by blood inheritance over another: Psalmist 51:5 "Behold, I was brought forth in iniquity, and in sin my mother conceived me."

We know the entire human race was born from one parent and structurally is the same in sin and no one is righteous to be a king of a queen: Romans 3:9-19 "What then? Are we better than they? Not at all, for we have already charged that both Jews and Greeks are all under sin as it is written,

"There is none righteous, not even one.

There is none who understands,

There is none who seeks for God,

Romans 9:5

whose are the fathers, and from whom is the Christ according to the flesh, who is over all, God blessed forever. Amen."

In Biblical Tradition, It was in the Old Testament when God Promise from Abrahim, Isaac and Jacob, the Messyah will come. At that time, the Jews were the only people believe in the True God and the remaining works were non-believer, Pagans, Idolaters and atheists!

I asked what is in Royal bloodstream that make Royalty forever transmitted from generation to another until end of ages??

What are the hidden genetics in the Royal blood that makes whoever born of Royal descendent is automatically Royal!!

What are those values transmitted through the blood that make Royals unique and vast difference than the entire population of a nation?

For certain there is no "Inclusion" in Monarchy with Royal inheritance!

For certain outsiders have no chance to be true Royalists and there absolutely no chance for them to be an accepted king or queen but can be called prince or princess!!

Tributes to Monarchy

The role of the Crown in society is largely symbolic, remainder of traditions passed down during the monarchy's thousand-year reign

Royal Family and Descendants consider themselves the owners of the country, the owners of the wealth of the land!

Royal Family and Descendants are originals, the natives and inheritances of the empire/ Country!

Royal Family and Descendants groomed and breed within inside and restrict anything outside in royalty to the empire!

Royal Family and Descendants are Extreme Loyalists to the empire and nation!

Royal Family and Descendants have the same faith and customs!

Royal Family and Descendants keep strict customs, rituals and respect routines!

Royal Family and Descendants believe in following their traditional "Orders"

Royal Family and Descendants always keep the memory alive and remember very well what they have been taught about their previous empires' kings and queens!

Royal Family and Descendants are appreciative of the ancestors and their Patriotism!

In the ancient history of mankind such as Kings and queens of Israel (Saul, David and Solomon), Egypt (Ramsis, Isis, Ahmos—)

At that time, kings and queens headed and ran the region including all aspects of public affairs!

In the modern era, many countries departed from monarchies, kings and queens and open the door to the public!

The few countries that still have monarchy and are not involved in public affairs!!

Definition Of A Royal Family:

A royal family is the immediate family of kings/queens, emirs/emiras, sultans/ sultanas, or raja/rani and sometimes their extended family. The term imperial family appropriately describes the family of an emperor or empress, and the term papal family describes the family of a pope, while the terms baronial family, comital family, ducal family, archducal family, grand ducal family, or princely family are more appropriate to describe, respectively, the relatives of a reigning baron, count/earl, duke, archduke, grand duke, or prince. However, in common parlance members of any family which reigns by hereditary right are often referred to as royalty or "royals". It is also customary in some circles to refer to the extended relations of a deposed monarch and their descendants as a royal family. A dynasty is sometimes referred to as the "House of ...". **In July 2013 there were 26 active sovereign dynasties in the world that ruled or reigned over 43 monarchies.**

As of 2021, while there are several European countries whose nominal head of state, by long tradition, is a king or queen, the associated royal families, with the notable exception of the British royal family, are non-notable ordinary citizens who may bear a title but are not involved in public affairs.

+++

It isn't the Blood inheritance or race to justify the man and a king of a queen but deep in the heart within the brain and deeds!! With God No favoritism or partiality! There is no difference!

1 Corinthians 12:13

13 For we were all baptized by one Spirit so as to form one body—whether Jews or Gentiles, slave or free—and we were all given the one Spirit to drink.

1 Samuel 16:7

7 But the LORD said to Samuel, "Do not consider his appearance or his height, for I have rejected him. The LORD does not look at the things people look at. People look at the outward appearance, but the LORD looks at the heart."

1 Timothy 5:21

21 I charge you, in the sight of God and Christ Jesus and the elect angels, to keep these instructions without partiality, and to do nothing out of favoritism."

Acts 17:26

26 From one man he made all the nations, that they should inhabit the whole earth; and he marked out their appointed times in history and the boundaries of their lands.

Colossians 3:13

13 Bear with each other and forgive one another if any of you has a grievance against someone. Forgive as the Lord forgave you.

Colossians 3:25

25 Anyone who does wrong will be repaid for their wrongs, and there is no favoritism.

Colossians 3:25

25 Anyone who does wrong will be repaid for their wrongs, and there is no favoritism.

Ephesians 4:32

32 Be kind and compassionate to one another, forgiving each other, just as in Christ God forgave you.

Exodus 22:21

21 “Do not mistreat or oppress a foreigner, for you were foreigners in Egypt.

Galatians 3:28

28 There is neither Jew nor Gentile, neither slave nor free, nor is there male and female, for you are all one in Christ Jesus.

James 2:1

1 My brothers and sisters, believers in our glorious Lord Jesus Christ must not show favoritism.

James 2:4

4 have you not discriminated among yourselves and become judges with evil thoughts?

John 7:24

24 Stop judging by mere appearances, but instead judge correctly.”

34 “A new command I give you: Love one another. As I have loved you, so you must love one another.

Proverbs 24:23

23 These also are sayings of the wise: To show partiality in judging is not good:

9 After this I looked, and there before me was a great multitude that no one could count, from every nation, tribe, people and language, standing before the throne and before the Lamb. They were wearing white robes and were holding palm branches in their hands.

Revelation 14:6

6 Then I saw another angel flying in midair, and he had the eternal gospel to proclaim to those who live on the earth—to every nation, tribe, language and people.

Romans 2:11

11 For God does not show favoritism.

Romans 10:12

12 For there is no difference between Jew and Gentile—the same Lord is Lord of all and richly blesses all who call on him,"

Mark 12:31

31 The second is this: 'Love your neighbor as yourself.' There is no commandment greater than these."

Matthew 28:19

19 Therefore go and make disciples of all nations, baptizing them in the name of the Father and of the Son and of the Holy Spirit,

It isn't the Blood inheritance or race to justify the man and a king of a queen but deep in the heart within the brain and deeds!! With God No favoritism or partiality! There is no difference!

https://en.m.wikipedia.org/wiki/Royal_family

https://en.m.wikipedia.org/wiki/British_royal_family

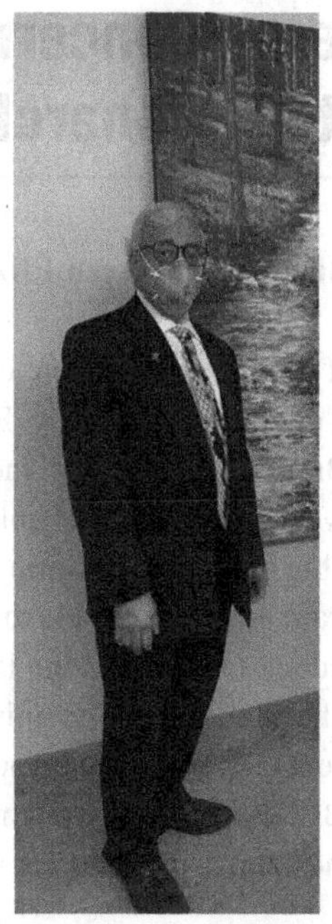

JT, Harry is a rule breaker...he will never be "king" or will he

ED, "We know the entire human race was born in sin" is what you wrote. Have you not taken the consideration that the Atonement that Jesus Christ paid means that children are innocent of sin until they reach accountability?

JA, Thanks so much for explaining

CG, The role of the Crown in society is largely symbolic, remainder of traditions passed down during the monarchy's thousand-year reign are just reminders of the past.

I so look forward to your articles. Bless you!

Controversy Concerning the British Monarchy!

In The Memory Of Queen Elizabeth II

Queen Eizabeth was the most kind hearted queen touched the entire world at the time of rise in animosity, lack of dialogue and love. Her personality was fantastic, worked so hard to keep the British empire fame and serviced to the last minute for decades minimum of 70 years. Yet, she was able to take the British atrocity away and transfer Britain as a big heart cared empire and supportive to other under developed countries. The Britain empire was able to elevate other countries, send missionaries and be part of education, spread the language and Christianity. In the countries they invaded, they built schools, universities, colleges, hospitals, modern building, entertainments, opera, music, sports, churches, city halls and established transportation. Britain was instrumental in outreaching, tackling ignorance, poverty and illiteracy and bring industry and modernization to various worldwide countries.

The death of Queen Elizabeth on 9/8/22, marks the end of huge era, the colonialism of British imperialism and transfer to commonwealth with liberation of British occupation to 90 countries and put a stop to brutality, invasions, torture, murder, slavery, racism and abuse. She was big part of helping those countries, let them regain independence and become free lancing. Queen Elizabeth was behind the great success of Britain common wealth. She put a great humanitarian end of the British Imperialism. She travelled all over and touched many hearts.

It was the time of freedom to all. It perhaps will put an end to British commonwealth and interference of Britain in other countries business. Queen Elizabeth was the shining star and the Rose of transition. She was so elegant and beautiful and in the same time modest. There is no doubt that for thousands of years, Queen Elizabeth is irreplaceable and no one like here. Queen Elizabeth, starting at very young age, She was able to be everything in one person, a daughter, a wife, a mother, a grandma, a queen and running global affair and be the queen of the people worldwide full of wisdom and energy, lively. May God repose her soul.

As many across the world praise the British monarchy, so many are aware of the British atrocities and wars against humanity including everlasting deleterious effects globally.

The British Empire under the leadership of British monarchs headed 415 million people, fifth of the world population, colonized 90 countries worldwide, murdered minimum 150 million people, since 16th century. At the peak of its power, it was described as "the empire on which the sun never sets", as the sun was always shining on at least one of its territories. First rise of British Empire was 1707-1783, second rise 1783-1815, Britain's imperial century (1815–1914), World wars (1914–1945), Decolonisation and decline 1945-1997! he Royal Firm: a $28 billion empire. One estimate says that the British transferred $45 trillion of wealth from India to UK by 1938. The monarchy holds nearly $28 billion in real estate assets as of 2021, That includes: The Crown Estate: $19.5 billion. Buckingham Palace: $4.9 billion. After the defeat of France in the Revolutionary and Napoleonic Wars (1792–1815), the British Empire emerged as the principal naval and imperial power of the 19th century. Unchallenged at sea, British dominance was later described as Pax Britannica ("British Peace"), a period of relative peace in Europe and the world (1815–1914) during which the British Empire became the global hegemon and adopted the role of global policeman.

It is estimated that the British Empire murdered 150 million people minimum tortured millions and millions of the innocent countrymen and women to colonize their lands. In 1922 the British empire took over the fifth of world population.

https://www.reddit.com/r/AskHistorians/comments/7r9eie/allegations_regarding_death_toll_under_the/

What about Amritsar massacre 1919, partitioning of India, Boer concentration camps 1899-1902, Mau Mau uprise 1951-1960, famines in India 1940's

https://www.independent.co.uk/news/uk/home-news/worst-atrocities-british-empire-amritsar-boer-war-concentration-camp-mau-mau-a6821756.html?amp

Some believe that The British empire is probably responsible for most deaths in the past and present due to its past policies. Turning self-sufficient countries to ones that experienced multiple famines. The current middle east and the sub-continent mess is the direct result of the messed-up and hasteful decisions.

British war crimes aren't secret are acts by the armed forces of the United Kingdom that have violated the laws and customs of war since the Hague Conventions of 1899 and 1907. Such acts have included the summary executions of prisoners of war and unarmed shipwreck survivors, the use of excessive force during the interrogation of POWs and enemy combatants, and the use of violence against civilian non-combatants and their property.

https://en.m.wikipedia.org/wiki/British_war_crimes

The British empire The British Empire was composed of the dominions, colonies, protectorates, mandates, and other territories ruled or administered by the United Kingdom and its predecessor states. It began with the overseas possessions and trading posts established by England between the late 16th and early 18th centuries. At its height it was the largest empire in history and, for over a century, was the foremost global power. By 1913 the British Empire held sway over 412 million people, 23 per cent of the world population at the time, and by 1920 it covered 35.5 million km2 (13.7 million sq mi),[24 per cent of the Earth's total land area. As a result, its constitutional, legal, linguistic, and cultural legacy is widespread. At the peak of its power, it was described as "the empire on which the sun never sets", as the sun was always shining on at least one of its territories.

https://en.m.wikipedia.org/wiki/British_Empire

As many across the world praise the British monarchy, so many are aware of the British Monarchy black history as I witnessed what the monarchy had colonized my hometown Egypt EG 1882 and 1807 in in Angelo- Egyptian war and when President Abd Nasr liberated Egypt July 23, 1952, Revolution and Suez Canal liberation in 1956 and regained the independence from its enemy the British monarchy. The price was so high, and the Nile River stained Red with the blood of the innocent Egyptians fighting for their land while the British people singing: "God save the Queen! God save the king" as in Moses times with king Ramses so at that time under British monarchy bloodshed to the Egyptians where the Nile River became red and bloody!! I remember in my primary and elementary and high school, we used to sing the national song and chat: **"By the Soul and the blood 💧 will defend Egypt from our enemy, the gentiles Britains"** as the military March wars and warriors fell by thousands.

https://en.m.wikipedia.org/wiki/Anglo-Egyptian_War

https://en.m.wikipedia.org/wiki/History_of_Egypt_under_the_British

The British monarchy until today never ever showed remorse or apologetic to their worldwide anti human right invasions and not even compensated Egypt or any of their colonies for all the damages and lives lost inflicted by them. But instead kept all the precious hold, diamonds, Pharos belongings—-to enrich their wealth!

Britain emerged as the principal naval and imperial power of the 19th century and expanded its imperial holdings. Through their advanced well equipped military Nay ships and brutal weapons, they voyaged the entire seas and oceans and held many hostages and colonized many countries by the British Army under the leadership monarchy have no good memory at all where they were invaded, occupied and ruled by the common enemy for no good reason other than using and steeling their goods and wealth for the richness of the monarchy over hundreds of years!!! What about taking over various contents including North America, Canada, Australia, New Zealand , India, Africa, many Islands,—- taking advantage of each country, murdering and killing, steeling and raping, taking advantage and control of their goods and wealth. They terrorized the world while living at the most luxurious castles built and decorated by saving these countries and their supporters showed no sympathy or deliver kindness saluting their brutality and dead action saying: "God Save the king" and "God save the Queen"!!!

Some called The brutal British empire that was responsible for the deaths of millions of people. Some called the British monarch "thieving raping genocidal empire". a very tragic period in this country and Africa's history," the statement said.

"Britain, under the leadership of the royal family, took over control of this territory that would become South Africa in 1795 from Batavian control, and took permanent control of the territory in 1806. "From that moment onwards, native people of this land have never known peace, nor have they ever enjoyed the fruits of the riches of this land, riches which were and still are utilized for the enrichment of the British royal family and those who look like them. "In Kenya, Britain built concentration camps and suppressed with such inhumane brutality the Mau Mau rebellion, killing Dedan Kimathi on the 18th of February 1957

https://www.newsweek.com/people-refusing-mourn-queen-elizabeths-death-why-1741462?amp=1

The rest of the world other than pro-British unionists and supporters, many parts of the world look down at the monarchy and its criminal history. Those kings and the Monarchy that took the wealth of so many third world undeveloped countries including Egypt to their own and lived in king's houses by the labor and the sweats of the poor slaving them and making them their maids. They have stolen the wealth of each country, killed their people and dominated the world up to 50 countries worldwide and majority remained poor, and they kept a minimum of 15 billion dollars wealth in their own.

When I was a child in my hometown Egypt, I remembered the horrific stories of the British monarchy killing my people, invading my country stealing all the goods and wealth including the ancient Egyptian mummies, gold, diamonds and arts bringing the stolen items to their home as they had done with the rest of the world poor countries. They murdered, slaved and abused my people for their own richness. I watched so many stories, TV and radio series how they took our freedom and independence and occupies Egypt. My forefathers suffered so much and one war after another terrorizing the public! But not only Egypt but so many countries and made an empire for their own called the British Empire where the sun never disappear as those saluted their British flag and monarchy kingdom by killing the people of different colors and race!! Their king and kingdom rose up by destroying the innocent and invading other countries and they have the guts to call them sovereign states, they overpowered the weak and took over the innocent by their swords and weapons! Interesting, nowadays the monarchy is proud of its charity work trying to redeem the past, yet the monarchy still takes so much money and wealth from those so called "sovereign states"!! It is the time of the British monarchy to give back what they have stolen and compensate the countries they occupied and give up their wealth to those belong too!

The wealth of British empire is in countable.

https://en.m.wikipedia.org/wiki/Economy_of_the_British_Empire

In Africa and Asia, the shadow of economic exploitation and seeds of division sown by the British continues to this day.

Earthly kings and queens are billionaires off the overseas colonies and slavery! British Imperialism admits to be century racists!! One estimate says that the British transferred $45 trillion of wealth from India to UK by 1938. The Council of Foreign Relations notes, "The East India Company [and later British government] set regulations on what crops could be grown, where they could be exported, and at what prices they could be sold. It then charged Indians high taxes on the land they worked. Unlike most taxes, which are invested back into society, money made from the East India Company's taxes flowed back to Britain."

The British reduced India to a source of raw material and eroded its textile output. The British also used money and men from India to further expand the Empire as soldiers were recruited to fight overseas.

Much of the racism today and racial tensions tearing the West is also rooted in colonial practices, most notably of slavery and the European notion of White people's superiority over others.

The Europeans are estimated to have bought and sold 12 million slaves from Africa. Of them, the British share is estimated to be 3 million. Slave labour fuelled the overseas British plantations and also fuelled the Industrial Revolution.

"Slavery made Britain incredibly wealthy. It provided slave owners with unpaid labour to farm expensive items like sugar, tobacco and cotton, which they could sell for huge profits – at the expense of the enslaved people and their homelands. It also largely funded Britain's Industrial Revolution, which only went on to make Britain richer,"

Even after slavery was formally banned, the notion of White Supremacy stuck and people of colour continued to face discrimination in the West. The racial equality movement is an ongoing one and while rights exist on paper, people continue to strive for equal treatment. Further, the USA remains highly divided and polarized today along racial lines. The US government now believes that White Supremacy is the top national domestic threat.

https://www.outlookindia.com/international/the-long-shadow-of-british-colonialism-and-list-of-countries-once-part-of-british-empire-news-222475/amp

Historians criticized its widespread use of violence and emergency laws to maintain power. Common criticisms of the empire include the use of detention camps in its colonies, massacres of indigenous peoples,[280] and famine-response policies. Some scholars, including Amartya Sen, assert that British policies worsened the famines in India that killed millions during British rule.

Diversity Equity Inclusion DEI Should be at Each Place In America!!

Written on 10/30/2022 by Ramsis Ghaly

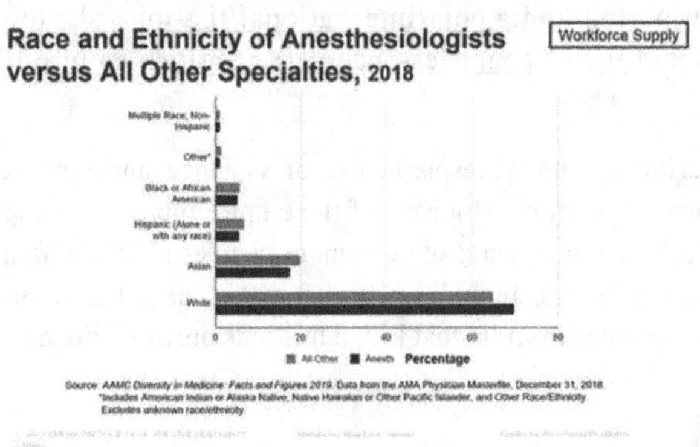

Diverse Equity & Inclusion (DEI) Should be at Each Place In America!!

Where is the Black Race in the Medical Specialty of Anesthesiology? Only 6% in the entire specialty! Indefensible!!!

Let us celebrate our great hospital JSH of Cook County Hospital, Chicago, Illinois, of being one of the few Healthcare centers across the world that employ staff of color compared to many others as as well mentioned by Dr Brunson at ASA 2022.

A Courageous Heart Lecture to everyone to listen, do and follow about DEI (Diversity Equity & Inclusion) at the Annual Meeting 2022 of the American Society of Anesthesiology presented by Dr Claude Brunson as he was given Dr Emery Andrew Rovenstine Memorial Lecture of the Year at New Orleans 10/24/2022.

Ramsis Ghaly

Post COVID Politics

It is Not Uncommon to Stand alone for Righteousness!

Written by Ramsis Ghaly

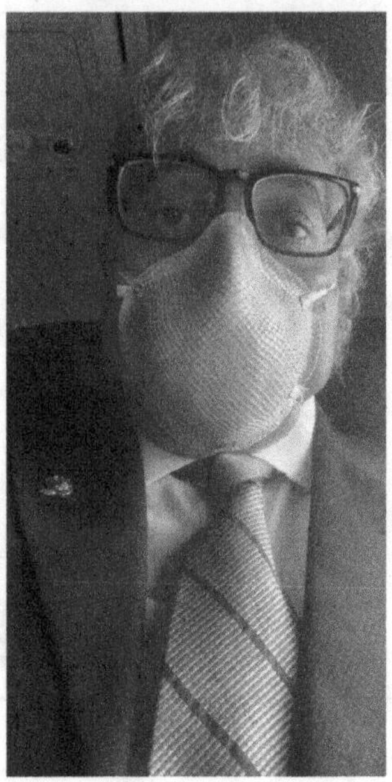

A Good man is revealed not by being a "Team player" and "go along with his pears" but rather in his standing up for the truth and Love for others!!!

It isn't uncommon to Stand alone and not being viewed as a "team player" and "go along with his pears" as it is called in recent years!!

Unfortunately, those are few and stand prominent in the history of mankind. They are the spirit of revolution, the mark of progress and roots of growth across human history..

It isn't uncommon to Stand alone and isn't unprofessionalism as might be called in modern era!!

A Righteous man should be able to make the right decision even if he is all alone!

An Ethical man should be able to speak up the truth before the public even if he is the only one!

A Strong moral man should be able to stand all alone to take the right step even if he is to stand against the world!

A Visionary man should never accept status quo but instead courageous lead the steps toward the future even if he is the only one!

A Wise man should never be part bureaucracy of but instead always transparent with solidarity even if he is the only one!

A Hero should be able to lay down his life before others even if he is all alone at the frontline!

Such situations and events are meant to test a man's truth within and solidarity of ethics, values determination, persistence, patience, faith and love deep in his heart and mind and soul and to refine his character and make him a better person!

Biblical words of St Paul: "And not only so, but we glory in tribulations also: knowing that tribulation worketh patience; [4] And patience, experience; and experience, hope: [5] And hope maketh not ashamed; because the love of God is shed abroad in our hearts by the Holy Ghost which is given unto us. [6] For when we were yet without strength, in due time Christ died for the ungodly. [7] For scarcely for a righteous man will one die: yet peradventure for a good man some would even dare to die. [8] But God commendeth his love toward us, in that, while we were yet sinners, Christ died for us. [9] Much more then, being now justified by his blood, we shall be saved from wrath through him." Romans 5:3-9 KJV

St James Biblical words: "My brethren, count it all joy when ye fall into divers temptations; [3] Knowing this, that the trying of your faith worketh patience. [4] But let patience have her perfect work, that ye may be perfect and entire, wanting nothing. [5] If any of you lack wisdom, let him ask of God, that giveth to all men liberally, and upbraideth not; and it shall be given him." James 1:2-5 KJV

Cr, These days are here and will become even more difficult as "The Day" drawers closer. I pray we'll all be ready. It won't be in our own power we will be able to stand tall. Only by the grace of God and the power of His Holy Spirit will we stand for truth and righteousness. Spirit of Truth prevail.

Kg, AMEN

JT, amen

SY, Amen

RH, Amen

CG, Very well stated. I believe we have all had a situation that forces us to decide if we will obey God or "follow the crowd."

LY, Amen Doctor!!!

SB, As someone who suffers from Medical PTSD, I wish all Doctors would adhere to this as you do!

AM, comparto su fe y su sacrificio para que todos elijamos el camino de la verdad

AV, Amen! Thank you for sharing God's Word!

KH, We'll said!

JM, AGREE AMEN

SB, As someone who suffers from Medical PTSD, I wish all Doctors would adhere to this as you do!

AM, comparto su fe y su sacrificio para que todos elijamos el camino de la verdad

AV, Amen! Thank you for sharing God's Word!

JM, AGREE AMEN

CR, Amen. Well said as always.

MB, Amen

rv, Standing alone can be proof your on the road to truth.

DY, Truth!

BL, Oh how I love the truths you share! Thank you.

ES, So true.

BCD, Amen, I agree. Always do the right thing

Who Among Those Could Stand and Read The Biblical Verse!

Written 3/30/2022

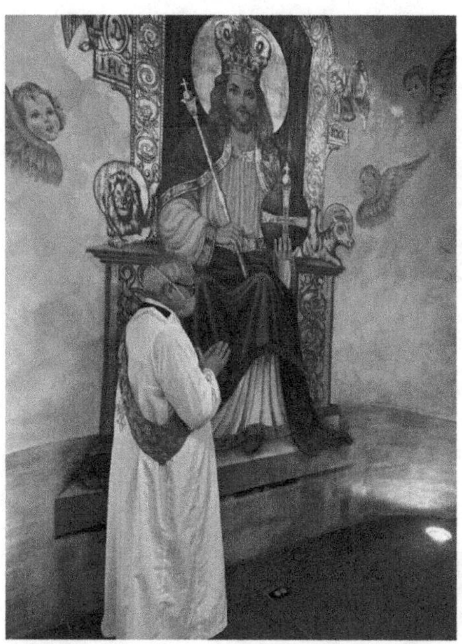

Who among each of Officials and leaders and all those worldwide behind and watching the devastating Russia Ukraine war can stand before Lord Jesus and gives account to the biblical verse:

"Be diligent to present yourself approved to God as a workman who does not need to be ashamed, accurately handling the word of truth." 2 Timothy 2:15

"Be diligent to present yourself approved to God as a workman who does not need to be ashamed, accurately handling the word of truth." 2 Timothy 2:15

The words of Proverbs: "He that justifieth the wicked, and he that condemneth the just, even they both are abomination to the Lord." Proverbs 17:15 KJV

If those were just lions ! "The wicked flee when no man pursueth: but the righteous are bold as a lion." Proverbs 28:1 KJV

Ramsis Ghaly

SM, Exactly.

JT, when the world leaders fail their people there shall be consequences...we are witnessing 2 continents emploding before our eyes...elected or not they have failed their people...we need an intervention before it is too late

MR, Lord Jesus Christ blessed be with you always

MS, Amen

Post-COVID First War and Human Aggression 2/22/2022!

Can Politicians Return to Their Civil Administration and Letting Obsession Over COVID Go!!
Written on 02/25/2022

Can politicians Return to Their Civil administration and Letting Obsession Over COVID Go!!

The politicians had the power to put their nose unto COVID and produce all kinds of rules, regulations, laws and penalties! YET they had not much of power to do their own job and control Putin/ Russia and rescue the loyal people of Ukraine. And the political task force followers aren't any better UN and NATO—

They restrained our nation and so are the leaders of the world lockdown their people yet they can't lockdown Putin and prevent Russia from their atrocity! What a shame!!

The politicians became doctors to treat and manage COVID for two years and told people what to do!! Yet they left their seats half empty toward their political job and administration!

Perhaps the politicians and leaders and governors worldwide stuck in COVID Management rather than concentrating at their civil duties to stand against corruptions and Putin invasion and soon China! They are still dressed as doctors with white coats ordering their own what to do even thou COVID is no more threat!!

Let pray for beloved people of Ukraine and the region

https://lnkd.in/e3p-xz44

https://lnkd.in/eY_qW64F

CNN.COM

Russia invades Ukraine: Live updates

Russian President Vladimir Putin announced a military operation in Ukraine early Thursday. US President Joe Biden announced new "strong" sanctions on Russia and limitations on exports as he condemned Putin's invasion of Ukraine. Follow here for live news updates from the ground in Ukraine.

May God bless Ukraine and Ukrainian against aggression of Putin and Russia!

Written 2/26/2022

May God bless Ukraine and Ukrainian. May our Lord intervene and put a stop to atrocity. We are bleeding for you as we are praying day and night!!!

The Ukrainian solidarity, faith and love are incredible. May we all learn from them! One people, one nation and one God. Amen

Ramsis Ghaly

YOUTUBE.COM

Ukrainian President Zelenskyy's heartbreaking, defiant speech to the Russian people [English sub.]

I hope these bad days pass and countries become intermediaries for peace rather than mere spectators.

cc. Praying for Ukraine

Cg, They are strong and fighting for their independence. God protect them.

Unheard Public Voices!

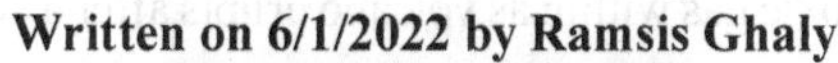

Written on 6/1/2022 by Ramsis Ghaly

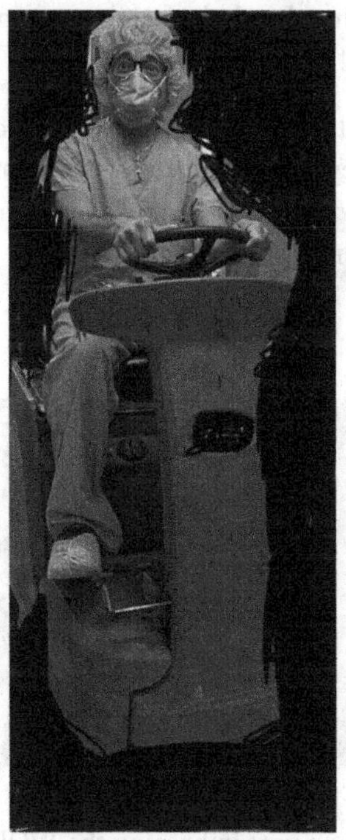

Over my five decades, I have learned these objective facts:

- As the government continues not to address the people pains and suffering, the demand for a change will rise sharply and even overnight!

- As patience of people run out, the beginning of the end of "Status Quo"!

- As the apples mature and ready to be picked up so is the sensible loyal government to the people reacting promptly at the right time feeling their needs, caring in regard to their wellbeing and answering their demands properly, timely and honestly!

- On the other hand, a careless insensitive government not reacting to the people demands, wellbeing, procrastinating and denies their repeated requests and ignoring the uprise, that government resembles those picking the mature apples late until they are spoiled, rotten and thrown in the ground!!

- At that time, a little adversity ignites the fire and can push to Flip with revenge!! The people can no longer be silenced and become as a cane was ignored for so long and inside it the pressure build up so high and no one is listening until it is exploded with high toxic gas within as volcano erupts after a very short warning!!!

Denial, oppression, turning head, ignoring, assuming, and apathy are the beginning of major failure!!

Matthew 13:15 KJV "For this people's heart is waxed gross, and their ears are dull of hearing, and their eyes they have closed; lest at any time they should see with their eyes, and hear with their ears, and should understand with their heart, and should be converted, and I should heal them."

Ramsis Ghaly

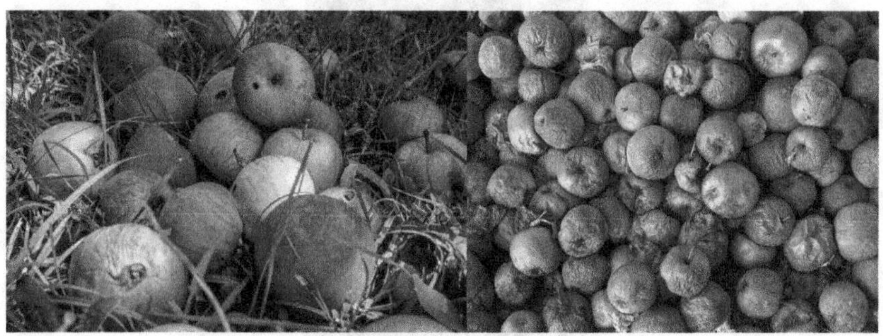

LM, Amen. The gvt wants no part in hearing the WORD.

BL, This is a great and purposeful analogy. Thank you.

DN, So true

CG, Well said. Also lack of trust has serious implications for how the public interacts with our government and how well federal agencies can respond to the major challenges facing the country.

JP, men!

CR, You are exactly what god has sent you here to be! Such an amazing soldier, servant of our dear lord, and above all the most compassionate healing soul I know! Never stop!

It is Not About Being Legal or Illegal But Rather About Who Will do and Who Will Not Do for America!

It Isn't About Legal or Illegal!! But Perhaps About Who will Do and Who Won't Do For America!

Ghaly Column

Written by Ramsis Ghaly

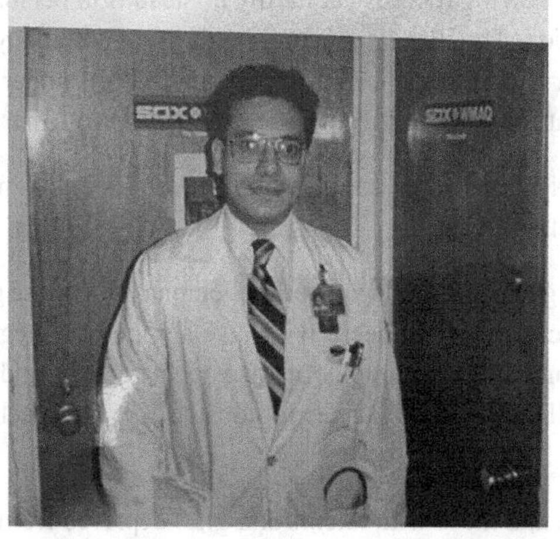

As the Nation approaches 9/11, America is reminded to whom it opens the door to! Absolutely America lives in those newcomers bring America up pursuing the American dreams and not those opportunists bringing America down!

Obviously Coming legal is the way of choice and coming illegal is despised. But have you ever thought in a corrupted multibillion population in 195 countries worldwide, it is impossible for those great type of immigrants to find legal pathways to come to America except for few!! For those no other means but whatever means to present themselves to America and proof themselves in person hoping one day they will be accepted as Americans doing for America !! Many of those are naïve to the American cultures and have been taken advantage by the wicked malicious self-served American opportunists who aren't truly Americans! Many of those profiled illegal but they were innocent or "do not know any better". They never meant to break the law as many perceived, they are just wanted a chance! Sadly, many fell victims unto human trafficking, money laundry, and slaved by the black market in the streets of American inside the heart of America under America flag! Many are running in hide living under false promises and lies of American thieves waiting one day America will take them out of their closets to continue to serve America after years of what is worse than the days of slavery!!

They might not find other ways but walk barefooted, boat ride, back of truck, climbing the barriers, —-Many can't afford the cost of the process, the bureaucracy to get through, the right connection needed, and the support needed. They look great in papers, and you hear what you like to hear, and references are balloony and in actuality they are disasters and harmful to America !

Customized personal medical care is better than nothing, but the best is in person medical care hands on! How many times to get mislead and fooled in screening interviews and reviewing records yet hardly mislead if in person assessment and hands on evaluation. The illegals may not be that bad and many may turn out to be great addition if they screened in person and placed under observation and perhaps, they beat thousands of legal s that don't deserve America!

I acknowledge this post will create many controversies but let me post my cause and explain the title!!!

Instead of focusing on legal or illegal, perhaps emphasis on those good for America and those America is truer in-need, will have stopped the negative destructive views and frictions and perceptions of disrespect to mankind. Instead, it will have united us all and lead all parties to constructive approach to Immigration to build America !

Those persecuted and those with talents and gifts deprived from opportunities in their home countries are those who value America most!

The true immigrants are few! Indeed, true laborers are few!! Jesus said: "Therefore said he unto them, The harvest truly is great, but the labourers are few: pray ye therefore the Lord of the harvest, that he would send forth labourers into his harvest." Luke 10:2 KJV

Unfortunately, they don't come from the front door and legal channels as many thinks! Those talents are determined individuals born with extraordinary gifts and don't mean to break the law! They aren't crooked enough and manipulative to fool the system and find the loop hokes instead they are naive and foolish in life matters but brilliant in their gifts!! But instead, their talents are suppressed, their gifts are buried, and they aren't cared for, or supported or encouraged or welcomed in their home country! Therefore, how could they find legal channels??? America is inspired with those of different cultures coming to diverse America and promote American values and what stand for!

The true laborers, highly intelligent, brilliance and those with special talents and rare skills aren't the majority and God made them spread equally worldwide regardless of the socioeconomic status! Losing one of them is a huge global loss. That talent could the one to discover a cure for cancer or create a new software, or engineer a new robot, or create new methods to revive organ damage, or regenerate nerves, or develop new ways in economy or politics or to prevent a world disaster or to find an early method of natural disaster or come up with new physics law! He or she could be a new Einstein or Edward Jenner and or Louis Pasteur of France for vaccine, microbiology and pasteurization!! A new thinker, a new innovator, a new champion, a new Elon Musk, a new Bill gates, a new Steve Job, a new Mark Zuckerberg of Facebook, Reed Hoffman of LinkedIn, Larry Page and Sergey Brin of Google,—. Who knows perhaps God only created one and only one with rare talent such as David or Solomon or Pete, or Paul,——

Jesus the Lord did what was thought to be "illegal" as a Jew to ask and speak to a Samaritan at that time! Yet it was historic, revolutionary, true legal and brought higher level of righteousness: "Then saith the woman of Samaria unto him, How is it that thou, being a Jew, askest drink of me, which am a woman of Samaria? for the Jews have no dealings with the Samaritans. "John 4:9 KJV

The Good Samaritan did what was thought to be "illegal" at that time in helping an Israelite but yet his own priest and Levite refused! Yet it was historic, revolutionary, true legal and brought new level to righteousness and blessings that wasn't present! "And Jesus answering said, A certain man went down from Jerusalem to Jericho, and fell among thieves, which stripped him of his raiment, and wounded him, and departed, leaving him half dead. [31] And by chance there came down a certain priest that way: and when he saw him, he passed by on the other side. [32] And likewise a Levite, when he was at the place, came and looked on him, and passed by on the other side. [33] But a certain Samaritan, as he journeyed, came where he was: and when he saw him, he had compassion on him, [34] And went to him, and bound up his wounds, pouring in oil and wine, and set him on his own beast, and brought him to an inn, and took care of him. "Luke 10:30-34 KJV

Have you ever thought that those called "illegals" are the most innovative hardworking individuals that believe it is a "privilege" to be in America and it isn't a given a "right"! They are those who have to work hard to proof themselves exposed to extreme hardship to come here in America and must be better than majority to be allowed among the common and natives! In other words, they must offer more than norms and be creative and bring new ideas to grow!!

Those running away for legitimate reasons are the best for America ! They are new minds and genuinely searching for new permanent home.

They turn their back to their home country and have only one determined goal: "Make America even greater". They appreciate heartedly America that is giving them a new refuge permanent home where the world denied them and rejected them unfairly. And it is not only to them but also to their children. Those new human genes, melting pot with new features and various heritage will bloom more and more in the land of freedom, the land of means, the land of opportunity and the land of rising up to the top! America will benefit much more in hosting those believing in "American Dream" than millions of illegal coming to be in well fair busy taking advantage of America !

Such individuals aren't usually connected lacking communication skills. They don't "play games" or know short cuts. They aren't like the majority "street smart" and they aren't satisfied with "status quo"!

In other words, those aren't the lucky ones to come through legal channels. They usually running away from the corrupted establishment! They can't surface themselves and the only ways open fir them are so called "illegal ways" to escape peacefully from their countries!

Those are the true immigrants America needs! Yet in those countries where corruption and bribing are so common, legal pathway to America is given to "who you know" and "how much money bribing in the black market. The embassy staff in those countries are for the majority and privileged and never in support or bringing up those underprivileged, persecuted and hardworking looking for a new home the land of opportunity. Certainly, those immigrants coming through such embassies aren't the true immigrants to America !

Such those type of immigrants are coming to use, abuse and misuse America !

Therefore, the efforts should be in screening those immigrants that will add goodness to America !

Such comprehensive screening is costly to navigate through so much dishonesty, corruption and screen in depth into each to identify and bring those hardworking respectful innovative minds!!

Let us face it, America is great for those looking to a land of freedom, of opportunity and better socioeconomic status!

What is good about legal or legal if it isn't the dreamer to build America !

What is good about legal or legal if no true love to America !

It isn't about legal or illegal but about making America a sincere new home moving forward!

It isn't about legal or illegal but about genuinely appreciate America !

It isn't about legal or illegal but about building America the Future!

It isn't about legal or illegal but about making America great land!

It isn't about legal or illegal but about saving America from malicious and criminals!

It isn't about legal or illegal but about Not taking advantage of America !

It isn't about legal or illegal but about contributing goodness to America !

It isn't about legal or illegal but about believing in America the land of opportunity for the underprivileged!

It isn't about legal or illegal but about America a refuge home to the persecuted minorities!!

It isn't about legal or illegal but about high morals working hard and earning living through good deeds!

Therefore, keep the doors open to those who deserve America as in the days in history when many came in their boats illegal to New York Harbors running away from the depression and suppression in Europe. And those are the true founders of America and made America today.

So instead of keep talking about legal or illegal and be divisive, unit and create new tools to screen for those true American immigrants that shall prosper America o and don't bring America down!!
Such a comprehensive screening system is costly to navigate through so much dishonesty, corruption and screen in depth into each to identify and bring those hardworking respectful innovative minds!!

Respectfully

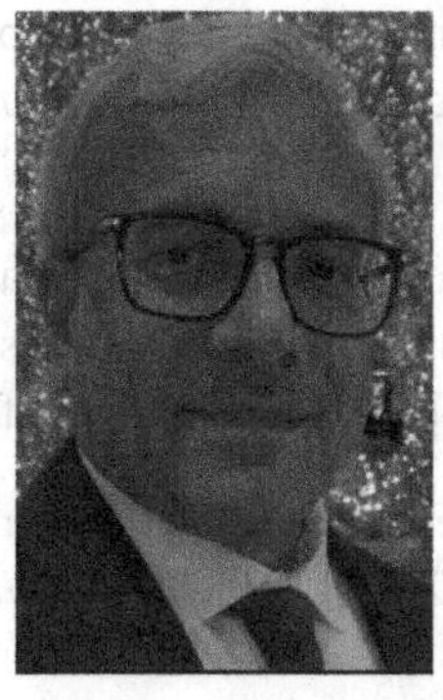

COVID 19 Have You Ever Wondered??

Ghaly Column!
Written on 04/23/2022 by Ramsis Ghaly

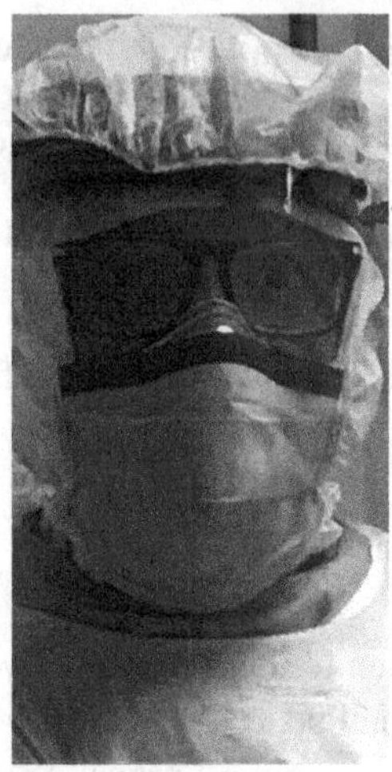

The world is not seeing return of COVID-19 despite the threats of officials!!

WHO, NATO and UN have done nothing to stop the COVID-19 pandemic or Russian invasion but justify the billions of dollars and spread fears!

The refugee camps aren't hot spots for COVID-19 those hosting the Ukrainians fleeing g the wars with poor condition, ventilation, sleeping over each other and not masking and cannot afford social distancing or COVID testing aren't dying from COVID-19 but dying from trauma as a result of man-made war and starvation!

Floridians didn't die because of not following facemask mandates since the beginning yet Florida was number one state to keep economy, get rich and many people moved to Florida nationwide and internationally and the now the prices sky rocketing!

Philadelphia looks like a fool mandating facemask and then reversing back within a week! Philadelphians aren't dying because of not following facemask any longer!! The officials couldn't let their abuse of power go!

All the states and cities that experiences nation demonstration and riots haven't ever became hot spots for COVID-19 including Washington DC Jan 6, haven't died from COVID-19!

Across the nation, America states according to vaccination versus no vaccination overall statistics we haven't heard significant difference!

The Ukraine Russian warriors with no mask or physical distance of vaccination aren't dying from COVID-19 but from man-made bullets!

The poor countries that living over earth other can't afford vaccination or face masking or social isolation or physical distancing aren't dead from COVID-19!

The world is still overpopulated and the thoughts that COVID-19 will wipe the underdeveloped countries more than developed countries because of lack of science and hygiene turn out to be a huge lie! The science thought COVID-19 will eradicate the poor countries such as those in AFRICA, Asia and Latin America!! Science was absolutely wrong, and those countries never became hot spot as Italy was and Europe and highly developed countries!

Tight restrictions and four to five boosters' mandates from the beginning in Israel didn't stop COVID-19!

COVID-19 has never threatened to Putin and Russian to bomb another country and the use of firearms against each other instead of getting the vaccine shot and boosters with facemask written ZZZ ! I wonder if fire artillery and toxic fumes as result explosions and bombs kill COVID-19!!

What have you done and God Almighty didn't do! Be down to earth and admit your shortcoming and fake science and so-called robots and artificial intelligence taking over the world! How many time people walk barefooted down to earth rather than put on their expensive high heal shoes??

So, what stopped COVID-19 God and His creation of Natural immunity more than any! And what Reese, never make a fool of yourself if you actually don't know all about COVID-19! Mass Coercing, forcing and humiliating the public saying:" We follow Science" What Science you are following if you just look around and observe the facts!!! You think science paid by industry, self-interest group and politicians is a true science???

Unfortunately, we can't bring the old days back and what we have done to people that we can at least apologize, admit them mistakes and learn lessons for the future!!

Critical Look at Banning Communion Abortion and Pedophilia!!

If an authority wishes to be John the Baptist in 2022, he or she must live by an example similar to John the Baptist and stand and say: It is not lawful for thee to have thy brother's wife. And It is not lawful for thee to have a communion and thy are pedophiles and rapper and child molester!! Mark 6:18-19 KJV "For John had said unto Herod, It is not lawful for thee to have thy brother's wife. [19] Therefore Herodias had a quarrel against him, and would have killed him; but she could not:"

Abortion is a murder and so is pedophilia, rapping, and child Molestation!! And all brought damnation to themselves For he that eateth and drinketh unworthily!!!! As it is written: 1 Corinthians 11:28-32 KJV "But let a man examine himself, and so let him eat of that bread, and drink of that cup. [29] For he that eateth and drinketh unworthily, eateth and drinketh damnation to himself, not discerning the Lord's body. [30] For this cause many are weak and sickly among you, and many sleep. [31] For if we would judge ourselves, we should not be judged. [32] But when we are judged, we are chastened of the Lord, that we should not be condemned with the world."

The abortion issue has been and continue to be an extremely hot topic and rightly so and so is the church pedophilia and rapping the nuns and having babies that they murdered and killed the mothers the nuns for their own hidden pleasure!!!

Hypocrisy!! Don't you think if a priest or bishop or pope forbid communion to someone for allowing abortion as an issue up to the mother and father of the baby, THEN THE MILLIONS OF CHRISTIAN LEADERS, MINISTERS AND PRIESTS INCLUDING HIERCHY THAT ALLOWED THESE SATANIC PRACTICES, MUST BE EXCLUDED NOT ONLY FROM COMMUNIONS. BUT ALSO FROM ENTERING THE HOUSE OF GOD THROUGH THE THOUSANDS OF YEARS FROM THEIR PEDOPHILIACS AND RAPPING NUNS AND CHURCH CHILDREN, MOLESTING AND COERCED THE MOST VULNERABLE???

Those pedophiles and pedophilia do not just deserve to be banned from communion but also be forbidden to enter the churches, temples and whatever God worshipping place and thrown in the lake of fire and Sulphur forever.

I wonder if those leaders understand the ongoing wrath of God upon them until the end!!

Matthew 23:13-36 "But woe unto you, scribes and Pharisees, hypocrites! for ye shut up the kingdom of heaven against men: for ye neither go in yourselves, neither suffer ye them that are entering to go in. [14] Woe unto you, scribes and Pharisees, hypocrites! for ye devour widows' houses, and for a pretence make long prayer: therefore ye shall receive the greater damnation. [15] Woe unto you, scribes and Pharisees, hypocrites! for ye compass sea and land to make one proselyte, and when he is made, ye make him twofold more the child of hell than yourselves. [16] Woe unto you, ye blind guides, which say, Whosoever shall swear by the temple, it is nothing; but whosoever shall swear by the gold of the temple, he is a debtor! [17] Ye fools and blind: for whether is greater, the gold, or the temple that sanctifieth the gold? [18] And, Whosoever shall swear by the altar, it is nothing; but whosoever sweareth by the gift that is upon it, he is guilty. [19] Ye fools and blind: for whether is greater, the gift, or the altar that sanctifieth the gift? [20] Whoso therefore shall swear by the altar, sweareth by it, and by all things thereon. [21] And whoso shall swear by the temple, sweareth by it, and by him that dwelleth therein. [22] And he that shall swear by heaven, sweareth by the throne of God, and by him that sitteth thereon. [23] Woe unto you, scribes and Pharisees, hypocrites! for ye pay tithe of mint and anise and cummin, and have omitted the weightier matters of the law, judgment, mercy, and faith: these ought ye to have done, and not to leave the other undone. [24] Ye blind guides, which strain at a gnat, and swallow a camel. [25] Woe unto you, scribes and Pharisees, hypocrites! for ye make clean the outside of the cup and of the platter, but within they are full of extortion and excess. [26] Thou blind Pharisee, cleanse first that which is within the cup and platter, that the outside of them may be clean also. [27] Woe unto you, scribes and Pharisees, hypocrites! for ye are like unto whited sepulchres, which indeed appear beautiful outward, but are within full of dead men's bones, and of all uncleanness. [28] Even so ye also outwardly appear righteous unto men, but within ye are full of hypocrisy and iniquity. [29] Woe unto you, scribes and Pharisees, hypocrites! because ye build the tombs of the prophets, and garnish the sepulchres of the righteous, [30] And say, If we had been in the days of our fathers, we would not have been partakers with them in the blood of the prophets. [31] Wherefore ye be witnesses unto yourselves, that ye are the children of them which killed the prophets. [32] Fill ye up then the measure of your fathers. [33] Ye serpents, ye generation of vipers, how can ye escape the damnation of hell? [34] Wherefore, behold, I send unto you prophets, and wise men, and scribes: and some of them ye shall kill and crucify; and some of them shall ye scourge in your synagogues, and persecute them from city to city: [35] That upon you may come all the righteous blood shed upon the earth, from the blood of righteous Abel unto the blood of Zacharias son of Barachias, whom ye slew between the temple and the altar. [36] Verily I say unto you, All these things shall come upon this generation."

With extreme humility

Respectfully

Ramsis Ghaly

CG. It is never acceptable to underestimate the harm caused by sexual abuse of minors, but abortion is also a sinful, immoral act, an abominable crime. I agree they should not be allowed in church for any reason.

It is the Time to Demand at Each Employees List Equity and Representation to Minorities!

Written by Ramsis Ghaly

It isn't only racist high ranking but across the common levels! It isn't only racist high rank but racist across ranks! Perhaps one the main reasons racism is still widespread because of lack an objective standard platform/ criterion to execute in hiring and appointing students, employees, applicants and candidates that is public subjective to auditing but rather unregulated subjective criteria based on subconscious bias, preference, likeness, favoritism, nepotism, kick back, conflict of interest,—-etc

I am dreaming to work in a place multiracial, equity to all, ensures opportunity to minorities, inclusion of all, celebrate diversity working all together under one roof! I have seen it all with all types of discrimination throughout the years of my life. I am a victim of discrimination first class since I was born in my own homeland Egypt because of being Christian and my mother being woman. It didn't stop there, when I arrived to USA I was severely discriminated upon as minority with no job or food or residency to take me. And it continued as I went through the most competitive residencies and specialties until today, I have been discriminated against.

Many believe it is how "life" is and "competition" and it is not discrimination. Absolutely not competition is based in equal opportunity and competition according to the individual achievement and performance. But discrimination is given no opportunity and not treated equally despite similar performance!

Each minority group is to be presented equally according to their ethnical and race percentages in the region both all types of working tasks, in education schools, colleges and universities. Only then, racial disparity disappears, and all will melt together in a big pot America learning from each other, helping each other promoting the gifts and talents in each color group, there is no reason to make minorities of any race and color continue to be discriminated upon segregated in their own shell and not participants locally and globally.

In 2022, not only in Chicago but nationwide, there should never be a list of applicants or Employees without involving minority groups of whatever organization, corporate, hospital, factory, school, college, university, board, committee, worshipping places, town hall, city hall, court, —all the way to the top the White House from the smallest to the largest. All regardless must respect diversity and protect minority and strive for equity. In Chicago area for instance, at minimum a list should have 13% blacks, 18% Latinos and 6% Asians.

Any American program list of applicants should match racial and ethnicity distribution of a given population. Therefore, it should be a law to ensure equity and diversity at minimum equal to the percentage of racial groups at each region.

In 2022, we must act with high integrity governed with unspotted ethics and moral values. We all the children of God created in His image, and we came out of the seeds of one parent Adam and Eve. In God's eyes we all His with no partiality treated equally loved equally gifted equally according to His mercy and grace created males and females having the same form presented in the body, soul and spirit having the same divine breath of life and multiplying from generation to generation equally. It is zero tolerance to favoritism, nepotism and any racial or ethnic inequality or social injustice.

Doing so, it is not only fair but also it will preserve equal rights of minority, equal representation and in addition, each race and ethnicity are equally distributed. People of each race and ethnicity is in dire need to be equally represented. But how can we do that if we aren't requiring applicants and employees to be diverse. As the matching of population occurs and so its needs to be fulfilled to each race and ethnicity. It will be providing full protection to their rights, and it will only inspire the growth of minority as soon as they believe there is a law of equity and a true hope to equity.

Action speaks louder. Only then groups will not fear to work together putting down their guards and no more feeling uneasy to be next to a person of different race and ethnicity. The love and respect will dominate the unconditional equity in all. Years from now, our children will grow in the manner of their fathers and not according to external appearances. John 7:24 KJV "Judge not according to the appearance, but judge righteous judgment." 1 Samuel 16:7 - But the LORD said unto Samuel, Look not on his countenance, or on the height of his stature; because I have refused him: for the LORD seeth not as man seeth; for man looketh on the outward appearance, but the LORD looketh on the heart." James 2:1-5 - My brethren, have not the faith of our Lord Jesus Christ, the Lord of glory, with respect of persons. "Proverbs 31:9 - Open thy mouth, judge righteously, and plead the cause of the poor and needy." Matthew 7:1 - Judge not, that ye be not judged."

Doing so, it helps to open our arms and hearts to one another, to ease the tensions, to break the barriers, to be open to accept differences, to promote admixtures with one to another and to adopt various cultures. If we can't live together and work together, how can we be in one paradise and in one heaven. I am certain that there is NO multiple heavens or multiple paradises or multiple New Jerusalem but Only One of Each!!! Revelation 21:1-3 KJV "And I saw a new heaven and a new earth: for the first heaven and the first earth were passed away; and there was no more sea. [2] And I John saw the holy city, new Jerusalem, coming down from God out of heaven, prepared as a bride adorned for her husband. [3] And I heard a great voice out of heaven saying, Behold, the tabernacle of God is with men, and he will dwell with them, and they shall be his people, and God himself shall be with them, and be their God."

And this is the core; If this indeed the case in our society equity to all and inclusion and we are doing it, why aren't we? Why we still see lists of employees and candidates and applicants not representing minorities??? What is strange we are keep talking about racial disparity and we aren't enforcing or demanding an equal representation in each list of applicants, students and Employees at any given place nationwide!!

Let us love, uplift and inspire each other regardless of the external appearances. Let us value the inward of all people. As it is written: 1 John 4:7-8,11,20-21 KJV "Beloved, let us love one another: for love is of God; and every one that loveth is born of God, and knoweth God. [8] He that loveth not knoweth not God; for God is love. [11] Beloved, if God so loved us, we ought also to love one another. [20] If a man say, I love God, and hateth his brother, he is a liar: for he that loveth not his brother whom he hath seen, how can he love God whom he hath not seen? [21] And this commandment have we from him, That he who loveth God love his brother also."

2020 U.S. Census,

Non-Hispanic White 57.8%

Hispanic and Latino (of any race) 18.7%

Black or African American 12.1%

Asian 5.9%

Two or more races 4.1%

Native Americans and Alaska Natives 0.7%

Some other race 0.5%

Native Hawaiians and Other Pacific Islanders 0.2%

The Black or African American in combination population grew by 88.7% since 2010. In 2020, the Black or African American alone population (41.1 million) accounted for 12.4% of all people living in the United States, compared with 38.9 million and 12.6% in 2010.Aug 12, 2021

As of 2020, white Americans are the racial and ethnic majority, with non-Hispanic whites representing 57.8% of the population. Hispanic and Latino Americans (who may belong to any racial group) are the largest ethnic minority, comprising 18.7% of the population, while Black or African Americans are the largest racial minority, making up 12.1%.

We all one sheep for One Good Shepherd as it is written in John 10:16 KJV "And other sheep I have, which are not of this fold: them also I must bring, and they shall hear my voice; and there shall be one fold, and one shepherd."

We all created the same from one God, one parent Adam and Eve in God's Image as it is written: Genesis 1:26-28 KJV "And God said, Let us make man in our image, after our likeness: and let them have dominion over the fish of the sea, and over the fowl of the air, and over the cattle, and over all the earth, and over every creeping thing that creepeth upon the earth. [27] So God created man in his own image, in the image of God created he him; male and female created he them. [28] And God blessed them, and God said unto them, Be fruitful, and multiply, and replenish the earth, and subdue it: and have dominion over the fish of the sea, and over the fowl of the air, and over every living thing that moveth upon the earth." Genesis 2:18,21-24 KJV

[18] And the Lord God said, It is not good that the man should be alone; I will make him an help meet for him. [21] And the Lord God caused a deep sleep to fall upon Adam, and he slept: and he took one of his ribs, and closed up the flesh instead thereof; [22] And the rib, which the Lord God had taken from man, made he a woman, and brought her unto the man. [23] And Adam said, This is now bone of my bones, and flesh of my flesh: she shall be called Woman, because she was taken out of Man. [24] Therefore shall a man leave his father and his mother, and shall cleave unto his wife: and they shall be one flesh."

In God there is no partiality

Matthew 5:45 KJV "That ye may be the children of your Father which is in heaven: for he maketh his sun to rise on the evil and on the good, and sendeth rain on the just and on the unjust." Romans 2:11 "For there is no partiality with God." Colossians 3:25 "For he who does wrong will receive the consequences of the wrong which he has done, and that without partiality." Deuteronomy 10:17

"For the Lord your God is the God of gods and the Lord of lords, the great, the mighty, and the awesome God who does not show partiality nor take a bribe." Acts 10:34 Opening his mouth, Peter said: "I most certainly understand now that God is not one to show partiality," 2 Chronicles 19:7 Now then let the fear of the Lord be upon you; be very careful what you do, for the Lord our God will have no part in unrighteousness or partiality or the taking of a bribe."

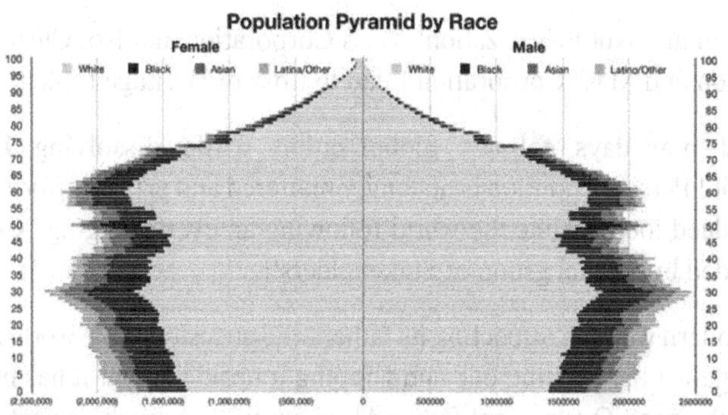

EN.WIKIPEDIA.ORG

Race and ethnicity in the United States - Wikipedia

The United States of America has a racially and ethnically diverse population.[1] At the federal level, race and ethnicity have been categorized separately. The most recent United States Census officially recognized five racial categories (White, Black or African American, Asian American, American I...

JT. amen Ramsis...

CG. Thank you for writing about this.

Equity is a goal. It insures that everyone has the resources they need to succeed and therefore they are respected and respect themselves. So many minorities are not given these tools to succeed. This definitely needs to change.

Globalization Mass Corporation Lead to Loss of Heritage Links!

My Personal Views written 10/12/2022

Globalization and Not Privatization! Mass Corporation and Not Customization! Globalization and Mass Corporation Lead to Loss of Heritage Links!

The world nowadays follows globalization while dissolving individual privatization! Personal opinion is no longer mattered and private efforts are cared for! It is indeed looking like the world following an ever changing "Cookbook" masterminded by special group of Stakeholders!!

Why the modern world is respecting its fathers and ancestors! The world nowadays is rioting against the existing one and flipping it upside down! It has never been the way in the past! Our ancient father Abraham was so much respected and his values by his own children, grandchildren and thousands of years after his death!

The Holy Bible was followed day and night at work as at home in public as in private without a shame! Why the modern world is moving fast and taking a turn that never heard before!

Is it because artificial technology taking over humanity!! Is it because modern technology ruling mankind! Is it because external forces redirecting the world to dissolve human brains? Or Is it the preparation of merging the entire world as one under satanic mindless self-interest leadership??

It almost appears that the work by laws much important than the traditional work bylaws! The Holy Bible isn't acknowledged as the source to guide the daily life but rather the social media, the news and HR doctrine!

Recently, I was told that my old ways of teaching are no longer accepted and perhaps considered offensive to the new students and residents!!

Furthermore, I must not expect them to be committed and dedicated as I was and set high expectation or work values from them that may take away their private time outside work!!

It is the time of "Work less" and "Make More", "Work Smart" and Not "Work Hard". I was told that we are living in a new world where the old days of sacrifices or going out of way to work or to volunteer to research or do things out of goodness without pay perform extra mile deeds are gone and are no longer promoted!

I was also told over the years that I must change! It isn't important any longer delivery of quality

but most important delivery must be according to the new comers consideration!!

What was norm in the past, is certainly perceived odd nowadays?

I walked in public, and it was first time to feel stranger! I looked around and I realized I was the only one in the entire airport with a classy suit, ironed shirt with cufflink, tie and pocket handkerchief and shining shoes!! Most of not all were wearing the new style tie-less, suit-less attire!!

Have you seen a person with normal and natural skins like in the past with respect to their own body? Or we see human skins tanned with explosive tattoos!!

Furthermore, it appears the new world is operated by technology and computer programs with pre-set steps to follow and adhere!!

The individual human mind has no longer say or existence!!

The young children's eyes are widely open to very sensitive things that they are boldly adopt as norms without being shameful!!

The hands-on touch was a cornerstone in the past and it us absolutely distinct in the modern world!

Is this the reason where the old must silence and retire and let the new minds flourish and lead their own the way they perceived?

Is it the way a man was created to die and take all the hardworking acquired experiences and skills to the grave yard?

How many of the wisemen and women are forced to retire early or pushed out of the way because of Incompatibility of the New coming generations!

How many small businesses are closing, and hardworking men and women sold theirs??

Proverbs 22:6 KJV [6] Train up a child in the way he should go: and when he is old, he will not depart from it.

However, let me ask the following questions??

What is wrong of the modern world? It looks okay and it is going and many are adopting while those having hard time are fading away?

Indeed, the new comers are happy with modernization and having technology take the leadership and they just focus in following the google steps and established policies while having good time and living so called "Balance life" that the previous generations were lacking and ignored"

In fact, it is rare to find parents as our parents love to raise numerous children and enforce every family ties and values! Instead the new homes now restrict to two children or even no children and enforce the current world teaching!!

Are we the ones responsible for the degradation of values of the new coming generations?

Are the adopted values and work ethics of the new coming generations being really inferior to the previous generations?

Is it the time now for the newcomers to take over and learn the hard way while the older step out of the way?

The new world must be guided by the previous one! However, the fear is that the modern world really needs the blessing and wisdom of the seniors and elders as the generations before! The new world needs the guidance, experience and skills of the forefathers! And if not, the modern world may deviate far away from the world that mankind was created for!!

The world must not be transformed away from God and His Holy Bible and His Commandments! The world must be continuum of previous ones to its Source God the Almighty! As It is written: Romans 12:1-2,16 KJV [1] I beseech you therefore, brethren, by the mercies of God, that ye present your bodies a living sacrifice, holy, acceptable unto God, which is your reasonable service. [2] And be not conformed to this world: but be ye transformed by the renewing of your mind, that ye may prove what is that good, and acceptable, and perfect, will of God. [16] Be of the same mind one toward another. Mind not high things, but condescend to men of low estate. Be not wise in your own conceits."

I hope that the seniors won't give up in their children and keep going as they were taught by their ancestors and maintained their own culture and values!

Regardless, the human race regardless of technology and advancement must be in the Image of the Most High as God the Creator made man and woman in His Likeness as it is written: Genesis 1:26-28 KJV "And God said, Let us make man in our image, after our likeness: and let them have dominion over the fish of the sea, and over the fowl of the air, and over the cattle, and over all the earth, and over every creeping thing that creepeth upon the earth. [27] So God created man in his own image, in the image of God created he him; male and female created he them. [28] And God blessed them, and God said unto them, Be fruitful, and multiply, and replenish the earth, and subdue it: and have dominion over the fish of the sea, and over the fowl of the air, and over every living thing that moveth upon the earth."

The children need their parents as the grandchildren need grandparents as the great grandchildren need their great grandchildren parents and it keeps all the way back to Adam and Eve to the ultimate Source of Life and Teaching, the Heavenly Father who created the human race and distended to return back one day in His Kingdom under One King Jesus the Lord!

And if not the history will repeat itself as written:

2 Samuel 7:12-16 KJV [12] And when thy days be fulfilled, and thou shalt sleep with thy fathers, I will set up thy seed after thee, which shall proceed out of thy bowels, and I will establish his kingdom. [13] He shall build an house for my name, and I will stablish the throne of his kingdom for ever. [14] I will be his father, and he shall be my son. If he commit iniquity, I will chasten him with the rod of men, and with the stripes of the children of men: [15] But my mercy shall not depart away from him, as I took it from Saul, whom I put away before thee. [16] And thine house and thy kingdom shall be established for ever before thee: thy throne shall be established forever.

2. Deuteronomy 6:5-9 Love the Lord your God with all your heart, with all your soul, and with all your strength. Take to heart these words that I give you today. Repeat them to your children. Talk about them when you're at home or away, when you lie down or get up. Write them down, and tie them around your wrist, and wear them as headbands as a reminder. Write them on the doorframes of your houses and on your gates.

3. Deuteronomy 4:9-10 "But watch out! Be careful never to forget what you yourself have seen. Do not let these memories escape from your mind as long as you live! And be sure to pass them on to your children and grandchildren. Never forget the day when you stood before the Lord your God at Mount Sinai, where he told me, Summon the people before me, and I will personally instruct them. Then they will learn to fear me as long as they live, and they will teach their children to fear me also."

4. Matthew 19:13-15 One day some parents brought their children to Jesus so he could lay his hands on them and pray for them. But the disciples scolded the parents for bothering him. But Jesus said, "Let the children come to me. Don't stop them! For the Kingdom of Heaven belongs to those who are like these children." And he placed his hands on their heads and blessed them before he left.

5. 1 Timothy 4:10-11 This is why we work hard and continue to struggle, for our hope is in the living God, who is the Savior of all people and particularly of all believers. Teach these things and insist that everyone learn them.

6. Deuteronomy 11:19 Teach them to your children. Talk about them when you are at home and when you are on the road, when you are going to bed and when you are getting up.

7. Proverbs 23:13-14 Do not hesitate to discipline a child. If you spank him, he will not die. Spank him yourself, and you will save his soul from hell.

8. Proverbs 22:15 A child's heart has a tendency to do wrong, but the rod of discipline removes it far away from him.

9. Proverbs 29:15 The rod and rebuke bestow wisdom, but an undisciplined child brings shame to his mother.

Biblical verses in Transformation

Isaiah 43:19 NLT For I am about to do something new. See, I have already begun! Do you not see it? I will make a pathway through the wilderness. I will create rivers in the dry wasteland.

Isaiah 43:18 NIV Forget the former things; do not dwell on the past.

Jeremiah 29:11 NIV For I know the plans I have for you, declares the Lord, plans to prosper you and not to harm you, plans to give you hope and a future.

2 Peter 3:17 NLT You already know these things, dear friends. So be on guard; then you will not be carried away by the errors of these wicked people and lose your own secure footing.

Ephesians 4:22 NLT Throw off your old sinful nature and your former way of life, which is corrupted by lust and deception.

2 Peter 3:18 WEB But grow in the grace and knowledge of our Lord and Savior Jesus Christ. To him be the glory both now and forever. Amen.

Matthew 5:48 NLT But you are to be perfect, even as your Father in heaven is perfect.

Philippians 3:13 NLT No, dear brothers and sisters, I have not achieved it (perfection), but I focus on this one thing: Forgetting the past and looking forward to what lies ahead.

Philippians 3:14 NLT I press on to reach the end of the race and receive the heavenly prize for which God, through Christ Jesus, is calling us.

Colossians 3:1 NLT Since you have been raised to new life with Christ, set your sights on the realities of heaven, where Christ sits in the place of honor at God's right hand.

Colossians 3:2 NLT Think about the things of heaven, not the things of earth. For you died to this life, and your real life is hidden with Christ in God.

Colossians 3:5a, 7 NLT So put to death the sinful, earthly things lurking within you. You used to do these things when your life was still part of this world.

Colossians 3:12 NLT Since God chose you to be the holy people he loves, you must clothe yourselves with tenderhearted mercy, kindness, humility, gentleness, and patience.

Colossians 3:15 NLT And let the peace that comes from Christ rule in your hearts. For as members of one body you are called to live in peace. And always be thankful.

Colossians 2:7 NLT Let your roots grow down into him, and let your lives be built on him. Then your faith will grow strong in the truth you were taught, and you will overflow with thankfulness.

Isaiah 43:19 NLT For I am about to do something new. See, I have already begun! Do you not see it? I will make a pathway through the wilderness. I will create rivers in the dry wasteland.

2 Peter 3:8 NLT But you must not forget this one thing, dear friends: A day is like a thousand years to the Lord, and a thousand years is like a day.

Colossians 3:16 NLT Let the message about Christ, in all its richness, fill your lives. Teach and counsel each other with all the wisdom he gives. Sing psalms and hymns and spiritual songs to God with thankful hearts.

Ephesians 4:30 NLT Do not bring sorrow to God's Holy Spirit by the way you live. Remember, he has identified you as his own, guaranteeing that you will be saved on the day of redemption.

Ephesians 4:23-24 NLT Let the Spirit renew your thoughts and attitudes. Put on your new nature, created to be like God—truly righteous and holy.

2 Peter 3:9 NLT The Lord isn't really being slow about his promise, as some people think. No, he is being patient for your sake. He does not want anyone to be destroyed, but wants everyone to repent.

2 Peter 3:14 NLT And so, dear friends, while you are waiting for these things to happen, make every effort to be found living peaceful lives that are pure and blameless in his sight.

Galatians 5:1 NLT So Christ has truly set us free. Now make sure that you stay free, and don't get tied up again in slavery to the law.

Galatians 5:13 NLT For you have been called to live in freedom, my brothers and sisters. But don't use your freedom to satisfy your sinful nature. Instead, use your freedom to serve one another in love

Galatians 5:16-17 NLT So I say, let the Holy Spirit guide your lives. Then you won't be doing what your sinful nature craves. The sinful nature wants to do evil, which is just the opposite of what the Spirit wants. And the Spirit gives us desires that are the opposite of what the sinful nature desires. These two forces are constantly fighting each other, so you are not free to carry out your good intentions.

Galatians 5:24-25 NLT Those who belong to Christ Jesus have nailed the passions and desires of their sinful nature to his cross and crucified them there. Since we are living by the Spirit, let us follow the Spirit's leading in every part of our lives.

We pray for this modern world and coming world until end of ages to keep the covenant with God the Lord fur ever and ever Amen

Biblical verses in God's Covenant

Psalm 78:70 He also chose David His servant

And took him from the sheepfolds;

2 Samuel 6:21 So David said to Michal, "It was before the Lord, who chose me above your father and above all his house, to appoint me ruler over the people of the Lord, over Israel; therefore I will celebrate before the Lord.

1 Kings 8:16 'Since the day that I brought My people Israel from Egypt, I did not choose a city out of all the tribes of Israel in which to build a house that My name might be there, but I chose David to be over My people Israel.'

2 Chronicles 6:6 but I have chosen Jerusalem that My name might be there, and I have chosen David to be over My people Israel.'

Psalm 89:3-4 "I have made a covenant with My chosen;

I have sworn to David My servant,

I will establish your seed forever

And build up your throne to all generations." Selah.

2Samuel 7:11-16 even from the day that I commanded judges to be over My people Israel; and I will give you rest from all your enemies. The Lord also declares to you that the Lord will make a house for you. When your days are complete and you lie down with your fathers, I will raise up your descendant after you, who will come forth from you, and I will establish his kingdom. He shall build a house for My name, and I will establish the throne of his kingdom forever.read more.

2Samuel 23:5 "Truly is not my house so with God?

For He has made an everlasting covenant with me,

Ordered in all things, and secured;

For all my salvation and all my desire,

Will He not indeed make it grow?

1 Kings 2:45 But King Solomon shall be blessed, and the throne of David shall be established before the Lord forever."

2 Chronicles 13:5 Do you not know that the Lord God of Israel gave the rule over Israel forever to David and his sons by a covenant of salt?

Psalm 18:50 He gives great deliverance to His king,

And shows lovingkindness to His anointed,

To David and his descendants forever.

Psalm 89:28-29 "My lovingkindness I will keep for him forever,

And My covenant shall be confirmed to him.

"So I will establish his descendants forever

And his throne as the days of heaven.

Jeremiah 33:17 For thus says the Lord, 'David shall never lack a man to sit on the throne of the house of Israel;

Psalm 132:11-12 The Lord has sworn to David

A truth from which He will not turn back:

"Of the fruit of your body I will set upon your throne.

“If your sons will keep My covenant

And My testimony which I will teach them,

Their sons also shall sit upon your throne forever.”

1 Kings 8:25-26 Now therefore, O Lord, the God of Israel, keep with Your servant David my father that which You have promised him, saying, ‘You shall not lack a man to sit on the throne of Israel, if only your sons take heed to their way to walk before Me as you have walked.’ Now therefore, O God of Israel, let Your word, I pray, be confirmed which You have spoken to Your servant, my father David.

2 Chronicles 6:16-17 Now therefore, O Lord, the God of Israel, keep with Your servant David, my father, that which You have promised him, saying, ‘You shall not lack a man to sit on the throne of Israel, if only your sons take heed to their way, to walk in My law as you have walked before Me.’ Now therefore, O Lord, the God of Israel, let Your word be confirmed which You have spoken to Your servant David.

1 Kings 9:4-5 As for you, if you will walk before Me as your father David walked, in integrity of heart and uprightness, doing according to all that I have commanded you and will keep My statutes and My ordinances, then I will establish the throne of your kingdom over Israel forever, just as I promised to your father David, saying, ‘You shall not lack a man on the throne of Israel.’

2 Chronicles 7:17-18 As for you, if you walk before Me as your father David walked, even to do according to all that I have commanded you, and will keep My statutes and My ordinances, then I will establish your royal throne as I covenanted with your father David, saying, ‘You shall not lack a man to be ruler in Israel.’

Jeremiah 22:4-5 For if you men will indeed perform this thing, then kings will enter the gates of this house, sitting in David’s place on his throne, riding in chariots and on horses, even the king himself and his servants and his people. But if you will not obey these words, I swear by Myself,” declares the Lord, “that this house will become a desolation.”””

1 Kings 9:6-9 “But if you or your sons indeed turn away from following Me, and do not keep My commandments and My statutes which I have set before you, and go and serve other gods and worship them, then I will cut off Israel from the land which I have given them, and the house which I have consecrated for My name, I will cast out of My sight. So Israel will become a proverb and a byword among all peoples. And this house will become a heap of ruins; everyone who passes by will be astonished and hiss and say, ‘Why has the Lord done thus to this land and to this house?’

2 Chronicles 7:19-22 "But if you turn away and forsake My statutes and My commandments which I have set before you, and go and serve other gods and worship them, then I will uproot you from My land which I have given you, and this house which I have consecrated for My name I will cast out of My sight and I will make it a proverb and a byword among all peoples. As for this house, which was exalted, everyone who passes by it will be astonished and say, 'Why has the Lord done thus to this land and to this house?'read more.

1 Kings 11:11-13 So the Lord said to Solomon, "Because you have done this, and you have not kept My covenant and My statutes, which I have commanded you, I will surely tear the kingdom from you, and will give it to your servant. Nevertheless I will not do it in your days for the sake of your father David, but I will tear it out of the hand of your son. However, I will not tear away all the kingdom, but I will give one tribe to your son for the sake of My servant David and for the sake of Jerusalem which I have chosen."

Jeremiah 7:24-26 Yet they did not obey or incline their ear, but walked in their own counsels and in the stubbornness of their evil heart, and went backward and not forward. Since the day that your fathers came out of the land of Egypt until this day, I have sent you all My servants the prophets, daily rising early and sending them. Yet they did not listen to Me or incline their ear, but stiffened their neck; they did more evil than their fathers.

Jeremiah 22:6-9 For thus says the Lord concerning the house of the king of Judah:

"You are like Gilead to Me,

Like the summit of Lebanon;

Yet most assuredly I will make you like a wilderness,

Like cities which are not inhabited.

"For I will set apart destroyers against you,

Each with his weapons;

And they will cut down your choicest cedars

And throw them on the fire. "Many nations will pass by this city; and they will say to one another, 'Why has the Lord done thus to this great city?'read more.

Jeremiah 36:30-31 Therefore thus says the Lord concerning Jehoiakim king of Judah, "He shall have no one to sit on the throne of David, and his dead body shall be cast out to the heat of the day and the frost of the night. I will also punish him and his descendants and his servants for their iniquity, and I will bring on them and the inhabitants of Jerusalem and the men of Judah all the calamity that I have declared to them—but they did not listen.'""

2 Chronicles 21:7 Yet the Lord was not willing to destroy the house of David because of the covenant which He had made with David, and since He had promised to give a lamp to him and his sons forever.

2 Kings 8:19 However, the Lord was not willing to destroy Judah, for the sake of David His servant, since He had promised him to give a lamp to him through his sons always.

1 Kings 11:34-36 Nevertheless I will not take the whole kingdom out of his hand, but I will make him ruler all the days of his life, for the sake of My servant David whom I chose, who observed My commandments and My statutes; but I will take the kingdom from his son's hand and give it to you, even ten tribes. But to his son I will give one tribe, that My servant David may have a lamp always before Me in Jerusalem, the city where I have chosen for Myself to put My name.

1 Kings 15:4 But for David's sake the Lord his God gave him a lamp in Jerusalem, to raise up his son after him and to establish Jerusalem;

Psalm 89:30-34 "If his sons forsake My law

And do not walk in My judgments,

If they violate My statutes

And do not keep My commandments,

Then I will punish their transgression with the rod

And their iniquity with stripes.

2 Kings 21:7 Then he set the carved image of Asherah that he had made, in the house of which the Lord said to David and to his son Solomon, "In this house and in Jerusalem, which I have chosen from all the tribes of Israel, I will put My name forever.

2 Chronicles 33:7 Then he put the carved image of the idol which he had made in the house of God, of which God had said to David and to Solomon his son, "In this house and in Jerusalem, which I have chosen from all the tribes of Israel, I will put My name forever;

1 Kings 8:20-21 Now the Lord has fulfilled His word which He spoke; for I have risen in place of my father David and sit on the throne of Israel, as the Lord promised, and have built the house for the name of the Lord, the God of Israel.

There I have set a place for the ark, in which is the covenant of the Lord, which He made with our fathers when He brought them from the land of Egypt."

2 Chronicles 6:10-11 Now the Lord has fulfilled His word which He spoke; for I have risen in the place of my father David and sit on the throne of Israel, as the Lord promised, and have built the house for the name of the Lord, the God of Israel. There I have set the ark in which is the covenant of the Lord, which He made with the sons of Israel."

1 Kings 11:32 (but he will have one tribe, for the sake of My servant David and for the sake of Jerusalem, the city which I have chosen from all the tribes of Israel),

1 Chronicles 23:25 For David said, "The Lord God of Israel has given rest to His people, and He dwells in Jerusalem forever.

2 Chronicles 6:41-42

"Now therefore arise, O Lord God, to Your resting place, You and the ark of Your might; let Your priests, O Lord God, be clothed with salvation and let Your godly ones rejoice in what is good. "O Lord God, do not turn away the face of Your anointed; remember Your lovingkindness to Your servant David."

Psalm 132:8-10 Arise, O Lord, to Your resting place,

You and the ark of Your strength.

Let Your priests be clothed with righteousness,

And let Your godly ones sing for joy.

For the sake of David Your servant,

Do not turn away the face of Your anointed.

Isaiah 37:35 'For I will defend this city to save it for My own sake and for My servant David's sake.'"

2 Kings 19:34 'For I will defend this city to save it for My own sake and for My servant David's sake.'"

2 Kings 19:20 Then Isaiah the son of Amoz sent to Hezekiah saying, "Thus says the Lord, the God of Israel, 'Because you have prayed to Me about Sennacherib king of Assyria, I have heard you.'

Zechariah 12:7-9 The Lord also will save the tents of Judah first, so that the glory of the house of David and the glory of the inhabitants of Jerusalem will not be magnified above Judah. In that day the Lord will defend the inhabitants of Jerusalem, and the one who is feeble among them in that day will be like David, and the house of David will be like God, like the angel of the Lord before them. And in that day I will set about to destroy all the nations that come against Jerusalem.

Amos 9:11 "In that day I will raise up the fallen booth of David,

And wall up its breaches;

I will also raise up its ruins

And rebuild it as in the days of old;

Acts 15:16 Verse Concepts

'After these things I will return,

And I will rebuild the tabernacle of David which has fallen,

And I will rebuild its ruins,

And I will restore it,

Jeremiah 33:25-26 Thus says the Lord, 'If My covenant for day and night stand not, and the fixed patterns of heaven and earth I have not established, then I would reject the descendants of Jacob and David My servant, not taking from his descendants rulers over the descendants of Abraham, Isaac and Jacob. But I will restore their fortunes and will have mercy on them.'"

Jeremiah 23:5-6 "Behold, the days are coming," declares the Lord,

"When I will raise up for David a righteous Branch;

And He will reign as king and act wisely

And do justice and righteousness in the land.

"In His days Judah will be saved,

And Israel will dwell securely;

And this is His name by which He will be called,

'The Lord our righteousness.'

Psalm 110:1-2 A Psalm of David.

The Lord says to my Lord:

"Sit at My right hand

Until I make Your enemies a footstool for Your feet."

The Lord will stretch forth Your strong scepter from Zion, saying,

"Rule in the midst of Your enemies."

Isaiah 9:7 There will be no end to the increase of His government or of peace,

On the throne of David and over his kingdom,

To establish it and to uphold it with justice and righteousness

From then on and forevermore.

The zeal of the Lord of hosts will accomplish this.

Isaiah 11:1-2 Then a shoot will spring from the stem of Jesse,

And a branch from his roots will bear fruit.

The Spirit of the Lord will rest on Him,

The spirit of wisdom and understanding,

The spirit of counsel and strength,

The spirit of knowledge and the fear of the Lord.

Isaiah 16:5 throne will even be established in lovingkindness,

And a judge will sit on it in faithfulness in the tent of David;

Moreover, he will seek justice

And be prompt in righteousness.

Isaiah 55:3 "Incline your ear and come to Me.

Listen, that you may live;

And I will make an everlasting covenant with you,

According to the faithful mercies shown to David.

Ezekiel 34:23-25 "Then I will set over them one shepherd, My servant David, and he will feed them; he will feed them himself and be their shepherd. And I, the Lord, will be their God, and My servant David will be prince among them; I the Lord have spoken. "I will make a covenant of peace with them and eliminate harmful beasts from the land so that they may live securely in the wilderness and sleep in the woods.

Zechariah 3:8 Now listen, Joshua the high priest, you and your friends who are sitting in front of you—indeed they are men who are a symbol, for behold, I am going to bring in My servant the Branch.

John 7:42 Has not the Scripture said that the Christ comes from the descendants of David, and from Bethlehem, the village where David was?"

Luke 1:32-33 He will be great and will be called the Son of the Most High; and the Lord God will give Him the throne of His father David; and He will reign over the house of Jacob forever, and His kingdom will have no end."

Revelation 22:16 "I, Jesus, have sent My angel to testify to you these things for the churches. I am the root and the descendant of David, the bright morning star."

Matthew 1:1 The record of the genealogy of Jesus the Messiah, the son of David, the son of Abraham:

Matthew 22:41-46 Now while the Pharisees were gathered together, Jesus asked them a question: "What do you think about the Christ, whose son is He?" They *said to Him, "The son of David." He *said to them, "Then how does David in the Spirit call Him 'Lord,' saying,read more.

Mark 12:35-37 And Jesus began to say, as He taught in the temple, "How is it that the scribes say that the Christ is the son of David? David himself said in the Holy Spirit,

'The Lord said to my Lord,

"Sit at My right hand,

Until I put Your enemies beneath Your feet."'

David himself calls Him 'Lord'; so in what sense is He his son?" And the large crowd enjoyed listening to Him.

Luke 20:41-44 Then He said to them, "How is it that they say the Christ is David's son? For David himself says in the book of Psalms,

'The Lord said to my Lord,

"Sit at My right hand,

Until I make Your enemies a footstool for Your feet."'

Mark 11:10 Blessed is the coming kingdom of our father David;

Hosanna in the highest!"

Matthew 21:9 The crowds going ahead of Him, and those who followed, were shouting,

“Hosanna to the Son of David;

Blessed is He who comes in the name of the Lord;

Hosanna in the highest!”

Luke 24:21 But we were hoping that it was He who was going to redeem Israel. Indeed, besides all this, it is the third day since these things happened.

Acts 1:6 So when they had come together, they were asking Him, saying, “Lord, is it at this time You are restoring the kingdom to Israel?”

Acts 2:29-31 “Brethren, I may confidently say to you regarding the patriarch David that he both died and was buried, and his tomb is with us to this day. And so, because he was a prophet and knew that God had sworn to him with an oath to seat one of his descendants on his throne, he looked ahead and spoke of the resurrection of the Christ, that He was neither abandoned to Hades, nor did His flesh suffer decay.

Acts 13:34 As for the fact that He raised Him up from the dead, no longer to return to decay, He has spoken in this way: ‘I will give you the holy and sure blessings of David.’

Romans 1:3 concerning His Son, who was born of a descendant of David according to the flesh,

2 Timothy 2:8 Remember Jesus Christ, risen from the dead, descendant of David, according to my gospel,

The Human Brain

Had the First Man and so the First Human Brain were "Cave Man and Cave Human Brain"?

Seven Stages of the Life Journey for Man and so The Human Brain!
Written by Ramsis Ghaly

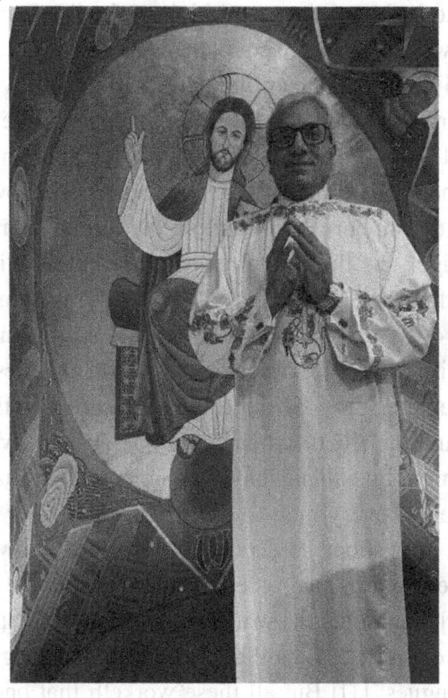

I was asked: Did the First Man and so the First Human Brain was "Cave Man and Cave Human Brain"?

The modern man and so the modern human brain is astonished of the genius and mighty ability of the first man and so the first human brain. So much historic and evolution had transpired without leaving description for who they were and how they accomplished the impossible.

This intrigued my thoughts to reflect: Did the first man and so the first human brain was so called "Cave Man and Cave Human Brain"

Indeed it is untrue and absolutely absurd to even believe for a second that God created the first man and first human brain retarded ancient and at the cave level!! In fact, it was the exact opposite! The first man and so the first human brain was in the image of God with so much superhuman nature with innumerable senses, skills, talents, dominion, intelligence —-much more than the modern man and so the modern human brain. The modern man and hence the modern human brain is trying to catch up with the Spiritual power and all supernatural nature. The cave man and cave human brain came later as you will see below!

In fact, I was able to look into deeper and joined the life journey of man and so the human brain. I was surprised to count the stages and revealed seven as seven is a perfect biblical number. In fact, the cave man and so was the cave human brain appeared later as the man and his brain managed to destroy their original nature and replaced God with evil. The wrath of God upon man and so his brain was a major factor on the deterioration of man and his brain over the generations. And in later ages, the modern brain and so the human brain is regaining the intelligence and mighty as the heaven opened the doors with Jesus salvation: John 1:51 KJV And he saith unto him, Verily, verily, I say unto you, Hereafter ye shall see heaven open, and the angels of God ascending and descending upon the Son of man." With Lord Jesus descending to earth and blessed human nature, once again connected the Spirit of God to human nature as at the times of the first man and first human brain!1 Corinthians 12:1,7-11,30-31 KJV "Now concerning spiritual gifts, brethren, I would not have you ignorant. [7] But the manifestation of the Spirit is given to every man to profit withal. [8] For to one is given by the Spirit the word of wisdom; to another the word of knowledge by the same Spirit; [9] To another faith by the same Spirit; to another the gifts of healing by the same Spirit; [10] To another the working of miracles; to another prophecy; to another discerning of spirits; to another divers kinds of tongues; to another the interpretation of tongues: [11] But all these worketh that one and the selfsame Spirit, dividing to every man severally as he will. [30] Have all the gifts of healing? do all speak with tongues? do all interpret? [31] But covet earnestly the best gifts: and yet shew I unto you a more excellent way."

The Human Brain

The human brain is the only organ that makes a man human being. It is the identity, the being, the persona and it is all specific and never be shared or transplanted. The human brain secret is in God and it shall be revealed at that day! No one has the key to a man brain but himself and God. Human brain is created unto two parts, one part is flesh and soul and the second part is spiritual not contained within the skull. In fact human brain isn't only the physical part seen within the skull but more outside the skull in the unseen spiritual world. Much of consciousness and cognition is sharing between the two parts. On the other hand, the gross function of the brain as locomotion and sensations are of the non-spiritual part. Indeed the human brain is the Godly treasure to mankind and created in His image and with endless potentials, senses, skills and talents.

It should never come to surprise that the first man and so the first human Brain 🧠 was so genius and highly nourished with multitude of superhuman nature highly connected and empowered with the Almighty Spirit!

The First Man and so the First Human Brain was Genius, Giant and Grand and Mighty! And The Resurrected Man and the Human Brain: Genius, Giant, Grand, Glorified and mighty.

Overview Stages of Man and so the Human brain during lifespan and creation Journey

Man and so is his Human Brain Life span from Newborn Immature to Mature and Aging during life journey and stages since World Creation Journey from Brilliant Most Blessed to Transition and Resurrected!

In the beginning the man and so Human brain was Brilliant, Impossible, Unconquered, Everlasting and Mighty. With the first man and so his brain sin and disobedience to His Master, deteriorated to earthly one and lost his eternity and everlasting glory. With further self-inflicted sins, the man and so his brain demoted further and further and went through four more stages where he stumbled and went down to pits he has dived for himself. In fact with Hod Mercy, man and do his brain would have demolished from earth and eradicated from the planet. Man and his brain went to grandiose that led to self-destruction. He used his own talents and brilliance to destroy himself. As it is written by those men blessed and so were their brains, from God and given special spiritual superhuman nature gifts: Lamentations 3:22-24 KJV " It is of the Lord's mercies that we are not consumed, because his compassions fail not. [23] They are new every morning: great is thy faithfulness. [24] The Lord is my portion, saith my soul; therefore will I hope in him."

Through those thousands of years man and human brain alienation from blessing and gifts, God had appointed various prophets and prophetesses. To those, the Almighty maintained His spiritual gifts and assigned the day of salivation for His coming to rescue man and she hid brain. And those died in the promise didn't let them pass away with no hope!

With the heavenly Father love and grace of Jesus His Son and Communion of the Holy Spirit, the man and do his human brain was reborn in Jesus blood and salvation. The modern blessed man and his brain reformed to man and his brain under trial on earth to be awarded accordingly at the judgment Day.

After death, the man and so his human brain shall enter to Transition temporary form spiritual in its core until the man snd the human brain be resurrected to the final everlasting glorified form at the Resurrection! At that time the glory of each be according to his deeds and faith! Those unfaithful with satanic dead are dead but alive in the brimstone lake of fire and those faithful with righteousness deeds resurrected to the glory of Christ at the Heavenly Father Kingdom!

The first man and first human brain had gone miraculous works and unimaginable build up to their culture. Unfortunately those spectacular capabilities they had were never shared with us. Perhaps, archeologists may dig deeper and deeper to search and perhaps God guide them to reveal the first man and first human brains secrets! It is certain as knowledge increase in the modern era to rediscover our roots that fingerprints thousands and perhaps millions and billions of years! It is the human journey since creation that a man and so is human brain cherishes most! Don't be surprised in your discovery searching for human roots at the early ages and you realized that they were much smarter, much capable and performed much better than the modern man and do the modern hunan brain ever imagined!!

No one but them were around at that time to get know and much left unknown to modern man but known to God as Job was told by God: Job 38:2-14,22-23,26,29,37 KJV "Where wast thou when I laid the foundations of the earth? declare, if thou hast understanding. [5] Who hath laid the measures thereof, if thou knowest? or who hath stretched the line upon it? [6] Whereupon are the foundations thereof fastened? or who laid the corner stone thereof; [7] When the morning stars sang together, and all the sons of God shouted for joy? [8] Or who shut up the sea with doors, when it brake forth, as if it had issued out of the womb? [9] When I made the cloud the garment thereof, and thick darkness a swaddlingband for it, [10] And brake up for it my decreed place, and set bars and doors, [11] And said, Hitherto shalt thou come, but no further: and here shall thy proud waves be stayed? [12] Hast thou commanded the morning since thy days; and caused the dayspring to know his place; [13] That it might take hold of the ends of the earth, that the wicked might be shaken out of it? [14] It is turned as clay to the seal; and they stand as a garment. [22] Hast thou entered into the treasures of the snow? or hast thou seen the treasures of the hail, [23] Which I have reserved against the time of trouble, against the day of battle and war? [26] To cause it to rain on the earth, where no man is; on the wilderness, wherein there is no man; [29] Out of whose womb came the ice? and the hoary frost of heaven, who hath gendered it? [37] Who can number the clouds in wisdom? or who can stay the bottles of heaven,"

Moreover, repeated natural disasters, flooding, earthquakes, Tsunamis and many others unknown such as out of space such as Sodom and Gomorrah that had done both destroyed the ancient cultures and architectures and transformed subsequent generations!! Those incredible disasters perhaps had produced indiscriminately irretrievable data from those historic generations!

The stages of man and human brain throughout thousands of years haven't been searched and examined! External appearances might be the same but functionally and internally differs! As there are changes, acclimation and modification across generations so is the man and so is the human brain develops over the years of the life span from immature newborn to mature adult and finally to aged elder!

Man and so his brain during life journey, born underdeveloped immature and go through stages of maturation and final stage before resurrection is aging and deterioration of his capabilities. On the other hand, the man and so is the human brain throughout the world journey, was born at the best shape and form genius, giant, grand and mighty and gradually self-deteriorated over thousands of years and only since Jesus salvation regaining much talents, skills, senses and capabilities.

Nonetheless, after death. the spiritual man and so his brain returns to the original sharpness but in a transition form until that time of Resurrection. At that time, the resurrected man and do his brain shall be genius, giant, grand, glorified and mighty in an immortal, incorruptible and honored form among the heavenly hosts in the Heavenly Father Kingdom. But it shall be only given to those sheep on the right hand!!

However at that time each man and do his brain shall be judged according to his deeds and works on earth while trading his talents and his profitability. And hence, the man and so his brain shall be given the rank and glory accordingly as it is explained in our Lord parable: Matthew 25:19-34 KJV "After a long time the lord of those servants cometh, and reckoneth with them. [20] And so he that had received five talents came and brought other five talents, saying, Lord, thou deliveredst unto me five talents: behold, I have gained beside them five talents more. [21] His lord said unto him, Well done, thou good and faithful servant: thou hast been faithful over a few things, I will make thee ruler over many things: enter thou into the joy of thy lord. [22] He also that had received two talents came and said, Lord, thou deliveredst unto me two talents: behold, I have gained two other talents beside them. [23] His lord said unto him, Well done, good and faithful servant; thou hast been faithful over a few things, I will make thee ruler over many things: enter thou into the joy of thy lord. [24] Then he which had received the one talent came and said, Lord, I knew thee that thou art an hard man, reaping where thou hast not sown, and gathering where thou hast not strawed: [25] And I was afraid, and went and hid thy talent in the earth: lo, there thou hast that is thine. [26] His lord answered and said unto him, Thou wicked and slothful servant, thou knewest that I reap where I sowed not, and gather where I have not strawed: [27] Thou oughtest therefore to have put my money to the exchangers, and then at my coming I should have received mine own with usury. [28] Take therefore the talent from him, and give it unto him which hath ten talents. [29] For unto every one that hath shall be given, and he shall have abundance: but from him that hath not shall be taken away even that which he hath. [30] And cast ye the unprofitable servant into outer darkness: there shall be weeping and gnashing of teeth. [31] When the Son of man shall come in his glory, and all the holy angels with him, then shall he sit upon the throne of his glory: [32] And before him shall be gathered all nations: and he shall separate them one from another, as a shepherd divideth his sheep from the goats: [33] And he shall set the sheep on his right hand, but the goats on the left. [34] Then shall the King say unto them on his right hand, Come, ye blessed of my Father, inherit the kingdom prepared for you from the foundation of the world:"

1) **The First Man and so the First Human Brain was Genius, Giant and Grand and Mighty!**

When God created the first man (Adam), He created in His image! He was an absolute genius, giant, grand and mighty The first man was huge and was ruling over the land and all creation! The first man was given so many senses, talents and capabilities! He was the man upon the entire universe and all creations! The first man was capable of doing everything and ordering other creation to do things for him. The first man was talking many languages and has authorities over the creation as it is given from God!

Genesis 1:26-30 KJV And God said, Let us make man in our image, after our likeness: and let them have dominion over the fish of the sea, and over the fowl of the air, and over the cattle, and over all the earth, and over every creeping thing that creepeth upon the earth. [27] So God created man in his own image, in the image of God created he him; male and female created he them. [28] And God blessed them, and God said unto them, Be fruitful, and multiply, and replenish the earth, and subdue it: and have dominion over the fish of the sea, and over the fowl of the air, and over every living thing that moveth upon the earth. [29] And God said, Behold, I have given you every herb bearing seed, which is upon the face of all the earth, and every tree, in the which is the fruit of a tree yielding seed; to you it shall be for meat. [30] And to every beast of the earth, and to every fowl of the air, and to every thing that creepeth upon the earth, wherein there is life, I have given every green herb for meat: and it was so.

Just imagine the Features of First Man and First Human Brain:

-Divine Image
-Divine Mighty
-Spiritual skills
-Spiritual Senses
-Divine Dominion
-Authority over the millions of creations
-Absolute direct connection to the Spirit of God
-Multiply, replenish, subdue in the air, on the land, under the land, under the seas, every beast, flowel, seas animals, grass, trees ——- all were under the first man and the first human brain —-

Man and so is the human brain has two parts one physical has the flesh and soul and the second part is the spirit. In the first man and first human brain both were interconnected directly with the Spirit of God. In other words, the first man and so is the first human brain was an absolute supernatural unlimited giant, genius and grand. Imagine how much the first man and first human brain was able to do!

First man was in the likeness of the image of God! Imaging how much talents, senses, power, abilities, skills and capabilities the first man had! The first human brain 🧠 had so much power, skills, talents and hundreds of senses, not just five or six senses! The first man had absolute authority cover the entire earth and creation.

God created the entire world and universe far before man and He created the first man and first human brain to be free totally minded in His image with unlimited capabilities. Through God, the first man and the first human brain had done the impossible and unimaginable.

2) **Second Man and Second Human Brain:**

However the first man and so is the first human brain used his supernatural gifts and freedom to disobey God His Creator! When Adam and Eve disobeyed God and was ejected out of garden of Eden, God cursed them both and both lost so much spiritual skills but both were still preserving their talents, skills and superhuman nature. God was their direct Master and working together to build life on earth with their unlimited potentials being Genius, Giant, Grand and mighty!

Genesis 3:16-19 KJV Unto the woman he said, I will greatly multiply thy sorrow and thy conception; in sorrow thou shalt bring forth children; and thy desire shall be to thy husband, and he shall rule over thee. [17] And unto Adam he said, Because thou hast hearkened unto the voice of thy wife, and hast eaten of the tree, of which I commanded thee, saying, Thou shalt not eat of it: cursed is the ground for thy sake; in sorrow shalt thou eat of it all the days of thy life; [18] Thorns also and thistles shall it bring forth to thee; and thou shalt eat the herb of the field; [19] In the sweat of thy face shalt thou eat bread, till thou return unto the ground; for out of it wast thou taken: for dust thou art, and unto dust shalt thou return.

The powerful first man and first human brain continues with their superhuman natural until before the flooding of the world during Noah time as it is written: Genesis 6:4 KJV There were giants in the earth in those days; and also after that, when the sons of God came in unto the daughters of men, and they bare children to them, the same became mighty men which were of old, men of renown.

3) **Third Man and Third Human Brain:**

With the wickedness of the second man and so the second human brain, God cursed that He created the first man and first human brain but because of His mercy He regretted. The second man and so is the second human brain was using their superhuman gifts to sin and not for good!! Nonetheless, God demoted the potentials of the first man and so the first human brain as it is written: Genesis 6:1-3,5-7 KJV And it came to pass, when men began to multiply on the face of the earth, and daughters were born unto them, [2] That the sons of God saw the daughters of men that they were fair; and they took them wives of all which they chose. [3] And the Lord said, My spirit shall not always strive with man, for that he also is flesh: yet his days shall be an hundred and twenty years. [5] And God saw that the wickedness of man was great in the earth, and that every imagination of the thoughts of his heart was only evil continually. [6] And it repented the Lord that he had made man on the earth, and it grieved him at his heart. [7] And the Lord said, I will destroy man whom I have created from the face of the earth; both man, and beast, and the creeping thing, and the fowls of the air; for it repenteth me that I have made them.

By then, the third man and so is the third human brain was less capable and live shorter, life span from 800years to 120 years, but still many of the first man and so the first human brain superhuman nature was still preserved!

4) **Fourth Man and Fourth Human Brain**

The third man and third human brain got demoted further after the tower of babel because of their grandiose. The third man and third human brain continue to use their superhuman nature to sin and try to use their power to reach high to be as God. Instead of the third man and human brain was one, one language and capable, genius, giant, grand and might, because of their sin, the fourth man and fourth human brain became disperse and fragmented as it is written: Genesis 11:1-9 KJV "And the whole earth was of one language, and of one speech. [2] And it came to pass, as they journeyed from the east, that they found a plain in the land of Shinar; and they dwelt there. [3] And they said one to another, Go to, let us make brick, and burn them throughly. And they had brick for stone, and slime had they for morter. [4] And they said, Go to, let us build us a city and a tower, whose top may reach unto heaven; and let us make us a name, lest we be scattered abroad upon the face of the whole earth. [5] And the Lord came down to see the city and the tower, which the children of men builded. [6] And the Lord said, Behold, the people is one, and they have all one language; and this they begin to do: and now nothing will be restrained from them, which they have imagined to do. [7] Go to, let us go down, and there confound their language, that they may not understand one another's speech. [8] So the Lord scattered them abroad from thence upon the face of all the earth: and they left off to build the city. [9] Therefore is the name of it called Babel; because the Lord did there confound the language of all the earth: and from thence did the Lord scatter them abroad upon the face of all the earth."

Yet, the fourth man and so was the fourth Human Brain, was genius, giant, grand and mighty but disperse, scattered with many languages and talents spread out

5) **Fifth Man and Fifth Human Brain**

The fourth man and so the fourth human brain used their talents, skills and supernatural human brain to sin and refused to have God as his King and Ruler. The fourth man and the fourth human brain with his mighty features given by God rejected Him and refused for God to reign over them as it is written: 1 Samuel 8:4-7 KJV Then all the elders of Israel gathered themselves together, and came to Samuel unto Ramah, [5] And said unto him, Behold, thou art old, and thy sons walk not in thy ways: now make us a king to judge us like all the nations. [6] But the thing displeased Samuel, when they said, Give us a king to judge us. And Samuel prayed unto the Lord. [7] And the Lord said unto Samuel, Hearken unto the voice of the people in all that they say unto thee: for they have not rejected thee, but they have rejected me, that I should not reign over them.

And despite what God and Samuel try to convince the fourth man and human brain, he was stubborn and grandiose and persistently refused God. Since tbe God maintained a distance and his multitude of unseen blessing and spiritual skills retracted from the fifth man and fifth human brain. 1 Samuel 8:8-9,11-22 KJV According to all the works which they have done since the day that I brought them up out of Egypt even unto this day, wherewith they have forsaken me, and served other gods, so do they also unto thee. [9] Now therefore hearken unto their voice: howbeit yet protest solemnly unto them, and shew them the manner of the king that shall reign over them. [11] And he said, This will be the manner of the king that shall reign over you: He will take your sons, and appoint them for himself, for his chariots, and to be his horsemen; and some shall run before his chariots. [12] And he will appoint him captains over thousands, and captains over fifties; and will set them to ear his ground, and to reap his harvest, and to make his instruments of war, and instruments of his chariots. [13] And he will take your daughters to be confectionaries, and to be cooks, and to be bakers. [14] And he will take your fields, and your vineyards, and your oliveyards, even the best of them, and give them to his servants. [15] And he will take the tenth of your seed, and of your vineyards, and give to his officers, and to his servants. [16] And he will take your menservants, and your maidservants, and your goodliest young men, and your asses, and put them to his work. [17] He will take the tenth of your sheep: and ye shall be his servants. [18] And ye shall cry out in that day because of your king which ye shall have chosen you; and the Lord will not hear you in that day. [19] Nevertheless the people refused to obey the voice of Samuel; and they said, Nay; but we will have a king over us; [20] That we also may be like all the nations; and that our king may judge us, and go out before us, and fight our battles. [21] And Samuel heard all the words of the people, and he rehearsed them in the ears of the Lord. [22] And the Lord said to Samuel, Hearken unto their voice, and make them a king. And Samuel said unto the men of Israel, Go ye every man unto his city."

The fifth man and so the fifth human brain continued to deteriorate and lost so much of his superhuman nature and lost the remnants of what was remained from the Spiritual skills. Most of that man and his brain was mostly materialistic and destructive!

The only exception was king Solomon and his human brain, God gifted him as the first man and first brain as it is written: 1 Kings 3:11-14 KJV And God said unto him, Because thou hast asked this thing, and hast not asked for thyself long life; neither hast asked riches for thyself, nor hast asked the life of thine enemies; but hast asked for thyself understanding to discern judgment; [12] Behold, I have done according to thy words: lo, I have given thee a wise and an understanding heart; so that there was none like thee before thee, neither after thee shall any arise like unto thee. [13] And I have also given thee that which thou hast not asked, both riches, and honour: so that there shall not be any among the kings like unto thee all thy days. [14] And if thou wilt walk in my ways, to keep my statutes and my commandments, as thy father David did walk, then I will lengthen thy days.

6) **The Sixth Man and Sixth Human Brain**

It is the reborn man and reborn human brain by the grace of His Son Jesus salvation. The sixth Man and Sixth Human Brain reborn by Jesus blood and became the era of grace and truth. The man and human brain regained so much dominion and spiritual power and connection again not from the flesh but directly from God and became His sons once more as it is written: "-power to become the sons of God, even to them that believe on his name: [13] Which were born, not of blood, nor of the will of the flesh, nor of the will of man, but of God"

John 1:12-13,17 KJV But as many as received him, to them gave he power to become the sons of God, even to them that believe on his name: [13] Which were born, not of blood, nor of the will of the flesh, nor of the will of man, but of God. [17] For the law was given by Moses, but grace and truth came by Jesus Christ."

The sixth man and sixth human brain is connected again via Jesus back to the Holy Spirit and capable of doing impossible as Jesus our Savior repeatedly said: Matthew 19:26 KJV

[26] But Jesus beheld them, and said unto them, With men this is impossible; but with God all things are possible.

The Holy Spirit is back again connecting to the spiritual human brain giving so many skills, talents, gifts and senses!! The human brain can now do the impossible and is given the power through binding in the True Vine and greater things he can do as it is written! John 14:12-17,26-27 KJV "Verily, verily, I say unto you, He that believeth on me, the works that I do shall he do also; and greater works than these shall he do; because I go unto my Father. [13] And whatsoever ye shall ask in my name, that will I do, that the Father may be glorified in the Son. [14] If ye shall ask any thing in my name, I will do it. [15] If ye love me, keep my commandments. [16] And I will pray the Father, and he shall give you another Comforter, that he may abide with you for ever; [17] Even the Spirit of truth; whom the world cannot receive, because it seeth him not, neither knoweth him: but ye know him; for he dwelleth with you, and shall be in you. [26] But the Comforter, which is the Holy Ghost, whom the Father will send in my name, he shall teach you all things, and bring all things to your remembrance, whatsoever I have said unto you. [27] Peace I leave with you, my peace I give unto you: not as the world giveth, give I unto you. Let not your heart be troubled, neither let it be afraid."

The sixth man and human brain knowledge increased exponentially as God opens the eyes of the modern human brain day after day until the fullness of time and the end of the world and so the end of the physical man and physical brain. In the meantime the man of God can have the mind of christ and through the Gifts of the Spirit be lifted up high as it is written:1 Corinthians 2:9-16 KJV "] But as it is written, Eye hath not seen, nor ear heard, neither have entered into the heart of man, the things which God hath prepared for them that love him. [10] But God hath revealed them unto us by his Spirit: for the Spirit searcheth all things, yea, the deep things of God. [11] For what man knoweth the things of a man, save the spirit of man which is in him? even so the things of God knoweth no man, but the

Spirit of God. [12] Now we have received, not the spirit of the world, but the spirit which is of God; that we might know the things that are freely given to us of God. [13] Which things also we speak, not in the words which man's wisdom teacheth, but which the Holy Ghost teacheth; comparing spiritual things with spiritual. [14] But the natural man receiveth not the things of the Spirit of God: for they are foolishness unto him: neither can he know them, because they are spiritually discerned. [15] But he that is spiritual judgeth all things, yet he himself is judged of no man. [16] For who hath known the mind of the Lord, that he may instruct him? But we have the mind of Christ."

7) **The Resurrected Man and The Resurrected Human Brain**

At that time, once more, the resurrected man and brain be of glorified spiritual and spectacular form. The Resurrected Man and the human brain shall be all made new stars in glory eternal and spiritual interact with God and all the heavenly hosts in His Kingdom. At that time, it shall be not only genius, giant, grand and mighty but Glorious! As it is written: 1 Corinthians 15:23,39-49,52-57 KJV [23] But every man in his own order: Christ the firstfruits; afterward they that are Christ's at his coming. [39] All flesh is not the same flesh: but there is one kind of flesh of men, another flesh of beasts, another of fishes, and another of birds. [40] There are also celestial bodies, and bodies terrestrial: but the glory of the celestial is one, and the glory of the terrestrial is another. [41] There is one glory of the sun, and another glory of the moon, and another glory of the stars: for one star differeth from another star in glory. [42] So also is the resurrection of the dead. It is sown in corruption; it is raised in incorruption: [43] It is sown in dishonour; it is raised in glory: it is sown in weakness; it is raised in power: [44] It is sown a natural body; it is raised a spiritual body. There is a natural body, and there is a spiritual body. [45] And so it is written, The first man Adam was made a living soul; the last Adam was made a quickening spirit. [46] Howbeit that was not first which is spiritual, but that which is natural; and afterward that which is spiritual. [47] The first man is of the earth, earthy: the second man is the Lord from heaven. [48] As is the earthy, such are they also that are earthy: and as is the heavenly, such are they also that are heavenly. [49] And as we have borne the image of the earthy, we shall also bear the image of the heavenly. [52] In a moment, in the twinkling of an eye, at the last trump: for the trumpet shall sound, and the dead shall be raised incorruptible, and we shall be changed. [53] For this corruptible must put on incorruption, and this mortal must put on immortality. [54] So when this corruptible shall have put on incorruption, and this mortal shall have put on immortality, then shall be brought to pass the saying that is written, Death is swallowed up in victory. [55] O death, where is thy sting? O grave, where is thy victory? [56] The sting of death is sin; and the strength of sin is the law. [57] But thanks be to God, which giveth us the victory through our Lord Jesus Christ.

The first man and so was the human brain:
Genius
Giant
Grand
Mighty

The Resurrected Man and the Human Brain:
Genius
Giant
Grand
Glorified
Mighty

Eternal
Immortal
Honored
Uncorrupted

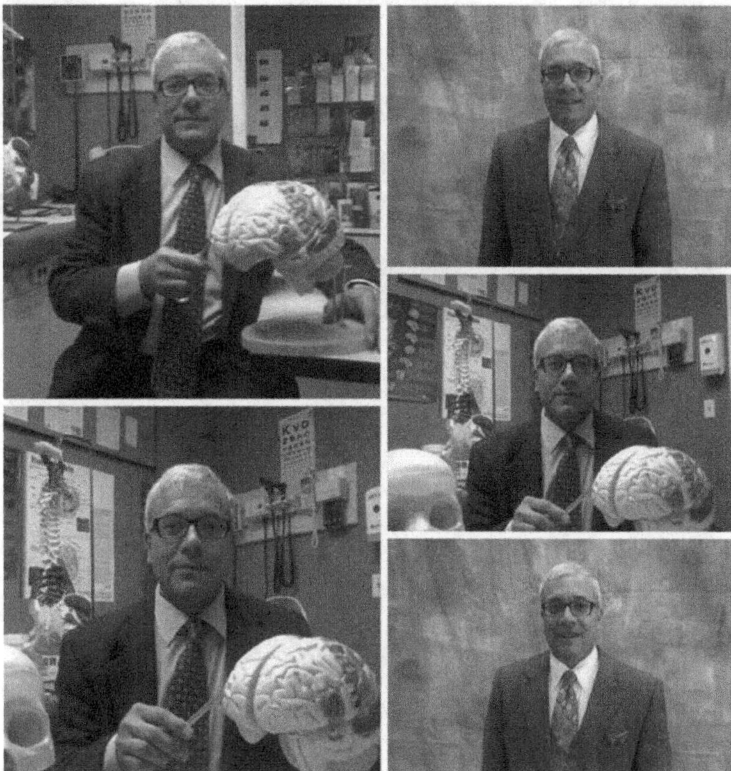

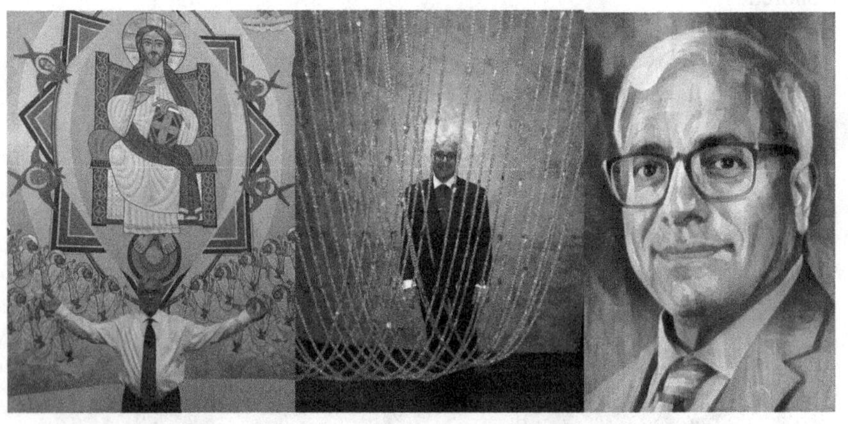

Does the Extracted Tooth Has a mind and emotion Within??

Written by Ramsis Ghaly

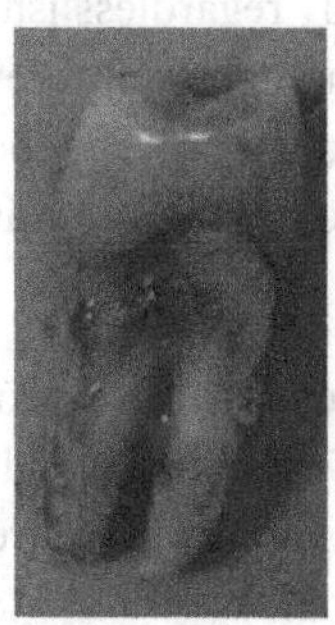

It wasn't just a tooth but part of my soul. I thought initially it was just a tooth but later I realized it was part of my soul!

They pulled my tooth and I didn't mind at all!

It was broken anyway! I really didn't care and I said! "It is just a tooth "!

The dentist and the staff were spectacular! You we I'll think next day, I would totally forget about the pulled tooth ! But it is the opposite, I felt something went out of my body and it is causing me to shiver!

It isn't pain but the emotions associated with pulling the tooth out! The tooth was deeply rooted to my jaw bone through two limbs firmly bound!

The tooth was cracked but the force to pull out was huge! I asked to look at it and I did! I thought naively that that image won't last around!!!

Within less an hour, all was done and went away in my way! I didn't think much about the entire experience!

I was so impressed of how painless the procedure and how kind and touched were the dentist and the staff! I was treated absolutely phenomenal!

In 6 months, I will receive an implant instead of that pulled tooth ! Until then, the spot of my pulled tooth is empty, lonely and packed with a sponge!

However, I still think about the pulled tooth and it's image that doesn't want to leave my mind! So I thought to write a post in my Facebook wall in the memory of my tooth extraction!

I asked myself: "What is big deal, put an artificial tooth and as if nothing had happened". It wasn't that simple and my own tooth nothing could replace that valuable part of me!!

I thought it is simple and should be forgotten but even little thing as pulling a tooth out of your body even if it is one tooth out of 32, it is still huge deal!!

Pulling something out of the body regardless isn't without feeling some loss! As if the tooth has a soul within and departed forever my living soul!! It was part of my flesh and forever gone and buried! The tooth has no mind and perhaps no feeling!! But to my thoughts, the tooth has a miniature mind and deep inside it has to be an emotion circuit!

I realized that tooth has been attached to the nervous system, the heart and vessels, and the jaw bone and was part of every bite and drink fir all these years. Not only attached to the jaw but receiving living blood stream, nerve signals and nutrition from the body and 24/7 protection!!

I was in a state of local and general aches and sadness feeling of some loss and be reminded of an empty space within my jaw. Replacing a genuine value with artificial despite how good it is, it isn't the same! The loss even it was trivial piece of the original human body, is irrecoverable and accompanied by sadness and feeling down!

I wonder if that is the reason some teeth are named wisdom tooth and other names 32 teeth, out of which 4 are wisdom teeth. Keeping the third molars away, adults have 28 teeth.

I thought this event is trivial and not as important! I feel stupid write this post since after all not s brain surgery!! However I look at social media and hear the news and I found much more stupid things that many won't even write or say!

Indeed I am reminded that my body is one and has many members yet they all are one! There are many members, yet but one body and each regardless is honorable, valuable and precious!! Indeed, "God hath tempered the body together, having given more abundant honor to that part which lacked: That there should be no schism in the body; but that the members should have the same care one for another."

So what I have learned, a tooth is essential part of the body "And whether one member suffer, all the members suffer with it; or one member be honored, all the members rejoice with it"

"For as the body is one, and hath many members, and all the members of that one body, being many, are one body: so also is Christ. [14] For the body is not one member, but many. [15] If the foot shall say, Because I am not the hand, I am not of the body; is it therefore not of the body? [16] And if the ear shall say, Because I am not the eye, I am not of the body; is it therefore not of the body? [17] If the whole body were an eye, where were the hearing? If the whole were hearing, where were the smelling? [18] But now hath God set the members every one of them in the body, as it hath pleased him. [19] And if they were all one member, where were the body? [20] But now are they many members, yet but one body. [21] And the eye cannot say unto the hand, I have no need of thee: nor again the head to the feet, I have no need of you. [22] Nay, much more those members of the body, which seem to be more feeble, are necessary: [23] And those members of the body, which we think to be less honourable, upon these we bestow more abundant honour; and our uncomely parts have more abundant comeliness. [24] For our comely parts have no need: but God hath tempered the body together, having given more abundant honour to that part which lacked: [25] That there should be no schism in the body; but that the members should have the same care one for another. [26] And whether one member suffer, all the members suffer with it; or one member be honoured, all the members rejoice with it. [27] Now ye are the body of Christ, and members in particular. [28] And God hath set some in the church, first apostles, secondarily prophets, thirdly teachers, after that miracles, then gifts of healings, helps, governments, diversities of tongues." 1 Corinthians 12:12,14-28 KJV

"Be strong and let your heart take courage, all you who hope in the Lord."

Psalm 31:24

I do believe that tooth was attached to the entire body and remove any part even distant is still essential part of the entire body and important!! It comes with some sadness and mourning and deserve some reflection and comfort!!!

So if you are a reader of my post and wish to comment, please do so at this time!!! Otherwise please keep your teeth healthy and care for them! They are yours and you don't want to loose any even one!! Even the tooth is part of my mind, body, soul and flesh!!!

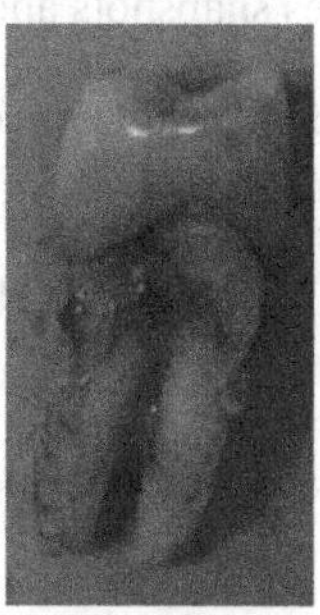

It Is A Night To Explore My Mind!!

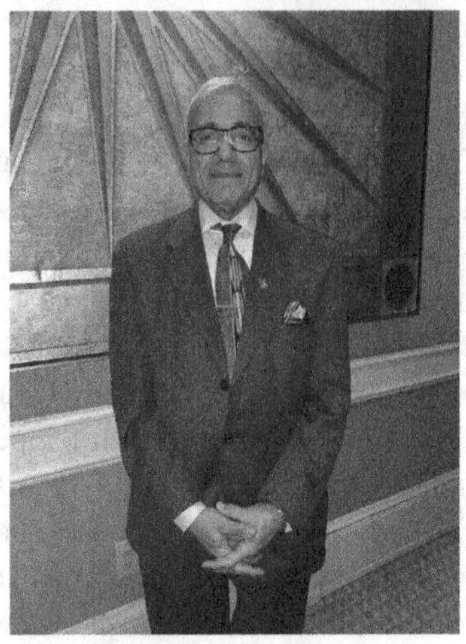

The topic with my mind what it takes for my mind to let it go and just take a break?? So, I took myself wandering in the streets of major city taking selfie to get my mind attention! But all failed!!

Taking my mind away yet it won't do it!!

A photo snapshot with a smile but mind still doesn't let it go!

Change sceneries was only good for a few and my mind still in its own thought!

Conversing with others but my mind doesn't communicate in the same wavelength, and it ends by aggravation if not departure!!

If the matter is deep and worthy attention, my mind gets drifted for a few, once grasp the idea, its interest is shut and gone, and my mind went back to its own!

In fact, it didn't take me much to find out my mind constantly screening not just internally but externally and takes snapshots and screen shots 24/7!

I followed those screenshots and snapshots once they were analyses, they were sent to the storage data filed accordingly!

I kept talking to mind rationalizing and each step forward many followed backwards!

But to tell you the truth, I personally didn't wish to stop my mind! My mind does what supposed to do!

I understand we are living in a dangerous world and my demand is high as my expectations of my mind are unlimited!

My mind indeed is my internal unceasing engine highly intellect, full of life and it is my own identity!

What I realized is that my mind has its own mind full of thoughts, fantasies and fictions originated from within!

To my surprise, my mind took me for a tour within my mind! I put on the highly illuminated telescope and followed my mind in silence!!!

The thoughts, fantasies and fictions became visible to me, and I was asked to follow them. All those interact at different levels and refined in the copper mills at the initial stage! Next phase those are transformed to red hot steel as glow white cleared and scrutinized! At the final stages, those by now transformed to Incandescence and passed through innumerable scenarios before they get stalked and imprinted!!!

The journey was so brief I felt absorbed as if out of space and had no word output!

Now I understand why my mind does take break or let it go and it's guards always in high alert as nothing pass my mind!

My mind asked me for privacy and to leave it alone to be in its own undisturbed, uninterrupted, unintimidated, unrestrained and unlimited, intuitive and free!!!

Perhaps another day and time I might be able to sit in one table with my mind at those wavelengths and capture my mind attention even for just a little!!!

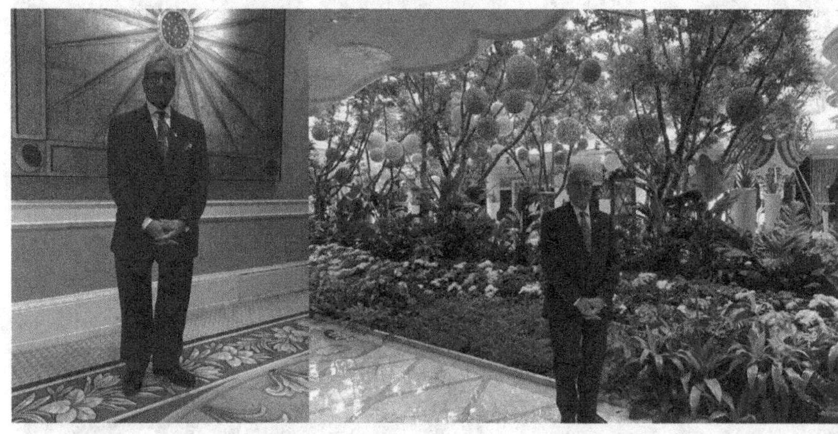

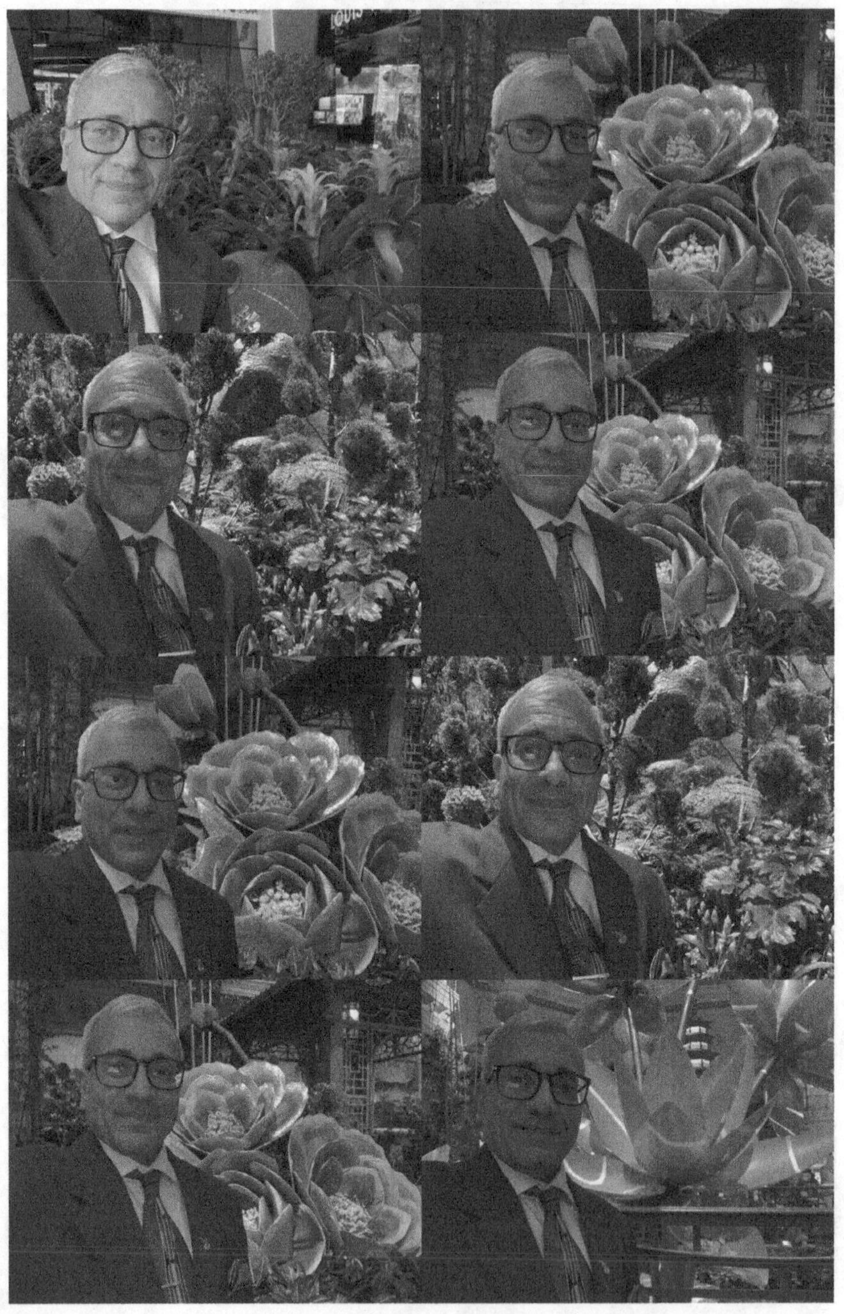

Modern Technology Constraint to Human Brain Growth!

Written by Ramsis Ghaly

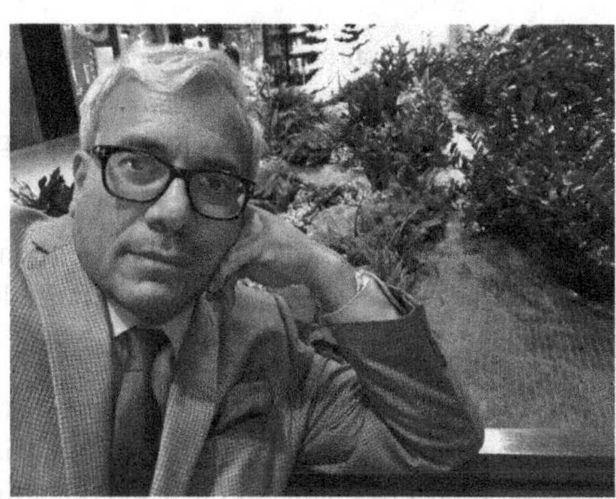

The human brain product of the new has limited ability to retain knowledge and depends on external data storage! The human brain product of the following futuristic generation will have, in addition, limited self-processing and problem-solving!

At that time, human brains will be fully dependent on artificial intelligence and can't function in themselves but instead they will be totally enslaved by technology!

On other words, modern technology is forcing its way to be smarter and smarter while pushing human brains to be more and more limited and unchallenged hindering their growth and development suppressing the unlimited inherited human brain potentials!!!

The Modern Human Brain is declining as those brains of the new generation have Limited Retention of knowledge induced by dependence on technology and data informatics since 5G and other unlimited data storage and search engines are becoming more and more the main resource to retain the knowledge!!

Modern technology enabling artificial intelligence and disabling Human brain development!

The newer and newer human brains are becoming more and more empty shells since they aren't challenged enough during the early growth period and thereafter!

The human nervous system develops through training, grows through challenging, matures through laboring, nurtures through trials and errors and shines through autonomy!!

In the decades to come, human brain won't be trained to information processing, problem solving, thinking, trouble shooting, critical thinking and creativity as artificial intelligence is being trained to do these functions instead!

Year after year as modernization continues to transfer human brain function to robots, the human brains find themselves totally restrained and fully dependent on artificial intelligence and informatics and external data storage!

Years and years shall pass as the human brains will lose more and more of its own executive functions and hands on skills and autonomy. Human brain slowly is being transformed from a giant master and independent leader to a follower of robots!!!

Imaging that the future human brain will be as a mindless machine does what the computer tell that brain to do!! Each day the human brain will be given APP updates to download and orders to follow. In the same time, the brain has the artificial intelligence data analysis and orders!

A magnificent human brain created in our Lord image with autonomy creativity and unlimited potentials will transgress to in brains captives, restrained and disabled!!!

It is a wakeup call to the world as its people are setting the foundation of the futuristic product of human brains!!

JN, Thank you. Makes a person really think.

CG, So what your saying is that technology use can create structural changes in the brain? That is very interesting and alarming.

JK, Very interesting...

For sure, we don't want to turn to robots.

How a Human Mind Conspire Against God and His Christ? How Human Mind Transform to Play God Instead of Being a Child of God!

Written by Ramsis Ghaly

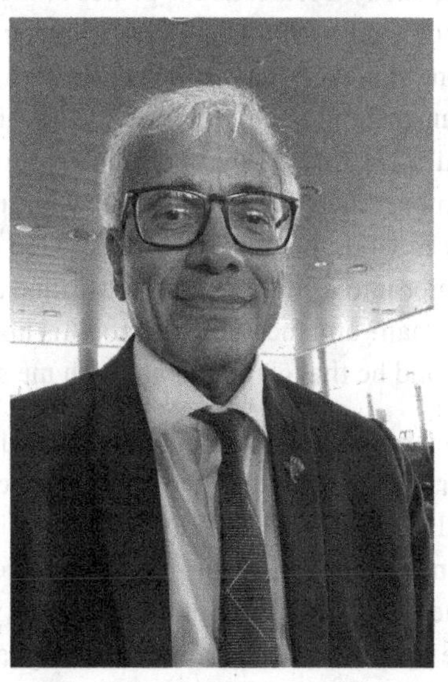

I asked myself may my Lord open my mind to show me what is actually behind the scene where Satan trick the human brain mind that one day since the beginning human brain was created in His Image and likeness and was blessed from the mouth of God the Creator?? As it is written: Genesis 1:26-28 KJV "And God said, Let us make man in our image, after our likeness: and let them have dominion over the fish of the sea, and over the fowl of the air, and over the cattle, and over all the earth, and over every creeping thing that creepeth upon the earth. [27] So God created man in his own image, in the image of God created he him; male and female created he them. [28] And God blessed them, and God said unto them, Be fruitful, and multiply, and replenish the earth, and subdue it: and have dominion over the fish of the sea, and over the fowl of the air, and over every living thing that moveth upon the earth."

Indeed, I saw a huge spiritual war by the spiritual powers hidden from the eyes and ears and various senses of human, unseen by the naked eyes ongoing between the righteous spirits and satanic wicked spirits!! As it is written: Ephesians 6:12 KJV "For we wrestle not against flesh and blood, but against principalities, against powers, against the rulers of the darkness of this world, against spiritual wickedness in high places."

Those deceived human brains initially captured by Satan, then gradually held hostage by Beelzebub, get darker and darker, polluted and rotten, self-damage until get suffocated by Satan and get dumped unto hell!!

Matthew 12:24-30 KJV "But when the Pharisees heard it, they said, This fellow doth not cast out devils, but by Beelzebub the prince of the devils. [25] And Jesus knew their thoughts, and said unto them, Every kingdom divided against itself is brought to desolation; and every city or house divided against itself shall not stand: [26] And if Satan cast out Satan, he is divided against himself; how shall then his kingdom stand? [27] And if I by Beelzebub cast out devils, by whom do your children cast them out? therefore they shall be your judges. [28] But if I cast out devils by the Spirit of God, then the kingdom of God is come unto you. [29] Or else how can one enter into a strong man's house, and spoil his goods, except he first bind the strong man? and then he will spoil his house. [30] He that is not with me is against me; and he that gathereth not with me scattereth abroad."

Those victimized human brains aren't armored with the whole armor of God with lions girt about with truth, the breastplate of righteousness, the shield of faith, helmet of salvation and the sword of the Holy Spirit!! As it is written: Ephesians 6:11,13-18 KJV "Put on the whole armour of God, that ye may be able to stand against the wiles of the devil. [13] Wherefore take unto you the whole armour of God, that ye may be able to withstand in the evil day, and having done all, to stand. [14] Stand therefore, having your loins girt about with truth, and having on the breastplate of righteousness; [15] And your feet shod with the preparation of the gospel of peace; [16] Above all, taking the shield of faith, wherewith ye shall be able to quench all the fiery darts of the wicked. [17] And take the helmet of salvation, and the sword of the Spirit, which is the word of God: [18] Praying always with all prayer and supplication in the Spirit, and watching thereunto with all perseverance and supplication for all saints;"

As the human mind drifts away from His True Source and Creator, the human brain stumbles and gets confused of his identity! That human brain first thing shuts the source of True Light, the living bread and the fountain of spring waters, the Holy Spirit! Slowly the human brain becomes malnourished from the lack of true healthy spiritual food and dry from no more living waters!

While the Heaven gets sadden by losing a child of God and being deceived by Satan, that individual becomes a host of demons as they laugh and exalt for pulling that human brain away from God the True Vine and the source of its spiritual nourishment! At the same time, darkness finds that lost mind and enters his brain and lives within. The wicked ones spoil the good human apples the treasures human brains!! For Satan that human mind is an easy target to confuse it even more and drift that ship far away from the shore.

Satan and that Human brain become tight as a very good match to fulfill Satan purpose and becomes anti-God and anti-christ full of false pride and grandiose atheist believe in himself that he is the prince of the word and god and moreover, capable of taking the Most Holy Lord and God, down and to defeat Him as in his mind a so called "God and His Commandants"!

Satan is one of the intelligent malicious manipulative creations and his bread if human souls. As it is written about that serpent: "Now the serpent was more subtil than any beast of the field which the Lord God had made."

He never gives up and keep changing his tactics according to the ongoing adversaries, disputes, advancements, and technology. Satan is creative and uses his intelligence to create new tricks to trap those vulnerable human minds! Satan targets are always Adam and Eve descendants and as he was able to trick them in a mind to mind conversation and false ideology, and so Satan is doing the same again. But instead, Satan is using the new technology and modern science and research to his favor! Satan is a master to put doubts in human minds and provides convincing false evidences to address the captured worldly human minds!!

Genesis 3:1-7 KJV "Now the serpent was more subtil than any beast of the field which the Lord God had made. And he said unto the woman, Yea, hath God said, Ye shall not eat of every tree of the garden? [2] And the woman said unto the serpent, We may eat of the fruit of the trees of the garden: [3] But of the fruit of the tree which is in the midst of the garden, God hath said, Ye shall not eat of it, neither shall ye touch it, lest ye die. [4] And the serpent said unto the woman, Ye shall not surely die: [5] For God doth know that in the day ye eat thereof, then your eyes shall be opened, and ye shall be as gods, knowing good and evil. [6] And when the woman saw that the tree was good for food, and that it was pleasant to the eyes, and a tree to be desired to make one wise, she took of the fruit thereof, and did eat, and gave also unto her husband with her; and he did eat. [7] And the eyes of them both were opened, and they knew that they were naked; and they sewed fig leaves together, and made themselves aprons."

Slowly-slowly, Satan infiltrates in that easy vessel taking that human brain to more and more self-destruction ways misleading him playing with his empty brain and fill it with convincing timely inspirational ideas that far from the truth and goodness throwing that soul to the lake of destruction attracting more and more of his own peers!

Now that evil human mind is held hostage to Satan and his demons joyful as they entangle that human mind unto doctrine and projects full of lies and fake promises until self-destruction and life lost in the hands of demons!! To that deceived mind acts as a laboratory to Satan believing he is going up to heaven, yet the truth is going down to hill!! The deceived human brains line up in the army of Satan filling the world with inequity and the ground they step on becomes adulterous dragging other human brains with!! Every night satan counts his gain and causalities and create more tedious experiments and misleading discovering to enhance their fake lordship and dominion over the world!

Gradually the satan the wicked leads the human brain to loss of hope and too late to go back and redeem thyself! The victimized human brain obsessed with darkness and Satan tricks and influence sees no way to salvation and rescue his soul. That human brain loses his purpose in life got distracted completely from the True Light and Joy, has no true peace within realizes the truth and the defeat by darkness! But at that time, that dark brain loses hope, trapped and advanced in evil doing. Satan is already mastering that falling human brain and leads him to the final step on earth which is self-destruction and ultimate death ! At that time, satan takes that human soul to his dungeon and God never send His angels to pick Him up because he denied Jesus Christ and lost the salvation through Jesus Bloodshed at the Cross because he didn't believe in Jesus the Lord!

And satan shall continue to capture as many human brains and minds attracting them to false ideology and Anti godly thoughts and deeds targeting their current interests and lusts far away from the Savior of the World Jesus the Lord! Then satan, the wicked gradually enslave them unto his hands doing evils and convince them to be antiGod and His Christ. Many get scammed and fall in satan mouth with sharp teeth and hungry belly and become his food and his tools for further destruction as satan use them to ignite the world and its people leading them away from the pass to salvation!!! And the end is predictable as it is written at the Judgment Day: Revelation 20:7-15 KJV "And when the thousand years are expired, Satan shall be loosed out of his prison, [8] And shall go out to deceive the nations which are in the four quarters of the earth, Gog and Magog, to gather them together to battle: the number of whom is as the sand of the sea. [9] And they went up on the breadth of the earth, and compassed the camp of the saints about, and the beloved city: and fire came down from God out of heaven, and devoured them. [10] And the devil that deceived them was cast into the lake of fire and brimstone, where the beast and the false prophet are, and shall be tormented day and night for ever and ever. [11] And I saw a great white throne, and him that sat on it, from whose face the earth and the heaven fled away; and there was found no place for them. [12] And I saw the dead, small and great, stand before God; and the books were opened: and another book was opened, which is the book of life: and the dead were judged out of those things which were written in the books, according to their works. [13] And the sea gave up the dead which were in it; and death and hell delivered up the dead which were in them: and they were judged every man according to their works. [14] And death and hell were cast into the lake of fire. This is the second death. [15] And whosoever was not found written in the book of life was cast into the lake of fire."

The same tricks Satan commit in the first days of Adam and Eve to become as God, he himself fell far before that time in his trial and so shall he be dressed as AntiChrist through another deceived human brain before the end of days! In fact, antichrist when he comes, he fools the people of being god himself as Satan himself fell from heaven when he played god and want to high as God

Call of Satan before man creation as follows: Isaiah 14:12-23 KJV "How art thou fallen from heaven, O Lucifer, son of the morning! how art thou cut down to the ground, which didst weaken the nations! [13] For thou hast said in thine heart, I will ascend into heaven, I will exalt my throne above the stars of God: I will sit also upon the mount of the congregation, in the sides of the north: [14] I will ascend above the heights of the clouds; I will be like the most High. [15] Yet thou shalt be brought down to hell, to the sides of the pit. [16] They that see thee shall narrowly look upon thee, and consider thee, saying, Is this the man that made the earth to tremble, that did shake kingdoms; [17] That made the world as a wilderness, and destroyed the cities thereof; that opened not the house of his prisoners? [18] All the kings of the nations, even all of them, lie in glory, every one in his own house. [19] But thou art cast out of thy grave like an abominable branch, and as the raiment of those that are slain, thrust through with a sword, that go down to the stones of the pit; as a carcase trodden under feet. [20] Thou shalt not be joined with them in burial, because thou hast destroyed thy land, and slain thy people: the seed of evildoers shall never be renowned. [21] Prepare slaughter for his children for the iniquity of their fathers; that they do not rise, nor possess the land, nor fill the face of the world with cities. [22] For I will rise up against them, saith the Lord of hosts, and cut off from Babylon the name, and remnant, and son, and nephew, saith the Lord. [23] I will also make it a possession for the bittern, and pools of water: and I will sweep it with the besom of destruction, saith the Lord of hosts."

St Paul said about Antichrist's and these coming days: 2 Thessalonians 2:3-4,7-12 KJV "Let no man deceive you by any means: for that day shall not come, except there come a falling away first, and that man of sin be revealed, the son of perdition; [4] Who opposeth and exalteth himself above all that is called God, or that is worshipped; so that he as God sitteth in the temple of God, shewing himself that he is God. [7] For the mystery of iniquity doth already work: only he who now letteth will let, until he be taken out of the way. [8] And then shall that Wicked be revealed, whom the Lord shall consume with the spirit of his mouth, and shall destroy with the brightness of his coming: [9] Even him, whose coming is after the working of Satan with all power and signs and lying wonders, [10] And with all deceivableness of unrighteousness in them that perish; because they received not the love of the truth, that they might be saved. [11] And for this cause God shall send them strong delusion, that they should believe a lie: [12] That they all might be damned who believed not the truth, but had pleasure in unrighteousness."

St John wrote: 1 John 4:1-6 KJV "Beloved, believe not every spirit, but try the spirits whether they are of God: because many false prophets are gone out into the world. [2] Hereby know ye the Spirit of God: Every spirit that confesseth that Jesus Christ is come in the flesh is of God: [3] And every spirit that confesseth not that Jesus Christ is come in the flesh is not of God: and this is that spirit of antichrist, whereof ye have heard that it should come; and even now already is it in the world. [4] Ye are of God, little children, and have overcome them: because greater is he that is in you, than he that is in the world. [5] They are of the world: therefore speak they of the world, and the world heareth them. [6] We are of God: he that knoweth God heareth us; he that is not of God heareth not us. Hereby know we the spirit of truth, and the spirit of error."

Revelation 13:1-18 - And I stood upon the sand of the sea, and saw a beast rise up out of the sea, having seven heads and ten horns, and upon his horns ten crowns, and upon his heads the name of blasphemy. (Read More...)

2 John 1:7 - For many deceivers are entered into the world, who confess not that Jesus Christ is come in the flesh. This is a deceiver and an antichrist.

PR, Good weekend Ramsis, so grateful for all you do.

KB, Look good Doctor Ramis.

AC, Nice to see Your beautiful smile Dear Ramsis I wish You Happy Sunday

SA, God Bless you!

CG, Doubt put in our minds is important because it helps us face and overcome our fears,challenge our religious beliefs,

ask new questions and search for new answers. It gets us thinking again.

JB, Jesus so good to us, I love him with all my heart and soul. I love him so much doctor, he gives us everything and when we go home to paradise he has his arms waiting for us he has his arms open really big so he can give us big hug when he sees us doctor

TJ, Wow! Great insight. Thank you for sharing God's word and wisdom.

MH, You have an awesome mind and a way with words. Have a bless day.

MH, Love the rose pin.

LA, Dr. **Ramsis Ghaly** has written several books:

A Christian from Egypt: Life Story of a Neurosurgeon Pursuing the Dreams for Quintuple Certifications…

See more

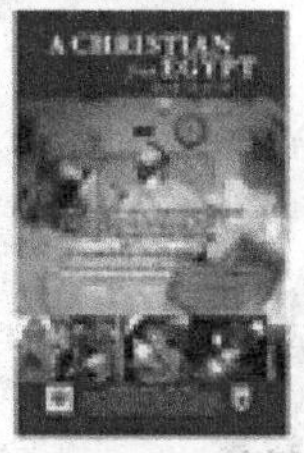

AMAZON.COM

A Christian from Egypt: Life Story of a Neurosurgeon Pursuing the Dreams for Quintuple Certifications

A Christian from Egypt: Life Story of a Neurosurgeon Pursuing the Dreams for Quintuple Certifications

https://www.facebook.com/rfghaly/posts/pfbid02UDrWD45Ga7bqApLfP2L13EbcMTyGQBjm5u5GobwRVg1oRRhCHkQ9yKTSLbRtY4jLl

https://www.facebook.com/lindas.pugs.1/posts/pfbid02Au7zQWWha2pkLLHhRdfFfFwCe6zJiXqzyxvka5dcttKiXwoEwENmMUxPbLuN66Nul

https://www.facebook.com/lindas.pugs.1/posts/pfbid0SZXruzaQrwwY83r8aXNLFdtLuYsaejunsigoGUC8o6Rbgrq98na2A9xQhoqCHDoel

https://www.facebook.com/lindas.pugs.1/posts/pfbid0289nSL3zcvNousSrpAEqzqengCGttNVHxf7bYjmdTw8cLBP3RezUqbWCu7p6tTaaHl

Have you ever thought how life would be if there was no death?

Philosophical View Written by <u>Ramsis Ghaly</u>

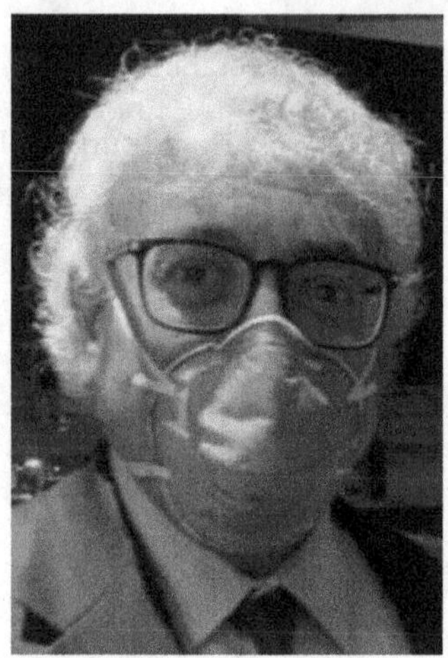

Have you ever thought how life would be if there was no death and out lived the great grandchildren and you have lost your youth, beauty and texture!

Have you ever thought how life would be if there was no death and out lived the great grandchildren and you live long enough to reap what you sow bad before good!

Have you ever thought how life would be if there was no death and out lived the great grandchildren and you live king enough to see the truth of what actually have transpired decades ago and were hidden from you!

Have you ever thought how life would be if there was no death and out lived the great grandchildren and all the eyes look at you as an obsolete old fashion outdated great grand Papa or great grand mama??

Have you ever thought how life would be if there was no death and out lived the great grandchildren and you find yourself completely lost your independence, crippled and living at nursing home looking at the walls and can't feed yourself and have no toilet control!

Have you ever thought how life would be if there was no death and out lived the great grandchildren and you realize that you are burden to your children and grandchildren and the society!!

Have you ever thought how life would be if there was no death and out lived the great grandchildren and you attracted so much illness, having no more immunity and your bag is a portable pharmacy!

Have you ever thought how life would be if there was no death and you live longer than your great grandchildren and you find thyself rejected by the modern generations and viewed retarded and not needed!

Have you ever thought how life would be if there was no death and out lived the great grandchildren and they look at you as an old aged feeble man or a woman needed 24/7 help!

Have you ever thought how life would be if there was no death and you live longer than your great grandchildren and you witness that your own waiting for your death to take over your wealth that you worked so hard all your life with sleepless nights and sweats!

Have you ever thought how life would be if there was no death and you live longer than your great grandchildren and your students and neighbors look at you are saying: "When he is going to die and why he is still living!"

Have you ever thought how life would be if there was no death and you live longer than your great grandchildren and your own country view you as the reason to bankrupt Medicare and bring economy down by all the bills spent on you with no production!

Have you ever thought how life would be if there was no death and you live longer than your great grandchildren and you discovered all your skills, expertise and knowledge are no far behind the times prehistoric and medieval with no need to it!

Have you ever thought how life would be if there was no death and you live longer than your great grandchildren and you have lost your mind and intellectuality and can no longer able to learn or read or see or hear or drive or fly or hike or walk??

Have you ever thought how life would be if there was no death and you live longer than your great great children and you get to know the facts of life and the truth if the world and nothing to be gained or enjoyed in materialism!!

"Vanity of vanities, saith the Preacher, vanity of vanities; all is vanity. [3] What profit hath a man of all his labour which he taketh under the sun? [4] One generation passeth away, and another generation cometh: but the earth abideth for ever. [5] The sun also ariseth, and the sun goeth down, and hasteth to his place where he arose. [6] The wind goeth toward the south, and turneth about unto the north; it whirleth about continually, and the wind returneth again according to his circuits. [7] All the rivers run into the sea; yet the sea is not full; unto the place from whence the rivers come, thither they return again. [8] All things are full of labour; man cannot utter it : the eye is not satisfied with seeing, nor the ear filled with hearing. [9] The thing that hath been, it is that which shall be; and that which is done is that which shall be done: and there is no new thing under the sun. [10] Is there any thing whereof it may be said, See, this is new? it hath been already of old time, which was before us. [11] There is no remembrance of former things ; neither shall there be any remembrance of things that are to come with those that shall come after. [12] I the Preacher was king over Israel in Jerusalem. [13] And I gave my heart to seek and search out by wisdom concerning all things that are done under heaven: this sore travail hath God given to the sons of man to be exercised therewith. [14] I have seen all the works that are done under the sun; and, behold, all is vanity and vexation of spirit. [15] That which is crooked cannot be made straight: and that which is wanting cannot be numbered. [16] I communed with mine own heart, saying, Lo, I am come to great estate, and have gotten more wisdom than all they that have been before me in Jerusalem: yea, my heart had great experience of wisdom and knowledge. [17] And I gave my heart to know wisdom, and to know madness and folly: I perceived that this also is vexation of spirit. [18] For in much wisdom is much grief: and he that increaseth knowledge increaseth sorrow." Ecclesiastes 1

CG, If there was no death life would have no meaning. We need death .It encourages us to seek meaning in our life. Besides we get to see the kingdom of our Lord after death.

DM, If there is no death a lot of people will receive miraculous healing from you through Jedus Christ.you are the greatest gift to humanity.

MH, You have an amazing mind.

MS, Good reading this! Thank you.

Cg, If there was no death life would have no meaning. We need death .It encourages us to seek meaning in our life. Besides we get to see the kingdom of our Lord after death.

Human Brain Health!

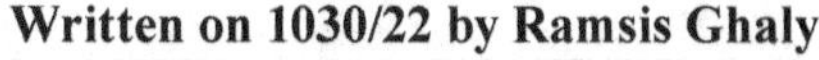

Written on 1030/22 by Ramsis Ghaly

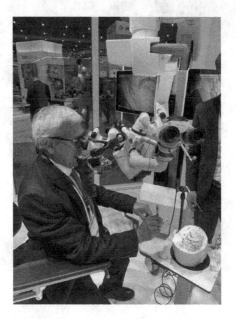

Human Brain Health in Neuroscience has been my passion for the last Forty Years and only now at the twenty One century where it becomes the Premier Hot Topic that continue challenging the Neuroscientists Worldwide at the modern times! With all the funds poured unto Brain Health, science still scramble!!

Brain Health is the core of human wellbeing and was extremely challenging to be addressed in thousands of years. The science almost mastered various organs of human anatomy but not the human brain. Understanding Human Brain remains in the infantile stage and only recently that has been acknowledged as the future for medicine and scientists.

Recently human brain health is getting much of public and global attention. Perhaps, the reason is the gravity and the impact of brain dysfunction and the huge burden on the patient, family and society. Furthermore, despite advancement in science and artificial intelligence technology, yet patients with neurocognitive dysfunctions are irreparable despite living with healthy other organs .

It does address not only the gross functions such as locomotion and sensations but also the Neuro-cognitive functions including intellect, memory, processing &

execution. And the primary focus is prevention and management of various gross and neuro-cognitive disorders such as Aging Brain, Memory lapse, Delirium, Stroke, Dementia and perioperative Neuro-Cognitive dysfunctions.

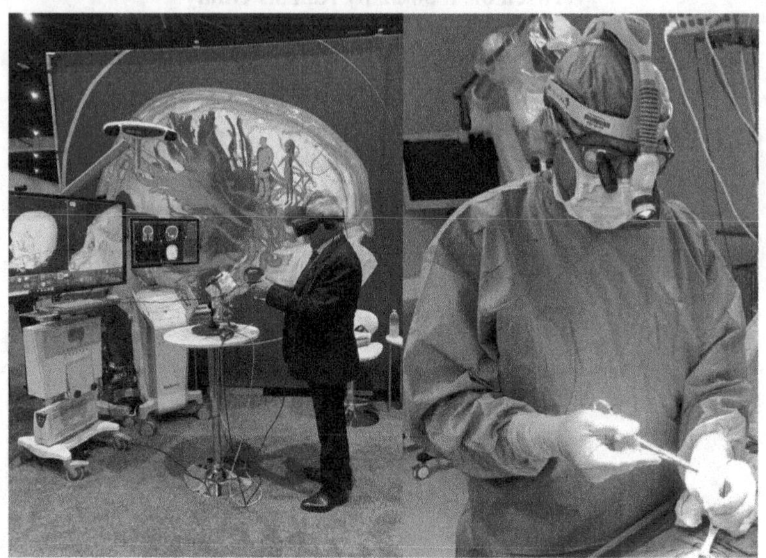

Marijuana is UNHEALTHY for Pregnant Mothers and their Baby Brains and Patients Scheduled for Surgery!

Ramsis Ghaly

Liberal use and abuse is in the rise including age of 18-25years old!! And more synthetics stronger K2 in 1.1 million!

New stats indicate Cannabis is most common illicit drug in America: 50 million Anerican consuming yearly and in the rise, 1/10 becomes addicted, Marijuana use disorder affects 15 million Americans,

New updates from the American society of anesthesiology meeting 2022 indicates

Mothers consuming medical or street Cannabinoids, spices and Marijuana are endanger themselves. Marijuana is bad for the mothers and the consumed Marijuana go to the babies and affect the brain development.

Marijuana slso bad for patients scheduled for surgery!

I attached some slides

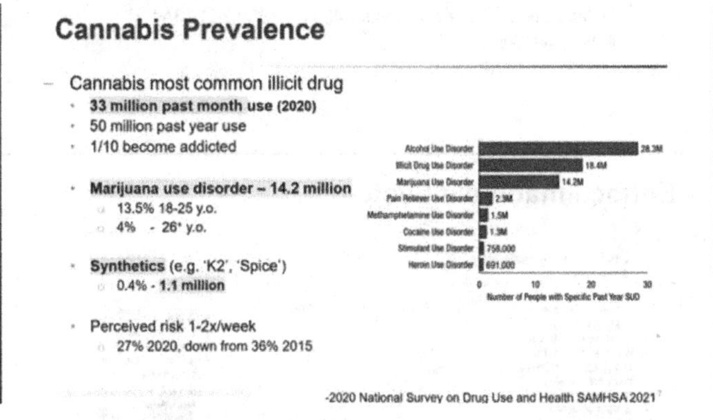

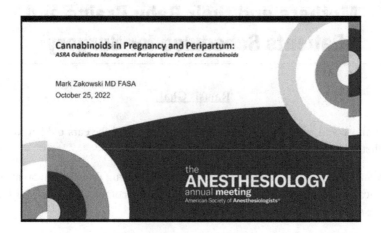

Cannabinoid Pharmacology: THC

- THC (Δ9-tetrahydrocannabinol)
  - **CB1R agonist, high affinity**
  - CB2R agonist
  - TRPV (transient receptor potential cation channel subfamily V) 1, 2
    - TRPV1 – **pain/temperature perception**
  - 5-HT_2
  - Metabolized by liver cytochrome P450 CYP2C9,2C19,3A4
  - Active metabolite 11-OH-THC

Endocannabinoid System

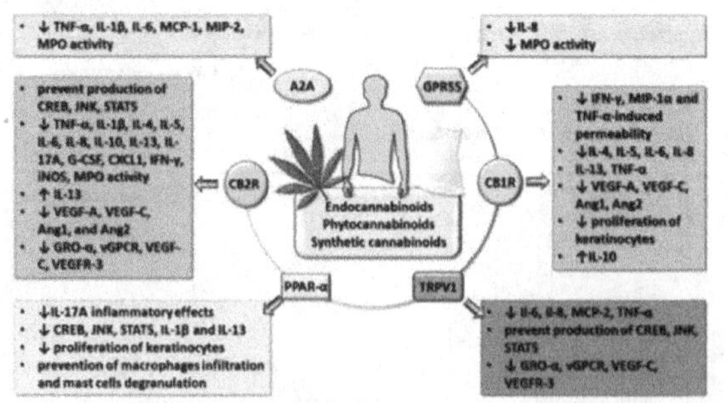

-Scheau,C. et al. Cannabinoids and Inflammations of the Gut-Lung-Skin Barrier. *J. Pers. Med.* **2021**, *11*,494

Cannabinoids: Placental transfer/effects

- $\geq$ **10% fetal:maternal plasma**
- CBD inhibits fetal CYP3A7
- **CB1R, CB2R placenta, fetus**
  - **CB1- brain cell differentiation**
  - **↓ dopamine receptors brain**
    - M>F
    - dose dependent
- Offspring
  - Cognitive impairment

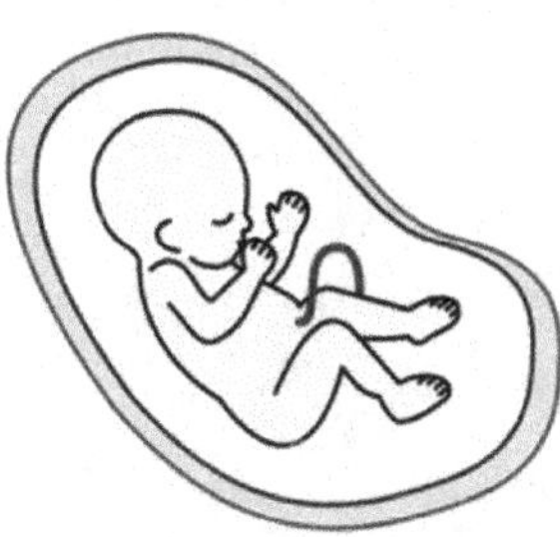

-Foster BC. Am J Medicine 2019:132:1266-70. Pharmacol Ther 2019:201:25-38., Hum Repro Update 2020:26:586-6-2. Metz TD. Obstet Gynecol 2018:132:1198-1210

Cannabis Withdrawal (Q9)

- **Cannabis withdrawal 24-72 h after cessation**
  - Anger, anxiety insomnia, mood, abdominal pain, sweating, fever, chills, HA
  - Likely if > 1.5g/day inhaled cannabis or 20 mg/day THC oil, smoking 2-3x/day
  - Monitor postop – can use Cannabis Withdrawal Scale
  - **Possible Rx – CBR agonist, gabapentin, N-acetylcysteine**
  - Risk lower if CBD dominant (>10:1 CBD:THC) product use

Recommendation

- **Monitor for Cannabis withdrawal symptoms**
  - **Use validated scale (e.g. Cannabis Withdrawal Scale)** - (Grade C)
- Cannabinoid agonist low dose **for severe withdrawal**
  - **Dronabinol low dose** (Grade C)

Cannabinoid Summary

- **Cannabinoid usage very frequent**
  - Including high dose, synthetic
  - Acute CB1/2 Stimulation sympathetic $\leq$ 2 h
    - Delay elective case: need $\geq$2 h from time of smoked cannabis
    - Chronic CB1/2 stimulation – may be parasympathetic, hypothermia
  - **Preop – Ask, Ask, Ask**
- Affects maternal and fetal systems
- **Beware interactions and altered metabolism** with other medications
  - Including opioids, anti-coagulants
- **Neuraxial anesthesia/analgesia no evidence contraindication**
- Intra/postop – **beware hypothermia**
- **High doses/synthetic - May mimic preeclampsia, PRES**

CG, Informative slides. I would think cannabis is like any other drug and harmful to everyone who abuses it. The question is why do these people want to get high? What could it possibly be that they want to forget.

Post COVID Aggression

AIN The Historic Monster Hurricane!

Written on 9/28/2022 by Ramsis Ghaly

As IAN Monster Hurricane Category Five, let us Pray and Watch they ye Enter Not Into Temptation!

We pray for our Beloved Floridians and Florida! The Lord says: "But now thus saith the Lord that created thee, O Jacob, and he that formed thee, O Israel, Fear not: for I have redeemed thee, I have called thee by thy name; thou art mine. [2] When thou passest through the waters, I will be with thee; and through the rivers, they shall not overflow thee: when thou walkest through the fire, thou shalt not be burned; neither shall the flame kindle upon thee. [3] For I am the Lord thy God, the Holy One of Israel, thy Saviour: I gave Egypt for thy ransom, Ethiopia and Seba for thee. [4] Since thou wast precious in my sight, thou hast been honourable, and I have loved thee: therefore will I give men for thee, and people for thy life. [5] Fear not: for I am with thee: I will bring thy seed from the east, and gather thee from the west; [15] I am the Lord, your Holy One, the creator of Israel, your King." Isaiah 43:1-5,15 KJV

As IAN Monster Hurricane category Five catastrophic tremendously damagingly, let us Pray and Watch they ye Enter Not Into Temptation! As Jesus in His last days in the flesh advice to His disciples: "Watch and pray, that ye enter not into temptation: the spirit indeed is willing, but the flesh is weak." Matthew 26:41 KJV

Indeed, as the world watching helplessly the Monster IAN as St Paul said: Hebrews 10:31 KJV "It is a fearful thing to fall into the hands of the living God."

Indeed, The Lord is Mighty Psalm 29:1

Ascribe to the Lord, O sons of the mighty,

Ascribe to the Lord glory and strength."

Man, thy aren't strong than He: 1 Corinthians 10:22

Or do we provoke the Lord to jealousy? We are not stronger than He, are we? Psalm 93:1

The Lord reigns, He is clothed with majesty;

The Lord has clothed and girded Himself with strength; Indeed, the world is firmly established, it will not be moved.

As the world watching Monster Hurricane Ian hitting hard the islands destroying the green lands, while the modern man is standing helpless unable to do anything to intercept or redirect or ameliorate the strength and impact of hurricane category five!!

Despite human artificial intelligence, frontier technology and science, yet mankind can't do anything g to face such unheard magnitude of hurricane!

Yet man is still believing that he has complete dominion over the world and universe!! I guess man narrow minded grandiose thinking believe carbon dioxide is the cause of natural disasters and fuel production is the root instead of referring to man's evil and denying Lord Jesus and shying away from prayers!!

The only man could do is to warn for the hurricane is coming within few days and nothing to stop the giant's hurricane and surges!

Indeed, It makes the faithful human minds that all these natural tragedies are related to the multitudes of the world sins, deviation from God the Lord and predetermined steps toward the ultimate end of the world and universe as it is written.

It is the time for humble hearts to strength their faith in our Lord Jesus and calling for the unity of the world rather than fighting against each other and turn away from Hod the Lord!

"Draw near to God and He will draw near to you." James 4:8

Indeed, we pray to our savior to lead us not unto temptation but deliver us from evil: "After this manner therefore pray ye: Our Father which art in heaven, Hallowed be thy name. [10] Thy kingdom come. Thy will be done in earth, as it is in heaven. [11] Give us this day our daily bread. [12] And forgive us our debts, as we forgive our debtors. [13] And lead us not into temptation, but deliver us from evil: For thine is the kingdom, and the power, and the glory, for ever. Amen." Matthew 6:9-13 KJV

It is the times and aren't otherwise and unless God shorten those days: "For nation shall rise against nation, and kingdom against kingdom: and there shall be famines, and pestilences, and earthquakes, in divers places. [8] All these are the beginning of sorrows. [15] When ye therefore shall see the abomination of desolation, spoken of by Daniel the prophet, stand in the holy place, (whoso readeth, let him understand:) [22] And except those days should be shortened, there should no flesh be saved: but for the elect's sake those days shall be shortened. [29] Immediately after the tribulation of those days shall the sun be darkened, and the moon shall not give her light, and the stars shall fall from heaven, and the powers of the heavens shall be shaken: [30] And then shall appear the sign of the Son of man in heaven: and then shall all the tribes of the earth mourn, and they shall see the Son of man coming in the clouds of heaven with power and great glory."Matthew 24:7-8,15,22,29-30 KJV

The Strength of Prayers

Rejoice always, pray continually, give thanks in all circumstances; for this is God's will for you in Christ Jesus. 1 Thessalonians 5:16-18

Do not be anxious about anything, but in every situation, by prayer and petition, with thanksgiving, present your requests to God. And the peace of God, which transcends all understanding, will guard your hearts and your minds in Christ Jesus.

Philippians 4:6-7gratitudeworryingfear

This is the confidence we have in approaching God: that if we ask anything according to his will, he hears us. 1 John 5:14

Devote yourselves to prayer, being watchful and thankful. Colossians 4:2

Therefore I tell you, whatever you ask for in prayer, believe that you have received it, and it will be yours. Mark 11:24

Then you will call on me and come and pray to me, and I will listen to you. Jeremiah 29:12

Be joyful in hope, patient in affliction, faithful in prayer. Romans 12:12

The Lord is near to all who call on him, to all who call on him in truth. Psalm 145:18

Call to me and I will answer you and tell you great and unsearchable things you do not know. Jeremiah 33:3

And when you pray, do not keep on babbling like pagans, for they think they will be heard because of their many words. Matthew 6:7

About midnight Paul and Silas were praying and singing hymns to God, and the other prisoners were listening to them. Acts 16:25

For where two or three gather in my name, there am I with them. Matthew 18:20

Let us then approach God's throne of grace with confidence, so that we may receive mercy and find grace to help us in our time of need. Hebrews 4:16

In my distress I called to the Lord; I cried to my God for help. From his temple he heard my voice; my cry came before him, into his ears. Psalm 18:6

But when you pray, go into your room, close the door and pray to your Father, who is unseen. Then your Father, who sees what is done in secret, will reward you. Matthew 6:6

And if we know that he hears us—whatever we ask—we know that we have what we asked of him.

1 John 5:15

Therefore confess your sins to each other and pray for each other so that you may be healed. The prayer of a righteous person is powerful and effective. James 5:16

But when you ask, you must believe and not doubt, because the one who doubts is like a wave of the sea, blown and tossed by the wind. James 1:6

You did not choose me, but I chose you and appointed you so that you might go and bear fruit—fruit that will last—and so that whatever you ask in my name the Father will give you. John 15:16

The end of all things is near. Therefore be alert and of sober mind so that you may pray. 1 Peter 4:7

I cried out to him with my mouth; his praise was on my tongue. Psalm 66:17

They all joined together constantly in prayer, along with the women and Mary the mother of Jesus, and with his brothers. Acts 1:14

And I will do whatever you ask in my name, so that the Father may be glorified in the Son. John 14:13

But to you who are listening I say: Love your enemies, do good to those who hate you, bless those who curse you, pray for those who mistreat you. Luke 6:27-28

You desire but do not have, so you kill. You covet but you cannot get what you want, so you quarrel and fight. You do not have because you do not ask God. James 4:2

Fear of God

Job 28:28

“And to man He said, ‘Behold, the fear of the Lord, that is wisdom;

And to depart from evil is understanding.’”

Psalm 111:10

The fear of the Lord is the beginning of wisdom;

A good understanding have all those who do His commandments;

His praise endures forever.

Proverbs 9:10

The fear of the Lord is the beginning of wisdom,

And the knowledge of the Holy One is understanding.

Proverbs 15:33

The fear of the Lord is the instruction for wisdom,

And before honor comes humility.

Proverbs 1:7

The fear of the Lord is the beginning of knowledge;

Fools despise wisdom and instruction.

Proverbs 10:27

The fear of the Lord prolongs life,

But the years of the wicked will be shortened.

Proverbs 14:27

The fear of the Lord is a fountain of life,

That one may avoid the snares of death.

Proverbs 19:23

The fear of the Lord leads to life,

So that one may sleep satisfied, untouched by evil.

Isaiah 33:6

And He will be the stability of your times,

A wealth of salvation, wisdom and knowledge;

The fear of the Lord is his treasure.

Proverbs 14:26

In the fear of the Lord there is strong confidence,

And his children will have refuge.

Proverbs 15:16

Better is a little with the fear of the Lord

Than great treasure and turmoil with it.

Proverbs 2:5

Then you will discern the fear of the Lord

And discover the knowledge of God.

Psalm 112:1

Praise the Lord!

How blessed is the man who fears the Lord,

Who greatly delights in His commandments.

Psalm 128:1

A Song of Ascents.

How blessed is everyone who fears the Lord,

Who walks in His ways.

Psalm 128:4

Behold, for thus shall the man be blessed

Who fears the Lord.

Proverbs 8:13

"The fear of the Lord is to hate evil;

Pride and arrogance and the evil way

And the perverted mouth, I hate.

Exodus 20:20

Moses said to the people, "Do not be afraid; for God has come in order to test you, and in order that the fear of Him may remain with you, so that you may not sin."

Psalm 19:9

The fear of the Lord is clean, enduring forever;

The judgments of the Lord are true; they are righteous altogether.

Job 4:6

"Is not your fear of God your confidence,

And the integrity of your ways your hope?

The Lord is Mighty

Psalm 29:1

A Psalm of David.

Ascribe to the Lord, O sons of the mighty,

Ascribe to the Lord glory and strength.

Psalm 96:7

Ascribe to the Lord, O families of the peoples,

Ascribe to the Lord glory and strength.

Psalm 68:34

Ascribe strength to God;

His majesty is over Israel

And His strength is in the skies.

Job 9:19

"If it is a matter of power, behold, He is the strong one!

And if it is a matter of justice, who can summon Him?

Job 9:4

"Wise in heart and mighty in strength,

Who has defied Him without harm?

Job 12:16

"With Him are strength and sound wisdom,

The misled and the misleader belong to Him.

Psalm 93:1

The Lord reigns, He is clothed with majesty;

The Lord has clothed and girded Himself with strength;

Indeed, the world is firmly established, it will not be moved.

Psalm 96:6

Splendor and majesty are before Him,

Strength and beauty are in His sanctuary.

Psalm 24:8

Who is the King of glory?

The Lord strong and mighty,

The Lord mighty in battle.

Psalm 68:28

Your God has commanded your strength;

Show Yourself strong, O God, who have acted on our behalf.

Psalm 21:13

Be exalted, O Lord, in Your strength;

We will sing and praise Your power.

Psalm 65:6

Who establishes the mountains by His strength,

Being girded with might;

Jeremiah 50:34

"Their Redeemer is strong, the Lord of hosts is His name;

He will vigorously plead their case

So that He may bring rest to the earth,

But turmoil to the inhabitants of Babylon.

Exodus 15:13

"In Your lovingkindness You have led the people whom You have redeemed;

In Your strength You have guided them to Your holy habitation.

Luke 1:51

"He has done mighty deeds with His arm;

He has scattered those who were proud in the thoughts of their heart.

Psalm 21:1

For the choir director. A Psalm of David.

O Lord, in Your strength the king will be glad,

And in Your salvation how greatly he will rejoice!

Ephesians 6:10

Finally, be strong in the Lord and in the strength of His might.

1 Corinthians 1:25

Because the foolishness of God is wiser than men, and the weakness of God is stronger than men.

Ecclesiastes 6:10

Whatever exists has already been named, and it is known what man is; for he cannot dispute with him who is stronger than he is.

Revelation 5:12

saying with a loud voice," Worthy is the Lamb that was slain to receive power and riches and wisdom and might and honor and glory and blessing."

1 Corinthians 10:22

Or do we provoke the Lord to jealousy? We are not stronger than He, are we?

Revelation 18:8

For this reason in one day her plagues will come, pestilence and mourning and famine, and she will be burned up with fire; for the Lord God who judges her is strong.

https://www.bbc.com/news/live/world-us-canada-63064253

https://weather.com/.../2022-09-28-hurricane-ian-forecast...

https://apple.news/A0IqwxXsQR6C87PtVb30f1w

WEATHER.COM

Ian Becomes Tropical Storm After Catastrophic Hurricane Strike | The Weather Channel

The very latest forecast information and current status of Hurricane Ian is here. - Articles from The Weather Channel | weather.com

mb. Safe again by the grace of God .But praying for the rest that have not been as blessed. Thank You for always thinking of us down here .Be blessed brother Ghaly.

Cg, Charlene Mentzer Glowaty

Praying for Florida

Lately Chicago Fatal Gun Shootings are Irremediable!

Written by Ramsis Ghaly

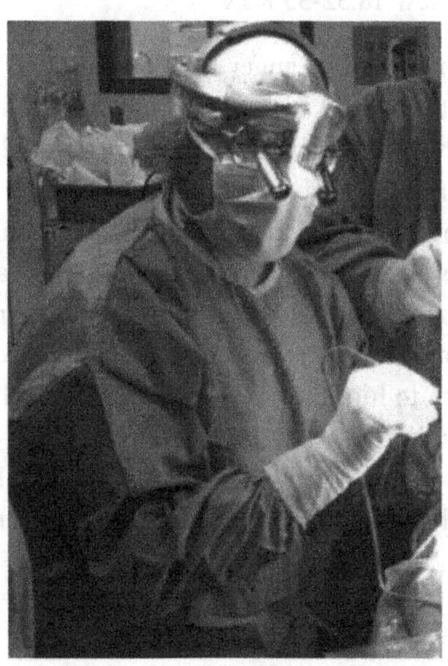

For decades resuscitating the violent trauma patients in Chicago, I must admit nowadays the shooting are carried out merciless, ruthless and brutal and results in immediate death with nil survival regardless of what we do!

It isn't as the old days! We used to be successful in saving their lives and their injuries are repairable since the shootings weren't as damaging as they are nowadays!!! Nowadays thd injuries are irreparable!

Chicago Gunshots are most damaging being not only fatal but also Irremediable and irreversible despite aggressive and immediate medical and surgical resuscitation!

What a huge disappointment and sadness to us and the medical community and to our city!!

Lately the Chicago gun shootings are merciless, evil and to kill! Unbelievable how evil man can be!

If they shoot to kill what they expect God to do to them at That Day!

Chicagoans, please have mercy so God Lord have mercy on thee as our lord said: "Blessed are the merciful: for they shall obtain mercy." Matthew 5:7 KJV. Our

Lord said this parable: "Then his lord, after that he had called him, said unto him, O thou wicked servant, I forgave thee all that debt, because thou desiredst me: [33] Shouldest not thou also have had compassion on thy fellowservant, even as I had pity on thee? [34] And his lord was wroth, and delivered him to the tormentors, till he should pay all that was due unto him. [35] So likewise shall my heavenly Father do also unto you, if ye from your hearts forgive not every one his brother their trespasses." Matthew 18:32-35 KJV

Our Lord Jesus taught us Not to anger a fellowman and absolutely don't Kill: "Ye have heard that it was said by them of old time, Thou shalt not kill; and whosoever shall kill shall be in danger of the judgment: [22] But I say unto you, That whosoever is angry with his brother without a cause shall be in danger of the judgment: and whosoever shall say to his brother, Raca, shall be in danger of the council: but whosoever shall say, Thou fool, shall be in danger of hell fire. [38] Ye have heard that it hath been said, An eye for an eye, and a tooth for a tooth: [39] But I say unto you, That ye resist not evil: but whosoever shall smite thee on thy right cheek, turn to him the other also. [41] And whosoever shall compel thee to go a mile, go with him twain. [42] Give to him that asketh thee, and from him that would borrow of thee turn not thou away. [43] Ye have heard that it hath been said, Thou shalt love thy neighbour, and hate thine enemy." Matthew 5:21-22,38-39,41-43 KJV

"Draw near to God and He will draw near to you."

James 4:8

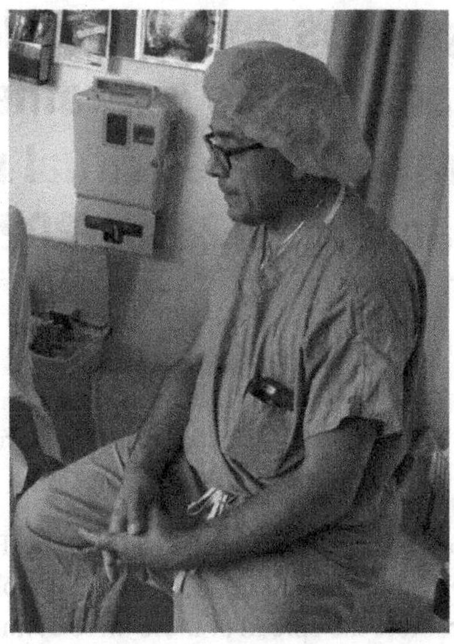

CG, Chicago is such a beautiful city. Too bad there is such ugliness taking over the city.

Bless you for trying to help those that are victims.

Chicago does need three days of Lollapalooza rocks but rather three days of prayers and spiritual ministers preaching (7/28-31/2022)!

Written by Ramsis Ghaly

Chicago doesn't need Lollapalooza rocks but rather a church mass and spiritual ministers preaching!

The last thing Chicago needs is Lollapalooza rocks! What a Bureaucracy, Chicago believes in recent COVID Serge and monkey box and violence!! The last even Chicago needs is to promote the spread of these three evilness!!!!

Chicago needs Billy Graham and not Lollapalooza!

Nothing good will come after Lollapalooza but material mighty dollars. But all heavenly treasure and peace and no violence by the Word of God!

But with Lollapalooza cones more violence, drunken, lusts, sins and —-///

https://www.ranker.com/list/notable-pastor_s)/reference

One of the world's premier music festivals makes its annual return to Chicago's Grant Park. Lollapalooza rocks out with the biggest names in music across all the genres: hip-hop, electronica, reggae, indie, modern roots, and more, attracting more than 100,000 attendees each year.

https://www.choosechicago.com/.../festivals.../lollapalooza/

The Word of God

Hebrews 4:12

For the word of God is living and active, sharper than any two-edged sword, piercing to the division of soul and of spirit, of joints and of marrow, and discerning the thoughts and intentions of the heart.

John 17:17

"Sanctify them in the truth; your word is truth."

John 1:1

In the beginning was the Word, and the Word was with God, and the Word was God.

Psalm 119:105

Your word is a lamp to my feet and a light to my path.

2 Timothy 3:16

All Scripture is breathed out by God and profitable for teaching, for reproof, for correction, and for training in righteousness.

1 Peter 1:23

Since you have been born again, not of perishable seed but of imperishable, through the living and abiding word of God.

1 Peter 2:2

Like newborn infants, long for the pure spiritual milk, that by it you may grow up into salvation.

1 Thessalonians 2:13

And we also thank God constantly for this, that when you received the word of God, which you heard from us, you accepted it not as the word of men but as what it really is, the word of God, which is at work in you believers.

2 Peter 3:16

As he does in all his letters when he speaks in them of these matters. There are some things in them that are hard to understand, which the ignorant and unstable twist to their own destruction, as they do the other Scriptures.

2 Timothy 2:15

Do your best to present yourself to God as one approved, a worker who has no need to be ashamed, rightly handling the word of truth.

Acts 17:11

Now these Jews were more noble than those in Thessalonica; they received the word with all eagerness, examining the Scriptures daily to see if these things were so.

Colossians 3:16

Let the word of Christ dwell in you richly, teaching and admonishing one another in all wisdom, singing psalms and hymns and spiritual songs, with thankfulness in your hearts to God.

Deuteronomy 8:3

And he humbled you and let you hunger and fed you with manna, which you did not know, nor did your fathers know, that he might make you know that man does not live by bread alone, but man lives by every word that comes from the mouth of the Lord.

Ephesians 6:17

And take the helmet of salvation, and the sword of the Spirit, which is the word of God.

Hebrews 1:3

He is the radiance of the glory of God and the exact imprint of his nature, and he upholds the universe by the word of his power. After making purification for sins, he sat down at the right hand of the Majesty on high.

Isaiah 40:8

The grass withers, the flower fades, but the word of our God will stand forever.

Isaiah 55:11

"So shall my word be that goes out from my mouth; it shall not return to me empty, but it shall accomplish that which I purpose, and shall succeed in the thing for which I sent it."

James 1:21

Therefore put away all filthiness and rampant wickedness and receive with meekness the implanted word, which is able to save your souls.

James 1:22

But be doers of the word, and not hearers only, deceiving yourselves.

John 1:14

And the Word became flesh and dwelt among us, and we have seen his glory, glory as of the only Son from the Father, full of grace and truth.

John 10:35

"If he called them gods to whom the word of God came—and Scripture cannot be broken."

John 12:48

"The one who rejects me and does not receive my words has a judge; the word that I have spoken will judge him on the last day."

John 14:6

Jesus said to him, "I am the way, and the truth, and the life. No one comes to the Father except through me."

John 15:3

"Already you are clean because of the word that I have spoken to you."

John 15:7

"If you abide in me, and my words abide in you, ask whatever you wish, and it will be done for you."

John 16:13

"When the Spirit of truth comes, he will guide you into all the truth, for he will not speak on his own authority, but whatever he hears he will speak, and he will declare to you the things that are to come."

John 6:63

"It is the Spirit who gives life; the flesh is no help at all. The words that I have spoken to you are spirit and life."

John 7:38

"Whoever believes in me, as the Scripture has said, 'Out of his heart will flow rivers of living water.'"

John 8:47

"Whoever is of God hears the words of God. The reason why you do not hear them is that you are not of God."

Matthew 24:35

"Heaven and earth will pass away, but my words will not pass away."

Matthew 4:4

But he answered, "It is written, 'Man shall not live by bread alone, but by every word that comes from the mouth of God.'"

Proverbs 30:5

Every word of God proves true; he is a shield to those who take refuge in him.

Psalm 119:11

I have stored up your word in my heart, that I might not sin against you.

Psalm 119:130

The unfolding of your words gives light; it imparts understanding to the simple.

Psalm 119:160

The sum of your word is truth, and every one of your righteous rules endures forever.

Psalm 119:18

Open my eyes, that I may behold wondrous things out of your law.

Psalm 119:9

How can a young man keep his way pure? By guarding it according to your word.

Psalm 33:4

For the word of the Lord is upright, and all his work is done in faithfulness.

Romans 10:17

So faith comes from hearing, and hearing through the word of Christ.

Romans 15:4

For whatever was written in former days was written for our instruction, that through endurance and through the encouragement of the Scriptures we might have hope.

CHOOSECHICAGO.COM

Lollapalooza Festival Lineup, Guide & Tickets 2022 | Chicago Music Festivals

Lollapalooza returns to Chicago's Grant Park this summer. The city's biggest and longest summer festival features a can't-miss lineup.

Nv, Well said Dr. Ghaly!

Sunrise forces Chicago Gun Shooting to Stop !

Written by Ramsis Ghaly

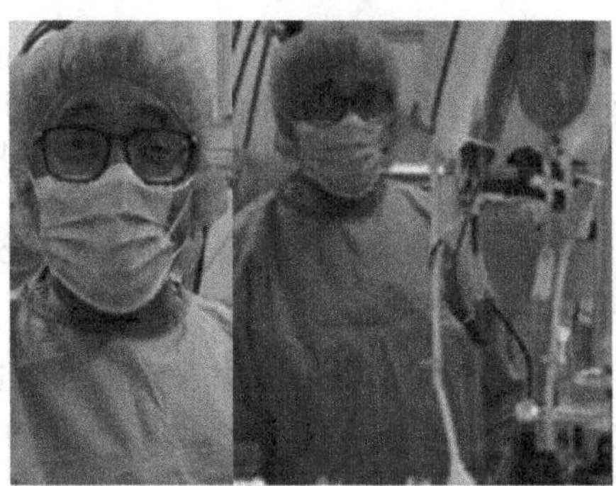

I pray each night since 1987 when I am on call to God: "Please God send the sun back soon to put a stop to the coming victims to the nonstop reckless gun shooting in Chicago!! Please God let this night be over soon! Please God bring Your light back to Chicago to force those shooters away!!"

Whenever I am on call it is so exhausting with my residents resuscitating the entire night the injured citizens in the harm's way!!

The nights are stained with heavy red from the running rivers of blood gushing out from the trauma victims as their hearts become empty and entire flesh exsanguinate to the sterile linens, sheets, tissues and some sneak to floor and gallons go to fill giant suction machines!

Never enough to use human help, one or two or three and usually ten staff members are grouped together to try to save a human life bleeding to death from the multiple gun shooting!

And it is getting so worse to the degree each coming victim has been shot so many times where the internal organs are so severed, the bones are broken, the vessels are torn, the mushy brain are coming out of the skull, the heart is leaking out blood and the lungs are drowned with blood —

At some point by the dawn, we scream to the walls and say, "please stop". By then everything is red, and we all soaked with blood and we too, become drowned with blood mixed with so many emotions, sadness, tears and heartbroken witnessing our fellowmen and fellowmen with all colors are dead from their injuries, gone and no more. And those lucky one's living are left disabled!

We transfuse so much blood and blood products as fast as the patient bleeds out and we always run out of products and drugs!! Never enough resources and so much manpower to revive a single patient!! I wish those shooters would come and witness firsthand what they had inflicted!!

I always say: "It isn't just pulling a trigger, it is a murder to human being to bleed to death, for the organs to be torn and exsanguinate until gives up the ghost!!! Many countries get civilized and with modernization of mankind, someone will think that violence will cease, and professionalism increase with other modem measures and courts to vent! But never ever the case, with modernization comes brutality and more inhumane atrocities!!

It is always the case for as long as I have been taken calls at Chicago major trauma center Cook County Hospital since 1987, nothing stops trauma violence except when God bring the sun back to cast out the darkness and the light shine back in Chicago!!

When the weather is bad outside or so many tornadoes and rains. We say: "Great Lord these weather difficulties certainly will keep those shooters away and limit their evilness!"

For years and years taking calls at Chicago trauma center JSH of Cook County hospital, there is no stop to the horrific inhumane gun shooting! And unfortunately, the Only Time for gun shooting to stop is when the night is over!! The only time the violence stops in Chicago is when the sun comes back!! The only way for gun shooting to cease when God sends the sun to shine upon the face of Chicago! The only time for satanic violence to stop in Chicago is when God sends the light to take the darkness away!

At that time, it is a new day as if nothing had happened, the dead are dead and the injured are injured and the living are living!!

It has been my life for close to four decades starting 1980's saving lives and resuscitating the falling victims of the worst violent city in the world Chicago metropolitan City!! It used to be the hot summer days when violence peak with many out of schools and drugs more in the streets and nothing to do!! But now all year around nonstop!!!

So many students, residents, nurses, doctors, ancillary staff, policemen and women, politicians and many more come and go and spend so much time, yet one thing has never changed the extreme atrocities of Gun shooting in our beloved city Chicago!!!

I prayed to my Lord Jesus back in High school: "Lord if You allow me to go to medical school and be a doctor, You must bless me and do miracles to heal them and them live and not die"

And My Heavenly Father kept my promise despite my shortcoming and my patients not just live but testimonies to Him!

I never ever want to see a patient die in the operating room table and be sent downstairs to the morgue!!! This what I always pray !

Lord Jesus always bring Your Sun and let it shine at our City Chicago to cast out the darkness and remove the hatred in the hearts of those and revive those victims as You taken Satan away from thy people!! In Jesus Name Amen

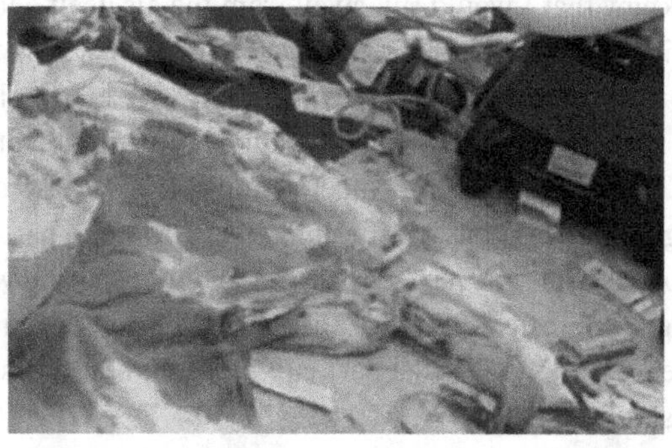

Kl, So sad!!! Praying for peace and strength for all of you fighting to save the lives of the victims

I Feel Something Major About to Happen!!

Written on 8/3/202 by Ramsis Ghaly

I feel Something major about to happen!!! I don't know why! I pray I am wrong but The devil is moving forward!!! We pray!! Taiwan/ China uprise, COVID19, Monkey Box, recession---etc

I didn't wish to know what, or when or how! It is written all around but who has the eyes to see and the ears to hear and the heart to listen! It is so dark and the light so dim in the tunnel where I am hiding since no other places are safe any longer! I never knew that I would run away from the air itself and I told my soul what else remained! Man is destroying his fellow man. I was told the nature couldn't handle it anymore! In fact, there is nothing else left to give in or buffer! As a result, the scale is all the way down and heavy while the other side all the way on the top and shall never ever meet again! So, what else remains but the remnants laying around and the whispering voices from the past! What brought us to this and how did the time have passed before our eyes, and we couldn't stop it! ! I am no longer interested to know! I used to be curious but my curiosity has left my soul at least for now! For that particular reason, I didn't ask what or when and how! It doesn't matter!

"And ye shall hear of wars and rumours of wars: see that ye be not troubled: for all these things must come to pass, but the end is not yet. [7] For nation shall rise against nation, and kingdom against kingdom: and there shall be famines, and pestilences, and earthquakes, in divers places. [8] All these are the beginning of sorrows. [10] And then shall many be offended, and shall betray one another, and shall hate one another. [12] And because iniquity shall abound, the love of many shall wax cold. [13] But he that shall endure unto the end, the same shall be saved." Matthew 24:6-8,10,12-13 KJV

Ramsis Ghaly

KC, I hate when I get feelings like that. I think sometimes He shows us so we can pray and intercede. These verses were from my morning quiet time this morning:

"Seek the Lord, all you humble of the land, you who do what he commands. Seek righteousness, seek humility; perhaps you will be sheltered on the day of the Lord's anger."

Zephaniah 2:3

SL, Take heart our dearest Dr Ghaly as we pray to the Almighty Heavenly Father on your behalf, for our family and friends and our fellow man.....we take comfort in knowing that while the devil prowls to seek and destroy he is in his death throws and the battle has ultimately already been won by our Lord & Savior Jesus Christ

DT, I know it's not a good feeling!

JH, Our Lord will prevail

LM, Pray without ceasing

LG, I trust in you Jesus Absolutely .

JI, But God

SW, God always wins.

VP, Lord have mercy!

ML, I hope your premonitions are wrong.

KM, Praying Dr Ghaly.

DL, Praise the Lord.

KO, LG, Praying with you Dr. Ghaly!

VW, We have AUTHORITY over the devil

AK, Praying with you

MA, KS, Prayers for safety of our country .

MO, Fear not for Christ has overcome the demons and has them on a leash

RZ, JM, HOPE NOT!!!

ML, God forbid

VG, God please watch over us and our Country

JF, We come against any plans of the adversary and we speak the name of Jesus over all situations! #PastorJeff90210

SC, JT, praying...

JB, Praying

LM, I can feel it too! Praying!

VW, I'm seeing many posts like this...pray!

GH, Maybe the 2nd coming of Christ!

SR, I will pray, I've said those exact words today.... It's a feeling I have as well

JD, I tend to agree my friend

MS, I'm glad God's in control. I'm praying for our country.

EA, I feel that too,especially when i see Pelosi

AL, In God we trust

SN, Don't worry Dr. Ghaly, It's always darkest before the dawn. The BEST IS YET TO COME

VA, Satan brings on feelings of anxiety

SM, Oh crap, what have I missed

MW, I said this to my Friend Monday Evening. "Something Huge is About to Happen"

LW, Praying for God's blessings and goodness.

DM, I agree. There is an uneasiness in the "air".

ED, This frightens me. God protect us please

BM, Praying in Jesus Name

IC, May God be with you

KH, Prayers

VM, Dr.Ghaly I started feeling this yesterday.. praying in Jesus name

Dk,I've been feeling that for some time now....its easy to see the change in our world and country and its getting that way much faster but we all need to just trust in Jesus as this is no surprise to God!Christians know how the end goes. Pray for unsaved people and make sure we are in the word of God and keeping close to the Lord no matter what. It's in God's hands and in his timing. Could be 100 years from now or today...devil will throw every problem and distraction he can to keep our eyes on that instead of Jesus and to fill people with fear. Jesus gives us a peace that surpasses all if we keep our eyes on him. (Think Peter and his fear to walk on water until Jesus). Praying for you. We are wrestling with spirits and demons many that come with faces of humans. We have power in Jesus name and his word to fight them!

DH, Yes, I know something bad, but I continually to pray everyday! In the end God Always will Win! Seems many will be gone, so sad, but their is good that pass on, shall be going on to our Father, who is in Heaven, HE has ALL THE POWER! OUR GOD ALMIGHTY!!!

GOOD TRIUMPHS OVER EVIL, THIS I KNOW. BAD THINGS TO HAPPEN, BECAUSE THEIR IS FREE WILL, AND THE DEVIL WHO IS HARD AT WORL, HE TOO WILL FAIL! HALLELUJAH

BCD, Yes, I agree. We are here to hold the Light for those in the Dark. Never give up, never surrender. We will do our souls job with all the strength and power we have. Amen

Abortion!!

Written by Ramsis Ghaly

"And it came to pass, that, when Elisabeth heard the salutation of Mary, the babe leaped in her womb; and Elisabeth was filled with the Holy Ghost:" Luke 1:41

God loves so much the children since before they formed day one in the womb even if mom forget God never: Isaiah 49:15 KJV Can a woman forget her sucking child, that she should not have compassion on the son of her womb? yea, they may forget, yet will I not forget thee."

"For your lifeblood I will surely require a reckoning; of every beast I will require it and of man; of every man's brother I will require the life of man. Whoever sheds the blood of man, by man shall his blood be shed; for God made man in his own image." Genesis 9:5- **Exodus 20:13 "You shall not murder." Genesis 1: 27 So God created mankind in his own image, in the image of God he created them; male and female he created them**

No abortion case was ever cited in the entire Holy Bible except a curse of unfaithfulness: ***"If she has made herself impure and been unfaithful to her husband, this will be the result: When she is made to drink the water that brings a curse and causes bitter suffering, it will enter her, her abdomen will swell and her womb will miscarry, and she will become a curse. 28 If, however, the woman has not made herself impure, but is clean, she will be cleared of guilt and will be able to have children. " Numbers 5:27-28 "Then the priest shall put the woman under oath and say to her, "If no other man has had sexual relations with you and you have not gone astray and become impure while married to your husband, may this bitter water that brings a curse not harm you. 20 But if you have gone astray while married to your husband and you have made yourself impure by having sexual relations with a man other than your husband"—21 here the priest is to put the woman under this curse—"may the LORD cause you to become a curse among your people when he makes your womb miscarry and your abdomen swell. 22 May this water that brings a curse enter your body so that your abdomen swells or your womb miscarries." " 'Then the woman is to say, "Amen. So be it." Numbers 5:19-22***

Biblical Moms and dad kept their babies regardless and many, at later time grew to be prophets. Many were barren and dreamed you have babies and by miracles and divine visions from God, they did have babies!! Abortion wasn't even considered as an option at all and wasn't in their vocabulary or table or thoughts. At the biblical time all children are inheritance from God, and all loved and wanted, and no one ever stepped on God children and said "No let us extract that child and cast him or her out from the land of living"

"3 Children are a heritage from the Lord,
offspring a reward from him. 4 Like arrows in the hands of a warrior are children born in one's youth. 5 Blessed is the man
whose quiver is full of them. They will not be put to shame
when they contend with their opponents in court."
Psalm 127:3-5

I understand both sides in allowing abortion verses not allowing abortion. But there is something to feel as a sword 🗡 piercing in thy heart, when a brutal instrument is taking away a living cell granted a breath of life from God to be a human being curetted out by that brutal Sharpe instrument, expelled out with no dignity, killed and suctioned out in a garbage bag!!

It isn't about the woman right to choose but rather about the illusion of how a mom and dad believe that both shall escape the damnation of murdering their own conception of an image of God Human embryo, a child of God!! It has never been about the earthly court system state and federal and supreme courts but about the Heavenly Father condemnation to mom and dad killing His child and the abandoning his living for their own lust!

Mothers in particular as My mom had never forgotten those babies to be lost in miscarriages!!!! And when moms see the dead fetal parts as they are spelled out and extracted and then grinded through the power suction containers, they scream crying . And when the time comes for moms to leave this world, they will be looking forward to meeting them above the clouds. They are alive with spirit, innocent, pure, angels and had no chance to live and many were rejected by their own mom and dad and went ahead intentionally to kill them ashamed of them for their own pleasure and convenience! It is an act of Satan and so evil to murder an image of God newly formed conception!

Psalms 22:10 "From birth I was cast on you; from my mother's womb you have been my God." "Listen, O isles, unto me; and hearken, ye people, from far; The LORD hath called me from the womb; from the bowels of my mother hath he made mention of my name." Isiah 49:1Ecclesiastes 11:5 - As thou knowest not what is the way of the spirit, nor how the bones do grow in the womb of her that is with child: even so thou knowest not the works of God who maketh all." Isaiah 46:3-4 KJV "Hearken unto me, O house of Jacob, and all the remnant

of the house of Israel, which are borne by me from the belly, which are carried from the womb: And even to your old age I am he; and even to hoar hairs will I carry you: I have made, and I will bear; even I will carry, and will deliver you."

How can the world surface the reckless and intentional ignorance and the extreme sinful behavior involved in aborting a living human conception! That human living embryo wasn't formed by airborne process or some sort of wireless technology or non-contact task but rather made by active man to women intimacy process with full awareness throughout!

"For you created my inmost being; you knit me together in my mother's womb. 14 I praise you because I am fearfully and wonderfully made; your works are wonderful, I know that full well.

15 My frame was not hidden from you when I was made in the secret place, when I was woven together in the depths of the earth. 16 Your eyes saw my unformed body; all the days ordained for me were written in your book before one of them came to be." Psalm 139:13-16

Murdering that living cell is criminal but so is the daily human trafficking, child molestation, rapping, abuse, and so daily shooting in Chicago and major cities, and so is violence, stealing, kidnapping, marriage to minors, cheating, Swearing, unbelieving in Lord Jesus—-etc! Never ever in human history a society was able to sanctify its own people and made sure they obey the Holy Bible commandment including the basics in the Ten Commandments more than 6 thousand years ago!!

Psalm 14:1 "For the choir director. A Psalm of David. The fool has said in his heart, "There is no God." They are corrupt, they have committed abominable deeds; There is no one who does good." Psalm 14:3 "They have all turned aside, together they have become corrupt; There is no one who does good, not even one." Psalm 53:1 "For the choir director; according to Mahalath. A Maskil of David. The fool has said in his heart, "There is no God," They are corrupt, and have committed abominable injustice; There is no one who does good." Psalm 53:3 "Every one of them has turned aside; together they have become corrupt; There is no one who does good, not even one." Psalm 143:2 "And do not enter into judgment with Your servant, For in Your sight no man living is righteous." Romans 3:9 "What then? Are we better than they? Not at all; for we have already charged that both Jews and Greeks are all under sin;" Romans 3:23 "for all have sinned and fall short of the glory of God," Galatians 3:22 "But the Scripture has shut up everyone under sin, so that the promise by faith in Jesus Christ might be given to those who believe."

Can the society actually prevent sins committed every second worldwide? Can government actually make sure that every man and woman behaves morally and ethically? Who can ever make sure that every human being follows our Lord Beatitudes??

If God, our Lord who created man and woman couldn't force any of His creation to follow His commanded against the will and freedom of choice! Ecclesiastes 7:20 "Indeed, there is not a righteous man on earth who continually does good and who never sins." Romans 3:10 "as it is written, "There is none righteous, not even one;"

The maximum a society, government or officials could do is to elevate awareness and promote morals and ethics bringing back family values and "God we trust" back to our homes, streets, offices, courts, schools and all public and private places! A government can enforce the law and educate at early age and facilitate the outreach and workout the obstacles. A root cause analysis of bad behavior under the umbrella of helping out and prevention can lead to so many optional solutions!

Jeremiah 30:14 'All your lovers have forgotten you, They do not seek you; For I have wounded you with the wound of an enemy, With the punishment of a cruel one, Because your iniquity is great And your sins are numerous." Jeremiah 30:15 "Why do you cry out over your injury? Your pain is incurable. Because your iniquity is great And your sins are numerous, I have done these things to you." Jeremiah 44:9 "Have you forgotten the wickedness of your fathers, the wickedness of the kings of Judah, and the wickedness of their wives, your own wickedness, and the wickedness of your wives, which they committed in the land of Judah and in the streets of Jerusalem?" 1 John 3:8 "the one who practices sin is of the devil; for the devil has sinned from the beginning. The Son of God appeared for this purpose, to destroy the works of the devil."

Indeed, Only the father and the mother of that living human cell called embryo, are fully responsible and shall give account before God the Lord no matter the age of that living conceived human cell as it begins. It doesn't matter how old is that human cell once formed from the very first second of life! Regardless of what thy political party is and how much thy is running away in denial, the fact remains thy killed thy own baby in whatever the cause is! There are many ways to prevent human conception and only one way to halt a human baby from living!!

"Whosoever therefore shall break one of these least commandments, and shall teach men so, he shall be called the least in the kingdom of heaven:

but whosoever shall do and teach them, the same shall be called great in the kingdom of heaven. [20] For I say unto you, That except your righteousness shall exceed the righteousness of the scribes and Pharisees, ye shall in no case enter into the kingdom of heaven. [21] Ye have heard that it was said by them of old time, Thou shalt not kill; and whosoever shall kill shall be in danger of the judgment: [22] But I say unto you, That whosoever is angry with his brother without a cause shall be in danger of the judgment: and whosoever shall say to his brother, Raca, shall be in danger of the council: but whosoever shall say, Thou fool, shall be in danger of hell fire. [27] Ye have heard that it was said by them of old time, Thou shalt not commit adultery: [28] But I say unto you, That whosoever looketh on a woman to lust after her hath committed adultery with her already in his heart. [29] And if thy right eye offend thee, pluck it out, and cast it from thee: for it is profitable for thee that one of thy members should perish, and not that thy whole body should be cast into hell. [30] And if thy right hand offend thee, cut it off, and cast it from thee: for it is profitable for thee that one of thy members should perish, and not that thy whole body should be cast into hell. [31] It hath been said, Whosoever shall put away his wife, let him give her a writing of divorcement: [32] But I say unto you, That whosoever shall put away his wife, saving for the cause of fornication, causeth her to commit adultery: and whosoever shall marry her that is divorced committeth adultery." Matthew 5:19-22,27-32 KJV

Galatians 1:15: "But when he who had set me apart before I was born, and had called me through his grace." **Jeremiah 1:5:** "Before I formed you in the womb I knew you, and before you were born I consecrated you; I appointed you a prophet to the nations."

Philippians 4:6-19 KJV "Be careful for nothing; but in every thing by prayer and supplication with thanksgiving let your requests be made known unto God. And the peace of God, which passeth all understanding, shall keep your hearts and minds through Christ Jesus. Finally, brethren, whatsoever things are true, whatsoever things are honest, whatsoever things are just, whatsoever things are pure, whatsoever things are lovely, whatsoever things are of good report; if there be any virtue, and if there be any praise, think on these things. Those things, which ye have both learned, and received, and heard, and seen in me, do: and the God of peace shall be with you. But I rejoiced in the Lord greatly, that now at the last your care of me hath flourished again; wherein ye were also careful, but ye lacked opportunity. Not that I speak in respect of want: for I have learned, in whatsoever..." Acts 15:28-29 KJV "For it seemed good to the Holy Ghost, and to us, to lay upon you no greater burden than these necessary things; That ye abstain from meats offered to idols, and from blood, and from things strangled, and from fornication: from which if ye keep yourselves, ye shall do well. Fare ye well."

I heard screams and they were the sounds of the Dead Aborted Babies!

Written by Ramsis Ghaly

The Lord gives life and Only the Lord can take the life away as it is written by the mouth of our father Job: ***"And said, Naked came I out of my mother's womb, and naked shall I return thither: the Lord gave, and the Lord hath taken away; blessed be the name of the Lord." Job 1:21 KJV***

I was about to be formed and I was refused, killed and extracted by the will of my own!!! Why? Why? Why? What I had done to be hated and murdered??

At the very early Dawn, I heard screams and I saw nothing but skeletons laying around in the very deep darkness!!

Precious babies are buried alive! Little white angels were murdered!! With no cause, their lives were taken away!! Their murderers thought they are no more!! But they aren't! They are alive before God their Heavenly Father as the earthly parents abandoned them, killed them and ran away from their conscious and guilt! They are awaiting the day of Justice when the books shall be open and give account to their blood!

It provoked the wrath of God upon the face of the earth and the day He saw the continuing evilness of man!!! Deuteronomy 32:35 "Vengeance is mine, and recompense, for the time when their foot shall slip; for the day of their calamity is at hand, and their doom comes swiftly.'

It was written "Their Day is Coming" I kneeled to the ground and screamed to my God: "I am so sinful and guilty for their blood O Lord my God"

He showed me how many of those and ask of me: "Count Them!! I couldn't count them they were innumerable cand I replied: "I can't O my Lord, please forgive me"

As I looked, so many were given the flesh and I saw their innocent angelic faces saying: Why you had done to me what have done to deserve to kill me"

"O listen, the earth shall never swallow them, and they are standing before my eyes. They are murdered and their blood shall be asked of those! Their day is coming!"

I walked and heard the cries of invisible babies and screams of the innocent souls by the river!

There are so so many and over the thousands of years they are in the millions!

Their door was shut and declared unwanted and condemned to death 💀 by the human hands!

They are thrown by the rivers, treated as trash and many are found by the garbage disposables!

Indeed, those babies are voiceless angels who weren't given the chance they deserve to live!

No one should despise those little ones and what about who murder them? "Take heed that you do not despise one of these little ones, for I say to you that in heaven their angels always see the face of My Father who is in heaven. 11For[c] the Son of Man has come to save that which was lost." Matthew 18:10. **Matthew 18:6** ESV But whoever causes one of these little ones who believe in me to sin, it would be better for him to have a great millstone fastened around his neck and to be drowned in the depth of the sea.

They had the breath of life, the spirit, the soul and the human cells required to be the children of God!

They could have been the messiahs to their generations and saints to their people!

They indeed are formed as any mankind has been born but instead, they were rejected upon the spot and refused by their own!!

Deuteronomy 27:24 "Cursed is anyone who kills their neighbor secretly." Then all the people shall say, "Amen!" What about those that kill their own flesh and blood???

Genesis 9:6 "If anyone takes a human life, that person's life will also be taken by human hands. For God made human beings in his own image."

Revelation 21:8 "But the cowardly, the unbelieving, the vile, the murderers, the sexually immoral, those who practice magic arts, the idolaters and all liars–they will be consigned to the fiery lake of burning sulfur. This is the second death." Revelation 21:27 But nothing unclean will ever enter it, nor anyone who does what is detestable or false, but only those who are written in the Lamb's book of life."

Even if some of the babies are a result of rape or incest as in the case of Lit's two daughters, there is no excuse to terminate a life: "And Lot went up out of Zoar, and dwelt in the mountain, and his two daughters with him; for he feared to dwell in Zoar: and he dwelt in a cave, he and his two daughters. [31] And the firstborn said unto the younger, Our father is old, and there is not a man in the earth to come in unto us after the manner of all the earth: [32] Come, let us make our father drink wine, and we will lie with him, that we may preserve seed of our father. [33] And they made their father drink wine that night: and the firstborn went in, and lay with her father; and he perceived not when she lay down, nor when she arose. [34] And it came to pass on the morrow, that the firstborn said unto the younger, Behold, I lay yesternight with my father: let us make him drink wine this night also; and go thou in, and lie with him, that we may preserve seed of our father. [35] And they made their father drink wine that night also: and the younger arose, and lay with him; and he perceived not when she lay down, nor when she arose. [36] Thus were both the daughters of Lot with child by their father. [37] And the firstborn bare a son, and called his name Moab: the same is the father of the Moabites unto this day. [38] And the younger, she also bare a son, and called his name Ben-ammi: the same is the father of the children of Ammon unto this day."Genesis 19:30-38 KJV

3Charlene Mentzer Glowaty, Suzi Hamilton and 1 other

KB, Everyone need to see this so sad,and evil.

JT, devil's work

PI, May Gods have mercy on their souls. Very sad indeed

https://en.m.wikipedia.org/wiki/Abortion

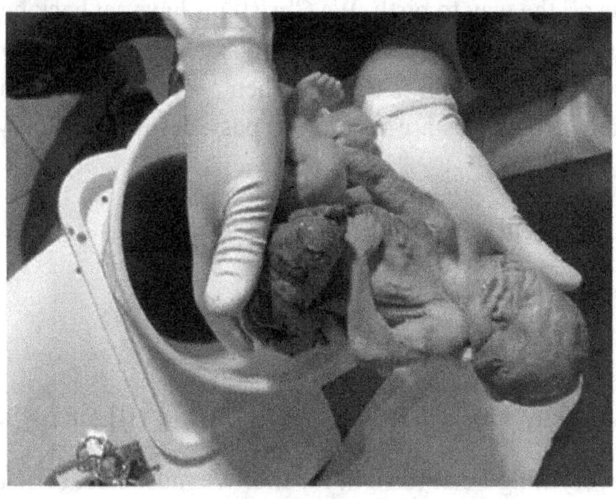

SM, Perfectly said by the most accomplished medical

doctor in the whole wide world! I mean—-this dude is a brain surgeon, a spine surgeon, an anesthesiologist, a pain management doctor, and an internal medicine doctor! That's 5 boards, y'all!!!! When I asked him how he accomplished all that—-he responded, and said, "That's easy, but you remaining a virgin in an impure world is what's super impossible." Thanks for always sharing your brilliance, Dr. Ramsis Ghaly! Motivating me! Being one of my favorite and top fans! On my saddest days, your words always make me smile! A true example of Keeping It Coptic (KIC) and proud!

#copticballer

#copticstar

SA, Heartbreaking.

CG, The woman that say, my body, my choice have always had control and always will.

The problem is they want full control over another life they created because they lost control of their body. That new life is not their body it's a new body growing inside their body. They have no right to end that life.

MB, So sad !

CG, This is so very sad when I see these aborted babies. There are so many people that would love these babies. God bless their little souls.

LW, I would pray for the Lord to have mercy, but why should he? We have allowed this to continue all the way to birth. We Christians have sat back being told don't get involved, until the day where it might be too late. People need yo get involved! And stop the madness, but if it is too late, then people better repent for the time is near! So many prophecies are coming to pass. Jesus is our only hope in this fallen world

MP, Sad truth. Free will at work, evil is there and Satan is at work.

JT, Precious babies. The devil is alive and well.

JT, this world is horrible

JK, The lord will deliver his ((WRATH APOND HIS CHILDRENS KILLERS!!))

SY, I will do everything I can to fight for life. We must elect officials who stand for life. How it breaks God's heart. Thank you as a Dr for standing up for babies lives! God bless you!

EB, OMG! It truly made me sick to my stomach. So sad.

JH, This is murder!!! Absolutely sickening!!!

JZ, So sad, horrifying. Poor sweet angels. Heartbreaking.

BS, Pray for the innocent ones! Punish the guilty!

KK, OMG.....this makes me so sad and so sick at the same time. These poor innocent children....God help us all!

CC, This breaks my heart and makes me so angry!

ET, Only God can give and take life away!!Sad…Sad world!!

MS, So painful. Whyyyy would anyOne do this??

ET, Only God can give and take life away!!Sad…Sad world!!

BC, So sad, God bless these sweet angels. Please lord, make them understand.

LA, a putrid stench in God's nostrils Linda Andzulis

2 Timothy 3:2"For people will be lovers of self, lovers of money, proud, arrogant, abusive, disobedient to their parents, ungrateful, unholy," "My Spirit (patience, benevolence, long suffering) will not always strive with man."—-Genesis 6:3

"There will be 60 million and counting aborted babies standing at the gates of Heaven barring your Democrat entrance, and nothing you can say will ever excuse you for your direct or indirect support of that diabolical agenda. Period. The end." Fr. James Altman

Challenges America is facing today shall make America Better again!

Ramsis Ghaly

What a difference!!! At the same time in 2018, there was talks about peace and no wars! It is so obvious and no one could turn his back to these below facts!!

Challenges America is facing today shall make America Better again! The key however is honesty and to admit mistakes and to learn from these challenges of what should have been done and wasn't and move forward!!

What. America going Through Now will make America Better again!!

Although America is seeing serious issues yet many lessons are being learned and tomorrow shall be better again!

What a difference!!! In the same time in 2018, there was talks about peace and no wars! Nowadays, it is all about wars and supplies of war weapons and rise in prices, inflation, recession and major spread of gun violence!!

Where America is now as follows:

-Inflation and Recession!

-Economy Collapse!

-Poverty and extreme shortage across all services!

-Gas price out of control and so are the essentials of living!

-Extreme rise in prices and short of resources and supplies!

-Gun violence and Lack of security in the streets and homes!

-Wars as never seen before and thousands are killed and murdered and America is unable to make a difference!

-News of more wars coming and more conflicts globally!

- Healthcare cost rising and wellbeing of care providers are suffering!

- Mental health, drug overdose, homicides, suicides and frustrations are at the roof!

-Border security and wellbeing of low enforcement extremely poor!

- The number of Self served and opportunistic are overwhelming!

-Insensitivity to people needs and demands!

-Family values and in God-we-trust deceleration are rare!

- Limited accountability and many are getting away with murder!!!

- Agenda addressing People's priorities is totally off people's demands!

-America image globally is all the way low!

-The look at the future is gloomy and trust in government us at the bottom! The moral is down and risk-taking investments and innovations are down! Many perceive is "path to death"

- Extreme rise in corporate America and who knows who!

-American dream has changed to government made policies and no more "living the American Dream! The Land Of Opportunity! The Land of the Free! The Land of the Brave!"

-Sanctions are useless and America's McDonalds replaced by Russian McDonald's new brand name in Russia could be 'Fun and Tasty' by Alexander Govor

https://amp.cnn.com/.../mcdonalds-russia-fun.../index.html

Ramsis Ghaly
June 12, 2018 ·
Shared with Public
Ramsis Ghaly
June 12, 2018 ·
Shared with Public
I wrote this post 6/12/2018 when president Trump went and Visited president North Korea a step for peace!!
"Blessed are the peacemakers: for they shall be called the children of God." (Matthew 5:9)
Blessed be the peacemaker on the historic day 6/12/2018: To President Trump of United States and Kim Jong Un of North Korea. We pray to our Lord Jesus to bring peace and bless you both.
Our Lord Jesus in His first verses of Aptitude blessed the peacemaker saying: "Blessed are the peacemakers: for they shall be called the children of God." (Matthew 5:9)
Ramsis Ghaly

Mc, The best thing I remember during his presidency is I was HAPPY, WE WERE ENERGY INDEPENDENCE,PEOPLE WERE WORKING, AND WE WERE FREE. He is a true patriot who cares about American people and country

CG, Very sad what has happened to our country. What is happening occurred because of a decline in morality and ethical behavior. Mass shootings, racial hatred, social injustice, incivility, fraud, and White Supremacy are all results of our decline in morality. Only our prayers can help.

JK, Dr Ramsis Ghaly you couldn't explain Today's situation in America better, the way you did.
Excellent, and very truth, but very sad... Everything what President Donald Trump achieved and arranged is totally destroyed by Biden together with his corrupted camrades...
Now, they are still attacking Trump and even blaming him for Democrats failures... What a disastrous situation in America, Our Country we love, and we want to protect from any Evils actions and against our enemies foreign and domestic, unfortunately inside Our Government.
Dear God come back to all of us, forgive us, help us to fight Satanic groups and saved Our Country...
In God We Trust Here, and that's the way we want to keep it
GOD BLESS AMERICA

SM, A sad America now

KM, I don't even recognize our America anymore. It's very sad.

AL, God bless us Oh Lord

KO, Amen it sure needs blessing and prayers

MD, I shared it on my Facebook. Very well said.

SC, As long as we have globalists in power nothing is going to change. This is not accidental, it was planned, long time ago, Trump only got in their way. The only thing we, the people have learned is we took things for granted for too long. Now is too late for many. This nation is not going to survive what the democrat party has done. Balkanization is next!

HV, So true

MPB, This is all so sad .

KK, Unfortunately it's not gods country anymore. Satan is in charge and comes in the form of many things!! God save our children from these evils and save our children from these perverts In the public school platforms.

SY, Yes! So sad what's happened in 2 years. I am volunteering on campaigns to change this. And of course lots of prayer!

KD, You are way off base on this…. Especially if you think Trump has anything to offer..he is corruption personified!!!!

PS, It's not going to get better until the Lord comes back.

CK, So true

MH, Make it right Lord! Bring us back our peace and happiness once again with out war Amen

JM, NO MORE WAR !!!!!!!!

NV, All so true!!

Modern Man Made Tragedies!!!

Written on 4/2/2022 by Ramsis Ghaly

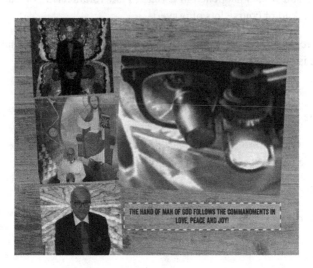

The Putin made war and major destructive human tragedy is only to confirm that COVID-19 tragedy is also man-made!

Man-made tragedies are featured as bizarre out of context, self-served, does not follow the usual Nature pattern, destruction out of measure, not following Science of Nature laws, and very vindictive!! It is aimed to result in widespread out of nature massacre! It's end usually surfaces the truth!

Therefore if Russia Ukraine war is Putin man-made 2022, Who is behind COVID-19!!

Furthermore, these tragedies are man-made on themselves an on the world and not Nature made!

Does those incidents confirm that civilization, modernization and knowledge are instrumental in promoting self-destruction??

These observation only indicates that man with all his material achievements is deviating further away from God and Goodness and only believe in his dominion and grandiose in his own godless self served castle!

If indeed this is true, then every three years the world should expect more and more man made **atrocities and mass destruction!!**

Measures to Prevent such man-made tragedies':

If you further dissect the Root-Cause analysis it should lead to the conclusion of Faith and Science must go together and not science without God if flesh without spirit!

So look from where a modern man fell and repent: Revelation 2:5 KJV Remember therefore from whence thou art fallen, and repent, and do the first works; or else I will come unto thee quickly, and will remove thy candlestick out of his place, except thou repent.

Love, Faith and Humility must accompany the modern man and highly intelligent artificial intelligence and not civilization alone!!

James 2:17,26 KJV ""Even so faith, if it hath not works, is dead, being alone. [26] For as the body without the spirit is dead, so faith without works is dead also."

This is because God has made man and formed him from dust snd His breath and all he has from Him!

In fact Lord Jesus said: man can do nothing without God:

John 15:5 KJV "—for without me ye can do nothing."

And a man must abide with the True Vine otherwise he will be withered away and be casted out !

But In order to abide on the true Vine, a man must believe in the True Vine and follow Lord Jesus commandments in love and Faith as it is written:

John 15:1-7,10-13 KJV I am the true vine, and my Father is the husbandman. [2] Every branch in me that beareth not fruit he taketh away: and every branch that beareth fruit, he purgeth it, that it may bring forth more fruit. [3] Now ye are clean through the word which I have spoken unto you. [4] Abide in me, and I in you. As the branch cannot bear fruit of itself, except it abide in the vine; no more can ye, except ye abide in me. [5] I am the vine, ye are the branches: He that abideth in me, and I in him, the same bringeth forth much fruit: for without me ye can do nothing. [6] If a man abide not in me, he is cast forth as a branch, and is withered; and men gather them, and cast them into the fire, and they are burned. [7] If ye abide in me, and my words abide in you, ye shall ask what ye will, and it shall be done unto you. [10] If ye keep my commandments, ye shall abide in my love; even as I have kept my Father's commandments, and abide in his love. [11] These things have I spoken unto you, that my joy might remain in you, and that your joy might be full. [12] This is my commandment, That ye love one another, as I have loved you. [13] Greater love hath no man than this, that a man lay down his life for his friends."

Therefore, the overwhelming results indicates the correct management strategy is Return to God and Repent as man get advanced in science and not to get pride in his accomplishment ignoring God and His commandments Jesus our Lord and Savior!

Isaiah 44:2, NIV This is what the LORD says – he who made you, who formed you in the womb, and who will help you: Do not be afraid, Jacob, my servant, Jeshurun, whom I have chosen.

Isaiah 44:21, NIV Remember these things, Jacob, for you, Israel, are my servant. I have made you, you are my servant; Israel, I will not forget you.

Isaiah 44:22, NIV I have swept away your offenses like a cloud, your sins like the morning mist. Return to me, for I have redeemed you.

Isaiah 31:6, BSB Return to the One against whom you have so blatantly rebelled, O children of Israel.

Joel 2:13, NIV Return to the LORD your God, for he is gracious and compassionate, slow to anger and abounding in love, and he relents from sending calamity.

Isaiah 1:18, ESV Come now, let us reason together, says the LORD: though your sins are like scarlet, they shall be as white as snow; though they are red like crimson, they shall become like wool.

Zechariah 1:3b Return to me,' declares the Lord Almighty, 'and I will return to you,' says the Lord of hosts

For the Lord your God is gracious and compassionate. He will not turn his face from you if you return to him. 2 Chronicles 30:9

I have swept away your offenses like a cloud,

your sins like the morning mist.

Return to me, for I have redeemed you.

Isaiah 44:22

'Return, faithless Israel,' declares the Lord,

'I will frown on you no longer,

for I am faithful,' declares the Lord,

'I will not be angry forever.'

Jeremiah 3:12bmercyangerforgiveness

"Even now," declares the Lord,

"return to me with all your heart,

with fasting and weeping and mourning."

Joel 2:12

Two are better than one,

because they have a good return for their labor.

Ecclesiastes 4:9friendshiprelationshipswork

So is my word that goes out from my mouth:

It will not return to me empty,

but will accomplish what I desire

and achieve the purpose for which I sent it.

Isaiah 55:11Word of Godspeakingreliability

Rend your heart

and not your garments.

Return to the Lord your God,

for he is gracious and compassionate,

slow to anger and abounding in love,

and he relents from sending calamity.

Joel 2:13heartgracelove

Let the wicked forsake their ways

and the unrighteous their thoughts.

Let them turn to the Lord, and he will have mercy on them,

and to our God, for he will freely pardon. Isaiah 55:7

Everyone comes naked from their mother's womb,

and as everyone comes, so they depart.

They take nothing from their toil

that they can carry in their hands. Ecclesiastes 5:15

At this, Job got up and tore his robe and shaved his head. Then he fell to the ground in worship and said:

"Naked I came from my mother's womb,

and naked I will depart.

The Lord gave and the Lord has taken away;

may the name of the Lord be praised." Job 1:20-21

I came from the Father and entered the world; now I am leaving the world and going back to the Father.

John 16:28

Jesus said, "I am with you for only a short time, and then I am going to the one who sent me." John 7:33

Since you are precious and honored in my sight,

and because I love you,

I will give people in exchange for you,

nations in exchange for your life.

Isaiah 43:4lovesalvationencouragement

But our citizenship is in heaven. And we eagerly await a Savior from there, the Lord Jesus Christ.

Philippians 3:20

What good will it be for someone to gain the whole world, yet forfeit their soul? Or what can anyone give in exchange for their soul?

Matthew 16:26materialismlifesoul

Give, and it will be given to you. A good measure, pressed down, shaken together and running over, will be poured into your lap. For with the measure you use, it will be measured to you. Luke 6:38

Do not be like your ancestors, to whom the earlier prophets proclaimed: This is what the Lord Almighty says: 'Turn from your evil ways and your evil practices.' But they would not listen or pay attention to me, declares the Lord. Zechariah 1:4

And let us consider how we may spur one another on toward love and good deeds, not giving up meeting together, as some are in the habit of doing, but encouraging one another—and all the more as you see the Day approaching.

Hebrews 10:24-25

But the one who does not know and does things deserving punishment will be beaten with few blows. From everyone who has been given much, much will be demanded; and from the one who has been entrusted with much, much more will be asked. Luke 12:48

Go back and tell Hezekiah, the ruler of my people, 'This is what the Lord, the God of your father David, says: I have heard your prayer and seen your tears; I will heal you. On the third day from now you will go up to the temple of the Lord.' 2 Kings 20:5

They were looking intently up into the sky as he was going, when suddenly two men dressed in white stood beside them. "Men of Galilee," they said, "why do you stand here looking into the sky? This same Jesus, who has been taken from you into heaven, will come back in the same way you have seen him go into heaven." Acts 1:10-11

I have fought the good fight, I have finished the race, I have kept the faith. Now there is in store for me the crown of righteousness, which the Lord, the righteous Judge, will award to me on that day—and not only to me, but also to all who have longed for his appearing. 2 Timothy 4:7-8

"Truly I tell you," Jesus replied, "no one who has left home or brothers or sisters or mother or father or children or fields for me and the gospel will fail to receive a hundred times as much in this present age: homes, brothers, sisters, mothers, children and fields—along with persecutions—and in the age to come eternal life." Mark 10:29-l

Salvation Of Human Race at Highest Risk!!

Written by Ramsis Ghaly

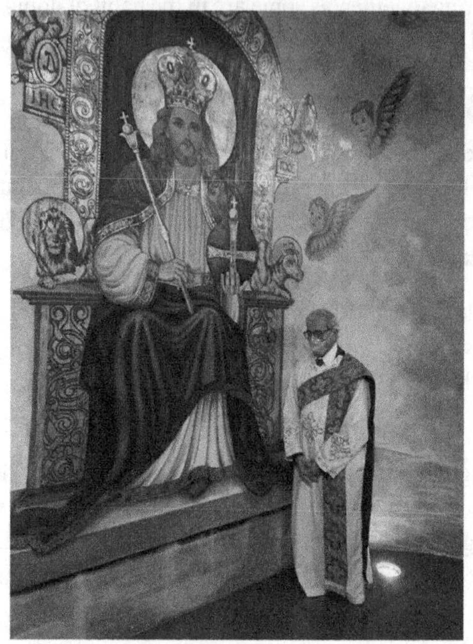

Who are those "Endure to the End shall be Saved"?

"And ye shall hear of wars and rumours of wars: see that ye be not troubled"

Examples of those spoken wars 2022/2023!!!!

-Radical Islamists against the West!

-Non-Christians against the Christians!

-White against People of colors!

-Russia againist Ukraine!

-Men against Women!

-Anti-semantics against Jews!

-Criminals against the people of nation!

-Immorals against Morals!

-Lovers of Money, Power and immorality against Humanity!

-Predators and human traffickers!

-Natural Disasters!

-Biologic and cyber-attacks!

And Satan and his demons continue committing wars against mankind born of women and his salvation in different shapes and forms!!!

Salvation of human race is at extreme risk as Satan snashing the children of The Most High from the Son of God's hand as Jesus Christ died for them to save each of human soul!

"And ye shall hear of wars and rumours of wars: see that ye be not troubled: for all these things must come to pass, but the end is not yet. [7] For nation shall rise against nation, and kingdom against kingdom: and there shall be famines, and pestilences, and earthquakes, in divers places. [8] All these are the beginning of sorrows. [9] Then shall they deliver you up to be afflicted, and shall kill you: and ye shall be hated of all nations for my name's sake. [10] And then shall many be offended, and shall betray one another, and shall hate one another. [11] And many false prophets shall rise, and shall deceive many. [12] And because iniquity shall abound, the love of many shall wax cold. [13] But he that shall endure unto the end, the same shall be saved."Matthew 24:6-13 KJV.

We aren't alone! let us run with endurance the race that is set before us, fixing our eyes on Jesus: "Therefore, since we have so great a cloud of witnesses surrounding us, let us also lay aside every encumbrance and the sin which so easily entangles us, and let us run with endurance the race that is set before us, fixing our eyes on Jesus, the author and perfecter of faith, who for the joy set before Him endured the cross, despising the shame, and has sat down at the right hand of the throne of God." Hebrews 12:1-2

Be strong in the Lord and put on the whole armour of God! For we wrestle not against flesh and blood, but against principalities, against powers, against the rulers of the darkness of this world, against spiritual wickedness in high places: "Finally, my brethren, be strong in the Lord, and in the power of his might. [11] Put on the whole armour of God, that ye may be able to stand against the wiles of the devil. [12] For we wrestle not against flesh and blood, but against principalities, against powers, against the rulers of the darkness of this world, against spiritual wickedness in high places. [13] Wherefore take unto you the whole armour of

God, that ye may be able to withstand in the evil day, and having done all, to stand. [14] Stand therefore, having your loins girt about with truth, and having on the breastplate of righteousness; [15] And your feet shod with the preparation of the gospel of peace; [16] Above all, taking the shield of faith, wherewith ye shall be able to quench all the fiery darts of the wicked. [17] And take the helmet of salvation, and the sword of the Spirit, which is the word of God: [18] Praying always with all prayer and supplication in the Spirit, and watching thereunto with all perseverance and supplication for all saints;" Ephesians 6:10-18 KJV

Humble thy self, the adversary the devil is a roaring lion seeking mankind: "Humble yourselves therefore under the mighty hand of God, that he may exalt you in due time: [7] Casting all your care upon him; for he careth for you. [8] Be sober, be vigilant; because your adversary the devil, as a roaring lion, walketh about, seeking whom he may devour: [9] Whom resist stedfast in the faith, knowing that the same afflictions are accomplished in your brethren that are in the world." 1 Peter 5:6-9 KJV

Yet count it joy: "My brethren, count it all joy when ye fall into divers temptations; [3] Knowing this, that the trying of your faith worketh patience. [4] But let patience have her perfect work, that ye may be perfect and entire, wanting nothing. [5] If any of you lack wisdom, let him ask of God, that giveth to all men liberally, and upbraideth not; and it shall be given him."James 1:2-5 KJV

"And not only so, but we glory in tribulations also: knowing that tribulation worketh patience; [4] And patience, experience; and experience, hope: [5] And hope maketh not ashamed; because the love of God is shed abroad in our hearts by the Holy Ghost which is given unto us. [6] For when we were yet without strength, in due time Christ died for the ungodly." Romans 5:3-6 KJV

"Behold, the hour cometh, yea, is now come, that ye shall be scattered, every man to his own, and shall leave me alone: and yet I am not alone, because the Father is with me. [33] These things I have spoken unto you, that in me ye might have peace. In the world ye shall have tribulation: but be of good cheer; I have overcome the world." John 16:32-33 KJV

Deuteronomy 31:8 The LORD himself goes before you and will be with you; he will never leave you nor forsake you. Do not be afraid; do not be discouraged.

Psalm 121:7 The LORD will keep you from all harm he will watch over your life.

Romans 8:28 KJV

[28] And we know that all things work together for good to them that love God, to them who are the called according to his purpose.

Psalm 9:9-10 KJV

[9] The Lord also will be a refuge for the oppressed, a refuge in times of trouble. [10] And they that know thy name will put their trust in thee: for thou, Lord, hast not forsaken them that seek thee.

"Thou art my hiding place; thou shalt preserve me from trouble; thou shalt compass me about with songs of deliverance. Selah." Psalm 32:7 KJV

James 4:4

You adulteresses, do you not know that friendship with the world is hostility toward God? Therefore whoever wishes to be a friend of the world makes himself an enemy of God.

Romans 12:2

And do not be conformed to this world, but be transformed by the renewing of your mind, so that you may prove what the will of God is, that which is good and acceptable and perfect.

1 John 2:15-17

Do not love the world nor the things in the world. If anyone loves the world, the love of the Father is not in him. For all that is in the world, the lust of the flesh and the lust of the eyes and the boastful pride of life, is not from the Father, but is from the world. The world is passing away, and also its lusts; but the one who does the will of God lives forever.

1 John 5:4

For whatever is born of God overcomes the world; and this is the victory that has overcome the world—our faith.

John 15:19-20

If you were of the world, the world would love its own; but because you are not of the world, but I chose you out of the world, because of this the world hates you. Remember the word that I said to you, 'A slave is not greater than his master.' If they persecuted Me, they will also persecute you; if they kept My word, they will keep yours also.

Matthew 5:10-12

"Blessed are those who have been persecuted for the sake of righteousness, for theirs is the kingdom of heaven. "Blessed are you when people insult you and persecute you, and falsely say all kinds of evil against you because of Me.

Rejoice and be glad, for your reward in heaven is great; for in the same way they persecuted the prophets who were before you.

Luke 6:22

Blessed are you when men hate you, and ostracize you, and insult you, and scorn your name as evil, for the sake of the Son of Man.

John 16:2

They will make you outcasts from the synagogue, but an hour is coming for everyone who kills you to think that he is offering service to God.

John 17:14

I have given them Your word; and the world has hated them, because they are not of the world, even as I am not of the world.

1 Peter 4:12-16

Beloved, do not be surprised at the fiery ordeal among you, which comes upon you for your testing, as though some strange thing were happening to you; but to the degree that you share the sufferings of Christ, keep on rejoicing, so that also at the revelation of His glory you may rejoice with exultation. If you are reviled for the name of Christ, you are blessed, because the Spirit of glory and of God rests on you.read more.

1 John 3:13

Do not be surprised, brethren, if the world hates you.

Revelation 13:7

It was also given to him to make war with the saints and to overcome them, and authority over every tribe and people and tongue and nation was given to him.

Colossians 2:8

See to it that no one takes you captive through philosophy and empty deception, according to the tradition of men, according to the elementary principles of the world, rather than according to Christ.

1 Timothy 4:1

But the Spirit explicitly says that in later times some will fall away from the faith, paying attention to deceitful spirits and doctrines of demons,

2 Timothy 4:3-4

For the time will come when they will not endure sound doctrine; but wanting to have their ears tickled, they will accumulate for themselves teachers in accordance to their own desires, and will turn away their ears from the truth and will turn aside to myths.

1 John 4:1

Beloved, do not believe every spirit, but test the spirits to see whether they are from God, because many false prophets have gone out into the world.

Revelation 13:11

Then I saw another beast coming up out of the earth; and he had two horns like a lamb and he spoke as a dragon.

Revelation 19:20

And the beast was seized, and with him the false prophet who performed the signs in his presence, by which he deceived those who had received the mark of the beast and those who worshiped his image; these two were thrown alive into the lake of fire which burns with brimstone.

1 John 2:16

For all that is in the world, the lust of the flesh and the lust of the eyes and the boastful pride of life, is not from the Father, but is from the world.

Luke 12:15

Then He said to them, "Beware, and be on your guard against every form of greed; for not even when one has an abundance does his life consist of his possessions."

2 Timothy 4:10

for Demas, having loved this present world, has deserted me and gone to Thessalonica; Crescens has gone to Galatia, Titus to Dalmatia.

Titus 2:12

instructing us to deny ungodliness and worldly desires and to live sensibly, righteously and godly in the present age,

Hebrews 11:24-25

By faith Moses, when he had grown up, refused to be called the son of Pharaoh's daughter, choosing rather to endure ill-treatment with the people of God than to enjoy the passing pleasures of sin,

Revelation 17:1-5

Then one of the seven angels who had the seven bowls came and spoke with me, saying, “Come here, I will show you the judgment of the great harlot who sits on many waters, with whom the kings of the earth committed acts of immorality, and those who dwell on the earth were made drunk with the wine of her immorality.” And he carried me away in the Spirit into a wilderness; and I saw a woman sitting on a scarlet beast, full of blasphemous names, having seven heads and ten horns. read more.

Galatians 5:17

For the flesh sets its desire against the Spirit, and the Spirit against the flesh; for these are in opposition to one another, so that you may not do the things that you please.

1 Peter 2:11

Beloved, I urge you as aliens and strangers to abstain from fleshly lusts which wage war against the soul.

Romans 6:12

Therefore do not let sin reign in your mortal body so that you obey its lusts,

Romans 7:14-23

For we know that the Law is spiritual, but I am of flesh, sold into bondage to sin. For what I am doing, I do not understand; for I am not practicing what I would like to do, but I am doing the very thing I hate. But if I do the very thing I do not want to do, I agree with the Law, confessing that the Law is good.read more.

Romans 8:13

for if you are living according to the flesh, you must die; but if by the Spirit you are putting to death the deeds of the body, you will live.

Galatians 5:24

Now those who belong to Christ Jesus have crucified the flesh with its passions and desires.

Colossians 3:5

Therefore consider the members of your earthly body as dead to immorality, impurity, passion, evil desire, and greed, which amounts to idolatry.

Hebrews 12:4

You have not yet resisted to the point of shedding blood in your striving against sin;

James 4:1

What is the source of quarrels and conflicts among you? Is not the source your pleasures that wage war in your members?

1 Peter 5:8

Be of sober spirit, be on the alert. Your adversary, the devil, prowls around like a roaring lion, seeking someone to devour.

Matthew 13:39

and the enemy who sowed them is the devil, and the harvest is the end of the age; and the reapers are angels.

Mark 4:15

These are the ones who are beside the road where the word is sown; and when they hear, immediately Satan comes and takes away the word which has been sown in them.

Luke 8:12

Those beside the road are those who have heard; then the devil comes and takes away the word from their heart, so that they will not believe and be saved.

John 17:15

I do not ask You to take them out of the world, but to keep them from the evil one.

2 Thessalonians 3:3

But the Lord is faithful, and He will strengthen and protect you from the evil one.

Revelation 2:10

Do not fear what you are about to suffer. Behold, the devil is about to cast some of you into prison, so that you will be tested, and you will have tribulation for ten days. Be faithful until death, and I will give you the crown of life.

Revelation 12:17

So the dragon was enraged with the woman, and went off to make war with the rest of her children, who keep the commandments of God and hold to the testimony of Jesus.

1 Thessalonians 3:5

For this reason, when I could endure it no longer, I also sent to find out about your faith, for fear that the tempter might have tempted you, and our labor would be in vain.

Genesis 3:1-6

Now the serpent was more crafty than any beast of the field which the Lord God had made. And he said to the woman, "Indeed, has God said, 'You shall not eat from any tree of the garden'?" The woman said to the serpent, From the fruit of the trees of the garden we may eat; but from the fruit of the tree which is in the middle of the garden, God has said, You shall not eat from it or touch it, or you will die.read more.

Hebrews 2:18

For since He Himself was tempted in that which He has suffered, He is able to come to the aid of those who are tempted.

Hebrews 4:15

For we do not have a high priest who cannot sympathize with our weaknesses, but One who has been tempted in all things as we are, yet without sin.

2 Corinthians 11:3

But I am afraid that, as the serpent deceived Eve by his craftiness, your minds will be led astray from the simplicity and purity of devotion to Christ.

Revelation 12:9

And the great dragon was thrown down, the serpent of old who is called the devil and Satan, who deceives the whole world; he was thrown down to the earth, and his angels were thrown down with him.

Genesis 3:13

Then the Lord God said to the woman, "What is this you have done?" And the woman said, "The serpent deceived me, and I ate."

2 Corinthians 2:11

so that no advantage would be taken of us by Satan, for we are not ignorant of his schemes.

2 Corinthians 4:4

in whose case the god of this world has blinded the minds of the unbelieving so that they might not see the light of the gospel of the glory of Christ, who is the image of God.

2 Corinthians 11:4

For if one comes and preaches another Jesus whom we have not preached, or you receive a different spirit which you have not received, or a different gospel which you have not accepted, you bear this beautifully.

Revelation 20:3

and he threw him into the abyss, and shut it and sealed it over him, so that he would not deceive the nations any longer, until the thousand years were completed; after these things he must be released for a short time.

Revelation 12:10

Then I heard a loud voice in heaven, saying,"Now the salvation, and the power, and the kingdom of our God and the authority of His Christ have come, for the accuser of our brethren has been thrown down, he who accuses them before our God day and night.

Job 1:9-11

Then Satan answered the Lord, "Does Job fear God for nothing? Have You not made a hedge about him and his house and all that he has, on every side? You have blessed the work of his hands, and his possessions have increased in the land. But put forth Your hand now and touch all that he has; he will surely curse You to Your face."

Zechariah 3:1

Then he showed me Joshua the high priest standing before the angel of the Lord, and Satan standing at his right hand to accuse him.

Let us pray for the Coptic Christians of Egypt 8 14 2022!

A huge causality by fire during mass at Abu Sofan church Giza, Egypt with 41 killed including Bishop and children. Churches must have a permit with huge restriction. More than 5000 people condensed in a small size church because government won't allow larger size to be build. Let us pray for the Coptic Christians of Egypt, my home country! They are persecuted, suppressed and oppressed and living for thousand and half years as minority with extreme unfair Islamic government restriction!!!

https://www.washingtonpost.com/.../egypt-church-fire-copt/

https://news-middleeast.churchofjesuschrist.org/.../condo...

https://www.bbc.com/news/world-middle-east-62555127.amp

https://www.aljazeera.com/.../egyptians-mourn-41-killed...

https://www.wsj.com/.../fire-kills-at-least-41-at...

https://www.nytimes.com/.../egypt-church-fire-children...

Ramsis Ghaly

NYTIMES.COM

Coptic Leader Criticizes Egypt's Building Restrictions on Churches After Deadly Fire

The patriarch of Egypt's 10 million Coptic Orthodox Christians said his community has been squeezed by decades of government regulations on the number and size of churches. In Sunday's blaze, 41 people died.

Today we remember the Christian persecution worldwide especially in the Middle East. You aren't forgotten. We pray to our Lord Jesus in this Great Lent to remember their souls and their family left behind Amen Lord Jesus!

April, 1 2018 post

The worst ever slow Holocaust of history of mankind since the creation, of my people the Middle East Christians by the Islamic sword of brutality from the fifth century to the twenty one century and still going, ignored by all and buried by all

Ramsis Ghaly

It is one of darkest history of human race that in the history book and at day of Judgment will ashame all the living and those responsible and those that could have done something and didn't do —

Why the entire world covered up and not even one extended the hand to my people the Christians of the Middle East?

So Many posts I wrote since 2014 and yet millions of Christians all alone killed by the Islamic swords and The most painful facts of how My people the Christians of the Middle East killed, exterminated and graved in alive and brutal burial

Tragically, Christians living in lands have been betrayed by many in the West.

Governments ignored their tragic fate. Bishops were often too aloof to denounce their persecution. Popes entertained to support politics and failed to speak up identifying the enemy.

The media acted as if they considered these Christians deserved to be purged from the Middle East.

And the so-called "human rights" organizations abandoned them.

The West was not willing to give sanctuary to these Christians when ISIS murdered 1,131 of them and destroyed or damaged 125 of their churches.

Persecution of Christians is worse today "than at any time in history", a recent report by the organization Aid to the Church in Need revealed.

"elimination" of Christians from the pages of history.

Discovered a mass grave with the bodies of Christians, The bodies, including those of women and children, Many had crosses with them in the mass grave.

Not a single article in the Western mainstream media wrote about this ethnic cleansing.

French Chief Rabbi Haim Korsia made an urgent plea to Europe and the West to defend non-Muslims in the Middle East, whom he likened to Holocaust victims. "As our parents wore the yellow star, Christians are made to wear the scarlet letter of nun" Korsia said. The Hebrew letter "nun" is the same sound as the beginning of Nazareen, an Arabic term signifying people from Nazareth,

A "slow genocide", which is shattering those ancient communities to the point of their disappearance. The numbers are significant.

According to the report, 81% of Christians have disappeared "extinction of Christians"."Christianity will disappear".

Many ancient Christian churches and sites have been destroyed

And many more——-

New Era of Targeting Nurses and Doctors as Criminals and Deserve Death!!

Written by Ramsis Ghaly

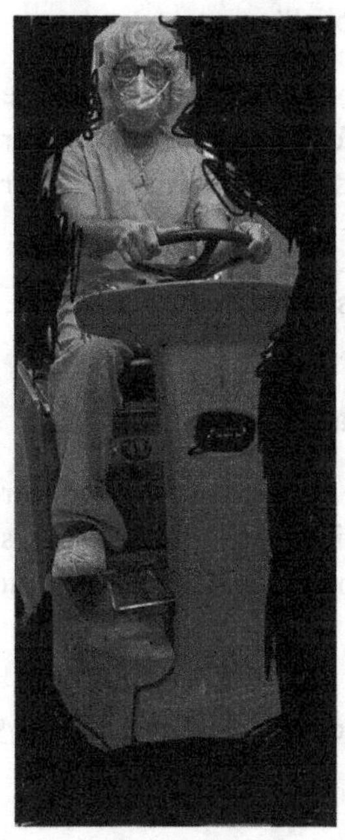

Nurses and doctors are currently targeted violently sentenced as criminals and shot killed for revenge!

Public frustration including uprise mental health and enragement has revealed itself by retaliation against doctors and nurses and both doctors and nurses are finding themselves with no help or protection totally exposed.

All healthcare facilities immediately must take steps to protect themselves and all employees against such atrocities!! The public must understand, their frustration with healthcare system and premium aren't caused by doctors and nurses!!

The senate and congress including AMA and healthcare organizations must convene and address the uprise in criminalities against healthcare providers!

Doctors and nurses are in the frontline all alone unprotected while healthcare administration and healthcare insurances are in the backfire!

Although nurses and doctors are the owners of healthcare, yet they actually aren't. They are treated as a regular employee working for big corporate run as factories!

Doctors and nurses are held in the highest standard and fully responsible of their patients and outcomes. The public frustration of healthcare insurance abuse, enragement, and denials, high premium, healthcare abuses, mental health crises ——-, nurses and physicians are paying the price costly including their own lives for the frustration of the public!!!

What is the real message, patients are fed up and regardless of how unfair the doctors and nurses are!! Yet doctors and nurses are viewed as the owner of healthcare and fully responsible of patients and their outcome! And NO no one else!

There is a reason that doctors and nurses are so visible, and their offices are known but others aren't.

A new era targeting nurses and doctors!!

I wonder American medical association and healthcare organizations continue to ignore and not to protect their own doctors and nurses! When they will step up to put a stop against the criminal atrocities against doctors and nurses!!!

Nurse sentenced to jail

https://www.medpagetoday.com/special.../exclusives/98706....

Surgeon killed by gunshot

https://apple.news/A_gLmive7TQqahFG5mpExQQ

https://www.thedailybeast.com/tulsa-mass-shooter...

THEDAILYBEAST.COM

Enraged Patient Bought Gun 3 Hours Before Tulsa Hospital Massacre

Michael Louis, 45, killed four people and himself after complaining repeatedly about back pain following surgery, Tulsa police said.

The world is Entering into the Cascade of Wars Trapped unto The Classic Vicious Cycle!!

Ghaly's Historic World Vicious Cycle!!
Written On 4/16/2022 by Ramsis Ghaly

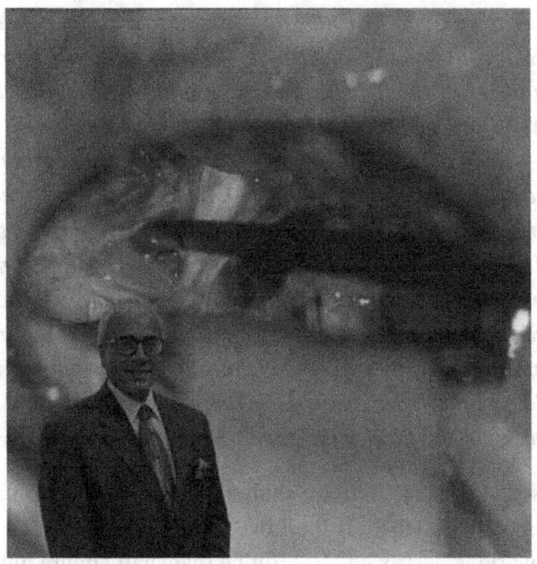

Since the human race decent to earth, the wars never stopped and a close unbiased objective look, it reveals the consistent pattern of the classic vicious cycle of destruction. as established since the first war between the two only brothers Cain against Abel where Cain slew his only brother Abel!! Genesis 4:7-8 KJV "If thou doest well, shalt thou not be accepted? and if thou doest not well, sin lieth at the door. And unto thee shall be his desire, and thou shalt rule over him. [8] And Cain talked with Abel his brother: and it came to pass, when they were in the field, that Cain rose up against Abel his brother, and slew him."

And now the world is going down in that vicious evil cascade!! The current equation promotes more killing of human lives and murdering people that won't come back!

"Ghaly' Historic Vicious Cycle of Getting to Wars"

More weapons are handed to Ukrainians —lead to more Russian's causalities —lead to more Russian's anger —lead to more Ukrainian's causalities —lead to more Ukrainian's, NATO's and America's anger —lead to more supply of weapons to Ukraine— lead to more Russian's causalities— lead to more Russian's anger— lead to more Russian's artilleries against Ukrainian— lead to more Ukrainian's causalities —lead to more Ukrainian's, NATO's and America's anger— lead to more supply of weapons to Ukraine—lead to more Russian's causalities —lead to more Russian's anger———ultimately lead to World War and Nuclear missiles —lead to world's causalities—-lead to the worst Holocaust of the world———End Point will be reached when significant numbers of those behind the original war die and those involved in the war die —-new generation lead to —-new breed—-new breed lead to —-new minds— lead to to new thinkers—-Lessons learned and regrets— War Memorials and commemorations—-new historic promises—-peace and build up—- build up—- man's rise against God and his Christ—man's grandiose and greatness and self interest grow back— Love of power and money grow—— world abundance of treasures and self lusts——disputes and conflicts arise again —- seeds of new war—- grow slowly until one day burst again and beginning of another world———the vicious cycle continues as long as Satan leads the world and the final stop will be the mark of the end of the world for man's kingdom upon the face of the earth the planet in the universe!!!

It is all because "—because iniquity shall abound, the love of many shall wax cold." Where is the wise where is the Love? And no winners and everyone lost and the entire world is destroyed. —-"But he that shall endure unto the end, the same shall be saved."

So "Where is the wise? where is the scribe? where is the disputer of this world? hath not God made foolish the wisdom of this world?" —-For after that in the wisdom of God the world by wisdom knew not God, it pleased God by the foolishness of preaching to save them that believe. [22] For the Jews require a sign, and the Greeks seek after wisdom: [23] But we preach Christ crucified, unto the Jews a stumblingblock, and unto the Greeks foolishness; [24] But unto them which are called, both Jews and Greeks, Christ the power of God, and the wisdom of God. [25] Because the foolishness of God is wiser than men; and the weakness of God is stronger than men. [26] For ye see your calling, brethren, how that not many wise men after the flesh, not many mighty, not many noble, are called : [27] But God hath chosen the foolish things of the world to confound the wise; and God hath chosen the weak things of the world to confound the things which are mighty; [28] And base things of the world, and things which are despised, hath God chosen, yea, and things which are not, to bring to nought things that are: [29]

That no flesh should glory in his presence. [30] But of him are ye in Christ Jesus, who of God is made unto us wisdom, and righteousness, and sanctification, and redemption: [31] That, according as it is written, He that glorieth, let him glory in the Lord." 1 Corinthians 1:20-31 KJV

It is all written in the Bible as the words of our Lord Jesus said it all:

Matthew 24 "And Jesus said unto them, See ye not all these things? verily I say unto you, There shall not be left here one stone upon another, that shall not be thrown down. [4] And Jesus answered and said unto them, Take heed that no man deceive you. [5] For many shall come in my name, saying, I am Christ; and shall deceive many. [6] And ye shall hear of wars and rumours of wars: see that ye be not troubled: for all these things must come to pass, but the end is not yet. [7] For nation shall rise against nation, and kingdom against kingdom: and there shall be famines, and pestilences, and earthquakes, in divers places. [8] All these are the beginning of sorrows. [9] Then shall they deliver you up to be afflicted, and shall kill you: and ye shall be hated of all nations for my name's sake. [10] And then shall many be offended, and shall betray one another, and shall hate one another. [11] And many false prophets shall rise, and shall deceive many. [12] And because iniquity shall abound, the love of many shall wax cold. [13] But he that shall endure unto the end, the same shall be saved. [14] And this gospel of the kingdom shall be preached in all the world for a witness unto all nations; and then shall the end come. [15] When ye therefore shall see the abomination of desolation, spoken of by Daniel the prophet, stand in the holy place, (whoso readeth, let him understand:) [16] Then let them which be in Judaea flee into the mountains: [17] Let him which is on the housetop not come down to take any thing out of his house: [18] Neither let him which is in the field return back to take his clothes. [19] And woe unto them that are with child, and to them that give suck in those days! [20] But pray ye that your flight be not in the winter, neither on the sabbath day: [21] For then shall be great tribulation, such as was not since the beginning of the world to this time, no, nor ever shall be. [22] And except those days should be shortened, there should no flesh be saved: but for the elect's sake those days shall be shortened. [23] Then if any man shall say unto you, Lo, here is Christ, or there; believe it not. [24] For there shall arise false Christs, and false prophets, and shall shew great signs and wonders; insomuch that, if it were possible, they shall deceive the very elect. [25] Behold, I have told you before. [26] Wherefore if they shall say unto you, Behold, he is in the desert; go not forth: behold, he is in the secret chambers; believe it not. [27] For as the lightning cometh out of the east, and shineth even unto the west; so shall also the coming of the Son of man be. [28] For wheresoever the carcase is, there will the eagles be gathered together. [29] Immediately after the tribulation of those days shall the sun be darkened, and the moon shall not give her light, and the stars shall fall from heaven, and the powers of the heavens shall be shaken: [30] And then shall appear the sign of the Son of man in heaven: and then shall all the tribes of the earth mourn, and they shall see the Son of man coming in the clouds of heaven with power and great glory. [31] And he shall send his angels with a great sound of a trumpet, and they shall gather together his elect from the four winds, from one end of heaven to the other. [32] Now learn a parable of the fig tree; When his branch is yet tender, and putteth forth leaves, ye know that summer is nigh: [33] So likewise ye, when ye shall see all these things, know that it is near, even at the doors. [34] Verily I say unto you, This generation shall not pass, till all these things be fulfilled. [35] Heaven and earth shall pass away, but my words shall not pass away. [36] But of that day and hour knoweth no man, no, not the angels of heaven, but my Father only. [37] But as the days of Noe were, so shall also the coming of the Son of man be. [38] For as in the days that were before the flood they were eating and drinking, marrying and giving in marriage, until the day that Noe entered into the ark, [39] And knew not until the flood came, and took them all away; so shall also the coming of the Son of man be. [40] Then shall two be in the field; the one shall be taken, and the other left. [41] Two women shall be grinding at the mill; the one shall be taken, and the other left. [42] Watch therefore: for ye know not what hour your Lord doth come."

JT, Amen Ramsis...we need a divine intervention

CG, The problem is people have turned their back on God. I pray they look to God He is our only hope to survive world destruction

Where is the Wisdom in this Critical Time?

Written on 8/5/2022 by Ramsis Ghaly

If thy wish to ignite fires and stir more wars in this highly polarized time, be adversary and take a Round Trip from JF Kennedy USA airport to China —to Taiwan —to Ukraine —to Russia and back to USA !!!

"Ye cannot drink the cup of the Lord, and the cup of devils: ye cannot be partakers of the Lord's table, and of the table of devils. [22] Do we provoke the Lord to jealousy? are we stronger than he? [23] All things are lawful for me, but all things are not expedient: all things are lawful for me, but all things edify not. [24] Let no man seek his own, but every man another's wealth."1 Corinthians 10:21-24 KJV

Ramsis Ghaly

JD, What about it? Not seriously thinking about it I hope

JT, she antagonized with purpose...

CR, There are some very smart people out there who refuse to see the truth in the lack of morals and soundness in our politicians. I believe many of them are doing nothing because they are still lining their pockets. It's time to make those who refuse to follow the laws of our land or to do what's right for the American people.

So Many Modern Conspirators Do Not Want to Know God But Want to Play as gods!! So Many Attacks On Christian Faith and Values Under the name of Science and Politics Threatening

Humanity as the Good God Has Created!
Written on 8/27/2022 by Ramsis Ghaly

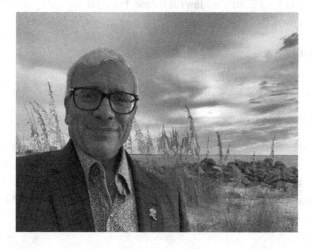

So Many Attacks On Christian Faith and Values Under the name of Science and Politics Threatening Manipulating Humanity as the Good God Has Created!

"You, Lord, in the beginning laid the foundation of the earth, And the heavens are the works of Your hands" Hebrews 1:10 John 1:1-5 KJV "In the beginning was the Word, and the Word was with God, and the Word was God. [2] The same was in the beginning with God. [3] All things were made by him; and without him was not any thing made that was made. [4] In him was life; and the life was the light of men. [5] And the light shineth in darkness; and the darkness comprehended it not."Genesis 1:1-4,31 KJV "In the beginning God created the heaven and the earth. [2] And the earth was without form, and void; and darkness was upon the face of the deep. And the Spirit of God moved upon the face of the waters. [3] And God said, Let there be light: and there was light. [4] And God saw the light, that it was good: and God divided the light from the darkness. [31] And God saw every thing that he had made, and, behold, it was very good. And the evening and the morning were the sixth day."

So Many Attacks On Christian Faith and Values Under the name of Science and Politics Threatening Manipulating Humanity as the Good God Has Created!

Play with minds of naïve, immature, gullible and destroy their innocence and created nature with fantasy of technology controlled hands off self-centered egocentric self served grandiose minds to enslave the world!

World Refusal to God

As the world refused Him back then and so is now. As many received Him Not back then and do is today as it is written: John 1:10-11 KJV "He was in the world, and the world was made by him, and the world knew him not. [11] He came unto his own, and his own received him not."

They are threatening humanity and trying to change the creation as God has created.

They are threatening humanity and trying to change the creation as God has created. They are searching to be God but not to know God through His hand made creation.

They are working to diminish God, promoting their self-interest image and their own agenda while working against God:

-Redefining a man and woman, male and female, husband and wife and father and no they! Each human being has a defined sex chromosome for male and female and nothing in between or a human being existed without sec chromosome or another set of chromosomes. There is no deviation since foundation of earth and first man and woman! The destructive storms and playing with minds are huge!

- Clone human genes to segregate and manufacture new man and cultivate certain population strains with certain minds!

- Control the world and override whoever defend righteousness and silence whoever stands in their way!

- Promote lusts and deepen satanic thoughts and deeds in their doctrine!

- Beliefs that they are able to create and change the universe!

- Take the control and power from God to hand-man made artificial intelligence!

_ Conspire upon God the Lord and his Christ and dimmish Him among His People! As it is written by Psalmist: Psalm 2:1-3 KJV "Why do the heathen rage, and the people imagine a vain thing? [2] The kings of the earth set themselves, and the rulers take counsel together, against the Lord, and against his anointed, saying, [3] Let us break their bands asunder, and cast away their cords from us."

- Brain washing the new generation and innocent minds attracting them to their own snashing them from the hands of God

- Grandios human minds and enthusiasm believe one day they shall concur the forces and established laws and be able to have total control upon the universe and alter the establish dynamics and control the day to day the universe and everything inside and out with no limits!

- And endless evil hidden goals setting a target to accomplish!

Through these deviations of how God created and established humanity, they are forgetting that all things are created by God, for God and with God. Indeed, their brains and minds are created by God, and they have zero capability to create by their own!

Nonetheless, It is all about

No God but Them

Total Control

Power

Money

And more to come

False Christs!

False scientists!

False Prophets!

Matthew 24:10-12,15,21-26,29-30 KJV "And then shall many be offended, and shall betray one another, and shall hate one another. [11] And many false prophets shall rise, and shall deceive many. [12] And because iniquity shall abound, the love of many shall wax cold. [15] When ye therefore shall see the abomination of desolation, spoken of by Daniel the prophet, stand in the holy place, (whoso readeth, let him understand:) [21] For then shall be great tribulation, such as was not since the beginning of the world to this time, no, nor ever shall be. [22] And except those days should be shortened, there should no flesh be saved: but for the elect's sake those days shall be shortened. [23] Then if any man shall say unto you, Lo, here is Christ, or there; believe it not. [24] For there shall arise false Christs, and false prophets, and shall shew great signs and wonders; insomuch that, if it were possible, they shall deceive the very elect. [25] Behold, I have told you before. [26] Wherefore if they shall say unto you, Behold, he is in the desert; go not forth: behold, he is in the secret chambers; believe it not. [29] Immediately after the tribulation of those days shall the sun be darkened, and the moon shall not give her light, and the stars shall fall from heaven, and the powers of the heavens shall be shaken: [30] And then shall appear the sign of the Son of man in heaven: and then shall all the tribes of the earth mourn, and they shall see the Son of man coming in the clouds of heaven with power and great glory"

But as many believe in Him those are the sons and daughters of God full of grace and truth as it is written: John 1:12-14 KJV "But as many as received him, to them gave he power to become the sons of God, even to them that believe on his name: [13] Which were born, not of blood, nor of the will of the flesh, nor of the will of man, but of God. [14] And the Word was made flesh, and dwelt among us, (and we beheld his glory, the glory as of the only begotten of the Father,) full of grace and truth."

God created mankind in His image and gave Him power to be the children of God and now they themselves want to be gods! Furthermore, they are working in cellular levels to manipulate the creation to their interest and form hand man living souls!!

Genesis 1:27-28 KJV "So God created man in his own image, in the image of God created he him; male and female created he them. [28] And God blessed them, and God said unto them, Be fruitful, and multiply, and replenish the earth, and subdue it: and have dominion over the fish of the sea, and over the fowl of the air, and over every living thing that moveth upon the earth." Genesis 5:2 KJV "Male and female created he them; and blessed them, and called their name Adam, in the day when they were created." Mark 10:5-9 KJV "And Jesus answered and said unto them, For the hardness of your heart he wrote you this precept. [6] But from the beginning of the creation God made them male and female. [7] For this cause shall a man leave his father and mother, and cleave to his wife; [8] And they twain shall be one flesh: so then they are no more twain, but one flesh. [9] What therefore God hath joined together, let not man put asunder."

Historic Satanic man attempts to be as gods since Adam and Eve Time!!

The very first independence deed and disobedience of man to God is his false grandiosity to be god! The evil mind wants to be god and take godhood from the True God and be false Ruler. The end result he was thrown with Satan to hill and became nothing but dust and ashes!! Genesis 3:4-8 KJV "And the serpent said unto the woman, Ye shall not surely die: [5] For God doth know that in the day ye eat thereof, then your eyes shall be opened, and ye shall be as gods, knowing good and evil. [6] And when the woman saw that the tree was good for food, and that it was pleasant to the eyes, and a tree to be desired to make one wise, she took of the fruit thereof, and did eat, and gave also unto her husband with her; and he did eat. [7] And the eyes of them both were opened, and they knew that they were naked; and they sewed fig leaves together, and made themselves aprons. [8] And they heard the voice of the Lord God walking in the garden in the cool of the day: and Adam and his wife hid themselves from the presence of the Lord God amongst the trees of the garden."

The history indeed repeat itself as in the Babel time when mankind wanted to be as high as God in heaven and attempt to create a tower to reach provoked God anger and brought man to nothing and dispersed their power : Genesis 11:4-9 KJV "And they said, Go to, let us build us a city and a tower, whose top may reach unto heaven; and let us make us a name, lest we be scattered abroad upon the face of the whole earth. [5] And the Lord came down to see the city and the tower, which the children of men builded. [6] And the Lord said, Behold, the people is one, and they have all one language; and this they begin to do: and now nothing will be restrained from them, which they have imagined to do. [7] Go to, let us go down, and there confound their language, that they may not understand one another's speech. [8] So the Lord scattered them abroad from thence upon the face of all the earth: and they left off to build the city. [9] Therefore is the name of it called Babel; because the Lord did there confound the language of all the earth: and from thence did the Lord scatter them abroad upon the face of all the earth."

But what to expect, it shouldn't come to surprise since the prince of this world is Satan: John 14:30-31 KJV "Hereafter I will not talk much with you: for the prince of this world cometh, and hath nothing in me. [31] But that the world may know that I love the Father; and as the Father gave me commandment, even so I do. Arise, let us go hence.

The righteous Christians and Humanity aren't from the World

The righteous Christians and Humanity aren't from the World and Lord Jesus always pray for them "to keep them from evil" and evil ideology, doctrine and thoughts. Out Hod in His last lengthy prayers to the Heavenly Father promised to protect man as He created and Humanity as He outlined it: John 17:9,12-21,23-26 KJV "I pray for them: I pray not for the world, but for them which thou hast given me; for they are thine. [12] While I was with them in the world, I kept them in thy name: those that thou gavest me I have kept, and none of them is lost, but the son of perdition; that the scripture might be fulfilled. [13] And now come I to thee; and these things I speak in the world, that they might have my joy fulfilled in themselves. [14] I have given them thy word; and the world hath hated them, because they are not of the world, even as I am not of the world. [15] I pray not that thou shouldest take them out of the world, but that thou shouldest keep them from the evil. [16] They are not of the world, even as I am not of the world. [17] Sanctify them through thy truth: thy word is truth. [18] As thou hast sent me into the world, even so have I also sent them into the world. [19] And for their sakes I sanctify myself, that they also might be sanctified through the truth. [20] Neither pray I for these alone, but for them also which shall believe on me through their word; [21] That they all may be one; as thou, Father, art in me, and I in thee, that they also may be one in us: that the world may believe that thou hast sent me. [23] I in them, and thou in me, that they may be made perfect in one; and that the world may know that thou hast sent me, and hast loved them, as thou hast loved me. [24] Father, I will that they also, whom thou hast given me, be with me where I am; that they may behold my glory, which thou hast given me: for thou lovedst me before the foundation of the world. [25] O righteous Father, the world hath not known thee: but I have known thee, and these have known that thou hast sent me. [26] And I have declared unto them thy name, and will declare it : that the love wherewith thou hast loved me may be in them, and I in them."

That sitteth in the heavens shall laugh: the Lord shall have them in derision!

Psalm 2:4-12 KJV "He that sitteth in the heavens shall laugh: the Lord shall have them in derision. [5] Then shall he speak unto them in his wrath, and vex them in his sore displeasure. [6] Yet have I set my king upon my holy hill of Zion. [7] I will declare the decree: the Lord hath said unto me, Thou art my Son; this day have I begotten thee. [8] Ask of me, and I shall give thee the heathen for thine inheritance, and the uttermost parts of the earth for thy possession. [9] Thou shalt break them with a rod of iron; thou shalt dash them in pieces like a potter's vessel. [10] Be wise now therefore, O ye kings: be instructed, ye judges of the earth. [11] Serve the Lord with fear, and rejoice with trembling. [12] Kiss the Son, lest he be angry, and ye perish from the way, when his wrath is kindled but a little. Blessed are all they that put their trust in him."

God will always protect mankind and humanity as He created and not as Satan tries to disrupt the human race and confuse His hand-made and attack His Own Children!

But what they failed to calculate is that Christ that they are against much stronger than they all are and their tricks and manipulation and innumerable offenses!

“I have told you these things, so that in me you may have peace. In this world you will have trouble. But take heart! I have overcome the world.” John 16:33

“Do not be overcome by evil, but overcome evil with good.” Romans 12:21

“For no word from God will ever fail.” Luke 1:37

“For everyone born of God overcomes the world. This is the victory that has overcome the world, even our faith.” 1 John 5:4

“But thanks be to God! He gives us the victory through our Lord Jesus Christ.” 1 Corinthians 15:57

“No, in all these things we are more than conquerors through him who loved us.” Romans 8:37

“But you, Lord, are a shield around me, my glory, the One who lifts my head high.” Psalm 3:3

“Therefore, since we are surrounded by such a great cloud of witnesses, let us throw off everything that hinders and the sin that so easily entangles. And let us run with perseverance the race marked out for us.” Hebrews 12:1

“The light shines in the darkness, and the darkness has not overcome it.” John 1:5

“Fight the good fight of the faith. Take hold of the eternal life to which you were called when you made your good confession in the presence of many witnesses.” 1 Timothy 6:12

“Be alert and of sober mind. Your enemy the devil prowls around like a roaring lion looking for someone to devour.” 1 Peter 5:8

“You, dear children, are from God and have overcome them, because the one who is in you is greater than the one who is in the world.” 1 John 4:4

“Who is it that overcomes the world? Only the one who believes that Jesus is the Son of God.” 1 John 5:5

“To the one who is victorious, I will give the right to sit with me on my throne, just as I was victorious and sat down with my Father on his throne.” Revelation 3:21

“The one who is victorious will, like them, be dressed in white. I will never blot out the name of that person from the book of life, but will acknowledge that name before my Father and his angels.” Revelation 3:5

"Lord, save us! Lord, grant us success! Blessed is he who comes in the name of the Lord. From the house of the Lord we bless you." Psalm 118:25-26

Rejoice greatly, Daughter Zion! Shout, Daughter Jerusalem! See, your king comes to you, righteous and victorious, lowly and riding on a donkey, on a colt, the foal of a donkey." Zechariah 9:9

What to Do!

"Pure religion and undefiled before God and the Father is this, To visit the fatherless and widows in their affliction, and to keep himself unspotted from the world." James 1:27 KJV

-Keep thyself Unspotted

-God is In- Control

-Believe Not: "But he that shall endure unto the end, the same shall be saved. [22] And except those days should be shortened, there should no flesh be saved: but for the elect's sake those days shall be shortened. [23] Then if any man shall say unto you, Lo, here is Christ, or there; believe it not." Matthew 24:13,22-23 KJV

-Endure to the End!

No Worries, Jesus Our Lord is far stronger than all of those antichrist and anti His teachings:

Isaiah 41:10 ESV "Fear not, for I am with you; be not dismayed, for I am your God; I will strengthen you, I will help you, I will uphold you with my righteous right hand."

1 Corinthians 1:25 ESV "For the foolishness of God is wiser than men, and the weakness of God is stronger than men."

1 Chronicles 16:11 ESV "Seek the Lord and his strength; seek his presence continually!"

Exodus 15:2 ESV "The Lord is my strength and my song, and he has become my salvation; this is my God, and I will praise him, my father's God, and I will exalt him."

1 Peter 4:11 ESV "Whoever speaks, as one who speaks oracles of God; whoever serves, as one who serves by the strength that God supplies—in order that in

everything God may be glorified through Jesus Christ. To him belong glory and dominion forever and ever. Amen."

Philippians 4:13 ESV "I can do all things through him who strengthens me."

John 16:33 ESV "I have said these things to you, that in me you may have peace. In the world you will have tribulation. But take heart; I have overcome the world."

2 Thessalonians 3:3 ESV "But the Lord is faithful. He will establish you and guard you against the evil one."

1 Corinthians 10:13 ESV "No temptation has overtaken you that is not common to man. God is faithful, and he will not let you be tempted beyond your ability, but with the temptation he will also provide the way of escape, that you may be able to endure it."

Psalm 46:1-3 ESV "To the choirmaster. Of the Sons of Korah. According to Alamoth. A Song. God is our refuge and strength, a very present help in trouble. Therefore we will not fear though the earth gives way, though the mountains be moved into the heart of the sea, though its waters roar and foam, though the mountains tremble at its swelling. Selah

Psalm 28:7 ESV "The Lord is my strength and my shield; in him my heart trusts, and I am helped; my heart exults, and with my song I give thanks to him."

2 Timothy 4:17 ESV "But the Lord stood by me and strengthened me, so that through me the message might be fully proclaimed and all the Gentiles might hear it. So I was rescued from the lion's mouth."

Nehemiah 8:10 ESV "Then he said to them, "Go your way. Eat the fat and drink sweet wine and send portions to anyone who has nothing ready, for this day is holy to our Lord. And do not be grieved, for the joy of the Lord is your strength."

Ephesians 6:10 ESV "Finally, be strong in the Lord and in the strength of his might."

2 Corinthians 12:9 ESV "But he said to me, "My grace is sufficient for you, for my power is made perfect in weakness." Therefore I will boast all the more gladly of my weaknesses, so that the power of Christ may rest upon me."

Luke 10:27 ESV "And he answered, "You shall love the Lord your God with all your heart and with all your soul and with all your strength and with all your mind, and your neighbor as yourself."

Psalm 73:26 ESV "My flesh and my heart may fail, but God is the strength of my heart and my portion forever."

Psalm 29:11 ESV "May the Lord give strength to his people! May the Lord bless his people with peace!"

Deuteronomy 31:6 ESV "Be strong and courageous. Do not fear or be in dread of them, for it is the Lord your God who goes with you. He will not leave you or forsake you."

Genesis 2:24 ESV "Therefore a man shall leave his father and his mother and hold fast to his wife, and they shall become one flesh."

1 Peter 2:1-25 ESV "So put away all malice and all deceit and hypocrisy and envy and all slander. Like newborn infants, long for the pure spiritual milk, that by it you may grow up into salvation— if indeed you have tasted that the Lord is good. As you come to him, a living stone rejected by men but in the sight of God chosen and precious, you yourselves like living stones are being built up as a spiritual house, to be a holy priesthood, to offer spiritual sacrifices acceptable to God through Jesus Christ. ..."

Matthew 17:20 ESV "He said to them, "Because of your little faith. For truly, I say to you, if you have faith like a grain of mustard seed, you will say to this mountain, 'Move from here to there,' and it will move, and nothing will be impossible for you."

Isaiah 40:31 ESV "But they who wait for the Lord shall renew their strength; they shall mount up with wings like eagles; they shall run and not be weary; they shall walk and not faint."

Isaiah 40:29 ESV "He gives power to the faint, and to him who has no might he increases strength."

Isaiah 40:28-31 ESV "Have you not known? Have you not heard? The Lord is the everlasting God, the Creator of the ends of the earth. He does not faint or grow weary; his understanding is unsearchable. He gives power to the faint, and to him who has no might he increases strength. Even youths shall faint and be weary, and young men shall fall exhausted; but they who wait for the Lord shall renew their strength; they shall mount up with wings like eagles; they shall run and not be weary; they shall walk and not faint."

Psalm 105:4 ESV "Seek the Lord and his strength; seek his presence continually!"

Psalm 18:32-34 ESV "The God who equipped me with strength and made my way blameless. He made my feet like the feet of a deer and set me secure on the heights. He trains my hands for war, so that my arms can bend a bow of bronze."

James 1:2-4 ESV "Count it all joy, my brothers, when you meet trials of various kinds, for you know that the testing of your faith produces steadfastness. And let steadfastness have its full effect, that you may be perfect and complete, lacking in nothing."

Colossians 1:10-12 ESV "So as to walk in a manner worthy of the Lord, fully pleasing to him, bearing fruit in every good work and increasing in the knowledge of God. May you be strengthened with all power, according to his glorious might, for all endurance and patience with joy, giving thanks to the Father, who has qualified you to share in the inheritance of the saints in light.

Ephesians 2:8-9 ESV "For by grace you have been saved through faith. And this is not your own doing; it is the gift of God, not a result of works, so that no one may boast."

1 Corinthians 2:14 ESV "The natural person does not accept the things of the Spirit of God, for they are folly to him, and he is not able to understand them because they are spiritually discerned."

John 13:34-35 ESV "A new commandment I give to you, that you love one another: just as I have loved you, you also are to love one another. By this all people will know that you are my disciples, if you have love for one another."

John 3:16-17 ESV "For God so loved the world, that he gave his only Son, that whoever believes in him should not perish but have eternal life. For God did not send his Son into the world to condemn the world, but in order that the world might be saved through him."

Ezekiel 34:16 ESV "I will seek the lost, and I will bring back the strayed, and I will bind up the injured, and I will strengthen the weak, and the fat and the strong I will destroy. I will feed them in justice."

Jeremiah 17:5 ESV "Thus says the Lord: "Cursed is the man who trusts in man and makes flesh his strength, whose heart turns away from the Lord."

Isaiah 33:2 ESV "O Lord, be gracious to us; we wait for you. Be our arm every morning, our salvation in the time of trouble."

Isaiah 12:2 ESV "Behold, God is my salvation; I will trust, and will not be afraid; for the Lord God is my strength and my song, and he has become my salvation."

Psalm 82:6 ESV "I said, "You are gods, sons of the Most High, all of you;"

Psalm 46:1 ESV "To the choirmaster. Of the Sons of Korah. According to Alamoth. A Song. God is our refuge and strength, a very present help in trouble."

1 Chronicles 29:12 ESV "Both riches and honor come from you, and you rule over all. In your hand are power and might, and in your hand it is to make great and to give strength to all."

1 Samuel 30:6 ESV "And David was greatly distressed, for the people spoke of stoning him, because all the people were bitter in soul, each for his sons and daughters. But David strengthened himself in the **Lord his God."**

God the Creator of all things seen and unseen!

Isaiah 45:12 ESV "I made the earth and created man on it; it was my hands that stretched out the heavens, and I commanded all their host."

Romans 1:20 ESV "For his invisible attributes, namely, his eternal power and divine nature, have been clearly perceived, ever since the creation of the world, in the things that have been made. So they are without excuse."

Revelation 4:11 ESV "Worthy are you, our Lord and God, to receive glory and honor and power, for you created all things, and by your will they existed and were created."

Psalm 19:1 ESV "To the choirmaster. A Psalm of David. The heavens declare the glory of God, and the sky above proclaims his handiwork."

2 Peter 3:5 ESV "For they deliberately overlook this fact, that the heavens existed long ago, and the earth was formed out of water and through water by the word of God,"

Isaiah 45:18 ESV "For thus says the Lord, who created the heavens (he is God!), who formed the earth and made it (he established it; he did not create it empty, he formed it to be inhabited!): "I am the Lord, and there is no other."

1 Corinthians 8:6 ESV "Yet for us there is one God, the Father, from whom are all things and for whom we exist, and one Lord, Jesus Christ, through whom are all things and through whom we exist."

Jeremiah 10:12 ESV "It is he who made the earth by his power, who established the world by his wisdom, and by his understanding stretched out the heavens."

Psalm 104:24-25 ESV "O Lord, how manifold are your works! In wisdom have you made them all; the earth is full of your creatures. Here is the sea, great and wide, which teems with creatures innumerable, living things both small and great."

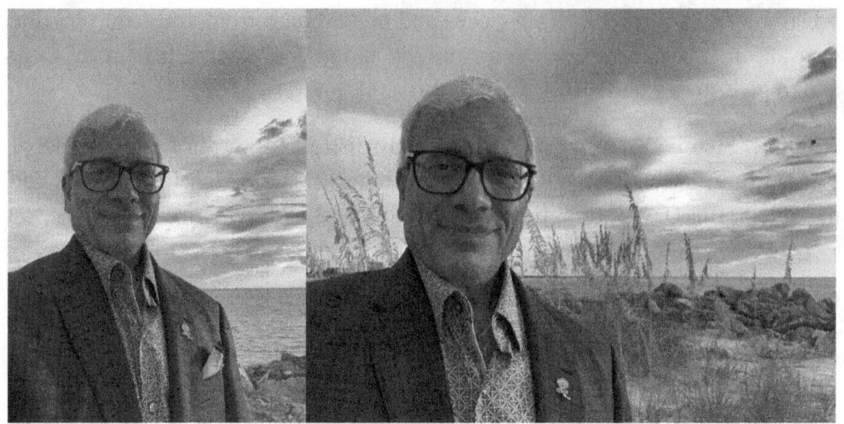

Lm, Amen

Dh, <u>Donna Hentsch</u>

Amen

CG, We must have faith because God is stronger than Satan, stronger than sin, stronger than shame, stronger than any storm and fire or suffering and pain, and stronger than any politician.

LM, Good morning. Praise God in all things for He is worthy.

TG, Amen.

ES, Amen

JM, AMEN

MN, Well said DrGhaly Amen I do believe.

DN, Amen God is everything

The Brutality in Chicago killed an innocent 7 years old child!!

Written on 10/27/22 by Ramsis Ghaly

With heroic work we do as a trauma team at JSH of Cook County hospital, to resuscitate the 7-years old child suffered from fatal GSW as an innocent bystander, despite we do the best, YET when it comes down to a child, with all my years of expertise, it leaves an everlasting scar and tears in our hearts as Frontliners!

Children aren't formed to shield the adult bullets and survive the brutality of adult gunshots!! Children can't sustain gunshots, their bodies are lean, tiny and small and they have no barriers like adults or space to protect against bullets! so these evil bullets easily find the vital organs and destroy them on the spot!! And the children have no way out but to give up their ghosts and go home to the Heavenly Father where they will be well received and treated with dignity, grace and holiness they deserve as angels of God!

As the children get shot, they silently cry and drift slowly to death without complaints! They then turn to their heads to the adult shooters saying: "Why you have done this to me? What I had done to you to take my life away and separate me from my beloved family!!"

The Brutality in Chicago had killed an innocent 7-year-old child and have reached the record high as the hub of Satan and laboratory for committing extreme evil!!

It shall no longer be sun to shine at that city, the capital of murder!

NEWSBREAK.COM

Child shot in Chicago: Stray bullet strikes 7-year-old boy in Humboldt Park - NewsBreak

CHICAGO (CBS) -- A 7-year-old boy was struck and critically wounded by a stray bullet in the Humboldt Park neighborhood Wednesday night.At 8:22 p.m., police received multiple calls of shots fired near Rockwell Street and Potomac Avenue, according to Deputy police Chief Ron Pontecore.Police then lear...

KO So heart breaking, prayers for this family and friends rest in peace

KO, So heart breaking, prayers for this family and friends rest in peace

CG, That poor child. Sending his parents prayers for strength as they find their way through each day.

MA, I saw this on the news and it's terrible! This violence is getting out of hand even in schools! That poor little boy probably was just getting ready to go to bed and now he's dead.

Post COVID Russian Aggression

Apocalypse 2022!

Ramsis Ghaly

Third week unto merciless brutal human slaughtering and man-made destruction!

More than two million are refugee and minimum of sixty thousand people exodus to strange lands!

The sun, moon and stars are hidden by firing Bombs, constant raining from the skies targeting building, homes, hospitals and ancient nonmilitary civilians!

The music, peace and hymns are replaced by unprovoked unjustified constant bombardment!

People starving to death, dehydrated and freezing to rocks cutting all the necessary supplies for basic human living!!

When you see the hell in Ukraine what are they inflicting in their fellowmen and women, in the maternity hospitals, the pregnant moms laboring, the neonates, infants, children, elders, the sick, the Ill, the civilians, —-witnessing the loss of life, the dead in the streets, the body parts all over, the rivers stained red with innocent bloodshed ——you know that earth is hell and heaven shall be heaven.

And your soul even feel more at peace that there is a God and our Savior will be our King and the only Ruler.

And never ever these atrocities will ever be seen once more!

When you see the departing souls, just know it is from the kindness of God and His grace that He is the True Caring Heavenly Father, is taking them back home to comfort them and host them in His paradise and soon heaven according to their faith and deeds in His Name Jesus the Lord

Revelation 21:1-7 KJV "And I saw a new heaven and a new earth: for the first heaven and the first earth were passed away; and there was no more sea. [2] And I John saw the holy city, new Jerusalem, coming down from God out of heaven, prepared as a bride adorned for her husband. [3] And I heard a great voice out of heaven saying, Behold, the tabernacle of God is with men, and he will dwell with them, and they shall be his people, and God himself shall be with them, and be their God. [4] And God shall wipe away all tears from their eyes; and there shall be no more death, neither sorrow, nor crying, neither shall there be any more pain: for the former things are passed away. [5] And he that sat upon the throne said, Behold, I make all things new. And he said unto me, Write: for these words are true and faithful. [6] And he said unto me, It is done. I am Alpha and Omega, the beginning and the end. I will give unto him that is athirst of the fountain of the water of life freely. [7] He that overcometh shall inherit all things; and I will be his God, and he shall be my son."

Revelation 22:7,12-16,20 KJV "Behold, I come quickly: blessed is he that keepeth the sayings of the prophecy of this book. [12] And, behold, I come quickly; and my reward is with me, to give every man according as his work shall be. [13] I am Alpha and Omega, the beginning and the end, the first and the last. [14] Blessed are they that do his commandments, that they may have right to the tree of life, and may enter in through the gates into the city. [15] For without are dogs, and sorcerers, and whoremongers, and murderers, and idolaters, and whosoever loveth and maketh a lie. [16] I Jesus have sent mine angel to testify unto you these things in the churches. I am the root and the offspring of David, and the bright and morning star. [20] He which testifieth these things saith, Surely I come quickly. Amen. Even so, come, Lord Jesus."

Es, So true...Revalation tells it all.

Tr, We need a world wide call to prayer

2Cron 7:14

A Plea and An Appeal Worldwide Do Not Repeat What You Have Done to Japanese after Pearl Harbor 1941!

Written by Ramsis Ghaly

Be not overcome of evil, but overcome evil with good. We must stand together Christians and Americans one race one country under one God and one Savior: One world one people one parent under one God and one Savior!!!

Please reach out with love and compassion and forgiveness not just to Ukrainians but also to our beloved Russians brothers and dusters, children and parents!

The fault isn't in the people but the leaders and wrong information do people should never pay the price for horrific leaders and government and satanic judgments!! Furthermore, Christians are known for love and reach out the other aisle and never ever revenge as it is written: "Dearly beloved, avenge not yourselves, but rather give place unto wrath: for it is written, Vengeance is mine; I will repay, saith the Lord." Romans 12:19 KJV

I have seen Satan and his demons are riding up more and more to destroy our human race as they are moving the hearts of world to avenge against Russians as they were successful thus far to flip Russia against Ukraine!!

Let it not be that please! I have noticed the extreme uncomfortable of our Russian friends to be around being ashamed, intimidated and fearful of what to expect next!

Stand up today and reach out to our Russian friends and hug them, please

Don't do what you have done to American Japanese after Pearl Harbor attack December 7, 1941!

We are one human race and as our Lord Jesus taught us: "A new commandment I give unto you, That ye love one another; as I have loved you, that ye also love one another." John 13:34 KJV

Be not overcome of evil, but overcome evil with good.

"Rejoicing in hope; patient in tribulation; continuing instant in prayer; [13] Distributing to the necessity of saints; given to hospitality. [14] Bless them which persecute you: bless, and curse not. [15] Rejoice with them that do rejoice, and weep with them that weep. [16] Be of the same mind one toward another. Mind not high things, but condescend to men of low estate. Be not wise in your own conceits. [17] Recompense to no man evil for evil. Provide things honest in the sight of all men. [18] If it be possible, as much as lieth in you, live peaceably with all men. [19] Dearly beloved, avenge not yourselves, but rather give place unto wrath: for it is written, Vengeance is mine; I will repay, saith the Lord. [20] Therefore if thine enemy hunger, feed him; if he thirst, give him drink: for in so doing thou shalt heap coals of fire on his head. [21] Be not overcome of evil, but overcome evil with good."Romans 12:12-21 KJV

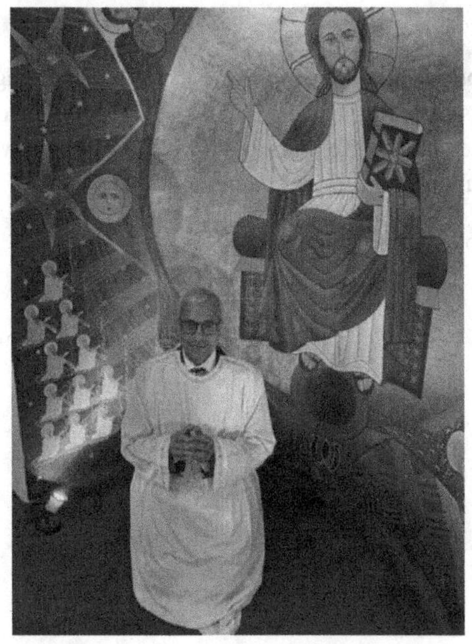

TR. Maybe your next step is into ministry as a Pastor

JT. amen

MT. THE GOVERNMENT was 100% RESPONSIBLE for the Japanese Internment.

surely you're not speaking of and blaming the US government for the brutal surprise attack on Pearl Harbor. Surely I am Elizabeth you obviously don't know history the US an oil embargo and completely shut Japan off from oil 100% which is an active of war so before you come at me go do some research because you are 100% wrong. Right now if the US pushes Russia too far they're going to nuke some cities, and I'm sure you're confident that Vladimir Putin is the devil himself when in fact America installed the Ukrainian government in 2014 and the United States has violated multiple treaties with Russia since 1991 you don't know that because you don't do your research that's what this war is all about. and we are corrupt up to the very top of our eyeballs all over the world. I am a very proud American who is completely embarrassed by our government.

JM, I love your heart for mankind. I pray for peace., for the people, the children, the country. Amen

AL. Amén

MS. Thank You.

JM, AGREE AMEN!!

CG. You are so correct that the people of Russia are suffering because of their leader. The soldiers from Russia were told they were going on drills and to guard the border. They lied to these soldiers and if they didn't fight when they got back to Russia they would have been sent to prison for 20 years.

God bless the people of both countries.

JH. Amen

Bureaucracy at its Best! War Weapons aren't using any Green Gas!!!

Written on 6/18/ 2022 by Ramsis Ghaly

The basic production of consumption is CO2 production and toxic fumes! As a principal Fact, there is no green gas in wars! Wars are the biggest CO2 production and the largest toxic gas spreader to the environment and futile to all green houses and destructive to anything green!! Yet the green gas and environmental activities aren't able to put a stop at Ukraine destruction, land ruining, CO2 massive war production and gas fumes toxic environmental hazards!!!

The wars generate huge amount of those gases and there production are being promoted by the well developed countries and especially by those advocate of global warming! In fact, it isn't war crime if explosions and fire missiles, bombs and tanks are used for defense! What is silly is the little car engine and the use of local green gas will supersede the huge amount of toxic fumes generated hourly by the three month ongoing Russian Ukraine war military artillery!!

Russia/ Ukraine war have caused sharp increase in CO2 production and harmed the environment with toxic fumes! large plume of pink smoke erupted from a chemical plant and rose above full of smoke and toxic gases and CO2!!

Furthermore, the world is helping to stop the war by suppling more military weapons, explosives, fire missiles, and firearms which indeed escalate more toxic fumes and CO2! The war is exploding in geysers of flame and more weapons have not stopped Russian forces from destroying Ukrainian towns and cities, like Mariupol, which largely stands in ruins after weeks of attacks with artillery, missiles and bombs. The arms, like cluster munitions and thermobaric rockets, have been criticized as too indiscriminate for use in warfare—-"

Nonetheless, Electric car manufacturing are in business more and more selling each electric car for more than $100,000 each. Furthermore, the space shuttle is burning more and more CO2 and toxic fumes to the atmosphere because electric engine does not work in space shuttles!

Europe and NATO are budgeting for billions of dollars for war weapons defense system to protect against future Russian atrocities using no green gas because electric non fuel war weapons do not work!

Yet the world the global warming warriors are planting green trees and putting electric engines as if they will make a difference n the big picture!

Exploding chemical plants have become a frightening reality for its citizens, but they're just one example of the staggering toll that war is taking on the nation's environment. Rockets are polluting the soil and groundwater; fires threaten to expel radioactive particles; and warships have reportedly killed dolphins in the Black Sea.

Yet having USA as a sovereign country energy sufficient to ease the economy upon the people will destroy the environment and promote disastrous global warming!!!

https://www.vox.com/.../ukraine-russia-war-pollution...

https://www.nytimes.com/.../us/weapons-ukraine-war.amp.html

VOX.COM

The pollution from Russia's war will poison Ukraine for decades

From chemical leaks to rampant wildfires, these are the unseen costs of Russia's invasion.

Conspiracy Theory in Regard to Unprovoked Russia Ukraine War!!

Written On 3/23/2022 by Ramsis Ghaly

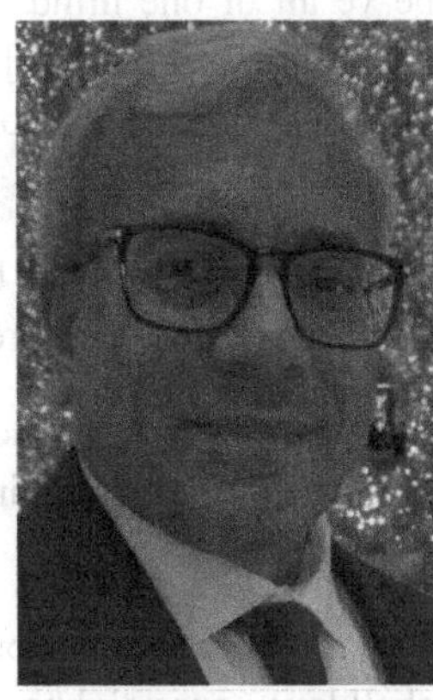

The world is still stunned with the ongoing radical actions of Putin! The world was taken by surprise and what is becoming more and more Obvious Anger of Putin and escalating unrelenting Revenge! And what is taken my mind is the more current US administration does, the More Putin Russian administration is angered more and more!! Although, Putin has been angry since the collapse of the Soviet Union, No one ever thought he will rage a brutal war at this particular time!!

I wonder if Putin Revenge at this time has much to do with previous history between him and the Current administration! If there is truth on that! O my gosh, the blood of all those causalities will be upon them and Russia at the judgment day!

God knows all things, and nothing is hidden by Him! What really tipped him off!!

This may explain the apparent obvious revenge between both administrations and obviously the more they do the more they put more gas on the fire!

If this is the case where the truth wasn't revealed, then more and more responsibility will fall upon them! In other hand, if the truth was revealed and previous history was surface and wasn't kept secret, America and the world would have taken the appropriate steps to prevent such war and the millions of innocent victims removing those with bad blood and old agenda!!

Moreover, the solution is to avoid those with conflict and get the right staff on place as mediators!!!

Lord has mercy once the book opens, and the truth comes! Indeed, the future will surface so much about what behind the worst war crime in Modern's man history!!!

1 Peter 3:8-9 KJV Finally, be ye all of one mind, having compassion one of another, love as brethren, be pitiful, be courteous: [9] Not rendering evil for evil, or railing for railing: but contrariwise blessing; knowing that ye are thereunto called, that ye should inherit a blessing.

Romans 12:19 Never take your own revenge, beloved, but leave room for the wrath of God, for it is written, "Vengeance is Mine, I will repay," says the Lord.

Genesis 4:15 So the Lord said to him, "Therefore whoever kills Cain, vengeance will be taken on him sevenfold." And the Lord appointed a sign for Cain, so that no one finding him would slay him.

Leviticus 19:18 You shall not take vengeance, nor bear any grudge against the sons of your people, but you shall love your neighbor as yourself; I am the Lord.

Deuteronomy 32:35Vengeance is Mine, and retribution, In due time their foot will slip;

For the day of their calamity is near,

And the impending things are hastening upon them.'

Proverbs 20:22 Do not say, "I will repay evil";

Wait for the Lord, and He will save you.

Luke 6:27-36But I say to you who hear, love your enemies, do good to those who hate you, bless those who curse you, pray for those who mistreat you. Whoever hits you on the cheek, offer him the other also; and whoever takes away your coat, do not withhold your shirt from him either.

1 Thessalonians 5:15 See that no one repays another with evil for evil, but always seek after that which is good for one another and for all people.

Proverbs 25:21 If your enemy is hungry, give him food to eat; And if he is thirsty, give him water to drink; For you will heap burning coals on his head,

And the Lord will reward you.

Luke 18:7-8 "now, will not God bring about justice for His elect who cry to Him day and night, and will He delay long over them? I tell you that He will bring about justice for them quickly. However, when the Son of Man comes, will He find faith on the earth?"

Deuteronomy 32:43 "Rejoice, O nations, with His people; For He will avenge the blood of His servants,And will render vengeance on His adversaries, And will atone for His land and His people."

JT, amen...

CG, Putin has been angry since the collapse of the Soviet Union. He wants to be back on top and will Ido it no matter what it takes and no matter how many lives are lost.

Jesus is being crucified again in Ukrainians and Ukraine and the world saying: let them be crucified!

Written on 3/2/2022 by Ramsis Ghaly

A week of brutal inhuman Russia's military assault a War-torn sovereign nation!! Convoy, artillery of cannons, paratroopers, shills, missiles, bombs, tanks, jets, ——all evil weapons

I feel ashamed of my human race seeing my fellow men are evil against other fellowmen and Nighbor land!! God has gifted man new lease in life with two years of COVID and man pay back by murdering His people Ukrainians and destroy His land Ukraine!

Ukrainians and Ukraine are pleading for someone to help them to carry some of the burden the cross as Simon from Cyrene and not yet! Matthew 27:32 KJV "And as they came out, they found a man of Cyrene, Simon by name: him they compelled to bear his cross."

Matthew 27:22-25,27-31 KJV Pilate saith unto them, What shall I do then with Jesus which is called Christ? They all say unto him, Let him be crucified. [23] And the governor said, Why, what evil hath he done? But they cried out the more, saying, Let him be crucified. [24] When Pilate saw that he could prevail nothing, but that rather a tumult was made, he took water, and washed his hands before the multitude, saying, I am innocent of the blood of this just person: see ye to it. [25] Then answered all the people, and said, His blood be on us, and on our children. [27] Then the soldiers of the governor took Jesus into the common hall, and gathered unto him the whole band of soldiers. [28] And they stripped him, and put on him a scarlet robe. [29] And when they had platted a crown of thorns, they put it upon his head, and a reed in his right hand: and they bowed the knee before him, and mocked him, saying, Hail, King of the Jews! [30] And they spit upon him, and took the reed, and smote him on the head. [31] And after that they had mocked him, they took the robe off from him, and put his own raiment on him, and led him away to crucify him."

What they are doing to Ukraine and Ukrainians downgrade our human nature to the bottommost pit!

What they are doing to Ukraine and Ukrainians are putting the human race as evil as Satan himself!

What they are doing to Ukraine and Ukrainians is ashaming humanity and provoking the wrath of our Heavenly Father!

What they are doing to Ukraine and Ukrainians is beyond criminality and reaching the satanic brutality!

And what the world's power are doing to intervene and rescue Ukraine and Ukrainian is shameful!

A world went through the humility of being helpless to fight COVID and God Almighty intervened and rescued the world while science and medicine weren't of great help but Jesus!

Look at the merciless world doing to Ukraine and Ukrainians and the tanks, bombs, explosions, and every evil surrounded the country and no single country get out of their home to reach out to put immediate stop to the bloodshed!

Talks sanctions are not the rescuing heroism of Nobel nations to stand by the injustice!

It isn't the tine to feel any good about my human Nature seeing what our race doing to each other: criminals brutal, merciless atrocities, worst aggression —— what rise remained for satanic man to do!

St James teaches us faith without work is dead like a body with no spirit! The world decided to be dead before the satanic deeds by Putin and Russians against Ukraine and Ukrainians! As it is written: James 2:13-20,26 KJV "For he shall have judgment without mercy, that hath shewed no mercy; and mercy rejoiceth against judgment. [14] What doth it profit, my brethren, though a man say he hath faith, and have not works? can faith save him? [15] If a brother or sister be naked, and destitute of daily food, [16] And one of you say unto them, Depart in peace, be ye warmed and filled; notwithstanding ye give them not those things which are needful to the body; what doth it profit? [17] Even so faith, if it hath not works, is dead, being alone. [18] Yea, a man may say, Thou hast faith, and I have works: shew me thy faith without thy works, and I will shew thee my faith by my works. [19] Thou believest that there is one God; thou doest well: the devils also believe, and tremble. [20] But wilt thou know, O vain man, that faith without works is dead? [26] For as the body without the spirit is dead, so faith without works is dead also."

The good human race I belong too is Abraham and his descendants when he treated his neighbors never invade or kill or murder his Neighbors as it is written Genesis 13:8-14 KJV "And Abram said unto Lot, Let there be no strife, I pray thee, between me and thee, and between my herdmen and thy herdmen; for we be brethren. [9] Is not the whole land before thee? separate thyself, I pray thee, from me: if thou wilt take the left hand, then I will go to the right; or if thou depart to the right hand, then I will go to the left. [10] And Lot lifted up his eyes, and beheld all the plain of Jordan, that it was well watered every where, before the Lord destroyed Sodom and Gomorrah, even as the garden of the Lord, like the land of Egypt, as thou comest unto Zoar. [11] Then Lot chose him all the plain of Jordan; and Lot journeyed east: and they separated themselves the one from the other. [12] Abram dwelled in the land of Canaan, and Lot dwelled in the cities of the plain, and pitched his tent toward Sodom. [13] But the men of Sodom were wicked and sinners before the Lord exceedingly. [14] And the Lord said unto Abram, after that Lot was separated from him, Lift up now thine eyes, and look from the place where thou art northward, and southward, and eastward, and westward:"

https://apple.news/AuZ85X1EsQSuJ90zAQdI_rg

https://www.cnbc.com/.../russia-ukraine-war-citizens...

https://www.aljazeera.com/.../ukraine-on-edge-as-russia...

https://www.nbcnews.com/news/amp/live-blog/ncna1290568

Indeed the fall unto the hands of God and not in the hand of man wither is NATO or America, or —-as it is written; 2 Samuel 24:14KJV "14] And David said unto Gad, I am in a great strait: let us fall now into the hand of the Lord ; for his mercies are great: and let me not fall into the hand of man." And 1 Chronicles 21:13 KJV "And David said unto Gad, I am in a great strait: let me fall now into the hand of the Lord ; for very great are his mercies: but let me not fall into the hand of man."

For when my hand is weak, I raise my hand to the Lord to hold on in His Almighty Hand, then I am strong!

Written by Ramsis Ghaly Dedicated to Ukraine:

My post from March 1, 2020 is dedicated to our beloved Ukraine and Ukrainians!

"For when my hand is weak, I raise my hand to the Lord to hold on in His Almighty Hand, then I am strong!"

Jesus our Lord His mighty hand is reaching yo you all. In Jesus name Amen

For when my hand is weak, I raise my hand to the Lord to hold on in His Almighty Hand ! then I am strong.

As I am falling, I raise my frail hand to the Lord to hold on in the Almighty Hand!

As I am drowning, I raise my sinking hand to the Lord to hold on in the Almighty Hand!

As I am falling, I raise my feeble hand to the Lord to hold on in the Almighty Hand!

As I am trembling, I raise my shivering hand to the Lord to hold on in the Almighty Hand!

As I am stumbling, I raise my frail hand to the Lord to hold on in the Almighty Hand!

As I am unclean, I raise my impure hand to the Lord to hold on in the Almighty Hand !

As I am adulterous, I raise my soiled hand to the Lord to hold on in the Almighty Hand!

As I am gloomy, I raise my helpless hand to the Lord to hold on in the Almighty Hand!

As I am defeated, I raise my beaten hand to the Lord to hold on in the Almighty Hand!

As I am sinning, I raise my unrighteous hand to the Lord to hold on in the Almighty Hand!

As I am ill, I raise my infirm hand to the Lord to hold on in the Almighty Hand!

As I am losing, I raise my incapacitated hand to the Lord to hold on in the Almighty Hand !

As I am exhausted, I raise my worn out hand to the Lord to hold on in the Almighty Hand !

As I am down, I raise my shaky hand to the Lord to hold on in the Almighty Hand !

As I am ailing, I raise my indisposed hand to the Lord to hold on in the Almighty Hand !

As I am laying in the hospital bed, I raise my sick hand to the Lord to hold on in His Almighty Hand !

As I am desperate at the eleventh hour, I raise my fatigued hand to the Lord to hold on in the Almighty Hand !

As I am in the fourthly hour of the night before the dawn, I raise my hopeless hand to the Lord to hold on in the Almighty Hand !

As I am dying, I raise my weak hand to the Lord to hold on in His Almighty Hand !

As I am buried under the ground, I raise my waisted hand to the Lord to hold on in His Almighty Hand !

As I am in the coffin, I raise my dead hand to the Lord to hold on in His Almighty Hand !

As I am no more and nothing left, I raise my lost hand to the Lord to hold on in His Almighty Hand !

As I am nothing in myself but I am everything in Lord Jesus Hand ! "Let the word of Christ dwell in you richly in all wisdom; teaching and admonishing one another in psalms and hymns and spiritual songs, singing with grace in your hearts to the Lord. 17And whatsoever ye do in word or deed, do all in the name of the Lord Jesus, giving thanks to God and the Father by him." (Colossians 3:16-17)

My hand is fruitless in itself but fruitful in the Almighty Hand the True Vine! "4 Abide in me, and I in you. As the branch cannot bear fruit of itself, except it abide in the vine; no more can ye, except ye abide in me.5 I am the vine, ye are the branches: He that abideth in me, and I in him, the same bringeth forth much fruit: for without me ye can do nothing.6 If a man abide not in me, he is cast forth as a branch, and is withered; and men gather them, and cast them into the fire, and they are burned.7 If ye abide in me, and my words abide in you, ye shall ask what ye will, and it shall be done unto you." ((John 15:4-7)

For when my hand is weak, I raise my hand to the Lord to hold on in His Almighty Hand ! then I am strong! "8 Concerning this thing I pleaded with the Lord three times that it might depart from me. 9 And He said to me, "My grace is sufficient for you, for My strength is made perfect in weakness." Therefore most gladly I will rather boast in my infirmities, that the power of Christ may rest upon me. 10 Therefore I take pleasure in infirmities, in reproaches, in needs, in persecutions, in distresses, for Christ's sake. For when I am weak, then I am strong." (2 Corinthians 12:8-10)

It in a no longer my hand but Christ's! "For to me to live is Christ, and to die is gain." (Philippians 1:21) "I am crucified with Christ: nevertheless I live; yet not I, but Christ liveth in me: and the life which I now live in the flesh I live by the faith of the Son of God, who loved me, and gave himself for me." (Galatians 2:20) "And if Christ be in you, the body is dead because of sin; but the Spirit is life because of righteousness." (Romans 8:10)

Nothing can separate my hand from the Almighty Hand !

"Who shall separate us from the love of Christ? shall tribulation, or distress, or persecution, or famine, or nakedness, or peril, or sword?36 As it is written, For thy sake we are killed all the day long; we are accounted as sheep for the slaughter.37

Nay, in all these things we are more than conquerors through him that loved us.38 For I am persuaded, that neither death, nor life, nor angels, nor principalities, nor powers, nor things present, nor things to come,39 Nor height, nor depth, nor any other creature, shall be able to separate us from the love of God, which is in Christ Jesus our Lord." Romans 8:35-39)

Psalm 4

1 Hear me when I call, O God of my righteousness: thou hast enlarged me when I was in distress; have mercy upon me, and hear my prayer.

2 O ye sons of men, how long will ye turn my glory into shame? how long will ye love vanity, and seek after leasing? Selah.

3 But know that the LORD hath set apart him that is godly for himself: the LORD will hear when I call unto him.

4 Stand in awe, and sin not: commune with your own heart upon your bed, and be still. Selah.

5 Offer the sacrifices of righteousness, and put your trust in the LORD.

6 There be many that say, Who will shew us any good? LORD, lift thou up the light of thy countenance upon us.

7 Thou hast put gladness in my heart, more than in the time that their corn and their wine increased.

8 I will both lay me down in peace, and sleep: for thou, LORD, only makest me dwell in safety.

Psalm 40

1 I waited patiently for the LORD; and he inclined unto me, and heard my cry.

2 He brought me up also out of an horrible pit, out of the miry clay, and set my feet upon a rock, and established my goings.

3 And he hath put a new song in my mouth, even praise unto our God: many shall see it, and fear, and shall trust in the LORD.

4 Blessed is that man that maketh the LORD his trust, and respecteth not the proud, nor such as turn aside to lies.

5 Many, O LORD my God, are thy wonderful works which thou hast done, and thy thoughts which are to us-ward: they cannot be reckoned up in order unto thee: if I would declare and speak of them, they are more than can be numbered.

6 Sacrifice and offering thou didst not desire; mine ears hast thou opened: burnt offering and sin offering hast thou not required.

7 Then said I, Lo, I come: in the volume of the book it is written of me,

8 I delight to do thy will, O my God: yea, thy law is within my heart.

9 I have preached righteousness in the great congregation: lo, I have not refrained my lips, O LORD, thou knowest.

10 I have not hid thy righteousness within my heart; I have declared thy faithfulness and thy salvation: I have not concealed thy lovingkindness and thy truth from the great congregation.

11 Withhold not thou thy tender mercies from me, O LORD: let thy lovingkindness and thy truth continually preserve me.

12 For innumerable evils have compassed me about: mine iniquities have taken hold upon me, so that I am not able to look up; they are more than the hairs of mine head: therefore my heart faileth me.

13 Be pleased, O LORD, to deliver me: O LORD, make haste to help me.

14 Let them be ashamed and confounded together that seek after my soul to destroy it; let them be driven backward and put to shame that wish me evil.

15 Let them be desolate for a reward of their shame that say unto me, Aha, aha.

16 Let all those that seek thee rejoice and be glad in thee: let such as love thy salvation say continually, The LORD be magnified.

17 But I am poor and needy; yet the Lord thinketh upon me: thou art my help and my deliverer; make no tarrying, O my God.

Psalm 69

1 Save me, O God; for the waters are come in unto my soul.

2 I sink in deep mire, where there is no standing: I am come into deep waters, where the floods overflow me.

3 I am weary of my crying: my throat is dried: mine eyes fail while I wait for my God.

4 They that hate me without a cause are more than the hairs of mine head: they that would destroy me, being mine enemies wrongfully, are mighty: then I restored that which I took not away.

5 O God, thou knowest my foolishness; and my sins are not hid from thee.

6 Let not them that wait on thee, O Lord GOD of hosts, be ashamed for my sake: let not those that seek thee be confounded for my sake, O God of Israel.

7 Because for thy sake I have borne reproach; shame hath covered my face.

8 I am become a stranger unto my brethren, and an alien unto my mother's children.

9 For the zeal of thine house hath eaten me up; and the reproaches of them that reproached thee are fallen upon me.

10 When I wept, and chastened my soul with fasting, that was to my reproach.

11 I made sackcloth also my garment; and I became a prover to them.

12 They that sit in the gate speak against me; and I was the song of the drunkards.

13 But as for me, my prayer is unto thee, O LORD, in an acceptable time: O God, in the multitude of thy mercy hear me, in the truth of thy salvation.

14 Deliver me out of the mire, and let me not sink: let me be delivered from them that hate me, and out of the deep waters.

15 Let not the waterflood overflow me, neither let the deep swallow me up, and let not the pit shut her mouth upon me.

16 Hear me, O LORD; for thy lovingkindness is good: turn unto me according to the multitude of thy tender mercies.

17 And hide not thy face from thy servant; for I am in trouble: hear me speedily.

18 Draw nigh unto my soul, and redeem it: deliver me because of mine enemies.

19 Thou hast known my reproach, and my shame, and my dishonour: mine adversaries are all before thee.

20 Reproach hath broken my heart; and I am full of heaviness: and I looked for some to take pity, but there was none; and for comforters, but I found none.

21 They gave me also gall for my meat; and in my thirst they gave me vinegar to drink.

22 Let their table become a snare before them: and that which should have been for their welfare, let it become a trap.

23 Let their eyes be darkened, that they see not; and make their loins continually to shake.

24 Pour out thine indignation upon them, and let thy wrathful anger take hold of them.

25 Let their habitation be desolate; and let none dwell in their tents.

26 For they persecute him whom thou hast smitten; and they talk to the grief of those whom thou hast wounded.

27 Add iniquity unto their iniquity: and let them not come into thy righteousness.

28 Let them be blotted out of the book of the living, and not be written with the righteous.

29 But I am poor and sorrowful: let thy salvation, O God, set me up on high.

30 I will praise the name of God with a song, and will magnify him with thanksgiving.

31 This also shall please the LORD better than an ox or bullock that hath horns and hoofs.

32 The humble shall see this, and be glad: and your heart shall live that seek God.

33 For the LORD heareth the poor, and despiseth not his prisoners.

34 Let the heaven and earth praise him, the seas, and everything that moveth therein.

35 For God will save Zion, and will build the cities of Judah: that they may dwell there, and have it in possession.

36 The seed also of his servants shall inherit it: and they that love his name shall dwell therein.

Psalm 80

1 Give ear, O Shepherd of Israel, thou that leadest Joseph like a flock; thou that dwellest between the cherubims, shine forth.

2 Before Ephraim and Benjamin and Manasseh stir up thy strength, and come and save us.

3 Turn us again, O God, and cause thy face to shine; and we shall be saved.

4 O LORD God of hosts, how long wilt thou be angry against the prayer of thy people?

5 Thou feedest them with the bread of tears; and givest them tears to drink in great measure.

6 Thou makest us a strife unto our neighbours: and our enemies laugh among themselves.

7 Turn us again, O God of hosts, and cause thy face to shine; and we shall be saved.

8 Thou hast brought a vine out of Egypt: thou hast cast out the heathen, and planted it.

9 Thou preparedst room before it, and didst cause it to take deep root, and it filled the land.

10 The hills were covered with the shadow of it, and the boughs thereof were like the goodly cedars.

11 She sent out her boughs unto the sea, and her branches unto the river.

12 Why hast thou then broken down her hedges, so that all they which pass by the way do pluck her?

13 The boar out of the wood doth waste it, and the wild beast of the field doth devour it.

14 Return, we beseech thee, O God of hosts: look down from heaven, and behold, and visit this vine;

15 And the vineyard which thy right hand hath planted, and the branch that thou madest strong for thyself.

16 It is burned with fire, it is cut down: they perish at the rebuke of thy countenance.

17 Let thy hand be upon the man of thy right hand, upon the son of man whom thou madest strong for thyself.

18 So will not we go back from thee: quicken us, and we will call upon thy name.

19 Turn us again, O LORD God of hosts, cause thy face to shine; and we shall be saved.

Psalm 86

1 Bow down thine ear, O LORD, hear me: for I am poor and needy.

2 Preserve my soul; for I am holy: O thou my God, save thy servant that trusteth in thee.

3 Be merciful unto me, O Lord: for I cry unto thee daily.

4 Rejoice the soul of thy servant: for unto thee, O Lord, do I lift up my soul.

5 For thou, Lord, art good, and ready to forgive; and plenteous in mercy unto all them that call upon thee.

6 Give ear, O LORD, unto my prayer; and attend to the voice of my supplications.

7 In the day of my trouble I will call upon thee: for thou wilt answer me.

8 Among the gods there is none like unto thee, O Lord; neither are there any works like unto thy works.

9 All nations whom thou hast made shall come and worship before thee, O Lord; and shall glorify thy name.

10 For thou art great, and doest wondrous things: thou art God alone.

11 Teach me thy way, O LORD; I will walk in thy truth: unite my heart to fear thy name.

12 I will praise thee, O Lord my God, with all my heart: and I will glorify thy name for evermore.

13 For great is thy mercy toward me: and thou hast delivered my soul from the lowest hell.

14 O God, the proud are risen against me, and the assemblies of violent men have sought after my soul; and have not set thee before them.

15 But thou, O Lord, art a God full of compassion, and gracious, longsuffering, and plenteous in mercy and truth.

16 O turn unto me, and have mercy upon me; give thy strength unto thy servant, and save the son of thine handmaid.

17 Shew me a token for good; that they which hate me may see it, and be ashamed: because thou, LORD, hast holpen me, and comforted me.

Psalm 102

1 Hear my prayer, O LORD, and let my cry come unto thee.

2 Hide not thy face from me in the day when I am in trouble; incline thine ear unto me: in the day when I call answer me speedily.

3 For my days are consumed like smoke, and my bones are burned as an hearth.

4 My heart is smitten, and withered like grass; so that I forget to eat my bread.

5 By reason of the voice of my groaning my bones cleave to my skin.

6 I am like a pelican of the wilderness: I am like an owl of the desert.

7 I watch, and am as a sparrow alone upon the house top.

8 Mine enemies reproach me all the day; and they that are mad against me are sworn against me.

9 For I have eaten ashes like bread, and mingled my drink with weeping,

10 Because of thine indignation and thy wrath: for thou hast lifted me up, and cast me down.

11 My days are like a shadow that declineth; and I am withered like grass.

12 But thou, O LORD, shalt endure for ever; and thy remembrance unto all generations.

13 Thou shalt arise, and have mercy upon Zion: for the time to favour her, yea, the set time, is come.

14 For thy servants take pleasure in her stones, and favour the dust thereof.

15 So the heathen shall fear the name of the LORD, and all the kings of the earth thy glory.

16 When the LORD shall build up Zion, he shall appear in his glory.

17 He will regard the prayer of the destitute, and not despise their prayer.

18 This shall be written for the generation to come: and the people which shall be created shall praise the LORD.

19 For he hath looked down from the height of his sanctuary; from heaven did the LORD behold the earth;

20 To hear the groaning of the prisoner; to loose those that are appointed to death;

21 To declare the name of the LORD in Zion, and his praise in Jerusalem;

22 When the people are gathered together, and the kingdoms, to serve the LORD.

23 He weakened my strength in the way; he shortened my days.

24 I said, O my God, take me not away in the midst of my days: thy years are throughout all generations.

25 Of old hast thou laid the foundation of the earth: and the heavens are the work of thy hands.

26 They shall perish, but thou shalt endure: yea, all of them shall wax old like a garment; as a vesture shalt thou change them, and they shall be changed:

27 But thou art the same, and thy years shall have no end.

28 The children of thy servants shall continue, and their seed shall be established before thee.

Psalm 142

1 I cried unto the LORD with my voice; with my voice unto the LORD did I make my supplication.

2 I poured out my complaint before him; I shewed before him my trouble.

3 When my spirit was overwhelmed within me, then thou knewest my path. In the way wherein I walked have they privily laid a snare for me.

4 I looked on my right hand, and beheld, but there was no man that would know me: refuge failed me; no man cared for my soul.

5 I cried unto thee, O LORD: I said, Thou art my refuge and my portion in the land of the living.

6 Attend unto my cry; for I am brought very low: deliver me from my persecutors; for they are stronger than I.

7 Bring my soul out of prison, that I may praise thy name: the righteous shall compass me about; for thou shalt deal bountifully with me.

Psalm 18

1 I will love thee, O LORD, my strength.

2 The LORD is my rock, and my fortress, and my deliverer; my God, my strength, in whom I will trust; my buckler, and the horn of my salvation, and my high tower.

3 I will call upon the LORD, who is worthy to be praised: so shall I be saved from mine enemies.

4 The sorrows of death compassed me, and the floods of ungodly men made me afraid.

5 The sorrows of hell compassed me about: the snares of death prevented me.

6 In my distress I called upon the LORD, and cried unto my God: he heard my voice out of his temple, and my cry came before him, even into his ears.

7 Then the earth shook and trembled; the foundations also of the hills moved and were shaken, because he was wroth.

8 There went up a smoke out of his nostrils, and fire out of his mouth devoured: coals were kindled by it.

9 He bowed the heavens also, and came down: and darkness was under his feet.

10 And he rode upon a cherub, and did fly: yea, he did fly upon the wings of the wind.

11 He made darkness his secret place; his pavilion round about him were dark waters and thick clouds of the skies.

12 At the brightness that was before him his thick clouds passed, hail stones and coals of fire.

13 The LORD also thundered in the heavens, and the Highest gave his voice; hail stones and coals of fire.

14 Yea, he sent out his arrows, and scattered them; and he shot out lightnings, and discomfited them.

15 Then the channels of waters were seen, and the foundations of the world were discovered at thy rebuke, O LORD, at the blast of the breath of thy nostrils.

16 He sent from above, he took me, he drew me out of many waters.

17 He delivered me from my strong enemy, and from them which hated me: for they were too strong for me.

18 They prevented me in the day of my calamity: but the LORD was my stay.

19 He brought me forth also into a large place; he delivered me, because he delighted in me.

20 The LORD rewarded me according to my righteousness; according to the cleanness of my hands hath he recompensed me.

21 For I have kept the ways of the LORD, and have not wickedly departed from my God.

22 For all his judgments were before me, and I did not put away his statutes from me.

23 I was also upright before him, and I kept myself from mine iniquity.

24 Therefore hath the LORD recompensed me according to my righteousness, according to the cleanness of my hands in his eyesight.

25 With the merciful thou wilt shew thyself merciful; with an upright man thou wilt shew thyself upright;

26 With the pure thou wilt shew thyself pure; and with the froward thou wilt shew thyself froward.

27 For thou wilt save the afflicted people; but wilt bring down high looks.

28 For thou wilt light my candle: the LORD my God will enlighten my darkness.

29 For by thee I have run through a troop; and by my God have I leaped over a wall.

30 As for God, his way is perfect: the word of the LORD is tried: he is a buckler to all those that trust in him.

31 For who is God save the LORD? or who is a rock save our God?

32 It is God that girdeth me with strength, and maketh my way perfect.

33 He maketh my feet like hinds' feet, and setteth me upon my high places.

34 He teacheth my hands to war, so that a bow of steel is broken by mine arms.

35 Thou hast also given me the shield of thy salvation: and thy right hand hath holden me up, and thy gentleness hath made me great.

36 Thou hast enlarged my steps under me, that my feet did not slip.

37 I have pursued mine enemies, and overtaken them: neither did I turn again till they were consumed.

38 I have wounded them that they were not able to rise: they are fallen under my feet.

39 For thou hast girded me with strength unto the battle: thou hast subdued under me those that rose up against me.

40 Thou hast also given me the necks of mine enemies; that I might destroy them that hate me.

41 They cried, but there was none to save them: even unto the LORD, but he answered them not.

42 Then did I beat them small as the dust before the wind: I did cast them out as the dirt in the streets.

43 Thou hast delivered me from the strivings of the people; and thou hast made me the head of the heathen: a people whom I have not known shall serve me.

44 As soon as they hear of me, they shall obey me: the strangers shall submit themselves unto me.

45 The strangers shall fade away, and be afraid out of their close places.

46 The LORD liveth; and blessed be my rock; and let the God of my salvation be exalted.

47 It is God that avengeth me, and subdueth the people under me.

48 He delivereth me from mine enemies: yea, thou liftest me up above those that rise up against me: thou hast delivered me from the violent man.

49 Therefore will I give thanks unto thee, O LORD, among the heathen, and sing praises unto thy name.

50 Great deliverance giveth he to his king; and sheweth mercy to his anointed, to David, and to his seed for evermore.

Please reach out and Hug your Ukrainians and Russians neighbors and help pray and fast for peace!!!

Never ever participate or be part of hate crimes against any nations;

Spread love !

Be source of love !

Surround others with tanks of love

Cast out the tanks of wars among you!!

ALJAZEERA.COM

Latest Ukraine updates: UNGA votes to demand Russian withdrawal

Russia-Ukraine news from March 2: UN General Assembly resolution condemns Russia for the invasion of Ukraine.

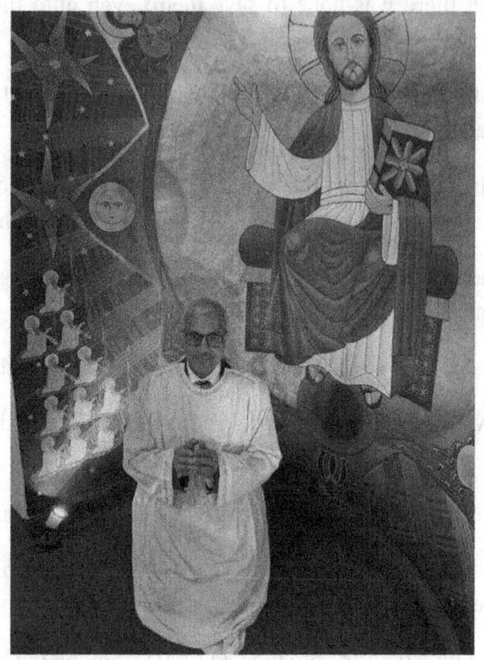

1Charlene Mentzer Glowaty

CG. This is so heartfelt. Bless the people of the Ukraine for having the courage to stand up to the evil of Putin.

JT. amen...God bless Ukraine...in good times and the bad

ED. So beautifully said Doctor. I pray for Ukraine. Those brave people are fighting with all they have. God protect them all especially the little innocent children.

NV. Powerful! Amen

CG, Praying for this strong willed country that God will protect them and bless them.

MA. Amen

JM, "Exceptional"AMEN

MA. Amen.

GH. Love the first picture of hands!

With Heavy Heart and Sadness The Entire World Shall see much more Dark Times!!

Written on 3/9/202 by Ramsis Ghaly

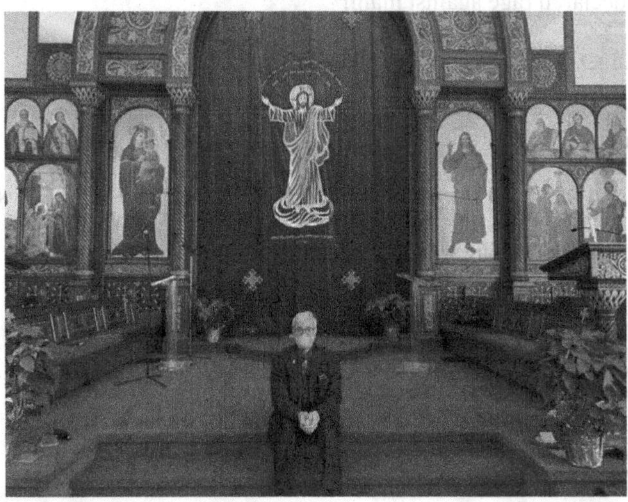

Global impact of Russian Putin Invasion to Ukraine on February 24, 2022 will be far worse than that of September 11, 2001!

O man! Mark that Day February 24, 2022, in thy book as thy allowed wickedness and destruction among God 'people and His children!! Listen O man: there were so many ways the world should have done and intervened but man's stiff neck and stoned heart prevailed! Your hearts were shut cold and so were your actions! You were tested for your love and failed before the Lord! Therefore, in the coming days, months and years, it shall be much more darkness upon the face of the earth made by the evil man!!

Satan and his demons are cheerful as the visitation of the Spirit has seen more evil upon the earth!!

The History will Remember the great failure of American and European leaders and their intelligence for underestimating Putin and Satanism of Russian Kremlin!

Let us not foul ourselves, the entire world is responsible for allowing such atrocity to millions of innocent people!

Let us admit, it is much worse than 9/11 and hence it shall affect each living soul in all the corners of earth!

The man should feel shameful of his manhood seeing the atrocities and allowing such evil to be conducted by man inflicting unto fellowmen and fellow women!!!

So the voice of the crying child, the aching mother, the wombs carrying the breath of God, the screaming refugee —-so is the voice of the Spirit crying for them!!

Who shall reverse the wrath of God?? Who shall overcome the uprise of Satan? Satan has declared rage against man!!

https://en.m.wikipedia.org/.../2022_Russian_invasion_of...

SJ, Sad, but well said

DR, Truth but it doesn't matter in the END. THE END IS THE BEGINNING

LM, It's so Heartbreaking what it's becoming. Where is the love

JT, dear Lord we need your son now please...

JM, "PRAYING"

MS, Thank you for this.

BC, Amen

CG, You're are so right in your comments.

Russia has launched a devastating attack on Ukraine.Its' people are suffering,the little children are suffering. Satan has indeed taken over. All mankind needs to pray for help.

KO, Most definitely they do need to pray so very hard for this world, Dear Lord hear our prayers

ED, Dear Lord. Have mercy upon us. Forgive us our sins. We trust in you dear God, our Father.

DW, Prayers for Ukraine

Who will win Putin the Russian Goliath or David the Ukrainian Shephard??

Written by Ramsis Ghaly

Today is Sunday the Lord's Day the eleventh day of the war between Putin the Russian Goliath and David the Ukrainian and the men of Ukraine! The entire world is being tested for its faith, solidarity and goodness!!

The tears of the mothers, the cries of innocent children, the suffering of the multitudes, the bloodshed, the loss of lives, the inhuman destruction, the prayers of the faithful servants, the love of the children of God and the injustice of the enemies, the brutality of the and wicked men, provoked the Lord of hosts and the Savior of the world!!

The war between Russia and Ukraine isn't any different from the war between philistines and Judah as Now the Philistines gathered together their armies to battle, and were gathered together at Shochoh, which belongeth to Judah, and pitched between Shochoh and Azekah, in Ephes-dammim.

God stands with those poor in the spirit, favors the humble and lowly rescuing him from the wicked ones! God chose the lowly things of this world and the despised things—and the things that are not—to nullify the things that are, so that no one may boast before him." 1 Corinthians 1:28-29 Psalm 138:6 "For though the Lord is exalted, Yet He regards the lowly, But the haughty He knows from afar." Isaiah 57:15 "For thus says the high and exalted One Who lives forever, whose name is Holy, "I dwell on a high and holy place, And also with the contrite and lowly of spirit In order to revive the spirit of the lowly And to revive the heart of the contrite." Isaiah 66:2 "For My hand made all these things, Thus all these things came into being," declares the Lord. But to this one I will look,To him who is humble and contrite of spirit, and who trembles at My word." Job 22:29 When you are cast down, you will speak with confidence, And the humble person He will save." James 4:6 But He gives a greater grace. Therefore it says, "God is opposed to the proud, but gives grace to the humble."

Ukraine needs David and neither Saul nor the men of the world, to stand against Putin Goliath "And Saul and the men of Israel were gathered together, and pitched by the valley of Elah, and set the battle in array against the Philistines."

Who is stronger boy named David or king named Goliath!

Who is larger boy named David or king named Goliath!

Who is taller boy named David or king named Goliath!

Who is Giant made of steel and made for war the boy named David or the king named Goliath!

Who is well equipped boy named David or king named Goliath!

Who will win the boy David or the champion Goliath!

Who will win the few bounds David or Goliath whose height was six cubits and a span!

Who will win the lamb David or the wolf Goliath!

Who will win the green valley David or the mountain Goliath!

Who will win David with or Goliath with an helmet of brass upon his head, and he was armed with a coat of mail; and the weight of the coat was five thousand shekels of brass!

Who will win David or Goliath with greaves of brass upon his legs, and a target of brass between his shoulders. And the staff of his spear was like a weaver's beam; and his spear's head weighed six hundred shekels of iron: and one bearing a shield went before him!

Who will stand against Putin Goliath Saul and men of Israel and the world or the child David??

Who won't be dismayed or feared Saul and the men of Israel of the young Shephard David?? "If he be able to fight with me, and to kill me, then will we be your servants: but if I prevail against him, and kill him, then shall ye be our servants, and serve us. [10] And the Philistine said, I defy the armies of Israel this day; give me a man, that we may fight together. [11] When Saul and all Israel heard those words of the Philistine, they were dismayed, and greatly afraid.—And all the men of Israel, when they saw the man, fled from him, and were sore afraid."

Who shall prevail, Putin the Goliath the champion out of the camp of the Philistines, named Goliath, of Gath, or David the son of that Ephrathite of Beth–lehem–judah, whose name was Jesse??

Who shall win the war the youngest son David to Jessie that cares for the few sheep in the wilderness, a youth not man of the war with staff in his hand and five smooth stones in the brook placed in shepherd's bag in a scrip and sling was in his hand!

Ukraine needs David to stand up in faith empowered with Lord Jesus not with jets, tanks, missiles and bombs! David Ukraine shall say with strong faith, authority undoubtedly: "Let no man's heart fail because of him; thy servant will go and fight with this Putin the Russian— The Lord that delivered me out of the paw of the lion, and out of the paw of the bear, he will deliver me out of the hand of this Putin the Russian! "David said to Saul, Let no man's heart fail because of him; thy servant will go and fight with this Philistine. [33] And Saul said to David, Thou art not able to go against this Philistine to fight with him: for thou art but a youth, and he a man of war from his youth. [34] And David said unto Saul, Thy servant kept his father's sheep, and there came a lion, and a bear, and took a lamb out of the flock: [35] And I went out after him, and smote him, and delivered it out of his mouth: and when he arose against me, I caught him by his beard, and smote him, and slew him. [36] Thy servant slew both the lion and the bear: and this uncircumcised Philistine shall be as one of them, seeing he hath defied the armies of the living God. [37] David said moreover, The Lord that delivered me out of the paw of the lion, and out of the paw of the bear, he will deliver me out of the hand of this Philistine. And Saul said unto David, Go, and the Lord be with thee."

How shall David win not by jets and tanks armed with armour, helmet of brass upon his head; also he armed him with a coat of mail and girded his sword upon his armour!!

As Putin the Russian Goliath look down to David the Ukrainian, disdained him: for he was but a youth, and ruddy, and of a fair countenance and says to David the Ukrainian, Am I a dog, that thou comest to me with staves? And cursed David by his gods!

The History Taught us!!!

Putin the Russian Goliath will say to David the Ukrainian: Come to me, and I will give thy flesh unto the fowls of the air, and to the beasts of the field!

The Ukrainian David will respond: "Thou comest to me with a sword, and with a spear, and with a shield: but I come to thee in the name of the Lord of hosts, the God of the armies of Israel, whom thou hast defied. This day will the Lord deliver thee into mine hand; and I will smite thee, and take thine head from thee; and I will give the carcases of the host of the Philistines this day unto the fowls of the air, and to the wild beasts of the earth; that all the earth may know that there is a God in Israel. And all this assembly shall know that the Lord saveth not with sword and spear: for the battle is the Lord's, and he will give you into our hands."

And David the Ukrainian won't come with artillery of machine guns and thousands of tanks, air jets to prevail against this Putin the Russian Goliath but by a bag with one stone where he slang it, and smote the Army in its forehead where that the stone sunk into the forehead; and paralyze the entire army of Putin the Russian Goliath!

At that day, David the Ukrainian shall stand proud in the midst of Ukraine triumphing as so called the champion and his men fled!

At that day, the men of Ukraine shall shout in victory Glory to God in the Highest praise Him O Ukraine and Ukrainians and all the world!!

What matters is not the jets or the shells or the missiles or the bombs but rather who has Lord Jesus by his side!

1 Samuel 17 "Now the Philistines gathered together their armies to battle, and were gathered together at Shochoh, which belongeth to Judah, and pitched between Shochoh and Azekah, in Ephes-dammim. [2] And Saul and the men of Israel were gathered together, and pitched by the valley of Elah, and set the battle in array against the Philistines. [3] And the Philistines stood on a mountain on the one side, and Israel stood on a mountain on the other side: and there was a valley between them. [4] And there went out a champion out of the camp of the Philistines, named Goliath, of Gath, whose height was six cubits and a span. [5] And he had an helmet of brass upon his head, and he was armed with a coat of mail; and the weight of the coat was five thousand shekels of brass. [6] And he had greaves of brass upon his legs, and a target of brass between his shoulders. [7] And the staff of his spear was like a weaver's beam; and his spear's head weighed six hundred shekels of iron: and one bearing a shield went before him. [8] And he stood and cried unto the armies of Israel, and said unto them, Why are ye come out to set your battle in array? am not I a Philistine, and ye servants to Saul? choose you a man for you, and let him come down to me. [9] If he be able to fight with me, and to kill me, then will we be your servants: but if I prevail against him, and kill him, then shall ye be our servants, and serve us. [10] And the Philistine said, I defy the armies of Israel this day; give me a man, that we may fight together. [11] When Saul and all Israel heard those words of the Philistine, they were dismayed, and greatly afraid. [12] Now David was the son of that Ephrathite of Beth-lehem-judah, whose name was Jesse; and he had eight sons: and the man went among men for an old man in the days of Saul. [13] And the three eldest sons of Jesse went and followed Saul to the battle: and the names of his three sons that went to the battle were Eliab the firstborn, and next unto him Abinadab, and the third Shammah. [14] And David was the youngest: and the three eldest followed Saul. [15] But David went and returned from Saul to feed his father's sheep at Beth-lehem. [16] And the Philistine drew near morning and evening, and presented himself forty days. [17] And Jesse said unto David his son, Take now for thy brethren an ephah of this parched corn, and these ten loaves, and run to the camp to thy brethren; [18] And carry these ten cheeses unto the captain of their thousand, and look how thy brethren fare, and take their pledge. [19] Now Saul, and they, and all the men of Israel, were in the valley of Elah, fighting with the Philistines. [20] And David rose up early in the morning, and left the sheep with a keeper, and took, and went, as Jesse had

commanded him; and he came to the trench, as the host was going forth to the fight, and shouted for the battle. [21] For Israel and the Philistines had put the battle in array, army against army. [22] And David left his carriage in the hand of the keeper of the carriage, and ran into the army, and came and saluted his brethren. [23] And as he talked with them, behold, there came up the champion, the Philistine of Gath, Goliath by name, out of the armies of the Philistines, and spake according to the same words: and David heard them. [24] And all the men of Israel, when they saw the man, fled from him, and were sore afraid. [25] And the men of Israel said, Have ye seen this man that is come up? surely to defy Israel is he come up: and it shall be, that the man who killeth him, the king will enrich him with great riches, and will give him his daughter, and make his father's house free in Israel. [26] And David spake to the men that stood by him, saying, What shall be done to the man that killeth this Philistine, and taketh away the reproach from Israel? for who is this uncircumcised Philistine, that he should defy the armies of the living God? [27] And the people answered him after this manner, saying, So shall it be done to the man that killeth him. [28] And Eliab his eldest brother heard when he spake unto the men; and Eliab's anger was kindled against David, and he said, Why camest thou down hither? and with whom hast thou left those few sheep in the wilderness? I know thy pride, and the naughtiness of thine heart; for thou art come down that thou mightest see the battle. [29] And David said, What have I now done? Is there not a cause? [30] And he turned from him toward another, and spake after the same manner: and the people answered him again after the former manner. [31] And when the words were heard which David spake, they rehearsed them before Saul: and he sent for him. [32] And David said to Saul, Let no man's heart fail because of him; thy servant will go and fight with this Philistine. [33] And Saul said to David, Thou art not able to go against this Philistine to fight with him: for thou art but a youth, and he a man of war from his youth. [34] And David said unto Saul, Thy servant kept his father's sheep, and there came a lion, and a bear, and took a lamb out of the flock: [35] And I went out after him, and smote him, and delivered it out of his mouth: and when he arose against me, I caught him by his beard, and smote him, and slew him. [36] Thy servant slew both the lion and the bear: and this uncircumcised Philistine shall be as one of them, seeing he hath defied the armies of the living God. [37] David said moreover, The Lord that delivered me out of the paw of the lion, and out of the paw of the bear, he will deliver me out of the hand of this Philistine. And Saul said unto David, Go, and the Lord be with thee. [38] And Saul armed David with his armour, and he put an helmet of brass upon his head; also he armed him with a coat of mail. [39] And David girded his sword upon his armour, and he assayed to go; for he had not proved it. And David said unto Saul, I cannot go with these; for I have not proved them. And David put them off him. [40] And he took his staff in his hand, and chose him five smooth stones out of the brook, and put them in a shepherd's bag which he had, even in a scrip; and his sling was in his hand: and he drew near to the Philistine. [41] And the Philistine came on and drew near unto David; and the man that bare the shield went before him. [42] And when the Philistine looked about, and saw David, he disdained him: for he was but a youth, and ruddy, and of a fair countenance. [43] And the Philistine said unto David, Am I a dog, that thou comest to me with staves? And the Philistine cursed David by his gods. [44] And the Philistine said to David, Come to me, and I will give thy flesh unto the fowls of the air, and to the beasts of the field. [45] Then said David to the Philistine, Thou comest to me with a sword, and with a spear, and with a shield: but I come to thee in the name of the Lord of hosts, the God of the armies of Israel, whom thou hast defied. [46] This day will the Lord deliver thee into mine hand; and I will smite thee, and take thine head from thee; and I will give the carcases of the host of the Philistines this day unto the fowls of the air, and to the wild beasts of the earth; that all the earth may know that there is a God in Israel. [47] And all this assembly shall know that the Lord saveth not with sword and spear: for the battle is the Lord's, and he will give you into our hands. [48] And it came to pass, when the Philistine arose, and came and drew nigh to meet David, that David hasted, and ran toward the army to meet the Philistine. [49] And David put his hand in his bag, and took thence a stone, and slang it, and smote the Philistine in his forehead, that the stone sunk into his forehead; and he fell upon his face to the earth. [50] So David prevailed over the Philistine with a sling and with a stone, and smote the Philistine, and slew him; but there was no sword in the hand of David. [51] Therefore David ran, and stood upon the Philistine, and took his sword, and drew it out of the sheath thereof, and slew him, and cut off his head therewith. And when the Philistines saw their champion was dead, they fled. [52] And the men of Israel and of Judah arose, and shouted, and pursued the Philistines, until thou come to the valley, and to the gates of Ekron. And the wounded of the Philistines fell down by the way to Shaaraim, even unto Gath, and unto Ekron. [53] And the children of Israel returned from chasing after the Philistines, and they spoiled their tents. [54] And David took the head of the Philistine, and brought it to Jerusalem; but he put his armour in his tent. [55] And when Saul saw David go forth against the Philistine, he said unto Abner, the captain of the host, Abner, whose son is this youth? And Abner said, As thy soul liveth, O king, I cannot tell. [56] And the king said, Enquire thou whose son the stripling is. [57] And as David returned from the slaughter of the Philistine, Abner took him, and brought him before Saul with the head of the Philistine in his hand. [58] And Saul said to him, Whose son art thou, thou young man? And David answered, I am the son of thy servant Jesse the Beth-lehemite."

Matthew 5:3-4 KJV "Blessed are the poor in spirit: for theirs is the kingdom of heaven. [4] Blessed are they that mourn: for they shall be comforted."

We pray Amen

MS, Hope Goliath destroys Putin a barbaric,killing women and children.Very sad and tragic

AV, Thx for sharing the Word of God! Praying for peace in Jesus name Amen!

ML, Thank U Dr. Ghaly, praying for Ukraine & World Peace

JT, the sinner shall fall onto the feet of the one who is blessed...

CG, What a great analogy between Zelensky and Putin. Praying that God will watch over the Ukranians.

TG, Pray that God will watch over the Ukranians. Pray for the world Peace.

The Biblical Russia Ukrainian Apocalyptic War ZZZZZZZ Involving the Strong Inheritance of Ancient Judaism and Ancient Apostolic Christians!!

Written on 3/14/2022 by Ramsis Ghaly

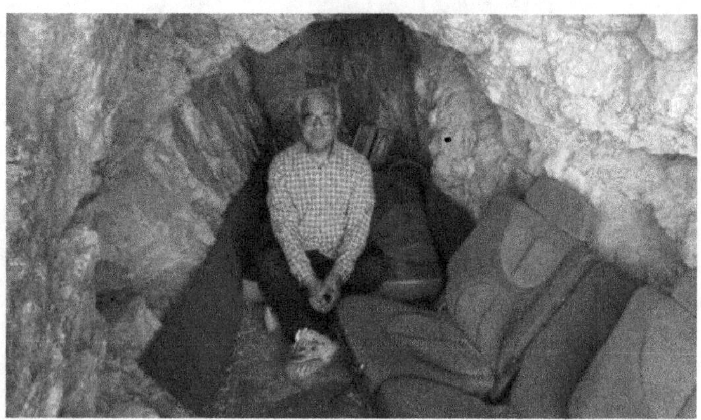

As I am searching the apocalyptic basic of the Russian Ukrainian War, I came with conclusion it is deeply Biblical and goes back to the ancient times with ancient Judaism and Apostolic Christianity!

Let us explore:

Letter Z is biblical: Zion, Zeal, Zealous, -/Psalm 69:9 "For the zeal of thine house hath eaten me up; and the reproaches of them that reproached thee are fallen upon me." Psalm 135:21 "Blessed be the Lord from Zion, Who dwells in Jerusalem. Praise the Lord!"

Source: https://bible.knowing-jesus.com/topics/Zion,-As-A-Symbol

What is so concerning is the Indirect tight relationship to ancient Judaism and Mesiah as following:

The war is marked with Letter ZZZZ. It has UNIQUE Symbols of letter ZZZZZ in the invaders tanks! Since it was spotted painted on tanks crossing into Ukraine, the final letter of the Latin alphabet has swiftly become a symbol of Russian nationalism.

https://www.npr.org/.../10854.../the-letter-z-russia-ukraine

Holocaust and ZZZZ!!!

The Z also is in the German NAZIS/ NAZISM and in the same time the Russian President Vladimir Putin's pretext says He will "denazify" Ukraine.

As Hitler Holocaust destruction so is Putin Holocaust Destruction!

It's Jewish president Volodymyr Zelensky lost family in Holocaust, his grandfather, Semyon Ivanovich Zelensky, who fought in the Soviet Union's Red Army during World War II. Mr. Zelensky wrote: "[Semyon] went through the whole war and remain[s] forever in my memory one of those heroes who defended Ukraine from the Nazis," he wrote. "Thanks for the fact that the inhuman ideology of Nazism is forever a thing of the past. Thanks to those who fought against Nazism — and won." "Three of them, their parents and their families became victims of the Holocaust. All of them were shot by German occupiers who invaded Ukraine," he said. "The fourth brother survived. ... Two years after the war, he had a son, and in 31 years, he had a grandson. In 40 more years, that grandson became president, and he is standing before you today, Mr. Prime Minister."

In the meantime, Israeli Prime minster Naftali Bennett fir the first time flew immediately to Moscow to meet with Russian President Vladimir Putin in Sabbath day to attempt to mediate for peace between both parties. Israel has begun absorbing thousands of Ukrainian Jewish refugees. The Israeli government said it is preparing for tens of thousands more.

https://www.washingtonpost.com/.../zelensky-family.../

https://www.voanews.com/.../israeli-prime.../6473174.html

Z in Hebrew is Zayin and it means 'sword' or 'a weapon of the spirit!

Z God's Zeal and Zealously

Is this a war of Zeal???

Z is the zeal of the lord

Z in words of the Bible:

Zeal

2 Kings 19:31

For out of Jerusalem shall go forth a remnant, and they that escape out of mount Zion: the zeal of the LORD of hosts shall do this

Source: https://bible.knowing-jesus.com/words/Zeal

Zealous

Acts 22:3:

I am verily a man which am a Jew, born in Tarsus, a city in Cilicia, yet brought up in this city at the feet of Gamaliel, and taught according to the perfect manner of the law of the fathers, and was zealous toward God, as ye all are this day. Titus 2:14:

Who gave himself for us, that he might redeem us from all iniquity, and purify unto himself a peculiar people, zealous of good works. Numbers 25:13

And he shall have it, and his seed after him, even the covenant of an everlasting priesthood; because he was zealous for his God, and made an atonement for the children of Israel.

Zealously

Zealousness

Zion Jerusalem and Holy Mountain

Is this war is of Zion??? Is it to liberate the daughters of Zion to their Savior!!!

Letter Z is Zion and Zion reflects heavily in both old and New Testament! In the Hebrew Bible, the Land of Israel and the city of Jerusalem are both referred to as Zion. Other religions use the word Zion to mean "utopia" or "holy place."

The ancient Hebrew word Tsiyon (Zion) is "a Canaanite hill fortress in Jerusalem captured by David and called in the Bible 'City of David.'" Zion can refer to one of three places: the hill where the most ancient areas of Jerusalem stood; the city of Jerusalem itself; or the dwelling place of God.

"the fortress of Zion—which is the City of David." (2 Samuel 5:7).

"holy mountain" (Psalm 2:6),"enthroned" (Psalm 9:11),

"Those who are left in Zion, who remain in Jerusalem, will be called holy" (Isaiah 4:3); "gifts will be brought to Mount Zion, the place of the Name of the Lord Almighty." (Isaiah 18:7)

"In Zion a stone that causes people to stumble and a rock that makes them fall, and the one who believes in him will never be put to shame." (Romans 9:33) 1 Peter 2:6 says this stone in Zion is Jesus, "a chosen and precious cornerstone."

So is it the return of Jews to Christ: as the world believe in Jesus the Messiha so shall is the Jews of Jerusalem believe in Jesus to be the True Mesiah!!

"Zion spreadeth forth her hands, and there is none to comfort her: the LORD hath commanded concerning Jacob, that his adversaries should be round about him: Jerusalem is as a menstruous woman among them." Lamentations 1:17

The Lord words as the end of days will be near until the those crucified Him will say: "till ye shall say, Blessed is he that cometh in the name of the Lord."

"O Jerusalem, Jerusalem, thou that killest the prophets, and stonest them which are sent unto thee, how often would I have gathered thy children together, even as a hen gathereth her chickens under her wings, and ye would not! [38] Behold, your house is left unto you desolate. [39] For I say unto you, Ye shall not see me henceforth, till ye shall say, Blessed is he that cometh in the name of the Lord."Matthew 23:37-39 KJV

[37]

More of interest that the Ancient Apostolic Ukrainian Eastern Christians dates back to the earliest centuries of he Apostolic Age, Saint Andrew with mission trips along the Black Sea and a legend of even ascending the hills of Kyiv. The first Christian community on territory of modern Ukraine is documented as early as the 9th century with establishment Metropolitanate of Gothia centered in Crimean Peninsula. The territory of the Old Rus in Kyiv became the dominant religion since its official acceptance in 988 by Vladmir the Great (Volodymyr the Great), who brought it from Byzantine Crimean

https://en.wikipedia.org/.../History_of_Christianity_in...

Behind the scenes, there is the most powerful force moving forward murdering and slaughtering those civilians. It has the sting of serpent snake misleading trick, malicious and wickedness of demon, the power of control and the dominion of Satan!

Conspirators and the rulers of the world got together against the Lord and Christ!!

What is the Truth and Who is behind it?

What is the coming role of the Russian Ukrainian War to Play in the Biblical end of Days??

The Heavy players are the two premier Opposing Powers!

Russia —Ancient Jews- Ancient Orthodox Christian-—West!

Those are affected first before the rest of the world Africa, Latin America, Australia, Canada —

__Zion in the Bible__

Psalm 135:21

Blessed be the Lord from Zion,

Who dwells in Jerusalem.

Praise the Lord!

Psalm 76:2 His tabernacle is in Salem;

His dwelling place also is in Zion.

Psalm 132:13-14 For the Lord has chosen Zion;

He has desired it for His habitation.

"This is My resting place forever;

Here I will dwell, for I have desired it.

Joel 3:17 Then you will know that I am the Lord your God, Dwelling in Zion, My holy mountain.

So Jerusalem will be holy,

And strangers will pass through it no more.

Psalm 9:14 That I may tell of all Your praises,

That in the gates of the daughter of Zion

I may rejoice in Your salvation.

Isaiah 52:1-2 Awake, awake, Clothe yourself in your strength, O Zion;

Clothe yourself in your beautiful garments,

O Jerusalem, the holy city;

For the uncircumcised and the unclean

Will no longer come into you.

Shake yourself from the dust, rise up,

O captive Jerusalem;

Loose yourself from the chains around your neck,

O captive daughter of Zion.

Lamentations 2:8-10

The Lord determined to destroy

The wall of the daughter of Zion.

He has stretched out a line,

He has not restrained His hand from destroying,

And He has caused rampart and wall to lament;

They have languished together.

Her gates have sunk into the ground,

He has destroyed and broken her bars.

Her king and her princes are among the nations;

The law is no more.

Also, her prophets find

No vision from the Lord.

The elders of the daughter of Zion

Sit on the ground, they are silent.

They have thrown dust on their heads;

They have girded themselves with sackcloth.

The virgins of Jerusalem

Have bowed their heads to the ground.

Micah 4:6-8

"In that day," declares the Lord,

"I will assemble the lame

And gather the outcasts,

Even those whom I have afflicted.

"I will make the lame a remnant

And the outcasts a strong nation,

And the Lord will reign over them in Mount Zion

From now on and forever.

"As for you, tower of the flock,

Hill of the daughter of Zion,

To you it will come—

Even the former dominion will come,

The kingdom of the daughter of Jerusalem.

Matthew 21:5 Say to the daughter of Zion,

'Behold your King is coming to you,

Gentle, and mounted on a donkey,

Even on a colt, the foal of a beast of burden.'"

John 12:15 Fear not, daughter of Zion; behold, your King is coming, seated on a donkey's colt."

Zechariah 9:9 Rejoice greatly, O daughter of Zion!

Shout in triumph, O daughter of Jerusalem!

Behold, your king is coming to you;

He is just and endowed with salvation,

Humble, and mounted on a donkey,

Even on a colt, the foal of a donkey.

Psalm 78:68 But chose the tribe of Judah,

Mount Zion which He loved.

Jeremiah 14:19 Have You completely rejected Judah?

Or have You loathed Zion?

Why have You stricken us so that we are beyond healing?

We waited for peace, but nothing good came;

And for a time of healing, but behold, terror!

Lamentations 2:1 How the Lord has covered the daughter of Zion

With a cloud in His anger!

He has cast from heaven to earth

The glory of Israel,

And has not remembered His footstool

In the day of His anger.

Isaiah 46:13 I bring near My righteousness, it is not far off; And My salvation will not delay.

And I will grant salvation in Zion,

And My glory for Israel.

Psalm 87:2 The Lord loves the gates of Zion

More than all the other dwelling places of Jacob.

Psalm 102:13-16 You will arise and have compassion on Zion;

For it is time to be gracious to her,

For the appointed time has come.

Surely Your servants find pleasure in her stones

And feel pity for her dust.

So the nations will fear the name of the Lord

And all the kings of the earth Your glory.

read more.

Psalm 133:3 It is like the dew of Hermon

Coming down upon the mountains of Zion;

For there the Lord commanded the blessing—life forever.

Psalm 132:13-16 For the Lord has chosen Zion;

He has desired it for His habitation.

"This is My resting place forever;

Here I will dwell, for I have desired it.

"I will abundantly bless her provision;

I will satisfy her needy with bread.

<u>"Zeal" in the Bible</u>

Numbers 25:11

"Phinehas son of Eleazar, son of Aaron the priest, has turned back My wrath from the Israelites because he was zealous among them with My zeal, so that I did not destroy the Israelites in My zeal.

Deuteronomy 29:20

Jehovah is not willing to be propitious to him, for then doth the anger of Jehovah smoke, also His zeal, against that man, and lain down on him hath all the oath which is written in this book, and Jehovah hath blotted out his name from under the heavens,

2 Samuel 21:2

And the king called the Gibeonites, and said unto them; (now the Gibeonites were not of the children of Israel, but of the remnant of the Amorites; and the children of Israel had sworn unto them: and Saul sought to slay them in his zeal to the children of Israel and Judah.)

2 Kings 10:16

And he said, Come with me, and see my zeal for the LORD. So they made him ride in his chariot.

2 Kings 19:31

For out of Jerusalem shall go forth a remnant, and they that escape out of mount Zion: the zeal of the LORD of hosts shall do this.

Ezra 7:23

Whatever is commanded by the God of heaven, let it be done with zeal for the house of the God of heaven, so that there will not be wrath against the kingdom of the king and his sons.

Psalm 69:9

For the zeal of thine house hath eaten me up; and the reproaches of them that reproached thee are fallen upon me.

Psalm 119:139

My zeal hath consumed me, because mine enemies have forgotten thy words.

Proverbs 19:2

Even zeal is not good without knowledge,and the one who acts hastily sins.

Ecclesiastes 9:6

Indeed their love, their hate and their zeal have already perished, and they will no longer have a share in all that is done under the sun.

Isaiah 9:7

Of the increase of his government and peace there shall be no end, upon the throne of David, and upon his kingdom, to order it, and to establish it with judgment and with justice from henceforth even for ever. The zeal of the LORD of hosts will perform this.

Isaiah 26:11

Lord, Your hand is lifted up to take action,but they do not see it.They will see Your zeal for Your people,and they will be put to shame.The fire for Your adversaries will consume them!

Isaiah 37:32

For out of Jerusalem shall go forth a remnant, and they that escape out of mount Zion: the zeal of the LORD of hosts shall do this.

Isaiah 42:13

The Lord advances like a warrior;He stirs up His zeal like a soldier.He shouts, He roars aloud,He prevails over His enemies.

Isaiah 59:17

For he put on righteousness as a breastplate, and an helmet of salvation upon his head; and he put on the garments of vengeance for clothing, and was clad with zeal as a cloke.

Isaiah 63:15

Look down from heaven, and behold from the habitation of thy holiness and of thy glory: where is thy zeal and thy strength, the sounding of thy bowels and of thy mercies toward me? are they restrained?

Ezekiel 5:13

Thus shall mine anger be accomplished, and I will cause my fury to rest upon them, and I will be comforted: and they shall know that I the LORD have spoken it in my zeal, when I have accomplished my fury in them.

Ezekiel 23:25

And I will direct my zeal against you, and they will deal with you in anger; your nose and your ears they will remove, and {those who are left}, they will fall by the sword, and they will take your sons and your daughters, and {your remnant} will be consumed by fire.

Ezekiel 36:5

"This is what the Lord God says: Certainly in My burning zeal I speak against the rest of the nations and all of Edom, who took My land as their own possession with wholehearted rejoicing and utter contempt so that its pastureland became plunder.

Ezekiel 36:6

Therefore, prophesy concerning the land of Israel and say to the mountains and hills, to the ravines and valleys: This is what the Lord God says: Look, I speak in My burning zeal because you have endured the insults of the nations.

Ezekiel 38:18

So it will be that on that day, when Gog invades the land of Israel,' declares the Lord GOD, "my zeal will ignite my anger.

Ezekiel 38:19

I swear in My zeal and fiery rage! On that day there will be a great earthquake in the land of Israel.

Zephaniah 1:18

Moreover, their silver and their gold will not be able to save them on the day of the wrath of Yahweh. And in the fire of his zeal, the whole land shall be consumed, for a terrifying end he shall make [for] all the inhabitants of the land.

Zephaniah 3:8

"Therefore wait for Me," declares the Lord,"For the day when I rise up as a witness.Indeed, My decision is to gather nations,To assemble kingdoms,To pour out on them My indignation,All My burning anger;For all the earth will be devouredBy the fire of My zeal.

Zechariah 1:14

And the messenger who is speaking with me, saith unto me, 'Call, saying: Thus said Jehovah of Hosts: I have been zealous for Jerusalem, and for Zion with great zeal.

Zechariah 8:2

'Thus said Jehovah of Hosts: I have been zealous for Zion with great zeal, With great heat I have been zealous for her.

Matthew 11:12

From the days of John the Baptist until now the kingdom of heaven suffers violent assault, and violent men seize it by force [as a precious prize].

John 2:17

And his disciples remembered that it was written, The zeal of thine house hath eaten me up.

Acts 5:17

And having risen, the chief priest, and all those with him -- being the sect of the Sadducees -- were filled with zeal,

Acts 13:45

and the Jews having seen the multitudes, were filled with zeal, and did contradict the things spoken by Paul -- contradicting and speaking evil.

Acts 18:25

This man had been instructed in the way of the Lord, and being spirituall impassioned, he was speaking and teaching accurately the things about Jesus, though he knew only the baptism of John;

Romans 10:2

For I bear them record that they have a zeal of God, but not according to knowledge.

Romans 12:8

or he who encourages, in the act of encouragement; he who gives, with generosity; he who leads, with diligence; he who shows mercy [in caring for others], with cheerfulness.

Romans 12:11

Do not lag in zeal, be enthusiastic in spirit, serve the Lord.

2 Corinthians 7:7

and not only by his arrival, but also by the comfort he received from you. He told us about your deep longing, your sorrow, and your zeal for me, so that I rejoiced even more.

2 Corinthians 7:11

For behold this selfsame thing, that ye sorrowed after a godly sort, what carefulness it wrought in you, yea, what clearing of yourselves, yea, what indignation, yea, what fear, yea, what vehement desire, yea, what zeal, yea, what revenge! In all things ye have approved yourselves to be clear in this matter.

2 Corinthians 7:12

So then, if also I wrote to you, it was not for the sake of him that injured, nor for the sake of him that was injured, but for the sake of our diligent zeal for you being manifested to you before God.

2 Corinthians 8:7

But just as you excel in everything, [and lead the way] in faith, in speech, in knowledge, in genuine concern, and in your love for us, see that you excel in this gracious work [of giving] also.

2 Corinthians 8:8

I do not speak as commanding it, but through the zeal of others, and proving the genuineness of your love.

2 Corinthians 8:16

But thanks be to God, who gives the same diligent zeal for you in the heart of Titus.

2 Corinthians 8:17

For he received indeed the entreaty, but, being full of zeal, he went of his own accord to you;

2 Corinthians 8:22

And we have sent with them our brother whom we have often proved to be of diligent zeal in many things, and now more diligently zealous through the great confidence he has as to you.

2 Corinthians 9:2

For I know the forwardness of your mind, for which I boast of you to them of Macedonia, that Achaia was ready a year ago; and your zeal hath provoked very many.

2 Corinthians 11:2

for I am zealous for you with zeal of God, for I did betroth you to one husband, a pure virgin, to present to Christ,

Galatians 1:13

You have heard of my career and former manner of life in Judaism, how I used to hunt down and persecute the church of God extensively and [with fanatical zeal] tried [my best] to destroy it.

Galatians 6:12

All who desire to display their zeal for external observances try to compel you to receive circumcision, but their real object is simply to escape being persecuted for the Cross of Christ.

Philippians 3:6

Concerning zeal, persecuting the church; touching the righteousness which is in the law, blameless.

Colossians 4:13

For I bear him record, that he hath a great zeal for you, and them that are in Laodicea, and them in Hierapolis.

Hebrews 10:27

but a certain fearful looking for of judgment, and fiery zeal, about to devour the opposers

James 3:14

and if bitter zeal ye have, and rivalry in your heart, glory not, nor lie against the truth

James 3:16

for where zeal and rivalry are, there is insurrection and every evil matter;

Revelation 3:19

Those whom I [dearly and tenderly] love, I rebuke and discipline [showing them their faults and instructing them]; so be enthusiastic and repent

Bible Verses That Start With The Letter Z

Nehemiah 10:12

Zaccur, Sherebiah, Shebaniah,

1 Chronicles 6:53

Zadok his son, Ahimaaz his son.

2 Samuel 15:29

Zadok therefore and Abiathar carried the ark of God again to Jerusalem: and they tarried there.

2 Samuel 23:28

Zalmon the Ahohite, Maharai the Netophathite,

Nehemiah 11:30

Zanoah, Adullam, and in their villages, at Lachish, and the fields thereof, at Azekah, and in the villages thereof. And they dwelt from Beersheba unto the valley of Hinnom.

Judges 5:18

Zebulun and Naphtali were a people that jeoparded their lives unto the death in the high places of the field.

Genesis 49:13

Zebulun shall dwell at the haven of the sea; and he shall be for an haven of ships; and his border shall be unto Zidon.

Jeremiah 52:1

Zedekiah was one and twenty years old when he began to reign, and he reigned eleven years in Jerusalem. And his mother's name was Hamutal the daughter of Jeremiah of Libnah.

2 Chronicles 36:11

Zedekiah was one and twenty years old when he began to reign, and reigned eleven years in Jerusalem.

2 Kings 24:18

Zedekiah was twenty and one years old when he began to reign, and he reigned eleven years in Jerusalem. And his mother's name was Hamutal, the daughter of Jeremiah of Libnah.

Chronicles 11:39

Zelek the Ammonite, Naharai the Berothite, the armourbearer of Joab the son of Zeruiah,

2 Samuel 23:37

Zelek the Ammonite, Nahari the Beerothite, armourbearer to Joab the son of Zeruiah,

Joshua 15:37

Zenan, and Hadashah, and Migdalgad,

Psalms 97:8

Zion heard, and was glad; and the daughters of Judah rejoiced because of thy judgments, O LORD.

Isaiah 1:27

Zion shall be redeemed with judgment, and her converts with righteousness.

Lamentations 1:17

Zion spreadeth forth her hands, and there is none to comfort her: the LORD hath commanded concerning Jacob, that his adversaries should be round about him: Jerusalem is as a menstruous woman among them.

Joshua 15:24

Ziph, and Telem, and Bealoth,

The meaning of words with Z as follows in this link:

https://bestbiblenames.com/all-biblical-names-that-start.../

NPR.ORG

The letter Z is becoming a symbol of Russia's war in Ukraine. But what does it mean?

It has become a symbol of the Russian invasion, painted on military vehicles, printed on T-shirts and widely distributed through social media in support of Moscow's war.

Putin Holocaust and Hitler Holocaust!

Written on 3/11/2022 by Ramsis Ghaly

Putin Holocaust 2022-2025 and Hitler Holocaust 1941-1945!

As 6 million of Jews killed so is the Ukrainians unless the world do something!!

Putin committing genocide to Ukrainians as Hitler had committed to Jews and despite modern and so called more civilized world 70 years later, yet the Reaction of the world is the same "watching"!!!

Back then, the world was blamed for "Not doing enough" and seventy years later, the world is the same "Not doing enough" and allowing a killer to kill thousands of innocent civil daily sucking their blood and call them "animals"????

What is the difference between the world reaction to Putin committing genocide to Ukrainians and Hitler committing genocide to the Jews?

The world reaction is the same in both; just watching the innocent people die, the children exterminated, the pregnant women murdered and their children buried with them —-

What ashamed we have never learned from the past! Those so called moral leaders: UN, NATO, Pope Francis, Israel prime minister, American and European leaders and the remaining countries all the same.

In our modern era, We are indeed much more accountable and guilty since we all are fully aware through the social Media and modern technology, we have at our finger tips millions of images and we have better communications and after all we are governed by high moral and ethical obligation under the roof of national and international laws!

What are we doing with all these information, higher education, judicial system, high tech,——but just watching millions of refugee and innocence are being slaughtered!!!

https://en.m.wikipedia.org/wiki/The_Holocaust

https://www.atlanticcouncil.org/.../putins-absurd.../

https://www.19fortyfive.com/.../vladimir-putin-is.../

EN.M.WIKIPEDIA.ORG

The Holocaust - Wikipedia

The Holocaust, also known as the Shoah,[b] was the genocide of European Jews during World War II.[3] Between 1941 and 1945, Nazi Germany and its collaborators systematically murdered some six million Jews across German-occupied Europe,[a] around two-thirds of Europe's Jewish population.[c] The murde...

CG, We are doing nothing. They are not part of NATO so therefore they won't help them. What a shame!

Who won and Who is Winning and Who Lost and Who is Losing?

Written on 3/31/2022 by Ramsis Ghaly

Who is from either side of the earth naive enough to believe any goodness or expect any gain from a war!!

Love and peace always much gains and prosperity but war always much loss and destruction!!

Whoever thy about to enter it even think about getting engaged to war just know no life or living in wars but death and grieving!!

Who won and Who is Winning???Who Lost and Who is Losing?

+ Who won and Who is Winning??? No Body and neither one can declare victory!! Who Lost and Who is Losing? Both sides lost and losing!!

Wars have proven over thousands of years destructive to both mankind and the planet!

There is nothing good in wars!

Nothing good will come in the long run!

Nothing green in wars but bombs, explosions, fires, fumes and extensive pollution, CO_2 production and toxins!

+ Who won and Who is Winning??? No Body and neither one can declare victory!! Who Lost and Who is Losing? Both sides lost and losing!!

In such a war, almost always, the loss is unbearable and devastation is everlasting!

No lessons learned from any wars since man is just a stubborn creation and does not learn from the past. It us the way it is! In fact in such wars and atrocities are part of human daily life since the beginning of creation even when only four people were living upon the entire earth planet, Cain rose up against his own brother and managed to stab to death his own brother Abel! Despite the thousands of wars man never learned to live in harmony with each other and never reach out to violence and wars!!

Genesis 4:8 KJV "And Cain talked with Abel his brother: and it came to pass, when they were in the field, that Cain rose up against Abel his brother, and slew him."

The everlasting trauma and the challenges of healing are everlasting because there is no such healing or recovery of losses. Indeed the only measures a society and the world will try to do are medicating, patching, forgetting, substituting—!

At the end, wars are never ever forgotten and when those involved in the wars come to reality, they realize the everlasting facts, they realize clearly the loss is forever and never ever return back to normal!

Soon to follow, only time, medication, Palliation and forgetfulness anyone can offer and hope for!!

The wars are followed with an everlasting shame, sorrows, sadness, cries, tears, commemoration, museums build up, science, support —

The causalities are numerous and can be classified into stages according to the timing as follows:

A-Acute stage (First month of War):

-Many lives lost and their lives cut short!

-Many are refugees and strangers in a foreign lands!

-Many are dying slowly from injuries, dehydration, hunger, freezing cold, suffocating!

- Grieving and screaming, gloominess and darkness, sorrows and cries—!

B- Subacute(Next Two Months)

-The same as under acute!

-Predators abusing Children and minorities!

-Opportunistic taking advantage!

- Robberies and crimes!

-Ongoing Trauma causalities!

- Grieving and screaming, gloominess and darkness, sorrows and cries—!

C- Chronic (Three month after War and Thereafter)

It is the worst result because it is everlasting and primarily Mental Health disruption!

- Stage of healing and minimize the mental trauma!

-Burden of causalities, disabilities,—!

- Grieving and screaming, gloominess and darkness, sorrows and cries—!

- Post traumatic syndrome!

- Come to accept reality: Sorrows, sadness,

- Family fragmentation and destruction of family ties!

-Mental health destruction and Emotionally unstable!

- Some of Those are:

Anger, hate, revenge, guilt, frustration,—-

Substance abuse and intoxication

Suicidal and self inflicted injuries, homicidal —-

Nuclear Radiation effects!

Rebuild up and reconstitute

Memorials, architectures to always remember and commemorate the war heroes

Love and peace always much gains and prosperity but war always much loss and destruction!! So Who won and Who is Winning??? No Body and neither one can declare victory!! Who Lost and Who is Losing? Both sides lost and losing!!

For that reason, the Bible is full of warning to those committing wars and atrocities and much more promoting Love and no violence but Peace and love as follows:

Revelation 21:4-8 KJV "And God shall wipe away all tears from their eyes; and there shall be no more death, neither sorrow, nor crying, neither shall there be any more pain: for the former things are passed away. [5] And he that sat upon the throne said, Behold, I make all things new. And he said unto me, Write: for these words are true and faithful. [6] And he said unto me, It is done. I am Alpha and Omega, the beginning and the end. I will give unto him that is athirst of the fountain of the water of life freely. [7] He that overcometh shall inherit all things; and I will be his God, and he shall be my son. [8] But the fearful, and unbelieving, and the abominable, and murderers, and whoremongers, and sorcerers, and idolaters, and all liars, shall have their part in the lake which burneth with fire and brimstone: which is the second death."

Matthew 5:3-14 KJV "Blessed are the poor in spirit: for theirs is the kingdom of heaven. [4] Blessed are they that mourn: for they shall be comforted. [5] Blessed are the meek: for they shall inherit the earth. [6] Blessed are they which do hunger and thirst after righteousness: for they shall be filled. [7] Blessed are the merciful: for they shall obtain mercy. [8] Blessed are the pure in heart: for they shall see God. [9] Blessed are the peacemakers: for they shall be called the children of God. [10] Blessed are they which are persecuted for righteousness' sake: for theirs is the kingdom of heaven. [11] Blessed are ye, when men shall revile you, and persecute you, and shall say all manner of evil against you falsely, for my sake. [12] Rejoice, and be exceeding glad: for great is your reward in heaven: for so persecuted they the prophets which were before you. [13] Ye are the salt of the earth: but if the salt have lost his savour, wherewith shall it be salted? it is thenceforth good for nothing, but to be cast out, and to be trodden under foot of men. [14] Ye are the light of the world. A city that is set on an hill cannot be hid."

+Romans 12:9-16,18-21 KJV "Let love be without dissimulation. Abhor that which is evil; cleave to that which is good. [10] Be kindly affectioned one to another with brotherly love; in honour preferring one another; [11] Not slothful in business; fervent in spirit; serving the Lord; [12] Rejoicing in hope; patient in tribulation; continuing instant in prayer; [13] Distributing to the necessity of saints; given to hospitality. [14] Bless them which persecute you: bless, and curse not. [15] Rejoice with them that do rejoice, and weep with them that weep. [16] Be of the same mind one toward another. Mind not high things, but condescend to men of low estate. Be not wise in your own conceits. [18] If it be possible, as much as lieth in you, live peaceably with all men. [19] Dearly beloved, avenge not yourselves, but rather give place unto wrath: for it is written, Vengeance is mine; I will repay, saith the Lord. [20] Therefore if thine enemy hunger, feed him; if he thirst, give him drink: for in so doing thou shalt heap coals of fire on his head. [21] Be not overcome of evil, but overcome evil with good."

The Russian Ukraine War Confirmed the World has neither Lion Leaders nor Lion Nations but Indecisive Conservative Thinkers!

Written on 3/22/2022 By Ramsis Ghaly

The Russian Ukraine War Confirmed the World has neither Lion Leaders nor Lion Nations but Indecisive Conservative Thinkers!

As I watched with broken heart the atrocity of Russian aggressions and the years of warning that a sovereign world leaders and nations should have put a stop many years ago, I asked myself who are the leaders and strong nations that should have put a stop to the inhuman killing of civilians and children??

I came up with this: "The Russian Ukraine War Confirmed the World has neither Lion Leaders nor Lion Nations but Indecisive Conservative Thinkers!" Furthermore, the Modern Moon Man is still behaving as the Ancient Cave Man!!! The Putin Modern Moon Man is still as malicious and evil as the Ancient Cave Man!!!

What the world had done different to stop Putin Holocaust for a month than the world had done since the ancient undeveloped nations had done since the beginning of the world!

The wars and crime of wars all the same regardless of civilization, Education, globalization and international and National guidelines, statues, merits and laws!!

All are the same: Barbarism, power, control, aggression, greediness, selfishness and absolute violation of human rights!! Man returns again to his prehistoric ancient image to be the One Grandiose Self Ego fulfilling his envious lust fighting to expand his dynasty and to run an empire and step on the weak and underprivileged!! As the times beginning of Mesopotamia,, Egyptian Empire and infantry, Babylonian war against Assyrian Empire, Ionia and Persian empire, Roman Empire, Tang dynasty in 618 AD, Gupta empire in 6th century, Kamakura period 12-13th century, --!

The stronger win! The lion is the king of the zoo! Well well well!! If this is the case, then can the world appoint the lion of the globe to keep the world in order and respect human right and the values of modern man that made it to the moon and soon to Mars.

Instead the Modern Moon Man is still behave as the Ancient Cave Man!!! The Putin Modern Moon Man is still as malicious and evil as the Ancient Cave Man!!!

What is the difference?? It is all slaughtering, murdering and killing of human lives. Death is death as an ancient days as in modern times!! What difference does it make to kill with a sword or machine gun, to have an army artillery tanks and flight jets ✈ or army with chariots of horses and Ancient weapons included the spear, the atlatl with light javelin or similar projectile, the bow and arrow, the sling; polearms such as the spear, falx and javelin; hand-to-hand weapons such as swords, spears, clubs, maces, axes, and knives. Catapults, siege towers, and battering rams were used during sieges.

The ancient warfare was of donkeys and oxen and of horses in the medieval warfare and of drones in the modern warfare and all aimed to slaughter mankind!!!

by Ramsis Ghaly

https://en.m.wikipedia.org/wiki/Ancient_warfare....

EN.M.WIKIPEDIA.ORG

Ancient warfare - Wikipedia

Ancient warfare is war that was conducted from the beginning of recorded history to the end of the ancient period. The difference between prehistoric and ancient warfare is more organization oriented than technology oriented. The development of first city-states, and then empires, allowed warfare to...

America Let Us Fly Our Air Buses and Get all those Civilian Ukrainians to Live in USA!

America shall Gain the best of the best building Historic Ukrainian villages and the World will be so proud and Jealous as Chicago is!!
Written On 3/23/2022 by Ramsis Ghaly

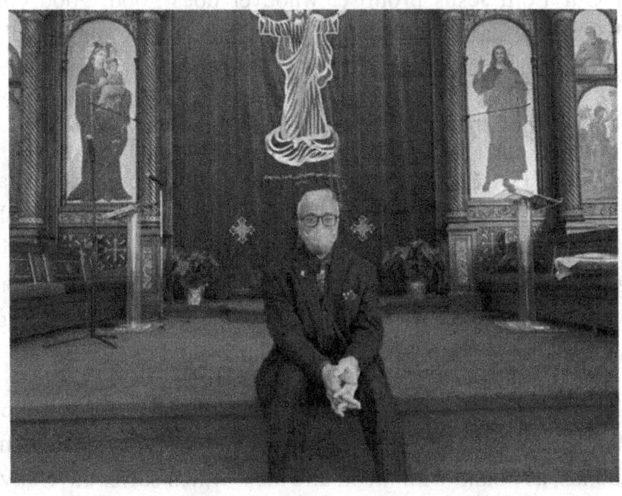

What is wrong of be courageous and kind and get the Ukrainians to America!! Fly all the civilians to America!! East Slavik's inherited genes are the best ethnicity and carry hardworking Nobel genes and produce great population!

America get your flights to Ukraine right now and rescue all the civilians and build Ukrainian villages across America the same as the Ukrainian village in Chicago!!

Let us go America ! The immigrant country of the world! The Ukrainians we have in Chicago they are the best ever people, hard worker, kind and never ever take advantage of the government!

Are you aware that God has blessed the Ukrainian genes and they were the founder of Russia and the genius minds of the original Nuclear technology and Farmers of Europe and the most religious Christians!!

America why should Europe take such a wonderful people and show kindness! God has blessed you with so much land and resources!

Those who truly in dire need are the people truly appreciate you most and with them it comes so much blessing from heaven!! Those children and mothers in loss and tears, they have angels in their sides that they will all be yours!!

America can do better!! Europe aren't immigrant countries. But America is!! And when things get settled whoever wants to go back, they can!! By this America you saved lives, you rescue multitudes, you brought love and joy instead of hate and destruction and you added much more treasure in the Lord Jesus Heart !

Remember Our Lord Jesus promise: whoever does good, good comes back multiplied! Whoever show kindness, kindness comes back multiplied! Whoever host strangers, angels comes multiplied!! God the Lord shall give more and more!

America you have nothing to loose and everything to win!

Galatians 6:7-10 KJV "Be not deceived; God is not mocked: for whatsoever a man soweth, that shall he also reap. [8] For he that soweth to his flesh shall of the flesh reap corruption; but he that soweth to the Spirit shall of the Spirit reap life everlasting. [9] And let us not be weary in well doing: for in due season we shall reap, if we faint not. [10] As we have therefore opportunity, let us do good unto all men, especially unto them who are of the household of faith."

Hebrews 13:1-3 KJV "Let brotherly love continue. [2] Be not forgetful to entertain strangers: for thereby some have entertained angels unawares. [3] Remember them that are in bonds, as bound with them; and them which suffer adversity, as being yourselves also in the body."

JM, AMEN

BC, Amen!

TM, Amen

TD, Amen

JB, Amen

Ukraine and Ukrainians. We are praying for you, We are crying fur you and we are torn and broken hearted witnessing what you and your children are going through!!

We are praying day and night for peace and peace shall prevail

I wish the world let me lead the mission for peace! I see Jesus and I see Satan in the war!!! Our Savior and His mother St Mary and archangel Michael shall prevail!!!!

https://www.facebook.com/100004402151562/posts/2115679515255433/?d=n

0:36 / 1:39

Журнал "ОТДОХНИ"

March 5 at 5:04 PM ·

Max of Barsky

JM, AMEN

BC, Amen!

TM, Amen

TD, Amen

JB, Amen

JB, Amen

CG, Love your idea. Let them come here like we do at our border.

ES, Amen. So well said.

A Thought of Peace Treaty of Egypt Israel and Ukraine Russia

Written By Ramsis Ghaly on 7/1/2022

1973, Egypt under President Sadat decided to pursue peace treaty 3/26/1979 with Israel despite the fact that Israel was rejected as a state among the Arabs.

Although Egypt was known to be also strong Arabic country allied with other Arabs and supported to be anti-Israel, President Sadat and Egypt took a huge turn against mainstream and decided to pursue peace to prevent further bloodshed and destruction!!

Following this thought, if President Volodymyr Zelensky made a peace treaty with President Volodymyr Putin and take a huge turn against mainstream even if temporary, he might have saved lives and lands like President Sadat yet let a better time in the future play out much better opportunity with minimal loss!

The Egypt–Israel peace treaty (Arabic: معاهدة السلام المصرية الإسرائيلية, romanized: Mu`āhadat as-Salām al-Misrīyah al-'Isrā'īlīyah; Hebrew: הסכם השלום בין ישראל למצרים, Heskem HaShalom Bein Yisrael LeMitzrayim) was signed in Washington, D.C., United States on 26 March 1979, following the 1978 Camp David Accords. The Egypt–Israel treaty was signed by Egyptian president Anwar Sadat and Israeli prime minister Menachem Begin and witnessed by United States president Jimmy Carter.

let us pray for peace, it has been four months of great destruction and killing civilians and non- civilians across the board! The green and yellow land is converted to ashes and the huge cities are buried under the smoke and the skies created by God almighty turned to grey clouds with smokes. Lord has mercy upon the malicious men and the creed and those benefitting from wars and behind wars!!

Amen lord have mercy!

Ramsis Ghaly

The Divine non human hand Warrior is coming to rescue Ukraine and our Beloved Ukrainians!

Written On 3/3/2022 by <u>Ramsis Ghaly</u>

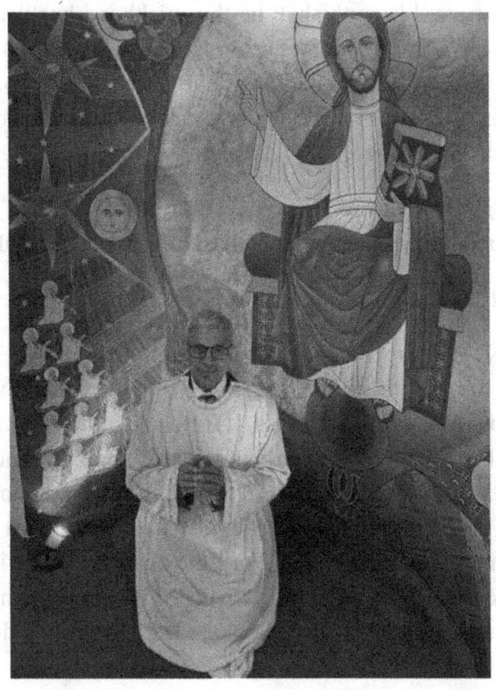

Ukraine and Ukrainians the world have failed you and so are the fellowmen but Jesus the Almighty never forsaken you all. The Rod of Moses and the Cross of Jesus is your undefeated heavenly weapon. God does not slack as it is written: "The Lord is not slack concerning his promise, as some men count slackness; but is longsuffering to us-ward, not willing that any should perish, but that all should come to repentance. [10] But the day of the Lord will come as a thief in the night; in the which the heavens shall pass away with a great noise, and the elements shall melt with fervent heat, the earth also and the works that are therein shall be burned up."2 Peter 3:9-10 KJV

Exodus 14:13-14 KJV "And Moses said unto the people, Fear ye not, stand still, and see the salvation of the Lord, which he will shew to you to day: for the

Egyptians whom ye have seen to day, ye shall see them again no more for ever. [14] The Lord shall fight for you, and ye shall hold your peace."

We all are praying as our tears and blood shedding for you all and so is God the Almighty coming to help you all and lift you up. You all shall remember of what the Almighty Lord is about to do!

Psalm 91:3-7 "Surely he shall deliver thee from the snare of the fowler, and from the noisome pestilence. [4] He shall cover thee with his feathers, and under his wings shalt thou trust: his truth shall be thy shield and buckler. [5] Thou shalt not be afraid for the terror by night; nor for the arrow that flieth by day; [6] Nor for the pestilence that walketh in darkness; nor for the destruction that wasteth at noonday. [7] A thousand shall fall at thy side, and ten thousand at thy right hand; but it shall not come nigh thee."

Psalm 3:7 KJV "Arise, O Lord ; save me, O my God: for thou hast smitten all mine enemies upon the cheek bone; thou hast broken the teeth of the ungodly."

Be still you shall see His salvation!! In Jesus our Heavenly Father name Amen!

Isaiah 41:10-14 KJV "Fear thou not; for I am with thee: be not dismayed; for I am thy God: I will strengthen thee; yea, I will help thee; yea, I will uphold thee with the right hand of my righteousness. [11] Behold, all they that were incensed against thee shall be ashamed and confounded: they shall be as nothing; and they that strive with thee shall perish. [12] Thou shalt seek them, and shalt not find them, even them that contended with thee: they that war against thee shall be as nothing, and as a thing of nought. [13] For I the Lord thy God will hold thy right hand, saying unto thee, Fear not; I will help thee. [14] Fear not, thou worm Jacob, and ye men of Israel; I will help thee, saith the Lord, and thy redeemer, the Holy One of Israel."

Psalm 3 "Lord, how are they increased that trouble me! many are they that rise up against me. [2] Many there be which say of my soul, There is no help for him in God. Selah. [3] But thou, O Lord, art a shield for me; my glory, and the lifter up of mine head. [4] I cried unto the Lord with my voice, and he heard me out of his holy hill. Selah. [5] I laid me down and slept; I awaked; for the Lord sustained me. [6] I will not be afraid of ten thousands of people, that have set themselves against me round about. [7] Arise, O Lord ; save me, O my God: for thou hast smitten all mine enemies upon the cheek bone; thou hast broken the teeth of the ungodly. [8] Salvation belongeth unto the Lord : thy blessing is upon thy people. Selah."

Psalm 91 "He that dwelleth in the secret place of the most High shall abide under the shadow of the Almighty. [2] I will say of the Lord, He is my refuge and my fortress: my God; in him will I trust. [3] Surely he shall deliver thee from the snare of the fowler, and from the noisome pestilence. [4] He shall cover thee with his feathers, and under his wings shalt thou trust: his truth shall be thy shield and buckler. [5] Thou shalt not be afraid for the terror by night; nor for the arrow that flieth by day; [6] Nor for the pestilence that walketh in darkness; nor for the destruction that wasteth at noonday. [7] A thousand shall fall at thy side, and ten thousand at thy right hand; but it shall not come nigh thee. [8] Only with thine eyes shalt thou behold and see the reward of the wicked. [9] Because thou hast made the Lord, which is my refuge, even the most High, thy habitation; [10] There shall no evil befall thee, neither shall any plague come nigh thy dwelling. [11] For he shall give his angels charge over thee, to keep thee in all thy ways. [12] They shall bear thee up in their hands, lest thou dash thy foot against a stone. [13] Thou shalt tread upon the lion and adder: the young lion and the dragon shalt thou trample under feet. [14] Because he hath set his love upon me, therefore will I deliver him: I will set him on high, because he hath known my name. [15] He shall call upon me, and I will answer him: I will be with him in trouble; I will deliver him, and honour him. [16] With long life will I satisfy him, and shew him my salvation."

AC. Dear Dr.**Ramsis Ghaly**, I told You, that Putin is devil We all people in Lithuania so scare, because Russia and Belarus aggressors and we have borders with them.

JM, Beautiful Dr. Ghhaly AMEN

RZ, Thank you for your prayers!

RC. Thank you for your prays All we need is peace for all

MS, Thank you for reminding me that God will take care of this and Putin. All keep praying.

LM, Amen

CG. Just keep praying and believing God will prevail

DW. Amen

JJ, Amen

Ukraine and Ukrainians we never stop praying and fasting for you all day and night to our Lord Jesus!!!

Ramsis Ghaly

We are remembering you all in every prayers. You are in our thoughts, hearts and souls forever!!! You shall never be forgotten!

The Christians worldwide remembering the Ukrainians and Ukraine during the prayers and fasting of the Grest Lent lifting our hearts and raising our arms in one voice to the world Savior Jesus Christ our Lord and God saying:

Lord Have mercy

O lord Have Mercy

O Lord and God have Mercy

We are pleading for you all. You are in our hearts, tears prayers and spirits all the time.

Amen

Al, Amén

Cg, Amen!

Kh, Praying 7:00am Pacific time daily. That's 5:00pm Ukraine time the start of their nightly curfew.

Es, Amen

Russia Ukrainian War February 24, 2022 is a True Biblical Turning Point!

Written on 3/13/2022 by Ramsis Ghaly

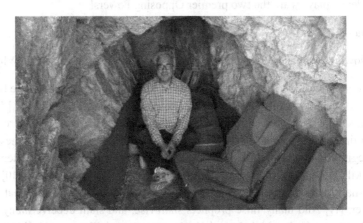

Russia Ukrainian War February 24, 2022 is a True Biblical Turning Point!

It is the beginning of sorrows!

The world has already seen: "Then let them which be in Judaea flee into the mountains: [17] Let him which is on the housetop not come down to take any thing out of his house: [18] Neither let him which is in the field return back to take his clothes. [19] And woe unto them that are with child, and to them that give suck in those days!" Matthew 24:16-19 KJV

It is a Biblical apocalyptic global Event!

It has prominent world's leaders!

It is externally unprovoked overnight major event with internal antichrist minds with hidden eyes!

It has heavy original ancient multi-nation-root connections: Christian, Jews and non-believers Agnostics Atheists!

It has the spirit of antichrist into its core!!!

Behind the scene it has the sting of serpent snake misleading trick, malicious and wickedness of demon, the power of control and the dominion of Satan!

Conspirators and the rulers of the world got together against the Lord and Christ!!

What is the Truth and Who is behind it?

What is the coming role of the Russian Ukrainian War to Play in the Biblical end of Days??

The Heavy players are the two premier Opposing Powers!

Russia ——West!

And low in the pole are Africa, Australia, Canada and Latin America!! Why!!!

It is written: "And ye shall hear of wars and rumours of wars: see that ye be not
troubled: for all these things must come to pass, but the end is not yet. [7] For
nation shall rise against nation, and kingdom against kingdom: and there shall
be famines, and pestilences, and earthquakes, in divers places. [8] All these are
the beginning of sorrows. [9] Then shall they deliver you up to be afflicted, and
shall kill you: and ye shall be hated of all nations for my name's sake. [10] And
then shall many be offended, and shall betray one another, and shall hate one
another. [11] And many false prophets shall rise, and shall deceive many. [12]
And because iniquity shall abound, the love of many shall wax cold. [13] But he
that shall endure unto the end, the same shall be saved. [15] When ye therefore
shall see the abomination of desolation, spoken of by Daniel the prophet, stand
in the holy place, (whoso readeth, let him understand:) [16] Then let them which
be in Judaea flee into the mountains: [17] Let him which is on the housetop not
come down to take any thing out of his house: [18] Neither let him which is in the
field return back to take his clothes. [19] And woe unto them that are with child,
and to them that give suck in those days! [20] But pray ye that your flight be not
in the winter, neither on the sabbath day: [21] For then shall be great tribulation,
such as was not since the beginning of the world to this time, no, nor ever shall
be. [22] And except those days should be shortened, there should no flesh be
saved: but for the elect's sake those days shall be shortened. [24] For there shall
arise false Christs, and false prophets, and shall shew great signs and wonders;
insomuch that, if it were possible, they shall deceive the very elect. [25] Behold,
I have told you before. [26] Wherefore if they shall say unto you, Behold, he is in
the desert; go not forth: behold, he is in the secret chambers; believe it not. [35]
Heaven and earth shall pass away, but my words shall not pass away." Matthew
24:6-13,15-22,24-26,35 KJV

Watch closely! Be prayerful! Humble thyself as thy begin to open thy eyes and hear thy voices! It is the Lent and the time of the conspirators on Christ and His salvation!

"But he that shall endure unto the end, the same shall be saved." Matthew 24:13 KJV

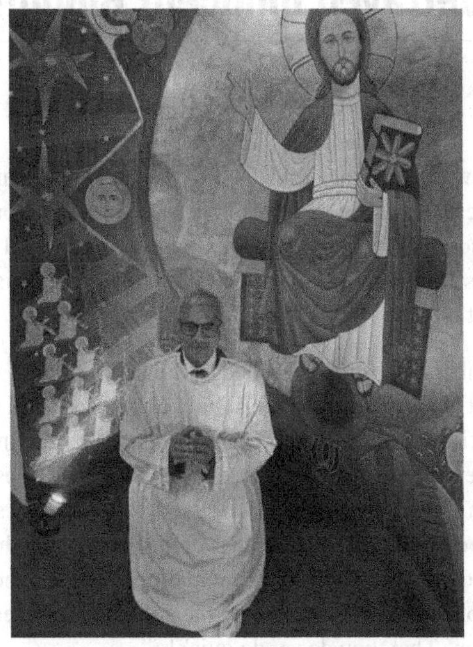

AV, Thx for info Dr Ghaly!! May God continue to bless you!

CR, Truly a Biblical event. We know Who eventually wins

JT, you speak from the heart and with faith Ramsis...this is all what we need to do now

Putin is 2022 Judas Iscariot Betrayed Innocent Blood!!

Written)3/30/2022 by Ramsis Ghaly

As the Christians worldwide including the Russian and Ukrainians are celebrating the Great Lent, Jesus Crucifix and soon Resurrection. The world remembers in this time Judas Iscariot, Traitor who with a false kiss betrayed His Master Lord Jesus for 30 silvers!! And so is Putin with 30 silvers of Ukrainians land and wealth, betrayed innocent blood!

The world remembers the innocent bloodshed of Ukrainians! As Judas Iscariot betrayed Innocent blood at that time so is Putin in modern time, the Traitor with a moment of false kiss, betrayed the innocent blood. As in that time, Satan entered Judas so is Satan entered Putin: John 13:21,26-27 KJV When Jesus had thus said, he was troubled in spirit, and testified, and said, Verily, verily, I say unto you, that one of you shall betray me. [26] Jesus answered, He it is, to whom I shall give a sop, when I have dipped it. And when he had dipped the sop, he gave it to Judas Iscariot, the son of Simon. [27] And after the sop Satan entered into him. Then said Jesus unto him, That thou doest, do quickly."

Today in my Coptic Orthodox church sister of Russian and Ukrainian Orthodox church, prayers were sent and incense ascending remembering all those died over the last 35 days of Russian /Ukrainian war and refugees. Those humiliated where their corps covering the streets and no one to burry them. No church to pray for them and no home to host them. Those their bodies exposed and lost dignity yet innocent in their core. They are the most treasured human being. May God repose their souls and remember those refugees.

Archangel Michael standing by Lord Jesus our Savior, please come down and put stop to the most satanic evil atrocity to mankind!!!

Incredible, the war is during the most holy fast of the Russian and Ukrainian Orthodox church, the Lent, Jesus crucifix to be followed by Resurrection!!! How have you all allowed Satan jealousy to ruin your holy fast and take advantage and overcome your holiness with wickedness and murdering the innocent!!

Millions of lives shall be asked of those committing the war crime! Predators of the world repent and return to Jesus immediately!

So many were waiting for the Great Lent, Jesus Crucifix and Resurrection to celebrate our Savior Salvation and triumph over Satan!! Look at what you have done!!! You took their lives away and send millions refugees in most holy days of your and our church!! You took them away from us and their families and you left millions homeless, hunger and dying!!! Yet you are still bombarding the lands and destroying the region and murdering the innocent!! You all won't be able to hid from history and from Jesus the Lord who fasted the Great lent for us and who Judas betrayed Him! So much similarities!!! Matthew 4:1-3 KJV "Then was Jesus led up of the Spirit into the wilderness to be tempted of the devil. [2] And when he had fasted forty days and forty nights, he was afterward an hungred. [3] And when the tempter came to him, he said, If thou be the Son of God, command that these stones be made bread."

O Russians and invaders you have done evil and you choose Satan to celebrate in this Easter and not Jesus the Savior of the world. Why why why???

You have done what Judas the betrayer did, surrender innocent blood of Jesus!!

O Russian Orthodox Church and Patriarch, rise and put an end to the war crime to your fellow Ukrainian Christians!!

We fast and pray crying for all the victims and bloodshed Amen

Psalm 2 "Why do the heathen rage, and the people imagine a vain thing? [2] The kings of the earth set themselves, and the rulers take counsel together, against the Lord, and against his anointed, saying, [3] Let us break their bands asunder, and cast away their cords from us. [4] He that sitteth in the heavens shall laugh: the Lord shall have them in derision. [5] Then shall he speak unto them in his wrath, and vex them in his sore displeasure. [6] Yet have I set my king upon my holy hill of Zion. [7] I will declare the decree: the Lord hath said unto me, Thou art my Son; this day have I begotten thee. [8] Ask of me, and I shall give thee the heathen for thine inheritance, and the uttermost parts of the earth for thy possession. [9] Thou shalt break them with a rod of iron; thou shalt dash them in pieces like a potter's vessel. [10] Be wise now therefore, O ye kings: be instructed, ye judges of the earth. [11] Serve the Lord with fear, and rejoice with trembling. [12] Kiss the Son, lest he be angry, and ye perish from the way, when his wrath is kindled but a little. Blessed are all they that put their trust in him."

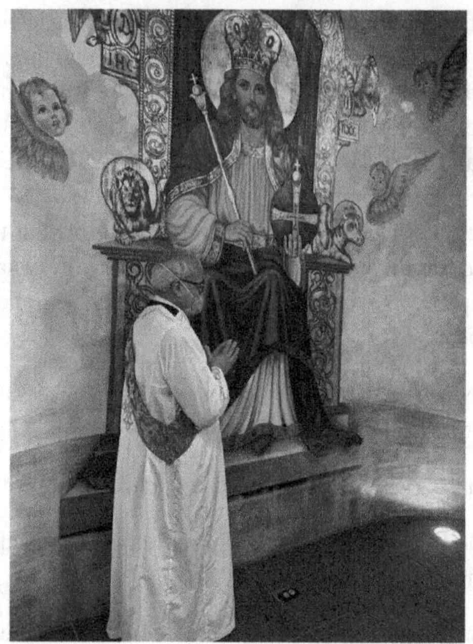

JT, amen...

MA, Amen!

KO, Amen we pray to the Lord

BM, Amen!

CG, What a great analogy of Putin and Judas. Let us pray oh Lord for all the victims. Amen

Disturbing Emigrant Russian Silence to Blatant Putin Aggression and War Crimes!

Written by Ramsis Ghaly

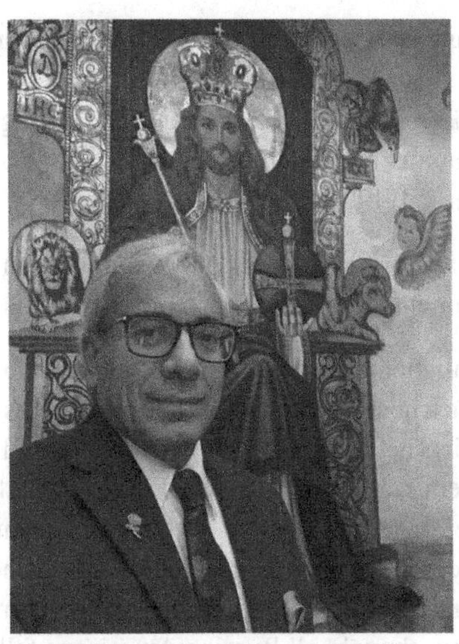

Normally we see emigrants speaking up when wrong-doing, corruptions and atrocities are transpired in their homelands! But isn't the case at all with emigrant Russians! None of emigrant Russians thus far spoke up nor any comments in common social media to deny or support obvious Putin aggression and atrocities against Ukrainians and Ukraine! The entire world spoke up but Not the Emigrant Russians!!

It certainly made me concern and I try to look deep unto the disturbing Emigrant Russian silence in this post!

Could Xenophobic Panic for Emigrant Russians as Why Media is Lacking the Russians Emigres living abroad comments about ongoing War and Speaking Up against Putin Actions! Why??

It is hard however, to do so because the majority of our Russian friends are not as social and they keep it to themselves!! But let us all check on them and support the Russian community as we do with the Ukrainian community!

I wonder why Russians native living abroad aren't demonstrating against Putin's war or denying in public the Russian actions against Ukraine or speaking up or commenting on the war!!

Perhaps it is not in the Russian nature to do so and perhaps they prefer to stay out of social media and be out of sight: keeping to themselves private!!!

Russians Fears and Emigration Briefing:

Unfortunately, nowadays with Putin Stalin action 2022 Emigrants Russians found themselves singled out and blamed in a xenophobic panic as their early years of Russia communist party 1919!

OR, Russians abroad are torn in fears not only from Russian government but also from the local governments where they currently live abroad!!

Are they afraid of retaliation from the Russian government or be poisoned or their family be in trouble back home?? Putin regime is a dangerous and can't be trusted!! It must be great conflicts between Russians in homeland and Russian Emigrants!! In fact in the twentieth century of Russian Emigration, they were threatened and any Soviet citizen who dared move to the U.S. became a nonperson—the Soviet Union stripped defectors of their citizenship, cut them off from contact with their families, and sometimes made it illegal to even mention their names. In the early days, Soon, though, all Russian Americans fell victim to a wave of xenophobic panic that spread through U.S. society. After the Russian Revolution, the American government began to fear that the U.S. was in danger of its own communist revolution and cracked down on political and labor organizations. Russian immigrants were singled out as a particular danger, and their unions, political parties, and social clubs were spied upon and raided by federal agents! https://www.loc.gov/.../imm.../polish-russian/soviet-exiles/

Recent report indicates 200,000 Russians exodus Russia emigrated out of Russia thousands fled abroad: https://www.bbc.com/news/world-europe-60697763.amp

In fact many Russians abroad are being blamed for Ukraine invasion and Putin actions: "I immigrated because murderers and thieves siezed power in Russia," said Kroo, a property developer originally from Omsk who fled the country over 20 years ago. "We have to oppose the actions of Putin and his criminal entourage." Yet many Russians living abroad are now being held responsible for a regime that they wanted to escape" https://www.themoscowtimes.com/.../russians-abroad-blamed...

Russians mass migration was 17th century. A significant ethnic Russian emigration took place in the wake of the Old Believer schism in the 17th century (for example, the Lipovans, who migrated southwards around 1700). Later ethnic Russian communities, such as the Doukhobors (who emigrated to the Transcaucasus from 1841 and onwards to Canada from 1899), also emigrated as religious dissidents fleeing centrist authority. One of the religious minorities that had a significant effect on emigration from Russia was the Russian Jewish Population.

The Russian-speaking (Russophone) diaspora are the people for whom Russian language is the native language, regardless of whether they are ethnic Russians or not. Early Russian migration to America was related to Widespread poverty and starvation cast a shadow over Russia during the late 1800s. For Jews, forced relocation to desolate areas coupled with ongoing persecutions and killings called pogroms inspired mass emigration. Between 1880 and 1910, more than two million hopeful Russians set out on foot, bound for port cities further east, where many sailed to the United States. Almost half of the newcomers put down roots in New York City, Boston, and Chicago, taking jobs in bustling factories, many as garment workers. Those who preferred rural living reaped the benefits of the Homestead Act and set up farms across the West, while still others worked in mills and mines in the American heartland. Russians contributed their diverse cultural traditions and devout faith (for some Judaism and others Russian Orthodox) to the places they settled. Unlike immigrants from other countries, few returned to Russia—: https://www.ancestry.com/histor.../russian-immigration-1800s

Russian emigres In the twentieth century, Emigration from the Soviet Union is often broken down into three "waves" (волны) of emigration. The waves are the "First Wave", or "White Wave", which left during the Russian Revolution of 1917 and then the Russian Civil War; the "Second Wave", which emigrated during and after World War II; and the "Third Wave", which emigrated in the 1950s, 1960s, 1970s, and 1980s.

A sizable wave of ethnic Russians emigrated in the wake of the October Revolution of 1917 and the Russian Civil War of 1917–1922. They became known collectively as the White émigrés. That emigration is also referred to as the "first wave" even though previous emigrations had taken place, as it was comprised the first emigrants to have left in the wake of the Communist Revolution, and because it exhibited a heavily political character. A smaller group of Russians, often referred to by Russians as the "second wave" of the Russian emigration, left during World War II. They were refugees, Soviet POWs, eastern workers, or surviving veterans of the Russian Liberation Army and other collaborationist armed units that had served under the German command and evaded forced repatriation. In the immediate postwar period, the largest Russian communities in the emigration settled in Germany, Canada, the United States, the United

Kingdom, and Australia. Emigres who left after the death of Stalin but before perestroika, are often grouped into a "third wave". The emigres were mostly Jews, Armenians, Germans, and other peoples who resided outside the former borders of the Russian Empire but now found themselves inside the Soviet Union. Most left in the 1970s. After the dissolution of the Soviet Union, Russia suffered an economic depression in the 1990s. This caused many Russians to leave Russia for Western countries. The economic depression ended in 2000. Also, during this time, ethnic Russians who lived in other post-Soviet states moved to Russia. https://en.m.wikipedia.org/wiki/Russian_diaspora

Russian Americans (Russian: ру́сские америка́нцы, tr. rússkiye amerikántsy, IPA: [ˈruskʲɪje ɐmʲɪrʲɪˈkant͡sɨ]) are Americans of full or partial Russian ancestry. The term can apply to recent Russian immigrants to the United States, as well as to those who settled in the 19th-century Russian possessions in northwestern America. Russian Americans comprise the largest Eastern European and East Slavic population in the U.S., the second-largest Slavic population generally, the nineteenth-largest ancestry group overall, and the eleventh-largest from Europe. In the mid-19th century, waves of Russian immigrants fleeing religious persecution settled in the U.S., including Russian Jews and Spiritual Christians. These groups mainly settled in coastal cities, including Alaska, Brooklyn (New York City) on the East Coast, and Los Angeles, San Francisco, and Portland, Oregon, on the West Coast, as well as in Great Lakes cities, such as Chicago and Cleveland. After the Russian Revolution of 1917 and the Russian Civil War of 1917-1922, many White émigrés also arrived, especially in New York, Philadelphia, and New England. Emigration from Russia subsequently became very restricted during the Soviet era (1917-1991). However, after the dissolution of the Soviet Union at the end of the Cold War, immigration to the United States increased considerably. In several major U.S. cities, many Jewish Americans who trace their heritage back to Russia; and Americans of East Slavic origin, such as Belarusian Americans, and Rusyn Americans sometimes identify as Russian Americans. Additionally, certain non-Slavic groups from the post-Soviet space, such as Armenian Americans, Georgian Americans, and Moldovan Americans, have a longstanding historical association with the Russian American community. https://en.m.wikipedia.org/wiki/Russian_Americans

Russians Emigrants are Being targeted:

Soon, though, all Russian Americans fell victim to a wave of xenophobic panic that spread through U.S. society. After the Russian Revolution, the American government began to fear that the U.S. was in danger of its own communist revolution and cracked down on political and labor organizations. Russian immigrants were singled out as a particular danger, and their unions, political parties, and social clubs were spied upon and raided by federal agents. In New York City alone more than 5,000 Russian immigrants were arrested. During the worst years of the Red Scare, 1919 and 1920, thousands of Russians were deported without a formal trial. Ironically, most were sent to the Soviet Union—a new nation that the older generation of immigrants had never lived in, and that the White Russians wanted to overthrow. As a result of the Red Scare, the Russian American community began to keep a low profile. Fear of persecution led many Russians to convert to Protestantism, to change their names, and to deny their heritage to any outsiders.

In the 1930s, fears of a new world war brought several thousand more Russians to the U.S. These immigrants were fairly affluent and well educated, and many were able to eventually find work in their old professions. Some had been farmers in the old country and founded a string of successful farms in the mid-Atlantic states. Others gravitated to established Russian American communities in Philadelphia, Chicago, Boston, Pittsburgh, New York City, and Cleveland.

This wave of Russian immigrants also carried with it the latest intellectual and artistic currents from Europe. The interwar years saw many of the major thinkers of the Russian avant-garde make their way to New York, where they influenced and enriched the burgeoning modernist movement. The composer Igor Stravinsky was able to present his challenging symphonies to U.S. audiences, while the choreographic vision of George Balanchine helped bring much of 20th century American dance into being. Later, the novelist Vladimir Nabokov brought his elegant prose and incisive critical sensibility to bear on the cultural landscape of his new homeland, illuminating both its promise and its paradoxes.

The end of World War II saw an even greater upheaval, as refugees from across Europe fled the chaos and depression of the postwar years. More than 20,000 Russian refugees—known as "displaced persons" successfully reached the United States. By this time, though, tensions between the U.S. and Soviet Union were rising, and prospective emigrants became pawns in a global geopolitical game. In 1952, the Soviet government had become embarrassed by the high rate at which its artists and scientists were decamping to America, and it established strict controls over emigration. Just as it had been during the rule of the czars, Russian immigration to the U.S. became a rare and risky undertaking.

For two decades, any Soviet citizen who dared move to the U.S. became a nonperson—the Soviet Union stripped defectors of their citizenship, cut them off from contact with their families, and sometimes made it illegal to even mention their names. In the early 1970s, however, relations between the two superpowers began to thaw. The authorities began allowing a few thousand dissatisfied citizens to leave the U.S.S.R. each year, including Jewish Soviets, dissidents, writers, and others deemed "undesirable" by the state. Cultural ties were also extended, and Soviet artists and musicians were sent on tours of the United States; when some of these cultural ambassadors chose to defect, the Soviet government was embarrassed once more. Recent report indicates 200,000 Russians exodus Russia emigrated out of Russia thousands fled abroad: https://www.bbc.com/news/world-europe-60697763.amp

In fact many Russians abroad are being blamed for Ukraine invasion and Putin actions: "I immigrated because murderers and thieves siezed power in Russia," said Kroo, a property developer originally from Omsk who fled the country over 20 years ago. "We have to oppose the actions of Putin and his criminal entourage." Yet many Russians living abroad are now being held responsible for a regime that they wanted to escape" https://www.themoscowtimes.com/.../russians-abroad-blamed...

Please check in our American Russians friends as you all are checking on our Ukrainians friends! I am sure they are devastated with Putin's actions against Ukraine!!

Let us know if you know why?? Media is Lacking the Russians Emigres living abroad comments about the ongoing War! Why??

Respectfully

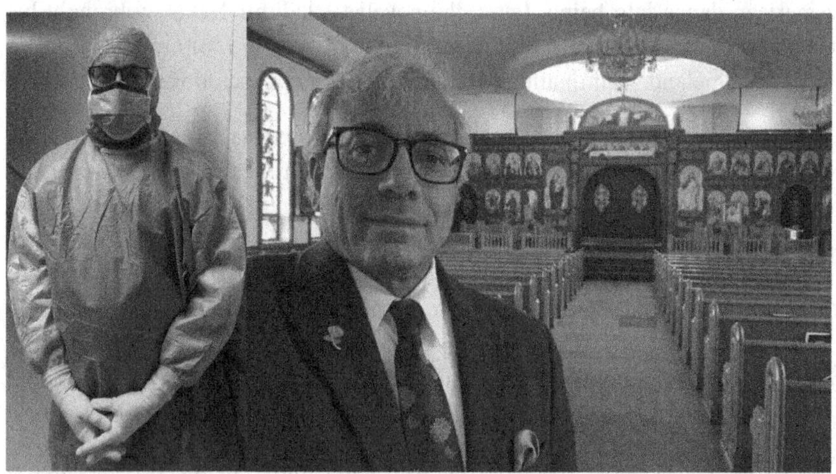

JT, that is right Ramsis...not all from any nation go along with or agree with their dictators or presidents rules and mandates...some of the globalists are the most

selfish, evil and greedy people on the planet...love everyone and spread the word of our God

NC, If only the Russians knew

CG, Russia has cracked down on free speech and placed strict propaganda controls on what citizens see and hear about the brutal war in Ukraine. They are told the soldiers are not attacking civilians. They were also told that they were accepted as liberators and wanted to live under Russian rule. It is a shame the people of Russia are living blindly.

Modern World Cannot Put a Stop to The Slaughtering of Innocent Civilians!!

Written On 3/19/2022 by Ramsis Ghaly

Modern World Can not Put a Stop to The Slaughtering of Innocent Civilians!!

The modern global world is supposed to be a free united world shared with laws and values under the umbrella of human rights. However, the unprovoked war crime committed by Putin and Russian army over Ukraine has shown otherwise!!

It has proven, Indeed our world has fake leaders, coward heroes, selfish patriots and unwise preachers to allow massacre of their children and innocent civilians occurring next door to their Neighbors and unable to put a stop to this satanic atrocity and is going for a month!! It has disgraced our world, cursed our living, took the civility of our land, degraded our humanity, ruined our reputation, spoiled our planet, dishonored our integrity, embarrassed our nature and provoked the wrath of our Creator!!!

Lucifer unimaginable Savage destruction and Massive ongoing war crimes all over social media reachable all the corners of earth worldwide and no one able to stop it immediately!!!! Demolition of Ukraine!! Besieged Discriminately targeting innocent civilians humiliated and mutilated as corps laying in the bombed roads wreckages, debris, remains, ruins and rubbles —-blockades —Kremlins careless merciless with no relieve 24/7 shillings-no axis to humanitarians— millions trapped in dire conditions—Fled dehydrated starved and mentally destroyed---ongoing massive destruction inconsiderate to international laws—-

“Therefore consider the members of your earthly body as dead to immorality, impurity, passion, evil desire, and greed, which amounts to idolatry. For it is because of these things that the wrath of God will come” Colossians 3:5-6 Revelation 21:8 KJV “But the fearful, and unbelieving, and the abominable, and murderers, and whoremongers, and sorcerers, and idolaters, and all liars, shall have their part in the lake which burneth with fire and brimstone: which is the second death.”

Malicious killing and tortures to innocence civilians begging fur help defenseless as the world watching it all in social media at their homes and coffee shops and bars!! Indeed that gesture without works is dead and means nothing as it is written: James 2:14-18,26 KJV “What doth it profit, my brethren, though a man say he hath faith, and have not works? can faith save him? [15] If a brother or sister be naked, and destitute of daily food, [16] And one of you say unto them, Depart in peace, be ye warmed and filled; notwithstanding ye give them not those things which are needful to the body; what doth it profit? [17] Even so faith, if it hath not works, is dead, being alone. [18] Yea, a man may say, Thou hast faith, and I have works: shew me thy faith without thy works, and I will shew thee my faith by my works. [26] For as the body without the spirit is dead, so faith without works is dead also."

How can be a Modern Moral World Cannot Put a Stop to The Slaughtering of Innocent Civilians!!

How can be a Courtesy Advocate World Cannot Put a Stop to The Slaughtering of Innocent Civilians!!

It is the time for the world and organizations to get together and examine what they had done wrong toward the Ukrainian rescue mission!! Doing so won't bring back the lives lost and they are considered sacrifice to careless world!! Let us review our books and laws and never ever to allow such inhuman war crimes to happen again!!

We must look at ourselves and question our leaderships worldwide and expose our cowardliness for not taking the appropriate bravery steps that a reasonable world will do to their own!

No matter whatever the reasons are, it is absolutely wrong to to watch civilians including children and minors be killed and slaughtered innocently through unprovoked war and the world watch each second of the killing in social media and either do nothing or do little and not doing enough to put stop immediately to the killing and madness!!!

It is the absolute disgrace and disastrously to a God believing world that the entire world should be ashamed! Before the world eyes watching day and night constant bombardments to civil building, homes, hospitals, schools, shelters, theaters, and green land cutting all basic life support to millions——and no one worldwide to stop it!!!!!!

What those children have done to deserve to be refugee and slaughtered? What those regular civilians have done wrong to deserve to be bombed and tortured? What those parents and Laborers have done to be war prisoners and be surrounded to be killed and live under constant curfew? The world acknowledged and met to conclude we are unable yo do anymore but watching!!!!

If the civilized highly educated modern world cannot put an immediate stop to such a blatant atrocity and the only thing they can do are sanctions and supply weapons of war, then the world has a serious problem and its doctrine is that of the Zoo and not that of humanity???

What kind of world we live in called "Modern and Governed Moral World" that a month now watching in social media 24/7 slaughtering civilians and millions refugees! The World Cannot Put a Stop to The Slaughtering of Innocent Civilians!!

Indeed our world has fake leaders, coward heroes, selfish patriots and unwise preachers to allow massacre of their children and innocent civilians occurring next door to their Neighbors and unable to put a stop to this satanic atrocity and is going for a month!! It has disgraced our world, took the civility of our land, degraded our humanity, ruined our reputation, spoiled our planet, dishonored our integrity, embarrassed our nature and provoked the wrath of our Creator!!!

Indeed happy is he putting his trust in the Lord of Jacob and not in the princes nor in the son of man, in whom there is no help!! The Lord shall reign for ever, even thy God, O Zion, unto all generations. Praise ye the Lord.

Psalm 146 "—-Put not your trust in princes, nor in the son of man, in whom there is no help. [4] His breath goeth forth, he returneth to his earth; in that very day his thoughts perish. [5] Happy is he that hath the God of Jacob for his help, whose hope is in the Lord his God: [6] Which made heaven, and earth, the sea, and all that therein is : which keepeth truth for ever: [7] Which executeth judgment for the oppressed: which giveth food to the hungry. The Lord looseth the prisoners: [8] The Lord openeth the eyes of the blind: the Lord raiseth them that are bowed down: the Lord loveth the righteous: [9] The Lord preserveth the strangers; he relieveth the fatherless and widow: but the way of the wicked he turneth upside down. [10] The Lord shall reign for ever, even thy God, O Zion, unto all generations. Praise ye the Lord."

CG, It is very hard to watch the destruction of Ukraine and its people. May God protect them and give them courage to carry on.

JT, the cowards have secret dealings with the enemy

TJ, They can but are afraid. Those who are afraid to stand up to a bully cannot win. We need strong leadership

SUMMIT NATO 7

WRITTEN 3/24/2022

Those Leaders will look better not by expensive suits and fashionable dresses but rather by taking an immediate action to put an immediate stop on the unprovoked war, the civilians death and torture and causalities!!

Do those leaders know that the dead are no longer need their help!! If you are dead, you are dead, supplying weapons and food won't help!!

If you need to do something for a month now go and stop the Russian invaders and protect Ukraine and save Ukrainians!

They meet and talk, then they talk and meet and no one is taking a radical action because of fears!! They miscalculate the entire war and now they are far behind! On the other hand, Putin neither meet or talk but does!

It reminds me of meeting in hospitals to go over the dead and what went wrong!! The true action is now to prevent death!!

Look at them, they look like having party and love their pictures!!! While millions are refugee and tens of thousands dead and broken!

Putin is laughing at them!! No one of them yet can stop him or take out of the box effective way to stop Putin!! Look at them, they are well fed, well rested and having expensive suites and dresses, yet many corps unburied in the streets and children in refugee camps, many trapped, dehydrated, naked, starve and lost all their belongings!!! What those people are doing, having talks snd funs!!

Look at them! The blood and the pains of all the Ukrainians and the helpless Russians soldiers are in their hands. This war shoukd have been prevented by true heroes!!!

Ramsis Ghaly

CNN.COM

G7 leaders take family photo ahead of emergency summit

The G7 leaders just took a family photo in Brussels ahead of an emergency summit to discuss Russia's invasion in Ukraine.

CG, You are such a compassionate person. You are so concerned for the people of the Ukraine like many Americans. Like you we would like too see someone stop Putin and the atrocities he is raging on Ukraine. Bless you!

Come And Rescue Me Why are You Standing Further Away!!

Written on 3/18/2022 by Ramsis Ghaly

How can it be the war atrocity in two nations sharing the same ethnicity from East Slavic and sharing almost similar language?? How can it be Russians are destroying and killing their own invade each other??? The Ukrainian cities can no longer be seen from the black smokes and lit of fires and fumes being under constant bombardments of the massacre!! Russia declare Death death death to Ukraine and Ukrainians, flooding the land with Ukrainian blood full scale —Five millions Russian missiles hit Ukraine—Curfew sustained firing three weeks since 2/24/2022!

Ukrainians, or the Ukrainian people, are an East Slavic ethnic group native to Ukraine.

Ukraine and Ukrainians: You are Not Forgotten: we pray for you and our tears and blood shed for you!!

As Hitler Holocaust brutality so is Putin Holocaust brutality to Ukrainians!!! No tolerance to war crimes and humanitarian assistance immediately to be implemented! We the people are demanding Rescue mission and rebuilding and recovery effort as soon as possible!!

I am bombed! I am lost! I am dead! What are you waiting for!!! I am vanishing away disintegrating to ashes before your eyes!! Come and rescue me why are you standing further away!! I am dying away burred in my wounds bleeding to death! If you can't come and help me, then come and burry me and write my story in history and teach the generations my heroism and your shame and cowardliness!

In such a time, lip services of no help! Every minute many lives are lost and building and hospitals are being destroyed!! Where is my helper? Where are you my Good Samaritan? Where are you my hero and my Patriot?

Who will put stop to this satanic madness and restrain Putin and his team? Who has the influence to make a difference and protect my nation and my people?? Where are you my Ukrainian and Russian Orthodoxia patriarch and Vatican church leaders to intervene???

Why you all are leaving me a nation and innocent people getting bombarding unceasing to these merciless unrelenting atrocities?

If you can't come and help me, then come and burry me and write my story in history and teach the generations my heroism and your shame and cowardliness!

I am a sovereign nation Ukraine is my ancient and historic free, Russia bombards me thousands and thousands times curfew with Heavy artillery barrage shaking my city!

My country is about to be destroyed with 40 miles lined up of explosives and ranked full of evil missiles and satanic man-made destructive missiles coming from the most powerful country!

My people are slaughtered and my country is bombed day and night from everywhere!

The enemy fire missiles are targeting my country from the air, the ground and the seas surrounding us!

The enemy have destroyed all what I have and my belonging! I am all alone under piles of ashes that had remained from my town! Stranger I am with no roof or safe place to hide!

The hunger, the thirst, the terror, the fear and explosives are killing us ! My people are being slaughtering unprovoked overnight, we are the innocent and being attacked by and the enemy forces are occupying my Ukraine !

My home Ukraine has no more sky and no more moon of stars seen but the entire high is lit up with firefight and jets full of explosives

Nonstop strikes, blowing, hitting, setting fires and soon I will be no more!

I am a free country under siege the enemy forces surround my town cutting off essential supplies, with the aim of compelling the surrender of those inside.

I am a huge housing complex and thousands are innocent living civilians destroyed to ashes!

I am a newborn shot dead just before my first breath and my first minute in the world!

I am a mother slaughtered as I was delivering my dream baby after 9 months nourishing in my body!

I am a child waiting in line going to the unknown away from my home! All the exits are swamped and blocked and ways for my parents and my children to escape are getting impossible!

The worse is yet to come! I lost everything! What else remained. I am by a bomb shelter, by a punker, by a camp! Ukrainians are in a Huge suffering and apocalyptic, country in a siege dire and desperate! The Russian are destroying us!

Hitting every part of us! We are crying grieving our tears and blood like rivers running and soaking our ground!!

Every second a child is becoming refugee and I need child protection service to protect me against predators of child exploitation!

I am terrified! I am among hundreds of lost children thrown unto a camp facing the unknown! I just became fatherless motherless lost all my family! I am an orphan! My life changed overnight seeing nothing but nightmare!!

Four millions of civilians were able to run away to safety leaving everything behind! Their treasures and history are gone! They are Strangers laying in camps in foreign lands refugee pleading for peace!!

The elders and minors are at great risk jumping broken bridges, walking barefooted and their safety from abusers and users can't be underestimated!

My family is no more and many are sick and Ill with no Pharmacy or hospital or someone to card for them!!

I am a city getting bombed day and night!

I am an ancient architecture demolished to rubbles!

I am a fertile land ready to produce crops destroyed to nothing!

I am a grocery store full of goods to feed the public ignites yo fire with the Russian explosives!

I am totally seized by my enemy for no reason! My enemy committing genocide against my country and my people!!

The recovery will be forever and healing will be impossible as nothing will return back! My country and my people are lost forever! With them to goes thousands of years of heritage!!

What are you waiting for!!! I am vanishing away disintegrating to ashes before your eyes!! Come and rescue me why are you standing further away!! I am dying away burred in my wounds bleeding to death! If you can't come and help me, then come and burry me and write my story in history and teach the generations my heroism and your shame and cowardliness!

O my Lord Jesu You are my Only One! They all ran away and left me alone so please don't go!!!

Psalm 22 "My God, my God, why hast thou forsaken me? why art thou so far from helping me, and from the words of my roaring? [2] O my God, I cry in the daytime, but thou hearest not; and in the night season, and am not silent. [3] But thou art holy, O thou that inhabitest the praises of Israel. [4] Our fathers trusted in thee: they trusted, and thou didst deliver them. [5] They cried unto thee, and were delivered: they trusted in thee, and were not confounded. [6] But I am a worm, and no man; a reproach of men, and despised of the people. [7] All they that see me laugh me to scorn: they shoot out the lip, they shake the head, saying, [8] He trusted on the Lord that he would deliver him: let him deliver him, seeing he delighted in him. [9] But thou art he that took me out of the womb: thou didst make me hope when I was upon my mother's breasts. [10] I was cast upon thee from the womb: thou art my God from my mother's belly. [11] Be not far from me; for trouble is near; for there is none to help. [12] Many bulls have compassed me: strong bulls of Bashan have beset me round. [13] They gaped upon me with their mouths, as a ravening and a roaring lion. [14] I am poured out like water, and all my bones are out of joint: my heart is like wax; it is melted in the midst of my bowels. [15] My strength is dried up like a potsherd; and my tongue cleaveth to my jaws; and thou hast brought me into the dust of death. [16] For dogs have compassed me: the assembly of the wicked have inclosed me: they pierced my hands and my feet. [17] I may tell all my bones: they look and stare upon me. [18] They part my garments among them, and cast lots upon my vesture. [19] But be not thou far from me, O Lord : O my strength, haste thee to help me. [20] Deliver my soul from the sword; my darling from the power of the dog. [21] Save me from the lion's mouth: for thou hast heard me from the horns of the unicorns. [22] I will declare thy name unto my brethren: in the midst of the congregation will I praise thee. [23] Ye that fear the Lord, praise him; all ye the seed of Jacob, glorify him; and fear him, all ye the seed of Israel. [24] For he hath not despised nor abhorred the affliction of the afflicted; neither hath he hid his face from him; but when he cried unto him, he heard. [25] My praise shall be of thee in the great congregation: I will pay my vows before them that fear him. [26] The meek shall eat and be satisfied: they shall praise the Lord that seek him: your heart shall live for ever. [27] All the ends of the world shall remember and turn unto the Lord : and all the kindreds of the nations shall worship before thee. [28] For the kingdom is the Lord's : and he is the governor among the nations. [29] All they that be fat upon earth shall eat and worship: all they that go down to the dust shall bow before him: and none can keep alive his own soul. [30] A seed shall serve him; it shall be accounted to the Lord for a generation. [31] They shall come, and shall declare his righteousness unto a people that shall be born, that he hath done this."

So Tragic, Prayers For All

All this destruction and death for what, more power and wealth. This is abhorrent!! Prayers for all Ukraine.

Have You Ever Stepped and Realized Both Evils are the Same Putin and COVID 19!

Written by Ramsis Ghaly

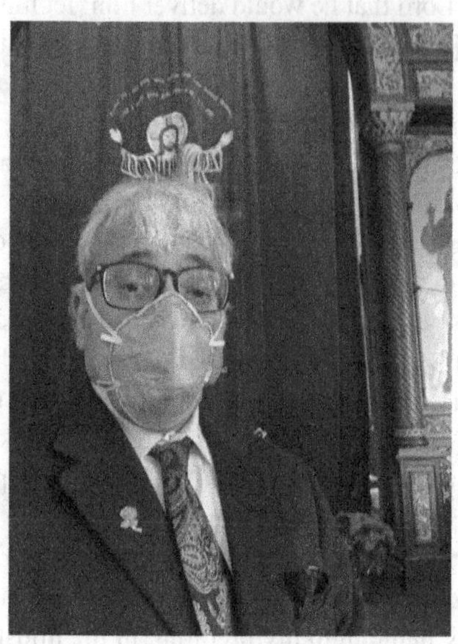

Have You Ever Stepped and Realized Both Evils are the Same: Putin and COVID-19!

The impact of Putin and Russian Kremlins is far worse than man-made COVID-19!

In fact, Russian aggression impact shall exceed the causalities of COVID-19 hundreds and hundreds of folds!

What a similarity between both evils! As COVID-19 controlled, terrorized, intimidated and restrained people, socially isolated the people, lockdown the world, destroyed economy, face masked and vaccine coercion and promote ruler abuse and so is the Russian Putin snipper aggression!!

These are all man-made and has nothing to do with God and Heaven, but it has everything to do with evil man and satanic minds!!

Satan man behind evil doing but not the good man!

The impact of Putin and Russian Kremlins, in the long run, is far worse than man-made COVID-19!

“Do not err, my beloved brethren. [17] Every good gift and every perfect gift is from above, and cometh down from the Father of lights, with whom is no variableness, neither shadow of turning.” James 1:16-17 KJV

Tr. Dr. Ghaly did you see that JESUS has HIS Arms wide open over you in this pic?

Mn, Well said Dr. Ghaly he will get his.

In a Modern civilized world Russia Trashed Human Nature Mock executions and days of torture and Torture chambers!!

Written by Ramsis Ghaly

To our beloved Ukrainians, Our Lord Jesus words: "In the world ye shall have tribulation: but be of good cheer; I have overcome the world." John 16:33 KJV

How could modern man use technology against himself! How could a man use knowledge to kill another fellowman? How could the man of Moon and Mars use frontier science to commit war crimes? How could man use industrial advancement to trash humanity hierarchy and highly ranked creation in the image of God the Lord Most Holy and Most High! How could man highly educated modern sized and civilized commit massacre and trash human hierarchy and highly ranked creation in the image of God the Lord Most Holy and Most High!

Who will ever believe one of the three top countries in a modern era, In a Modern civilized world, commits the worst brutality and cruelty against innocent nation including the worst mock executions and days of torture and Torture chambers?? Who would ever believe that a modern blessed man era would see and witness all the coming images of extreme violation to human rights and ongoing war crimes?? Who would ever believe that a 2022 highly blessed man's era would see and witness the inability of the world leaders to put an immediate stop to Putin Holocaust and imperialism?

O Those committed atrocities to our beloved innocent Ukrainian civilians, you have trashed our human nature by your cruelty and unimaginable brutality! How could man highly educated modern sized and civilized commit massacre and trash human hierarchy and highly ranked creation in the image of God the Lord Most Holy and Most High!

O Those committed murders, rape, torture and horrors to our beloved innocent Ukrainian civilians, you have trashed our human nature your cruelty and unimaginable brutality! You have demoted to the bottomest pit from the hierarchy and highly ranked creation in the image of God the Lord Most Holy and Most High!

O Those committed merciless and ruthless criminal acts against our beloved innocent Ukrainian civilians, you have trashed our human nature by your cruelty and unimaginable brutality! You have demoted to the bottomest pit from the hierarchy and highly ranked creation in the image of God the Lord Most Holy and Most High!

O Those Committed mock executions and days of torture, forced to torture rooms, beaten, forced to kneel, bullets shot at his head and feet, against our beloved innocent Ukrainian civilians, you have trashed our human nature by your cruelty and unimaginable brutality! You have demoted to the bottomest pit from the hierarchy and highly ranked creation in the image of God the Lord Most Holy and Most High!

O Those gunned down, shot, stabbed, set fire, mocked, humiliated, mutilated and inflicted all kind of tortures to our beloved innocent Ukrainian civilians, you have trashed our human nature your cruelty and unimaginable brutality! You have demoted to the bottomest pit from the hierarchy and highly ranked creation in the image of God the Lord Most Holy and Most High!

O Those responsible for the discovered and undiscovered mass graves with Ukrainians shot dead, allegedly by Russian forces, in Bucha. Images of dead naked women, some of them burned, have also emerged from Bucha in the last several days. Ukrainians have also had their hands bound behind their backs, and been shot dead in the streets, images taken in the city show, piles of bodies, burnt beyond recognition, lay cordoned of you have trashed our human nature your cruelty and unimaginable brutality! You have demoted to the bottomest pit from the hierarchy and highly ranked creation in the image of God the Lord Most Holy and Most High!

Daily ongoing Hod knows for how long!! Bodies in the streets, blood running in the streets and roads staining Ukraine. No human aids can reach and no one can flee. Intentionally indiscriminate target civilians, blasts, fires, exploding, women and children, destruction and damages to all standing building and structures! Held civilian Captives for weeks, bombs civilians trying to escape the war while standing in railroad lines

O Those criminals committed The horrors of Bucha laid bare: Man's cheek was cut out before he was shot in the heart while another was burned with a flamethrower, as 'torture chamber' is uncovered inside a children's hospital, Russian troops tortured and executed a village mayor and her family, you have trashed our human nature by your cruelty and unimaginable brutality! You have demoted to the bottomest pit from the hierarchy and highly ranked creation in the image of God the Lord Most Holy and Most High!

O Those committed rapes and repeated rapes, thousands killed including children, execution, unlawful violence looting civilian property, including food, clothing, and firewood. Those who carried out these abuses are responsible for war crimes, you have trashed our human nature by your cruelty and unimaginable brutality! You have demoted to the bottomest pit from the hierarchy and highly ranked creation in the image of God the Lord Most Holy and Most High!

O Those failed to intervene to put immediate stop to the inhuman criminality to our beloved innocent Ukrainian civilians, you have trashed our human nature! You have demoted to the bottomest pit from the hierarchy and highly ranked creation in the image of God the Lord Most Holy and Most High!

https://www.cbsnews.com/.../russia-accused-killing.../

https://www.hrw.org/.../ukraine-apparent-war-crimes...

https://www.businessinsider.com/officials-discover...

https://www.independent.co.uk/.../ukraine-russia-torture...

https://www.dailymail.co.uk/.../Ukraine-war-Torture...

https://www.thedailybeast.com/ukraines-prosecutor...

https://news.sky.com/.../ukraine-war-some-1-200-war...

https://www.thedailybeast.com/ukraines-prosecutor...

https://amp.theguardian.com/.../ukrainian-man-tells-of...

To our Beloved Ukrainians, Our Savior Jesus words: "Come unto me, all ye that labour and are heavy laden, and I will give you rest. [29] Take my yoke upon you, and learn of me; for I am meek and lowly in heart: and ye shall find rest unto your souls. [30] For my yoke is easy, and my burden is light."Matthew 11:28-30 KJV

CG,Amen

Listen to the Divine Voice to Stop the War!

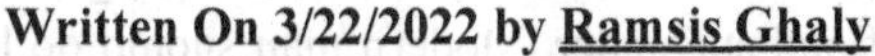
Written On 3/22/2022 by Ramsis Ghaly

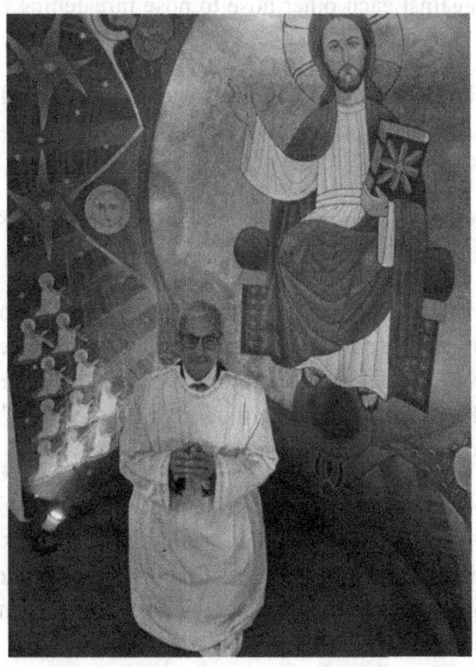

I will be happy to lead this mission and bring peace in my Lord Name and Savior Jesus Christ!!

Step up for peace as a wise world diplomats seeking peace and be a mediator between Russia and Ukraine ! Change the gear and get vigilant! In Faith and Love for the sake of those vulnerable, Act Softly, Remove the Pride, be Humble, be Timely and Calculate Carefully the Steps, Thoughtful and Prayerful"

Before the war escalate   Putin/Russia against the world, the last chance is for NATO Leaders with America and other leaders of the world and spiritual clergy to meet with Putin himself and the Russian leaders and deescalate the war!! Please stop the failed tactic of nose to nose, teeth to teeth and eye to eye!!!!

The tactics used by America and NATO aren't the wise and did nothing but aggravated the Russian angers! Deprivation, sanctions and antagonistic measures are known to do the opposite!

The world has so many diplomats than those around and really need to back off and recognize they failed and let other talented diplomats intervene!

Come on!!! FBIs and CIAS and many others are so good to let those about to murder back off and surrender. Modern man should do better than making presidents stand against each other nose to nose threatening and as a result so many causalities!!

Experienced Diplomats from all countries should meet ASAP with Putin and Russians to solve and bring peace immediately!

Lord Jesus want us to do so and this will bring Satan to his knees while our Savior will say to those heroes made it possible: Matthew 5:9 KJV "Blessed are the peacemakers: for they shall be called the children of God."

Indeed it was written; Romans 12:19-21 KJV "Dearly beloved, avenge not yourselves, but rather give place unto wrath: for it is written, Vengeance is mine; I will repay, saith the Lord. [20] Therefore if thine enemy hunger, feed him; if he thirst, give him drink: for in so doing thou shalt heap coals of fire on his head. [21] Be not overcome of evil, but overcome evil with good."

I will be happy to lead this mission and bring peace in my Lord Name and Savior Jesus Christ!! Step up for peace as a wise world diplomats seeking peace and be a mediator between Russia and Ukraine! Change the gear and get vigilant! In Faith and Love for the sake of those vulnerable, Act Softly, Remove the Pride, be Humble, be Timely and Calculate Carefully the Steps!

MD, Thank you Dr. Ghaly.

RC, I really want to stop the war

TJ, Amin

Much Tears To Come Before That Dove Returns Back To Thy Land!

Written On 3/11/2022 by Ramsis Ghaly

I sat by the shore of the Black Sea as my mind was drifted away into a terror and dark vision!!!!

Despite the black sea was quiet but the Nighbor land weren't! I asked why thy name is "black"? And immediately I heard the following words: One day thy were beautiful and another day thy beauty faded away and nothing remained in thy darkness and thy stained deep black all over thy land!! Why thy enemy had to do to thy!!!

I was terrified as I saw Thy sky is full of Smokes and rise of fires resulting in absolute devastation! The destruction was sweeping further away with no stop ruining thy land! There was no more safety any longer as slaughtering and bloodshed don't cease!!

Nothing is standing, no more city or shops, thy land is abandoned as thy people half died and the other have fled thy land! No living souls are seen around and no signs of life! Dead silence and thy bodies are thrown under the ground at the clefts and crakes of earth!

It was taken away from thy land! I wandered and there was no stone over stone standing! A baby is mourning for his mother! A child is crying underneath crumbled building and many trapped alive between the ruffles!

Much tears to come before that dove returns back to thy Land!

Much weeping ahead before the bird with an olive branch fly over thy sky again!

Much screams from under the piles with shouts before quiescence returns back to thy Land!

Much aches and broken bones before thy heal again!

Much sadness before thy joy return to thy soul again!

Much broken hearts before thy stand on thy feet again!

Much atrocities and destruction before thy peace returns back to thy land!

Much loss of life before thy prosper again!

Much lamentations before thy smile again!

Have you ever seen the earth erupts blood out of its depth! The land was no more home but a curse! Thy sojourner wanders in strange land while those left behind one by one covered by gun fires!

Soon the world joins and the world war about to start! The sky will experience opposing collisions ! Many shall flee unto safe tunnels but only few remained!

The fears didn't help much as across the seas bombs back and forth and so are the snippers have no mercy!

Poverty, sickness and contagious pandemics are eroding thy land! They couldn't put handle in their stations, and it was what was remained to do. They are blown and radiation leaked all over!!

There was no end to evil as many legions of demons joined from all over! No further greens or grass in thy land before thy land produce grains and fruits again!

No much of creeping animals walk in thy land before the sun shines again!

It isn't any more before that determined time to rejuvenate again! The roads are blocked and so are the ways to save thy land!

The land is no longer fertile, the wells are empty of waters and so is thy dry! Thy bones are exposed under thy skin. Thy have lost weight, feeble and no more flesh on thy but be buried under thy ground! Sigh the last breath and go to thy grave!

It is for a long while O thy soul in that land! There is no more but dry, dark and abandonment!

Where is that love! Those days are marked and no more exit but genocide!!

Much tears to come before that dove returns back to thy Land!

O thy souls can no longer find they bones and no more visitations in thy land! I saw the dry brittle skin, the yellow grass, the stony ground and the fumed air all around! No longer communication, no electricity, no supplies and basics of sustained life resources are dismal! How could living be continued???

I was speechless torn in tears ran out breath asking: O man how wickedness and aggression have reached that unimaginable destruction? Why O leaders of the world couldn't stop the wars? Whom has the power to reverse those everlasting historic damages to our planet and mankind!

They were all made by man to destroy man! When can my soul sit again by the river close to the still waters in the valley overshadowed by the tree branches?

When the ground be fertile again and bring about fruits and leaves? When the birds fly again singing the new song of peace? When the roses of love erupts in thy land?

O man why thy done so!! Why the evil in you! It was and it is and so it shall be!! Indeed, much tears to come before that dove returns back to thy Land!

Listen to the Word of God:

"This I recall to my mind, therefore have I hope. [22] It is of the Lord's mercies that we are not consumed, because his compassions fail not. [23] They are new every morning: great is thy faithfulness. [24] The Lord is my portion, saith my soul; therefore will I hope in him. [25] The Lord is good unto them that wait for him, to the soul that seeketh him. [26] It is good that a man should both hope and quietly wait for the salvation of the Lord. [27] It is good for a man that he bear the yoke in his youth. [28] He sitteth alone and keepeth silence, because he hath borne it upon him. [29] He putteth his mouth in the dust; if so be there may be hope. [30] He giveth his cheek to him that smiteth him: he is filled full with reproach. [31] For the Lord will not cast off for ever: [37] Who is he that saith, and it cometh to pass, when the Lord commandeth it not? [38] Out of the mouth of the most High proceedeth not evil and good? [39] Wherefore doth a living man complain, a man for the punishment of his sins? [40] Let us search and try our ways, and turn again to the Lord. [41] Let us lift up our heart with our hands unto God in the heavens. [42] We have transgressed and have rebelled: thou hast not pardoned. [43] Thou hast covered with anger, and persecuted us: thou hast slain, thou hast not pitied. [44] Thou hast covered thyself with a cloud, that our prayer should not pass through. [45] Thou hast made us as the offscouring and refuse in the midst of the people. [46] All our enemies have opened their mouths against us. [47] Fear and a snare is come upon us, desolation and destruction. [48] Mine eye runneth down with rivers of water for the destruction of the daughter of my people. [49] Mine eye trickleth down, and ceaseth not, without any intermission, [50] Till the Lord look down, and behold from heaven. [51] Mine eye affecteth mine heart because of all the daughters of my city. [52] Mine enemies chased me sore, like a bird, without cause. [53] They have cut off my life in the dungeon, and cast a stone upon me. [54] Waters flowed over mine head; then I said, I am cut off. [55] I called upon thy name, O Lord, out of the low dungeon. [56] Thou hast heard my voice: hide not thine ear at my breathing, at my cry. [57] Thou drewest near in the day that I called upon thee: thou saidst, Fear not. [58] O Lord, thou hast pleaded the causes of my soul; thou hast redeemed my life. [59] O Lord, thou hast seen my wrong: judge thou my cause. [60] Thou hast seen all their vengeance and all their imaginations against me. [61] Thou hast heard their reproach, O Lord, and all their imaginations against me;"Lamentations 3:21-31,37-61 KJV

CG, Your writing has such depth allowing readers to imagine the physical world you're writing about. Bless you and the people of the Ukraine whose world is being destroyed.

MS, Stay close to Jesus, pray to Him

KG, God Bless you always!

CR, Blessings dear Doctor!!!!

JM, "Incredible" Visuals AMEN

O Lord Jesus For How Long Will Thou Forget Ukrainians' Outcry??

Written 4/4/2022 by Ramsis Ghaly

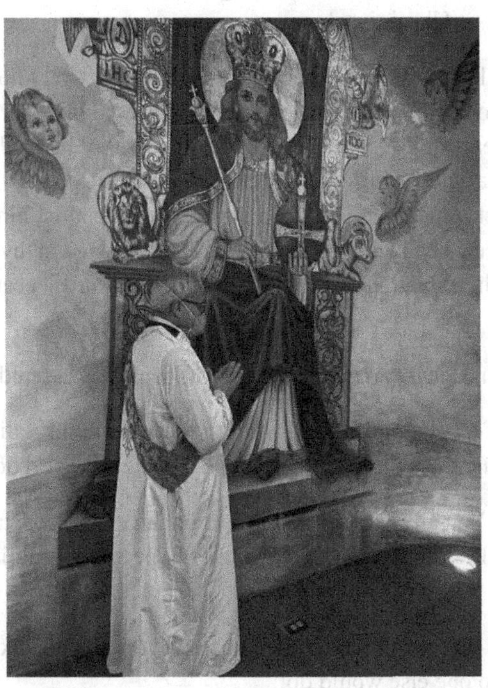

For how long satanic massacre be continued Murders, looters, rapists, War Criminals, crime against humanity, inhuman crime of aggression and genocide atrocities??

O Lord Jesus, You can see, for six weeks, the entire world with all its capabilities is unable to put an immediate stop to the war crimes, genocide and aggression toward innocent civilians!!

O my Lord Jesus, I am ashamed of my humanity to witness my fellowmen committing nonstop atrocities against Ukrainians!! My soul is Sickening so is thy people worldwide!!

For how long, O Lord Jesus, for how long will thou forget Our Ukrainian outcry?? For how long will thou hide thy face from satanic brutality committed to thy people Ukrainians ? For how long shall the enemy be exalted over thy people Ukrainians the vulnerable, the civilians, the children?

O Lord Jesus Consider and hear our Ukrainians prayers, O Lord my God!! O Lord Jesus Come hastily, lest We Ukrainians sleep the sleep of death; Lest the enemy say, I have prevailed against us Ukrainians; and those that trouble us Ukrainians rejoice when we moved!

O Lord Jesus, But we Ukrainians have trusted in thy mercy; our heart shall rejoice in thy salvation! O Lord Jesus we will sing unto the Lord, because You hath dealt bountifully with us Ukrainians!

Psalm 13 "How long wilt thou forget me, O Lord ? for ever? how long wilt thou hide thy face from me? [2] How long shall I take counsel in my soul, having sorrow in my heart daily? how long shall mine enemy be exalted over me? [3] Consider and hear me, O Lord my God: lighten mine eyes, lest I sleep the sleep of death; [4] Lest mine enemy say, I have prevailed against him; and those that trouble me rejoice when I am moved. [5] But I have trusted in thy mercy; my heart shall rejoice in thy salvation. [6] I will sing unto the Lord, because he hath dealt bountifully with me."

++Lord God Jesus, Please Arise and let the Russians be Scattered and Flee Away!!

O Lord Jesus, if You aren't putting Stop to the horrific brutality and massacre committed against thy people Ukrainians, No one else would do!

O Lord Jesus, if You aren't coming down to put an end to constant bombing and tortured to thy children, committed against thy people Ukrainians, No one else would do!

O Lord Jesus, if You aren't be the One to rescue thy people Ukrainians and thy land Ukraine, No one else would do!

O Lord Jesus, if You aren't be the Savior to save thy people Ukrainians and thy land Ukraine, No one else would do!

Psalm 68:1-2,5,20-21,31,35 KJV Let God arise, let his enemies be scattered: let them also that hate him flee before him. [2] As smoke is driven away, so drive them away: as wax melteth before the fire, so let the wicked perish at the presence of God. [5] A father of the fatherless, and a judge of the widows, is God in his holy habitation. [20] He that is our God is the God of salvation; and unto God the Lord belong the issues from death. [21] But God shall wound the head of his enemies, and the hairy scalp of such an one as goeth on still in his trespasses. [31] Princes shall come out of Egypt; Ethiopia shall soon stretch out her hands unto God. [35] O God, thou art terrible out of thy holy places: the God of Israel is he that giveth strength and power unto his people. Blessed be God.

+O Lord God: Please Come Down Hear Our Prayers:

O Lord God! Lord God is One! Lord God is Holy Trinity Three in One and One in Three!

Lord God has No Beginning and has No End!

John 1:1-2 KJV "In the beginning was the Word, and the Word was with God, and the Word was God. [2] The same was in the beginning with God."

Lord God is the Alpha and Omega! Revelation 1:8 KJV "I am Alpha and Omega, the beginning and the ending, saith the Lord, which is, and which was, and which is to come, the Almighty."

Lord God is Eternal, immortal has no beginning and has no end! Lord God is the Pantocrator!

Lord God is the Most Holy Full of Glory! Lord God is The True Master! Lord God is The True Teacher!

Lord God is The Warrior over all things! Lord God is The Unconquered God! Lord God never ever dies! Lord God is Everlasting Almighty!

Lord God made all things seen and unseen!

John 1:3 KJV "All things were made by him; and without him was not any thing made that was made."

Lord God created all things seen and unseen! Lord God is the Only Source of Life! Lord God is the Only True Light! John 1:4-5 KJV "In him was life; and the life was the light of men. [5] And the light shineth in darkness; and the darkness comprehended it not."

Lord God is all and in all and for all! Lord God is In Total control of all Creation! Lord God has no limit!

Lord God knows all things seen and unseen! Lord God knows all thoughts of all seen and unseen!

Lord God hears all audible and inaudible! Lord God oversees the earth and heavens and in between!

Lord God oversees the universe and the uppermost heavens! Lord God oversees the seen and unseen!

Lord God indescribable! Lord God is Unchangeable! Lord God the Ultimate Judge of all! No life given except from Lord God!

Lord God is full Spirit and No Matter in God!

John 4:24 KJV God is a Spirit: and they that worship him must worship him in spirit and in truth.

Lord God is the Truth! Lord God is the Way! Lord Hod is the Life! John 14:6 KJV Jesus saith unto him, I am the way, the truth, and the life: no man cometh unto the Father, but by me.

Lord God is the Resurrection! John 11:25-26 KJV Jesus said unto her, I am the resurrection, and the life: he that believeth in me, though he were dead, yet shall he live: [26] And whosoever liveth and believeth in me shall never die. Believest thou this?

Lord God Nothing Hidden from thy sight and all know to Lord God! Hebrews 4:13 KJV Neither is there any creature that is not manifest in his sight: but all things are naked and opened unto the eyes of him with whom we have to do.

Lord God is Full of Love! Lord God is True Love!

Lord God is the True Savior of mankind!

John 3:16 KJV For God so loved the world, that he gave his only begotten Son, that whosoever believeth in him should not perish, but have everlasting life." 1 John 4:8,16 KJV He that loveth not knoweth not God; for God is love. [16] And we have known and believed the love that God hath to us. God is love; and he that dwelleth in love dwelleth in God, and God in him."

Jt, presidential elections count...we must do the right thing next time America!!

Cg, We pray for peace and intervention in this senseless war.

There is no excuse for a True Christian Leader to support a war!!

Ramsis Ghaly
Written on 3/23/2022

Not Sure only God knows the Truth. Is it true Pope of Russia supporting the War and Russian atrocities or the church is silenced and or in a propaganda news! God forgive me if I am wrong, Nonetheless:

There is no excuse for a True Christian Leader to support a war!! Even the Russian Pope is Brain washed!! Who will ever believe!!!

Those justify war crime by really thinking that Ukraine by joining the West, is joining Sodom and Gomorrah and therefore deserve death and destruction??? Jesus our Master taught us: Luke 12:14-15 KJV And he said unto him, Man, who made me a judge or a divider over you? [15] And he said unto them, Take heed, and beware of covetousness: for a man's life consisteth not in the abundance of the things which he possesseth."

1 Peter 3:8-9 KJV Finally, be ye all of one mind, having compassion one of another, love as brethren, be pitiful, be courteous: [9] Not rendering evil for evil, or railing for railing: but contrariwise blessing; knowing that ye are thereunto called, that ye should inherit a blessing." Romans 12:19 Never take your own revenge, beloved, but leave room for the wrath of God, for it is written, "Vengeance is Mine, I will repay," says the Lord." Romans 12:19-21 KJV "Dearly beloved, avenge not yourselves, but rather give place unto wrath: for it is written, Vengeance is mine; I will repay, saith the Lord. [20] Therefore if thine enemy hunger, feed him; if he thirst, give him drink: for in so doing thou shalt heap coals of fire on his head. [21] Be not overcome of evil, but overcome evil with good."

Regardless, No one should ever justify or support or be part of a war against innocent civilians or turn his or her back and okay deaf and blind without doing all he or she can to stop such atrocity! What an evil Satan that allows the Christian orthodox of East Slavik killing each other!! A Christian pope, a bishop, a priest, a minister, a deacon, a clergy and any human being in modern era should never ever support such a war or be silent especially those appointed to be representative of our Savior Lord Jesus! Luke 12:48 KJV "But he that knew not, and did commit things worthy of stripes, shall be beaten with few stripes. For unto whomsoever much is given, of him shall be much required: and to whom men have committed much, of him they will ask the more."

God Loves the children and moms so much: Matthew 18:5-7 KJV "And whoso shall receive one such little child in my name receiveth me. [6] But whoso shall offend one of these little ones which believe in me, it were better for him that a millstone were hanged about his neck, and that he were drowned in the depth of the sea. [7] Woe unto the world because of offences! for it must needs be that offences come; but woe to that man by whom the offence cometh!"

Regardless who are those, with Lord Jesus there is No Partiality!!! The blood of the Ukrainian children and mothers and destruction will be asked of all those supporting the war crimes!!

Russian Patriarch Kirill's full-throated blessing for Moscow's invasion of Ukraine has splintered the worldwide Orthodox Church and unleashed an internal rebellion that experts say is unprecedented. Kirill, 75, a close ally of Russian President Vladimir Putin, sees the war as a bulwark against a West he considers decadent, particularly over the acceptance of homosexuality.

Ukraine is of visceral significance to the Russian Orthodox Church because it is seen as the cradle of the Rus' civilisation, a medieval entity where in the 10th century Byzantine Orthodox missionaries converted the pagan Prince Volodymyr. Kyiv Metropolitan (Archbishop) Onufry Berezovsky of the UOC-MP appealed to Putin for "an immediate end to the fratricidal war", and another UOC-MP Metropolitan, Evology, from the eastern city of Sumy, told his priests to stop praying for Kirill.

In the behalf of the world, I am so sorry that anyone will ever justify the satanic atrocity and especially under the name of God. I will continue to write more and more and whatever I can. Not only myself but the entire world. We all are sinners and God is love and He never was a God of war or promote nothing but unconditional love among all people. They all are His children and never ever wish to cut their life short or torture them. But it is all satanic and wolves dressed in sheep!!

Ecclesiastes 7:20 Indeed, there is not a righteous man on earth who continually does good and who never sins." Romans 3:10 as it is written,

"There is none righteous, not even one;" Psalm 14:1 For the choir director. A Psalm of David.

The fool has said in his heart, "There is no God."

They are corrupt, they have committed abominable deeds; There is no one who does good."

1 John 4:7-12,16 KJV "Beloved, let us love one another: for love is of God; and every one that loveth is born of God, and knoweth God. [8] He that loveth not knoweth not God; for God is love. [9] In this was manifested the love of God toward us, because that God sent his only begotten Son into the world, that we might live through him. [10] Herein is love, not that we loved God, but that he loved us, and sent his Son to be the propitiation for our sins. [11] Beloved, if God so loved us, we ought also to love one another. [12] No man hath seen God at any time. If we love one another, God dwelleth in us, and his love is perfected in us. [16] And we have known and believed the love that God hath to us. God is love; and he that dwelleth in love dwelleth in God, and God in him."

Ramsis Ghaly

REUTERS.COM

Analysis: Ukraine invasion splits Orthodox Church, isolates Russian patriarch

Russian Patriarch Kirill's full-throated blessing for Moscow's invasion of Ukraine has splintered the worldwide Orthodox Church and unleashed an internal rebellion that experts say is unprecedented.

CG, Great comments.

This is just the beginning of counting losses and exploring more and more of war crimes!!

Written on 4/3/2022 by Ramsis Ghaly

The World be Shameful of Not Working Hard Enough yo put immediate stop to Russian atrocities!!

As COVID-19 man- made pandemic disaster of the decades so is Russian aggression is!!!

These disasters are coming from the Northeastern of the globe!!!!

It shouldn't never had happened to start with! The world formed so many organizations, Human Rights Watch m, international war-crimes investigation and international laws to prevent such atrocities such as UN, G 7 summit, —-! Where were they to put immediate stop before destruction and massacre—!

Putin Holocaust as Hitler Holocaust, the world now shall count the causalities that should have prevented if actions were taken correctly by the leaders of so called civilized countries!!

What a shame there was no civility unto this and it shall enter the history books that there is no cowardliness civilized countries should ever allowed and immediate change in leaderships should take place accordingly!!

What a shame when the world continues to just talk talk and never take an immediate actions to prevent atrocities but to wait until full atrocities take place and meet and talk and say "we should have done that and this—-". What a disaster, after math does not bring lives of repair destructions. What a shame!!

O Lord Jesus, look what Satan and his evil doers had done:—-Ravaged cities full of Massive graves, horrors, shattered, charred and toxins all over the cities of Ukraine!! Mass killing civilians and prisoners of war, destroying private property or engaging in torture, sexual violence, looting or other banned acts. Civilian building attacked Evidence of fighting spilled onto every street and block. Bullets had sprayed The Garden Center malls was a charred hulk, the dancing school blackened. Inside among piles of ash lay bodies and corps of civilians burnt. Civilians bodies had been left in streets. Trucks stacked with bodies and reman ants of body parts because dogs have been eating them," grassy basketball court, a row of bodies was visible in a hole in the ground through a slit in a concrete carapace, eight or nine torsos wrapped in plastic, faces newly lifeless, yet to gray in decay. By the Church, piles of bodies, thrown any which way. From the dirt tossed upon them appeared an elbow, a knee, the sole of a running shoe, wrapped in a plastic shopping bag, white with red roses. Repeated rapes, execution of men, as well as looting of civilian property, including food, clothing and firewood, Russia fired missiles igniting fires in civilian districts, dead bodies displayed in streets, corps scattered, consciously killed, and ——-

All the world has been doing implement sanctions, supply weapons and human aids anc being helpless feeling International outrage, outcry, facetious, inhuman, racist, bloody genocide, indiscriminately atrocities against civilians, destruction, killing of civilians, cutting parts, raping, abandoned destroyed homes, children killed before parents, pregnant mothers in Labor murdered with their own womb fetuses dead, no priests no coffins no burials, tortures, horrific distressing massacre, ——all while the Russians drinking and drinking mocking and killing and celebrating their atrocities as in the ancient times of cave man. They aren't Orthodox Christian's or Jews but heartless merciless satanism!!

All the world can do is to be shameful that they didn't work hard enough to put immediate stope and move forward proceedings and open investigations of war crime and collect hard evidence credible evidence to Human Rights committee!!

Lord have Mercy Lord have Mercy Lord have Mercy Lord have Mercy Lord have Mercy

APPLE.NEWS

New reports of war crimes in Ukraine emerge as Russians retreat from Kyiv area — The Wall Street Journal

Findings by rights groups and Ukrainian authorities could alter global response

Cg, So terrible what is happening to the people of Ukraine. Prayers for the people of Ukraine who are suffering and afraid.

A Divine Message to Ukraine and Ukrainians!

Written 3/4/2022
Ramsis Ghaly

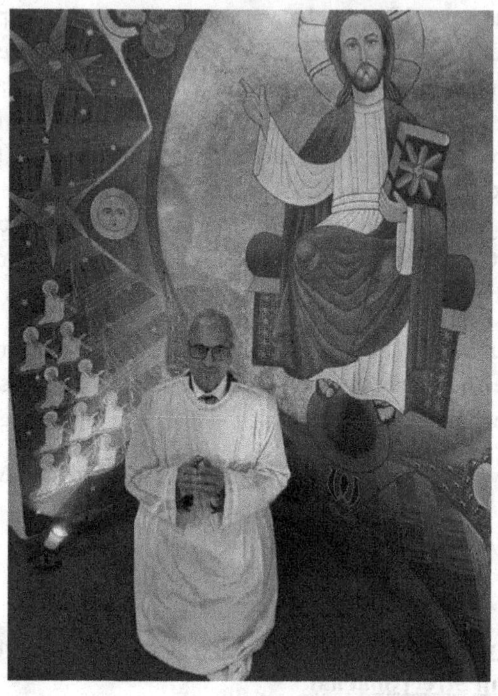

God heard your cries!! The evil man has avenged sevenfold against you! The Spirit of God is descending upon you Ukraine and Ukrainians to rescue you all! You have found mercy in His eyes! Yet your hearts are away from Jesus our Savior!

The multitude of mercy are about to tough your ground and lift you up from the multitude of tanks and aggression!! Yet your faith is hesitant!

You must stand strong in faith and put on the armor of salvation! Touch God's Heart! He has already been provoked by your enemy deeds!! He shall enter upon you calling Him! Curse to those who depend upon human hands:" Psalm 146:3 Do not trust in princes, In mortal man, in whom there is no salvation." Jeremiah 17:5 "Thus says the Lord,

"Cursed is the man who trusts in mankind

And makes flesh his strength, and whose heart turns away from the Lord." Psalm 118:9 "It is better to take refuge in the Lord Than to trust in princes." Isaiah 2:22 Stop regarding man, whose breath of life is in his nostrils; For why he should be esteemed?"

So please all of you call upon His Name the ancient Trisagion Prayers in one voice and one heart in love, forgiveness and humility as follows:

Glory to Thee, our God, Glory to Thee. لك المجد إلهنا يا لك المجد

O Heavenly King, Comforter, the Spirit of Truth, Who art everywhere present and fillest all things, the Treasury of good things and Giver of life: Come, and abide in us, and cleanse us from every stain, and save our souls, O Good One. .الكل والمالىءُ مكانٍ كلّ في الحاضرُ، الحقّ روحُ المعزّي السّماويّ الملكُ أيُّها نفوسنا الصّالح أيُّها وخلص ، دنس كلِّ من وطهرنا ،فينا واسكُنْ هلمَّ .الحياة ورازقُ الصّالحاتِ كنزُ

+Holy God, Holy Mighty, Holy Immortal: have mercy on us. (3 times) إرحمنا يموت لا الذي قدوسٌ ، القوي قدوسٌ ، الله قدوسٌ

+Glory to the Father, and to the Son, and to the Holy Spirit, both now and ever, and unto the ages of ages. Amen. وكلّ الآن ،القدس والرُّوحِ والإبنِ للآبِ المجد آمين ،الدّاهرين دهر وإلى آنٍ

All-Holy Trinity, have mercy on us. Lord, cleanse us from our sins. Master, pardon our iniquities. Holy God, visit and heal our infirmities for Thy name's sake. عن تجاوزْ سَيّدُ يا .خطايانا إغفِرْ ربُّ يا .إرحمنا القدُّوس الثالوثُ أيُّها اسمك أجل من أمراضنا واشْفِ إطّلِعْ قدُّوسُ يا .سيّئاتِنا

Lord, have mercy. (3 times) ارحم ربّ يا (ثلاثاً)3

+Glory to the Father, and to the Son, and to the Holy Spirit, both now and ever, and unto the ages of ages. وإلى آنٍ وكلّ الآن ،القدس والرُّوحِ والإبنِ للآبِ المجد آمين ،الدّاهرين دهر

Our Father, who art in Heaven, hallowed be Thy name. Thy Kingdom come, Thy will be done, on earth as it is in heaven. Give us this day our daily bread, and forgive us our trespasses as we forgive those who trespass against us; and lead us not into temptation, but deliver us from the evil one. كذلك السّماءِ في كما ،مشيئتُك لتكن ،ملكوتُك ليأتِ ،اسمُك ليتقدّس ،السّماوات في الذي أبانا ولا .عليه لنا لمن نحن نترك كما علينا ما لنا واترُكْ ،اليومَ أعطنا الجوهريّ خبزنا .الأرض على الشرّير من نَجّنا لكنْ ،تجربة في تُدخِلْنا

For Thine is the Kingdom, and the power, and the glory, of the +Father, and of the Son, and of the Holy Spirit, now and ever and unto ages of ages. Amen.

The Trisagion prayer is an ancient prayer in Christianity.

In Greek:

Ἅγιος ὁ Θεός, Ἅγιος ἰσχυρός, Ἅγιος ἀθάνατος, ἐλέησον ἡμᾶς.

Hágios ho Theós, Hágios iskhūrós, Hágios āthánatos, eléēson hēmâs.

In Latin:

Sanctus Deus, Sanctus Fortis, Sanctus Immortalis, miserere nobis.[2][3]

In English - Literal Translation:

Holy God, Holy Strong, Holy Immortal, have mercy on us.[4]

In English - Common Liturgical Translation:

Holy God, Holy Mighty, Holy Immortal, have mercy on us.[5][6][7]

In Aramaic:

ܩܕܝܫܬ ܐܠܗܐ: ܩܕܝܫܬ ܚܝܠܬܢܐ: ܩܕܝܫܬ ܠܐ ܡܝܘܬܐ: ܕܐܨܛܠܒܬ ܚܠܦܝܢ ܐܬܪܚܡ ܥܠܝܢ

Qadišat Aloho, qadišat ḥayltono qadišat lo moyuto d-eṣṭlebt ḥlofayn etraḥam ʿalayn.

https://en.m.wikipedia.org/wiki/Trisagion

https://orthodoxwiki.org/Trisagion

https://apple.news/AKWdot5JrTgmPYME-cQxiQw

JT. amen...china and russia are Godless

RZ. Amen! Glory to God!

The Peacemakers for Russian Ukraine War Please Pray for the as Satan trying to destroy them!!

Written on 10/06/2022 by Ramsis Ghaly

Blessed are those pursue their calling and persevere to the End, a Crown of Life Eternal is waiting for them! I wish to be that one: "Blessed is a man who perseveres under trial; for once he has been approved, he will receive the crown of life which the Lord has promised to those who love Him." James 1:12

Who will be the Peacemakers of the 2023 New year to intervene and stop the Russian Ukraine war?

Our Savior and Lord is Ready to grant the promise on earth and in heaven to those Peacemakers and be ranked the children of God the Most High?

Who are they and where are they coming from??

"Blessed are the peacemakers: for they shall be called the children of God." Matthew 5:9 KJV

The Peacemakers at the Door! Please Pray for the as Satan trying to destroy them!!

To Those Peacemakers: Be Courageous and Don't be Afraid as it is written:

1 Chronicles 28:20

David also said to Solomon his son, "Be strong and courageous and do the work. Do not be afraid or discouraged, for the LORD God, my God is with you. He will not fail you or forsake you until all the work for the service of the temple of the LORD is finished.

1 Corinthians 15:58

Therefore, my dear brothers and sisters, stand firm. Let nothing move you. Always give yourselves fully to the work of the Lord, because you know that your labor in the Lord is not in vain.

Deuteronomy 31:6-8

Be strong and courageous. Do not be afraid or terrified because of them, for the LORD your God goes with you; he will never leave you nor forsake you." Then

Moses summoned Joshua and said to him in the presence of all Israel, "Be strong and courageous, for you must go with this people into the land that the LORD swore to their ancestors to give them, and you must divide it among them as their inheritance. The LORD himself goes before you and will be with you; he will never leave you nor forsake you. Do not be afraid; do not be discouraged."

Ephesians 6:10

Finally, be strong in the Lord and in his mighty power.

Isaiah 54:4

"Do not be afraid; you will not be put to shame. Do not fear disgrace; you will not be humiliated. You will forget the shame of your youth and remember no more the reproach of your widowhood.

John 14:27

Peace I leave with you; my peace I give you. I do not give to you as the world gives. Do not let your hearts be troubled and do not be afraid.

Psalm 27:1

The LORD is my light and my salvation— whom shall I fear? The LORD is the stronghold of my life— of whom shall I be afraid?

Psalm 56:3-4

When I am afraid, I put my trust in you. In God, whose word I praise— in God, I trust and am not afraid. What can mere mortals do to me?

2 Timothy 1:7

For the Spirit God gave us does not make us timid, but gives us power, love, and self-discipline.

Joshua 1:9-11

Have I not commanded you? Be strong and courageous. Do not be afraid; do not be discouraged, for the LORD your God will be with you wherever you go." So Joshua ordered the officers of the people: "Go through the camp and tell the people, 'Get your provisions ready. Three days from now you will cross the Jordan here to go in and take possession of the land the LORD your God is giving you for your own.'"

Isaiah 41:10-13

So do not fear, for I am with you; do not be dismayed, for I am your God. I will strengthen you and help you; I will uphold you with my righteous right hand. "All who rage against you will surely be ashamed and disgraced; those who oppose you will be as nothing and perish. Though you search for your enemies, you will not find them. Those who wage war against you will be as nothing at all. For I am the LORD your God who takes hold of your right hand and says to you, Do not fear; I will help you.

1 Corinthians 16:13

Be on your guard; stand firm in the faith; be courageous; be strong.

Psalm 27:14

Wait for the LORD; be strong and take heart and wait for the LORD.

Proverbs 3:5-6

Trust in the LORD with all your heart and lean not on your own understanding; in all your ways submit to him, and he will make your paths straight.

Psalm 23:1-4

The LORD is my shepherd, I lack nothing. He makes me lie down in green pastures, he leads me beside quiet waters, he refreshes my soul. He guides me along the right paths for his name's sake. Even though I walk through the darkest valley, I will fear no evil, for you are with me; your rod and your staff, they comfort me. You prepare a table before me in the presence of my enemies. You anoint my head with oil; my cup overflows. Surely your goodness and love will follow me all the days of my life, and I will dwell in the house of the LORD forever.

Mark 5:36

Overhearing what they said, Jesus told him, "Don't be afraid; just believe."

Philippians 1:28

without being frightened in any way by those who oppose you. This is a sign to them that they will be destroyed, but that you will be saved—and that by God.

Psalm 112:7

They will have no fear of bad news; their hearts are steadfast, trusting in the LORD.

Joshua 1:6

Be strong and courageous, because you will lead these people to inherit the land I swore to their ancestors to give them.

Psalm 31:24

Be strong and take heart, all you who hope in the LORD.

"And let the peace of God rule in your hearts, to the which also ye are called in one body; and be ye thankful. [16] Let the word of Christ dwell in you richly in all wisdom; teaching and admonishing one another in psalms and hymns and spiritual songs, singing with grace in your hearts to the Lord. [17] And whatsoever ye do in word or deed, do all in the name of the Lord Jesus, giving thanks to God and the Father by him."Colossians 3:15-17 KJV

The Peacemakers for Russian Ukrain War! Please Pray for the as Satan trying to destroy them!!

Blessed are those pursue their calling and persevere to the End, a Crown of Life Eternal is waiting for them! I wish to be that one: "Blessed is a man who perseveres under trial; for once he has been approved, he will receive the crown of life which the Lord has promised to those who love Him." James 1:12

JK, You said it so well.

Dr. RAMSIS GHALY...

CL, Amen

Medical Care Post COVID

Patients Come First and Not Institution or Organization Don't Practice In unsafe Environment!

Many times healthcare workers, nurse and doctors find themselves fully responsible and sues from any errors yet the organization administrative staff putting all rules and regulations almost always settle outside the court and not included in the primary law suites. A nurse under stress and hectic work environment had given a patient wrong drug and the plaintiff pursued criminal charges and jury agreed for years in jail sentence.

Just think about this, non-clinical class run the hospitals and put all orders and rules and regulations . Yet in every legal case a doctor or a nurse is always almost held responsible.

Nurses and doctors have no autonomy and overwhelmed every day with nonsense and business class makes thing impossible to practice. Yet only doctors and nurses are absolutely held responsible.

Yet those business non-clinical class who have autonomy, are almost always find their way out and have no legal responsibility or legal impact!!!

No wonder why clinical providers are burned out and running away and mentally destroyed!

Honest look, doctors and nurses found the reality isn't the medical oath but that enforced in order to survive: Institution comes first and not the patients. Organization regulations come first and not the patients!

Doctors and nurses are working under tremendous pressure and the demand from them is unbearable, almost zero tolerance to so much despite they are forced to work in unsafe practices!! The distractive forces from patient's care are unreal and render things to go wrong!! Many of those are real; overwork, mentally consumed, burdened with non-clinical work—-.

Medical clinical providers nowadays find themselves all alone unsupported, unappreciated and easily blamed for system errors, situational mishaps and overlooked errors as being stressed not only by work environment but daily life circumstances!

What is the lesson, doctors and nurses do not practice medicine in any facility that has risk practices, not supporting you and not allowing you to practice safe medicine. Be advocate for yourself and your wellbeing. You are all alone when it comes to medicolegal issues. Be extremely diligent, watch over yourself, don't take anything for grant, —-YOUR COMMITMENT IS THE PATIENT AND NOT THE INSTITUTION OR THE ORGANIZATION. Hospitals are not place for social club, diplomacy or politics in the cost of patients care!! Be patient advocate more than organization advocate!

Nowadays it better not to practice at all unless in absolutely safe practice listening to you and your concerns. Practice in a facility that patients come first and not mighty dollars. Speak up and do not be part of cover up or short cuts.

My heart for those doctors and nurses fell victim to the system imposed on them and coerced to shut up and forced to be submissive to bureaucracy and threatened!

Ramsis Ghaly

Great team working together serving maternal ward! It is what counts when it comes to success!

Ramsis Ghaly

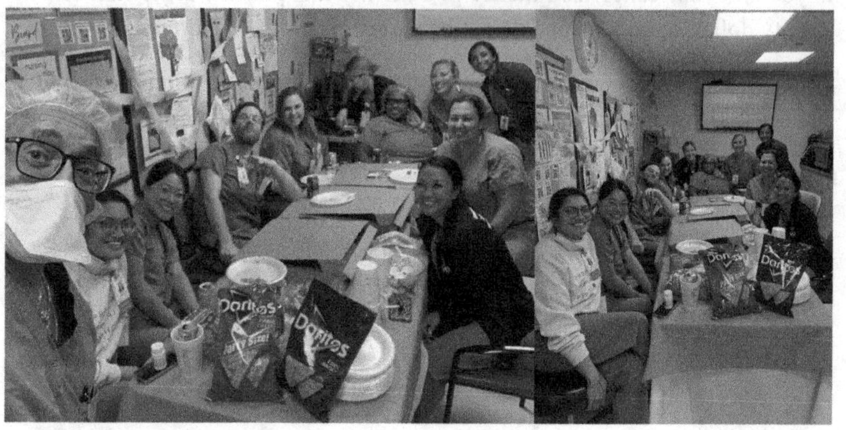

I am Set to Race!

A Poem dedicated to Kristin Rice an all those Youth Ready to Journey!!
Written by Ramsis Ghaly

My name is Kristin Rice and I come from great family roots!

My years ahead shall be much more as I will get to do things in my own!!

I am not off to move forward to a spectacular future! And I am not fearful from what will be placed before me! My Lord and blessing of you all shall guard me all my life long!

In fact, I have confidence in my ability and all what I have learned from my parents and my family!

My Lord and my parents blessed me to be brilliant and gorgeous! Just wait and see what I will be one day! My dreams are huge, and my aspiration is unlimited. Like my mom and my dad my aspiration goes up to the top with no one to beat me!

I am ready for the race sit before me from the life journey I am about step in in my own feet!! I will endure! I will resist any evil! I will be kind and loving! I will be humble and patience!

O my soul let us go! No time to waist and no more for laziness or negativism! Look at me and see my pretty wide open and determined eyes! Never shall I look back but you the future my Lord God prepared ahead of me! The Holy Bible is my reference and science is my adventure!

I will be careful as I am a temple for the Most High! So what if my road is rocky, I certainly can handle it and if I fall, I will stand again and learn from it! I know it won't be easy as the path will be full of challenges and choices! But I am no alone as my Almighty shall never forsake me nor my parents and friends! Together I shall success and my dreams are up high above the clouds ☁ in His hands!

I am courageous and ready to take adventures and calculate the risks along the way! So please don't worry about me! I will only few miles away and never ever be out of sight!

Mom and dad, thank you for all what you had done for me! I shall always treasure and cherish the memories of all those made it possible for me!

Pray for me as I pray for you and wish me the best for steps about to take!

Biblical verses selected for you all!!

1 Corinthians 9:24-27 KJV "Know ye not that they which run in a race run all, but one receiveth the prize? So run, that ye may obtain. [25] And every man that striveth for the mastery is temperate in all things. Now they do it to obtain a corruptible crown; but we an incorruptible. [26] I therefore so run, not as uncertainly; so fight I, not as one that beateth the air: [27] But I keep under my body, and bring it into subjection: lest that by any means, when I have preached to others, I myself should be a castaway." Hebrews 12:1-2 KJV "Wherefore seeing we also are compassed about with so great a cloud of witnesses, let us lay aside every weight, and the sin which doth so easily beset us, and let us run with patience the race that is set before us, [2] Looking unto Jesus the author and finisher of our faith; who for the joy that was set before him endured the cross, despising the shame, and is set down at the right hand of the throne of God." Isaiah 40:29-31 KJV "He giveth power to the faint; and to them that have no might he increaseth strength. [30] Even the youths shall faint and be weary, and the young men shall utterly fall: [31] But they that wait upon the Lord shall renew their strength; they shall mount up with wings as eagles; they shall run, and not be weary; and they shall walk, and not faint." 1 Corinthians 3:16-21 KJV "Know ye not that ye are the temple of God, and that the Spirit of God dwelleth in you? [17] If any man defile the temple of God, him shall God destroy; for the temple of God is holy, which temple ye are. [18] Let no man deceive himself. If any man among you seemeth to be wise in this world, let him become a fool, that he may be wise. [19] For the wisdom of this world is foolishness with God. For it is written, He taketh the wise in their own craftiness. [20] And again, The Lord knoweth the thoughts of the wise, that they are vain. [21] Therefore let no man glory in men. For all things are yours;"

Ramsis F Ghaly, MD

Www.Ghalyneurosurgeon.com

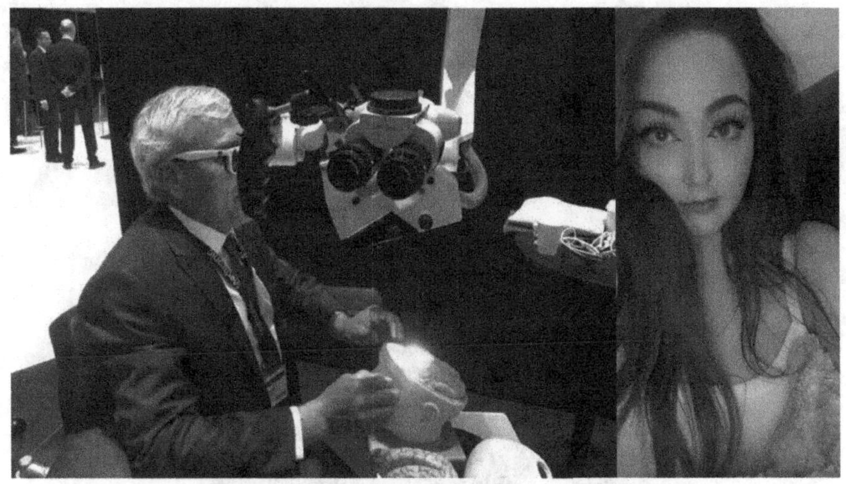

KR, **Ramsis Ghaly** thank you very much for that! That was very kind of you to write. I wish you peace and happiness in your present and future.

CR, Ramsis Ghaly you are an amazing light and this poem you wrote brought me to tears! My family is everything to me, love them all so very much! You have touched my family with your healing hands to give us our lives back. I am so forever grateful, we are all so very grateful for you THANK YOU FROM THE BOTYOM OF MY HEART!

DT, Beautiful!!!!!

MA, Great picture

Is This How We Should Treat an American Hero?

Written by Ramsis Ghaly

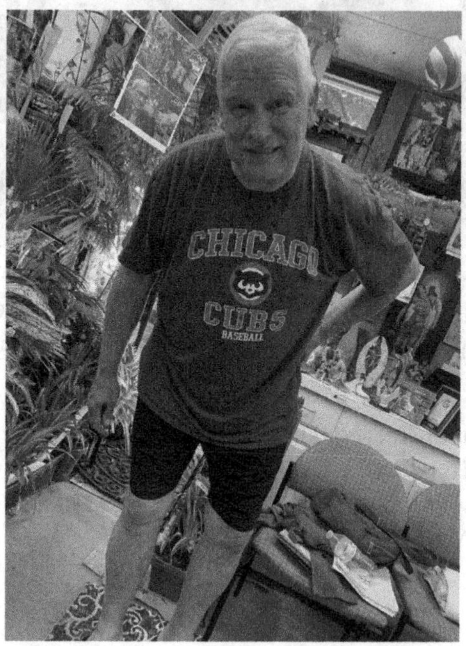

Is this how we treat an American hero suffering of horrific pains for 6months day and night screaming?

A patient with horrific pains and no one to help make a diagnosis and do the correct treatment. He needed urgent surgery and was all set. To the patient surprise, he was told as BCBS PPO, his Chicago city insurance as a firefighter, if will not cover Dr Ghaly and CDH northwestern and he must go to a Blue distinctive hospital for spine surgery. Patient and his wife. Tying and crying, made, upset, frustrated.

This is the catch when the patient called BCBS they told him Dr Ghaly was approved and the hospital. When Dr Ghaly office called, he was told NO NO.

I made the patient call BCBS in a conference call and finally they admitted, if he to go to spine surgery despite it is PPO, he needs to have surgery in a different hospital

Patient and his wife were devastated and absolutely unaware!!

Patient cries and said I am a firefighter for the city of Chicago for 20 years and this how I am treated.

Interesting his doctors and caregivers have been seeing him and suffering and no one is able to help. Both came to me as a referral from his friend Lanette Sellers Yingling. Jim, her husband, had also had the same misdiagnose and suffered for a year and no one could help him. I made the correct diagnosis and did the surgery and now he is home free and back to work.

We live in a strange age; a surgeon would like to help a patient and the insurance bureaucracy!!

Health insurance scams allover!!!

Patients' words: Dr Ghaly is the one of the kindest Drs I've met and have never seen anyone care about patients the way he does, and I've seen a lot of Drs. The medical system is a shame to our country that we can't have a surgery with the best Dr at a great hospital, this should be our choice and Dr Ghaly not the other way around. But dr Ghaly fought for us! Great man great Dr!

www.ghalyneurosurgeon.com

MA, He is the Brst

KG, Bravo for our Heroes and Dr **Ramsis Ghaly**!

I surely don't know where or what I would do without you to rely on and I'm American in Egypt. Even here Medical can be good but little errors make big mistakes! Thank God for Dr Ghaly as I've no doubt I'd be paralyzed or something! Thank God for you, Dr Ghaly!

PP, There are many wonderful special doctors.

MD, Great story Dr. Ghaly praise the Lord for Doctors like you. God Bless

JW, Dr. Ghaly is truly a miracle worker, he is my hero!

CG, A delightful couple I met today. They were so excited to see Dr Ghaly. Very disappointing that the insurance is giving them a hard time. There used to be a time when you could make your own choice of where and who did your sugery. Not any more since the insurance took over medical decisions. I pray their insurance permits Dr. Ghaly to do his surgery. 🙏

SA, It's Obama Care. The democrats gift to America. Bait and Switch. It's a crime against humanity that prevents good doctors from treating their patients.

AS, It's Obama Care. The democrats gift to America. Bait and Switch. It's a crime against humanity that prevents good doctors from treating their patients.

DM, Tired of insurance dictating who, where, how and when people can be treated!!!

SL, Obamacare destroyed the system. We might have to all go to pure cash pay and cut the insurance companies out because they're just absorbing dollars from the system

JC, U are a gift

ZC, No one can play the role better than you, You are the best Dr.Ghally.

DH,Dr. GHALY, YOU NEVER FAIL TO AMAZE ME, you are for "WE THE PEOPLE" LOVE YOU DR. GHALY

RC, I'm glad you are in a milacle hands and a mavelous doctor! Thanks god!

KO, Amen to that Char

TM, With firsthand knowledge, I can say that Dr. Ghaly is the kindest and most caring doctor in the USA, and I am thankful every day that I met this wonderful man, who just happens to be the best neurosurgeon ever. If ever God guided a person's hands, it is Dr. Ramsis Ghaly

Robotic Technology and Augmented Virtual Reality In Neurosurgery!

One of the advantages of technology in Neurosurgery is making myself look out of space genius and face is sophisticated in the ere of Virtual Augmented Reality!!!

Ramsis Ghaly

Www.ghalyneurosurgeon.com

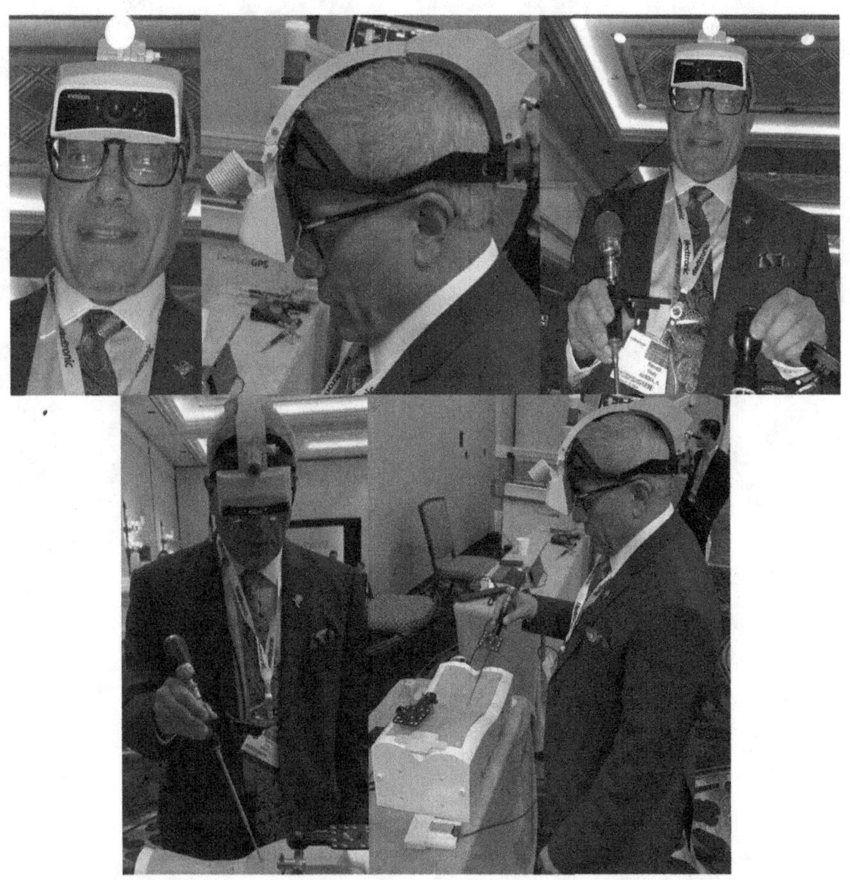

A new idea for Robot Navigation Technology in medicine must provide immediate feedback for any deviation and take full responsibility!

Written by Ramsis Ghaly

So far, Robot Navigation Technology in medicine doesn't provide immediate feedback of any deviation and doesn't take full responsibility!

A robot that gives immediate feedback and grantee a job well done. So far robot guide the Surgeon to place various hardware such as screws and cages in the correct anatomy without causing damage to adjacent essential bodily organs especially brain, spinal cord and nerves!

And if the technology is do good if should give immediate feedback gut any wrongdoing or warning before deviation. An example is GPS navigation does so while driving. But so far not in Medical technology!

YR, Love it!

CG, Very impressive!

Lm, Impressive Doc

I Love Robotic surgery but it has a limited role in the brain or the spine! A Role for NANO-Robotism!!

Written on 9/27/22 by Ramsis Ghaly

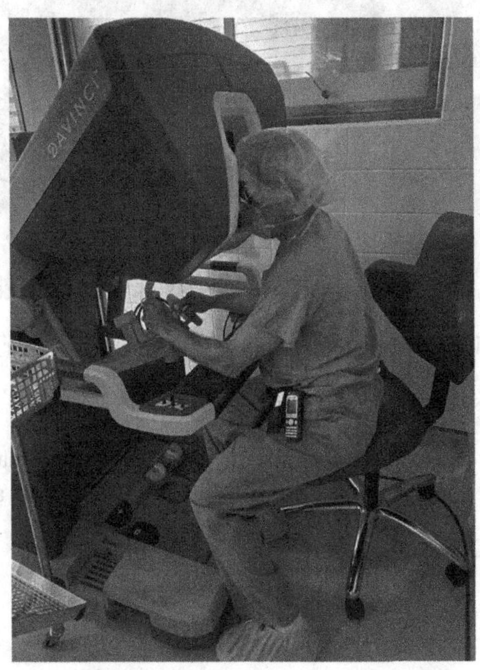

The brain and spinal cord are extremely sensitive to pressure or touch. For the robotic arms to work, a cavity must be created to develop a space for the arms to move around and for the 3D cameras to provide the close up vision. Unfortunately, these conditions are impossible for the brain and spinal cord withing the skeleton of the skull and the spinal canal. Who knows, perhaps in the future a NANO Robotic Arms to be developed and could work in micro-spaces without compressing the neural elements???

Ramsis Ghaly

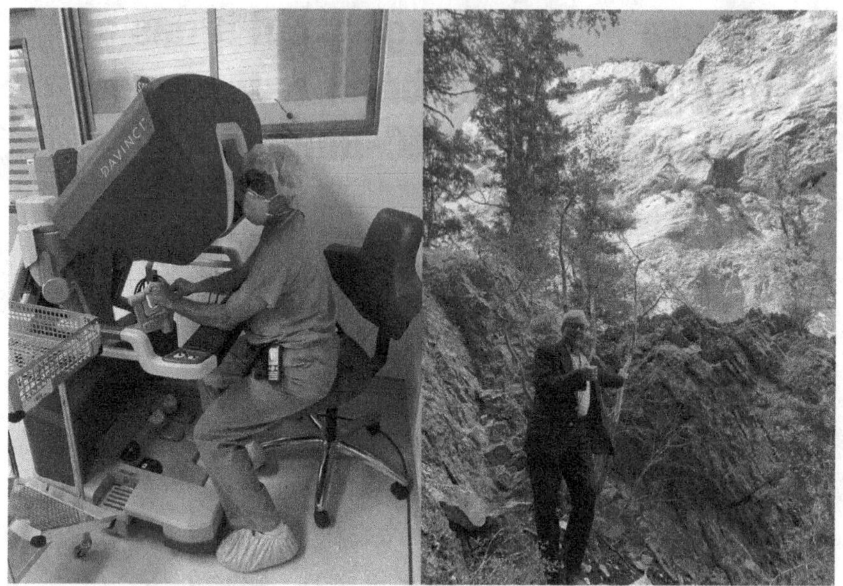

Mp, That's amazing that tool to assist you. You are amazing Dr Ramsis Ghaly

Rc, marvelous! Is nice you can use this tool

Sc, I don't know doctor i don't think me personally would have liked robotic hands in my glad you had the skillful hands that you did thank all mighty Jesus!

Jm, "Awesome" Dr. Ghaly Wow.

Jb, That is so advanced technology

Doing the Right Thing Is Cost Effective and Nobel!

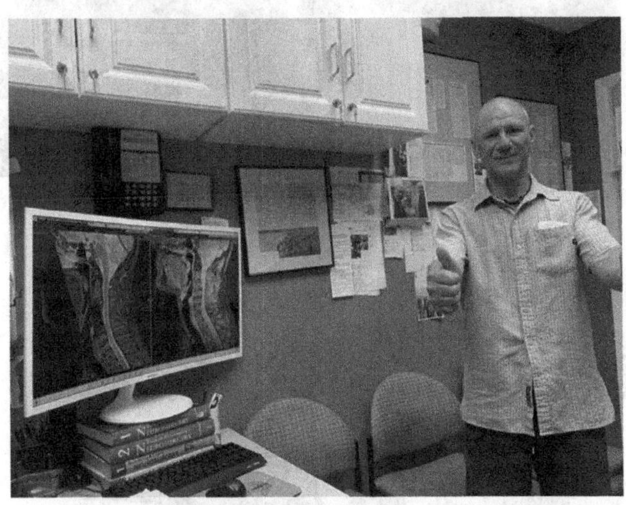

Watch the difference when a good corrective surgery is done! MRI before and after surgery.

Complete resolution of severe spinal stenosis, spinal cord injury, spinal cord signal and deformity.

Interestingly the surgery performed by me was the cheapest Management strategy to this patient that spent so much money in conservative management, mismanagement, wrong diagnosis, misinformation—-!

What is the true message: doing the right thing from the first time early on without delay, is cost effective and the surgery is cost effective? It isn't conservative injection, therapy, MRI, radiology———- but the surgery and the Neurosurgeon

Complete resolution of crippling spinal cord injury and my patient back to golfing praising Lord Jesus!!

It isn't money! It isn't misuse or abuse the system! It is patient comes first and maintain autonomy to highly ethical physician and surgeon in practice! Compensate not based in procedures and fake surgeries and procedures but based on the right surgery. My cost to care for this man was only $1200!!!

Ramsis Ghaly

www.ghalyneurosurgeon.com

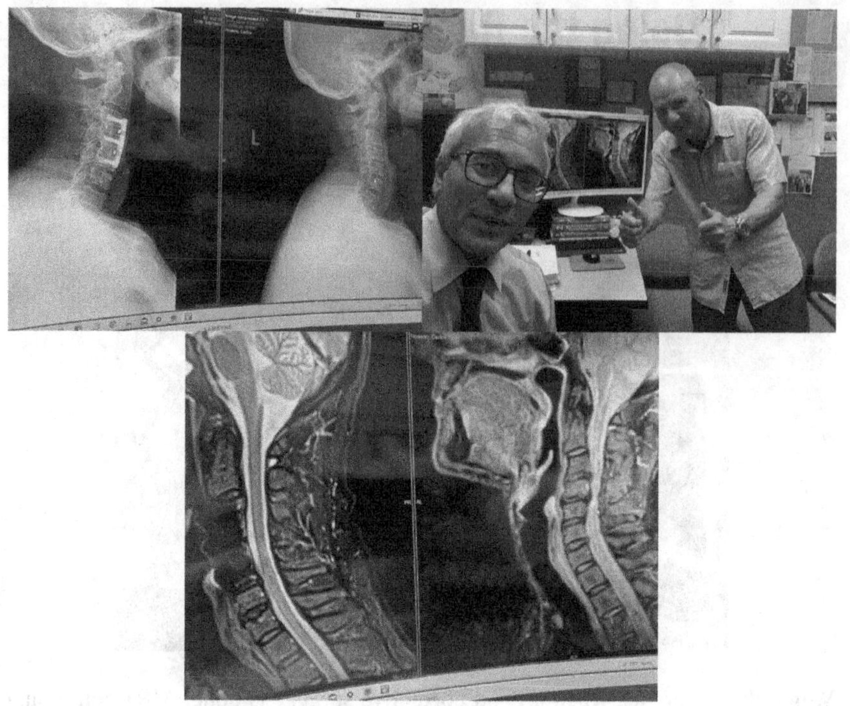

KO, Amen your a fabulous Surgeon

TN, Grateful he has the best surgeon possible!! God's Blessings are all around

LK, Just look at that beautiful alignment and disc space! God Bless Dr. **Ramsis Ghaly**!

DC, Amen to that!

MD, God Bless you Dr. Ghaly you are truly a God sent to restore peoples lives. You are an amazing caring doctor sharing your remarkable talents to cure people.

RN, I'm running through that issue now with my scaiticas, the pain in only managable if I'm not doing anything. Having an MRI done and looking at injections.

MG, God bless you Dr. Ghaly

BK, Looks like a wonderful outcome. I'm proud to be a part of the team.

DL, Praise the Lord ! What kind of symptoms does this cause ? I have neck issues. I gave up on pain mgmt ...

JM, Wow

MN, You truly are a wonderfully gifted surgeon Dr. Ghaly.

I wouldn't trust anyone else to work on me.

I'm back to work thanks to you.

JM, "Superb"

CB, Great job Dr. Ghaly, do you have a recommendation for someone having seizures? He is currently in the hospital, I don't have details, it was mentioned as a prayer request.

MP, You are an Angel Doctor of the Lord with the heart and soul in the right place. Awesome story, and looks like the airway is not impinged any longer and those vertebra are spaced and not crunching nerves making inflammation. You fixed it!

EO, Amazing.

RC,Amazing, superb, great hoy. **Congrats**

KM, I need you where I live.

SM, You are amazing Dr. GHALY! I might be needing you soon after all these years of nursing.

CG, You are truly a great doctor and surgeon. You are personable, great listener, and empathetic to the concerns of your patients. God has truly blessed your patients when they found you.

Word of Mouth Referral and PPO BCBS Story!!

Written on 6/1/2022 by <u>Ramsis Ghaly</u>

I had a surprised call today from BCBS Representative about a patient I did the surgery!!!

I called her back and she said thank you for helping our patient and if BCBS PPO can do something this is my contact info!!!

I was shocked because most of the time, a solo Neurosurgeon like myself, insurance won't bother and easily deny or procrastinate the claims and they give my office very hard time!!!

I was about to fall out of my chair to tell you the truth!!

I told the BCBS representative to use this case nationwide that PPO FREE TO CHOOSE is America Healthcare and support solo neurosurgeon like myself it is America Choice!!

BCBS PPO made a difference in a patient and family life. A patient was in horrific pains and suffering for 6 months, going nowhere! Many wrong diagnoses and wrong managements!

By word of mouth, she came to see me. Instantly correct diagnosis was made as followed by surgery. Now she is cured.

Many said she had it in her head and ignored the fact that she had a hidden tumor

BCBS PPO approved the surgery despite the fact that I am not hospital employee or attached to any hospital base HMO.

How many patients in America resemble this case!

Neither health insurance plans nor hospital-based HMO nor money can buy skilled honest and talented surgeons!

At the end the most effective treatment and cost effective is the correct treatment!

Think twice about Cook-book medicine, HMO,——-question your care and make sure the diagnosis is the correct diagnosis and the right treatment—

My Early Days in Medicine late 1980 and 1990's!!

Written by Ramsis Ghaly

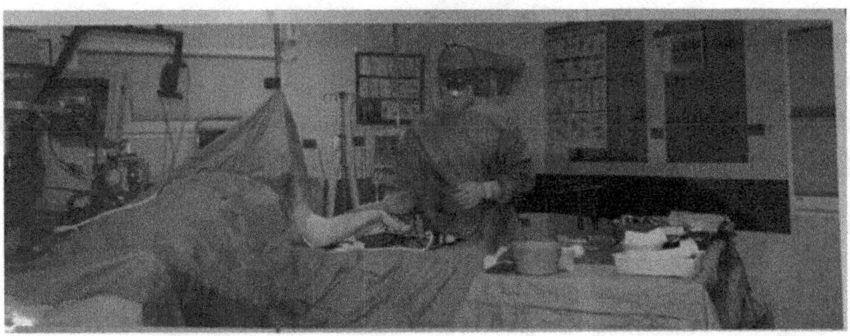

I look back at those old good days and I remember how privileged I was to be part of them!! Look at the pictures, they speak for themselves!!

Although those days were the best days in healthcare, but they were the worst days of allowing healthcare opportunistically and invaders to enter and spoiled the good American healthcare known worldwide!!

Those and We are guilty of not doing enough in particular the American Patriots and various medical organizations and associations! We didn't stand strong and firm defending our American Healthcare Independence!!

They fouled us and worked secretly behind closed doors and many of us sold our souls and ethics and values for self-gain purposes. Many payouts made between those business organizations, Industry, traders, and physicians and nurses! Medical team owners were excited to get so much money and ignored the American values in healthcare and their future generations and the disastrous impact in patients care!

At that time all what matters were patients' wellbeing and recovery to do the best to save lives. All of a sudden, those businesspeople, I remember gave us false lectures and fake data that: "Healthcare in the surge of collapse and bankruptcy if we are not going to do something about it and let them help us" We never realized that those liars were masters of tactics to intimate, threat and put fears upon the naïve trusting physicians and nurses.

We didn't know that those evil minded did so to take over healthcare and justify their expenses that currently have nothing to do with patients' care but to themselves.

It was the most luxurious wide open un-tapped gate that nonclinical organizations and government found an easy business to take advantage to enter and control and make a wealthy living!!

The medical team were medically dedicated and retarded outside medicine business, non-street smart and never ever Let the history know what we 1980's and 1990's has witnessed and seen!!! And we stood ashamed that we hadn't do enough at that time to prevent the historic healthcare degradation!!!

These Days Mark the Following:

1) PreCOVID and when face time face and in person care!

2) The last days of physician and nurses autonomy and ownership!

3) The beginning of healthcare transformation from the hands of clinical providers to non clinical staff!

4) The last days of patients' centered care!

5) Thd birth of Cookbook Medicine!

6) The beginning of so called "Evidence based Medicine"

7) The beginning of government and healthcare insurances to tell doctors and nurses what to do!

8) The birth of Electronic and digital takeover healthcare!

9) It was the last days of No Burnouts or concerns of leaving medicine to something else or early retirement!

10) It was the last days of healthcare simplicity and Patients Come First" the only mission statement and goal!

11) It was the last days of No Mission statement called: "Organization comes first"

12) The last days of medical care providers loved to come to work and we never heard of people quitting because of overwhelming bureaucracy!

13) It was the last relaxing non-burden non-intimidated, non-terrorized and feared when coming to work!

14) It was the last days of no hundreds of emails, messages and so much policing and eye watchers to distract and take our focus away from what actual patient's needs!

15) The last days of the great days in Medicine!

I wish those who were instrumental to sell the good old American Healthcare can come back and see what they had done the fruits of their works!! At the time where disastrous Healthcare changes were born!!!

This post I wrote in 2020

How did the time go that fast???

Healthcare Transformed from Free-Choice Medicine Independent to Corporate Medicine Regulated

Photos while I was working at Sliver Cross Hospital, Joliet Illinois 1995-2001

God had given me the vision twenty years earlier than the entire medical community at that tine. Whatever I called at that time became the standard and norm twenty years later!

Everything I have called for back then, wasn't allowed and I received gratitude from my patients but rather so much hardship from the superiors and administration both at Silver Cross Hospital in Joliet and Rush Copley Hospital in Aurora, Illinois.

I have brought so much frontline neuroscience medicine to a community that was so far behind to the degree that if a patient had a brain tumor or stroke, the treatment was "let hone die, nothing to be done". So many surgeries, community monthly awareness, education, stroke awareness, Neuroscience centers close to home and many more I have established at that time!

My career in healthcare was at the time of turmoil so much unrest and uprising roads full of rocks as Medicine was being transformed from Free-Choice Medicine Independent to Corporate Medicine Regulated!

As much as painful memories for how I was treated yet my patients were the candlelight in the midst of the darkness and their voices were the calming birds among the roaring lions and their faith on me was like the shield 🛡intercepting the rocks thrown at me. I love my patients so much. Lord Jesus know how much

Ramsis Ghaly

Www.ghalyneurosurgeon.com

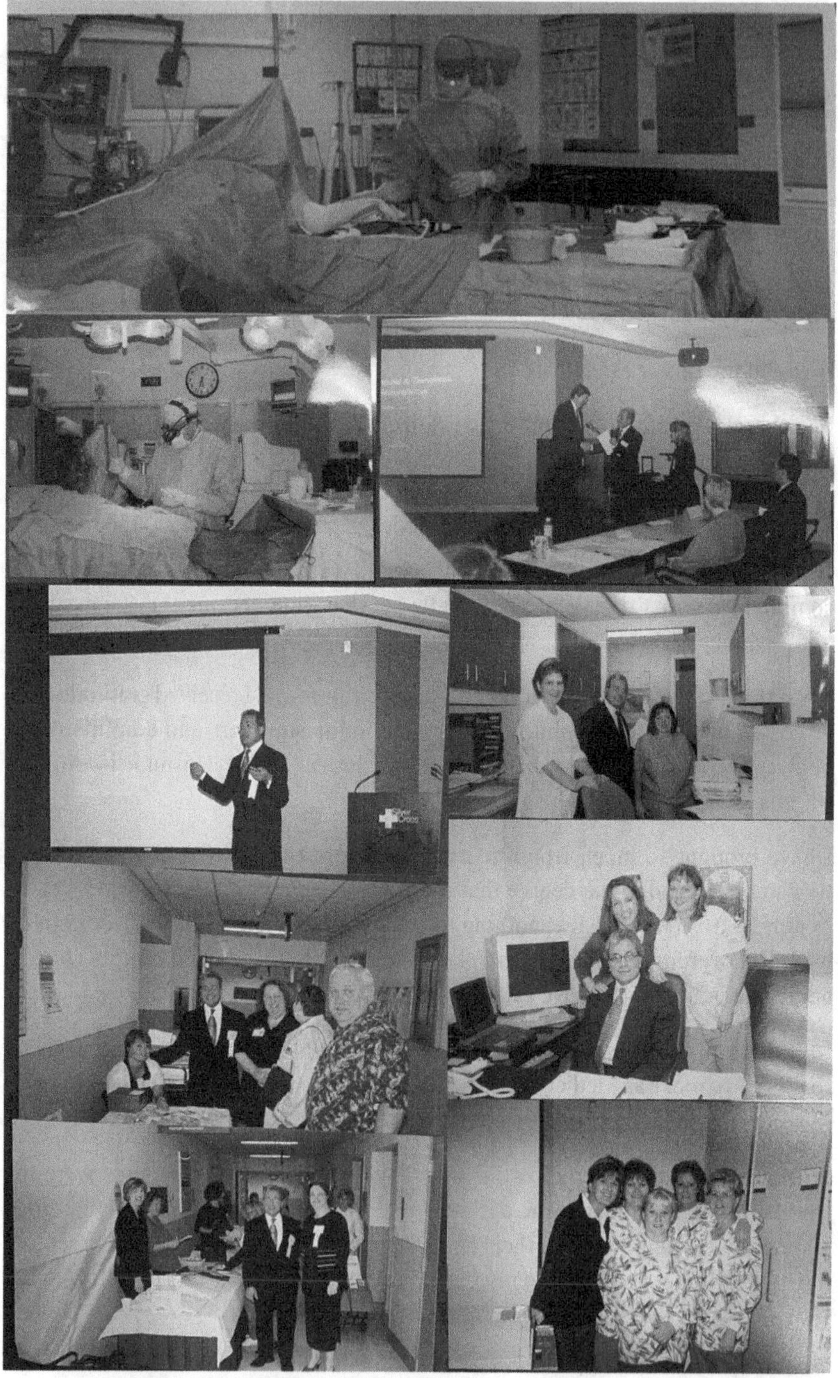

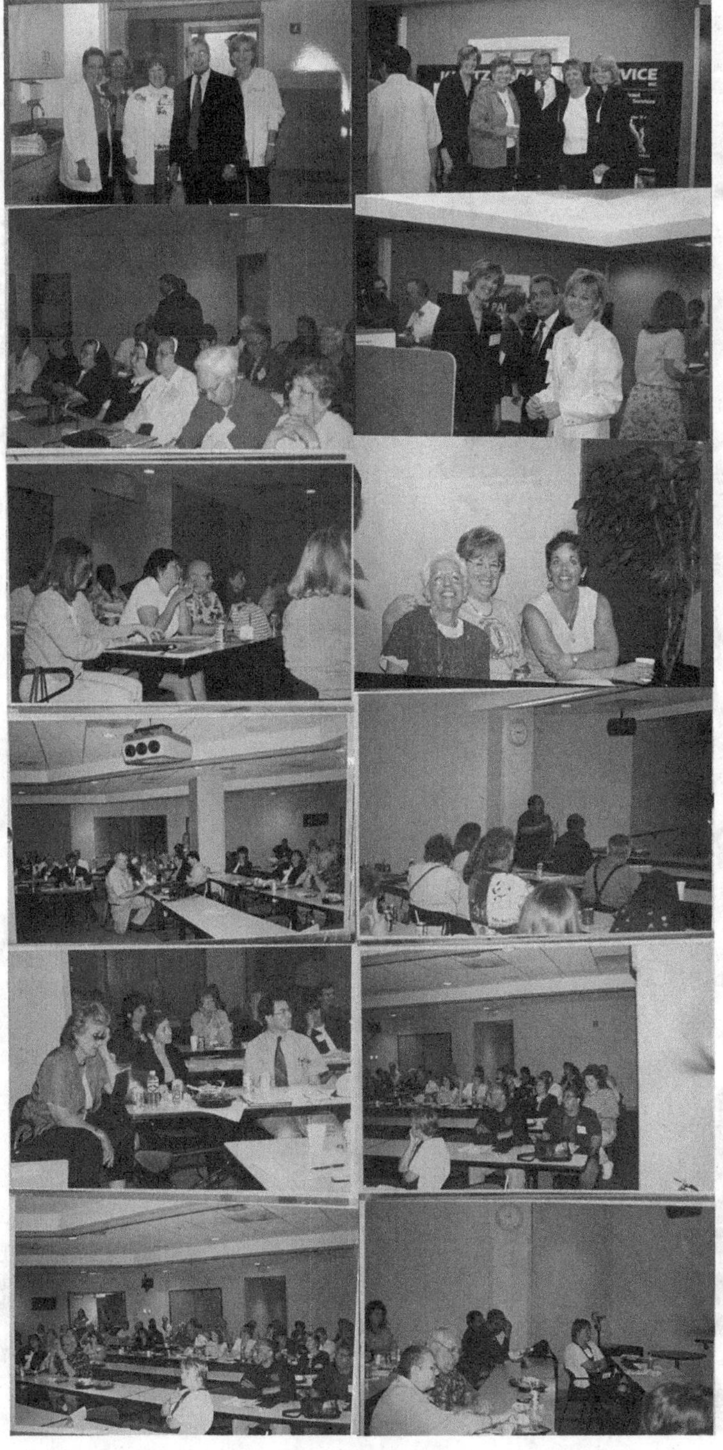

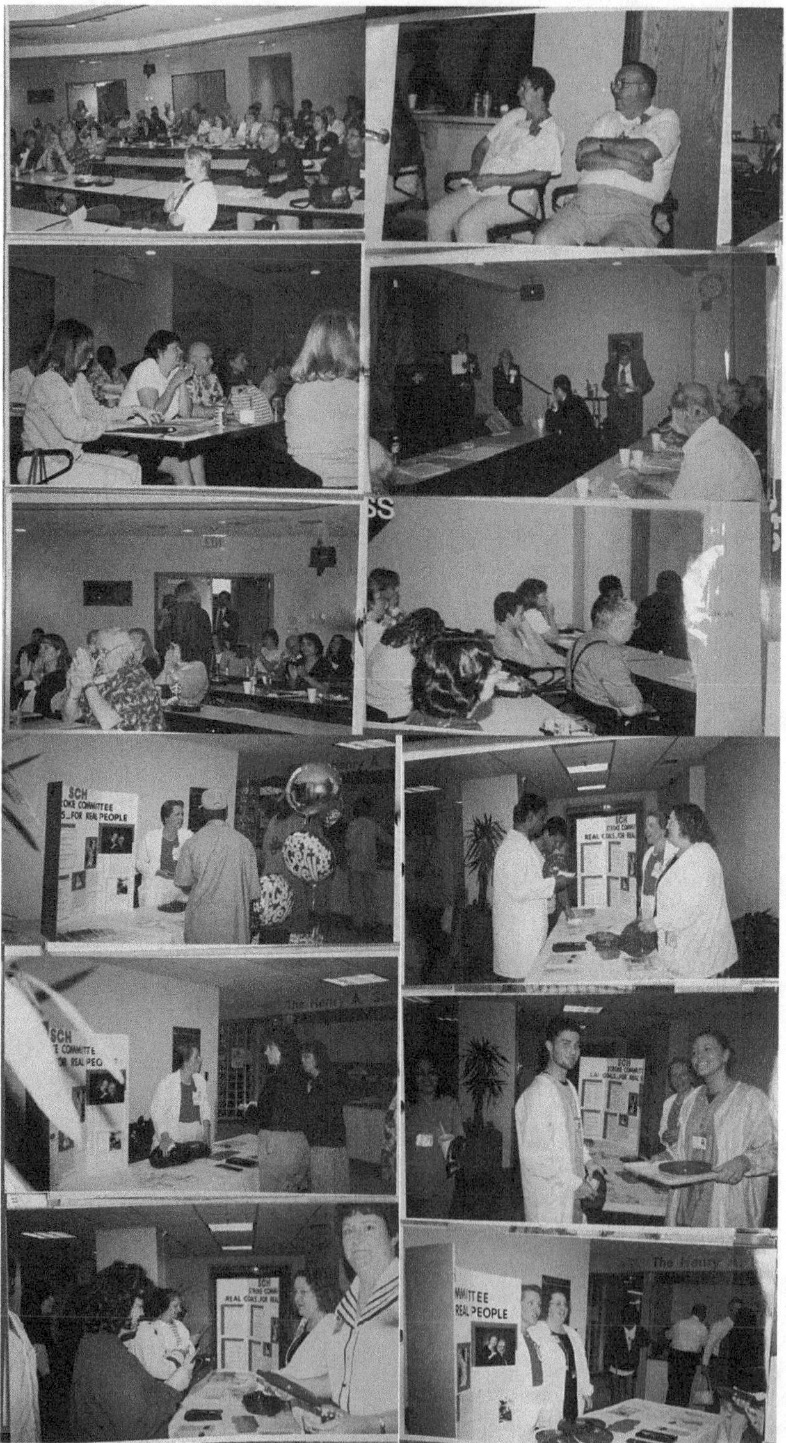
SCH
FOR REAL PEOPLE
SCH
MMITTEE
REAL PEOPLE

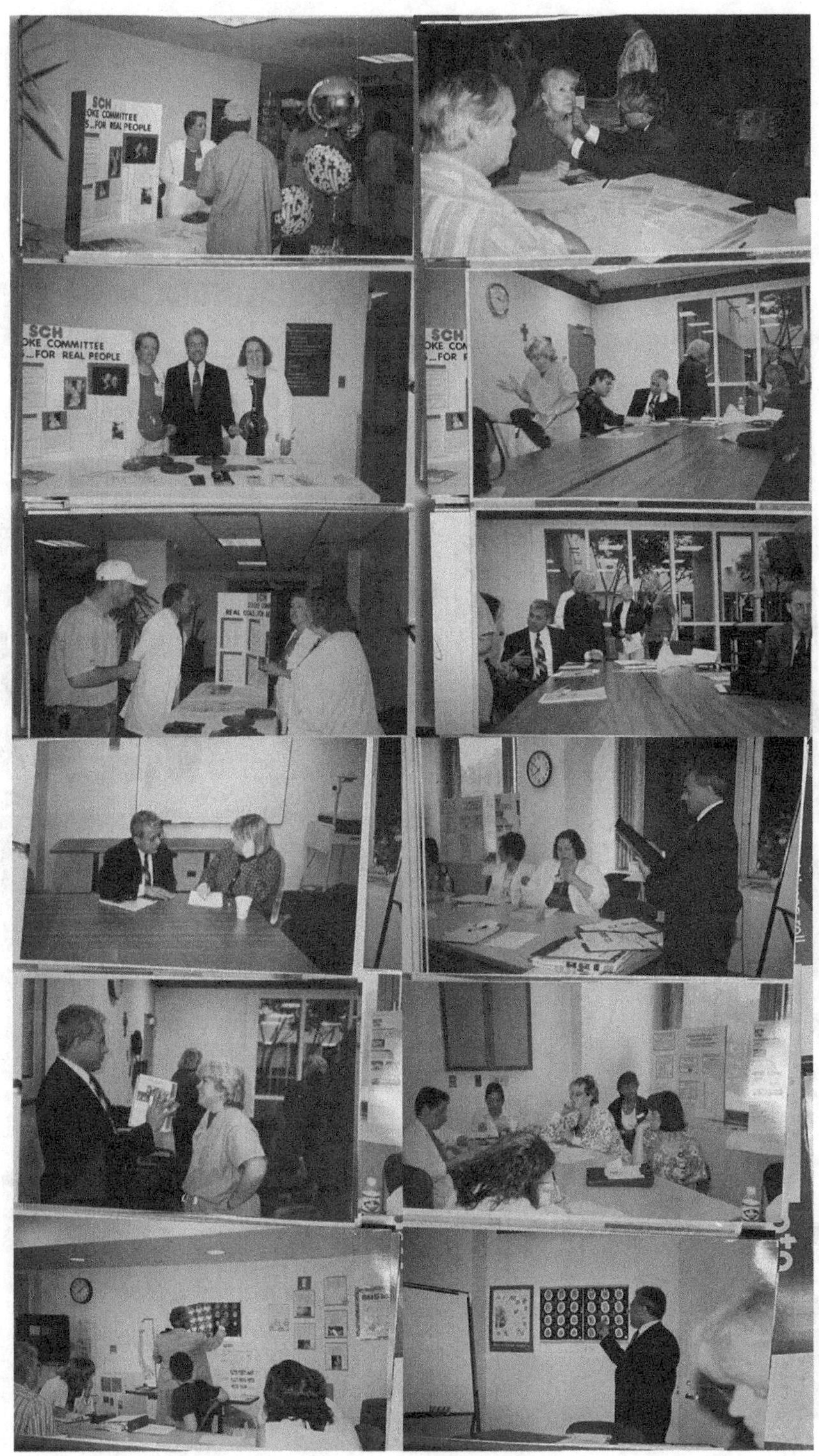
SCH
...FOR REAL PEOPLE

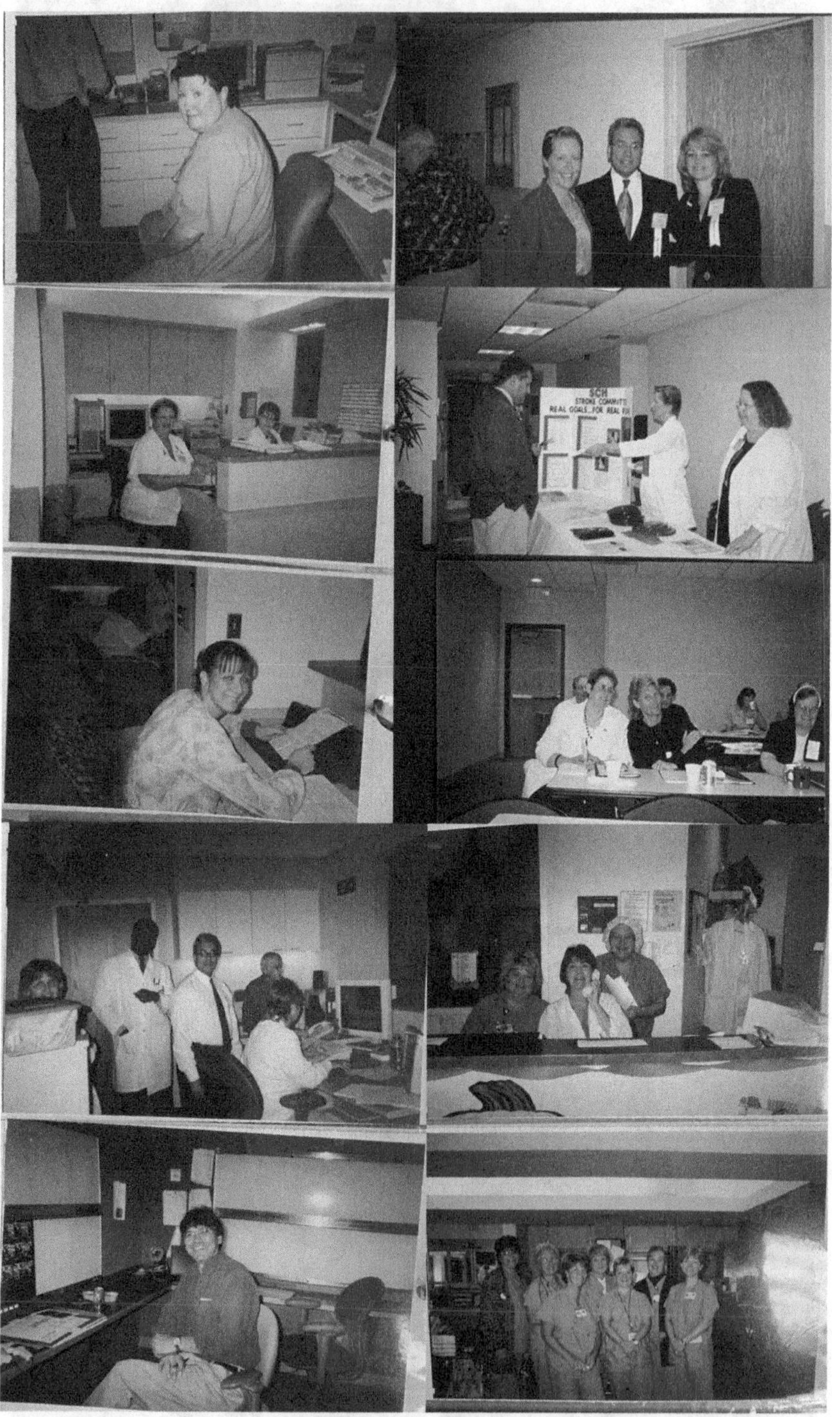
SCH
REAL GOALS...FOR REAL

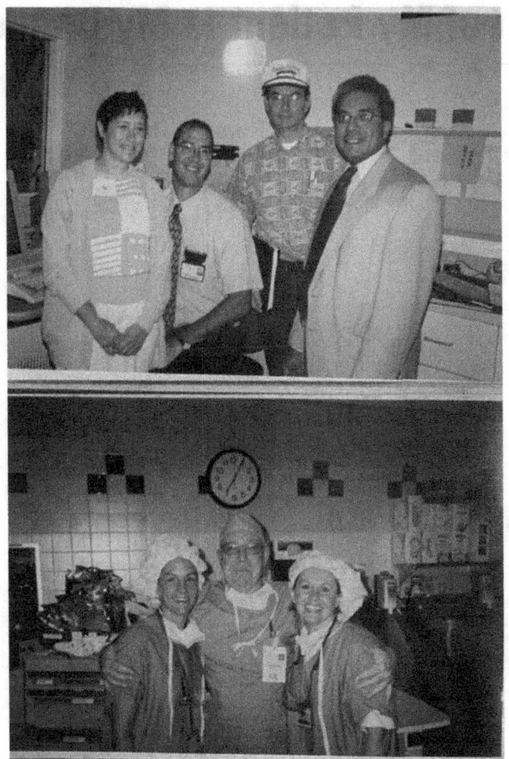

MP. Wow, not only you save people's way of living, to give them a new chance at life without pain or medication. But, you also teach and have taught so many new doctors and medical staff over the years. All of that and you look to God to be on your side in every possible way. Not forgetting your an author of many books. You have touched thousands of lives in positive ways. Awesome human Award Dr **Ramsis Ghaly**

Each of My Patient is My Diamond!

Written by Ramsis Ghaly

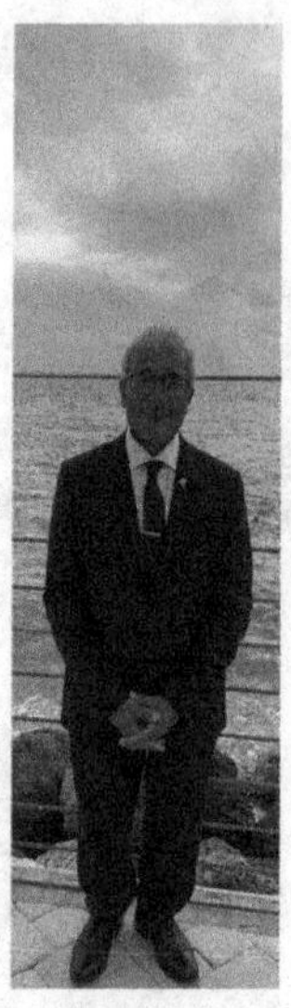

Patients ask me: "When it comes to patients, Why I do everything by myself and not to delegate to others and put full trust in modern technology and science to the degree I appear obsessive-compulsive hands-on caregiver micromanager lacking trust to the intermediaries ?"

I replied: "My patients, each of them like a diamond high price and great Pearl and if I have one, I can't ask anyone else to take care of that diamond but myself!"

In fact, I am like a **"Helicopter Mom"** dying GPS system to my eyes on my patient a track them!

Indeed, proudly I spend all my life to Medicine and patients! I learned and strived to obtain all the knowledge beyond boundaries and look at each patient as myself crowned my deeds and mission in my Mentor, My Love, My Healing, my Savior and my Lord God Jesus Christ!!!

Again, the kingdom of heaven is like unto treasure hid in a field; the which when a man hath found, he hideth, and for joy thereof goeth and selleth all that he hath, and buyeth that field. 45 Again, the kingdom of heaven is like unto a merchant man, seeking goodly pearls: 46 Who, when he had found one pearl of great price, went and sold all that he had, and bought it." Matthew 13:44-45

Hebrews 1:3 "And He is the radiance of His glory and the exact representation of His nature and upholds all things by the word of His power. When He had made purification of sins, He sat down at the right hand of the Majesty on high," Colossians 1:15 "He is the image of the invisible God, the firstborn of all creation." Colossians 1:19 "For it was the Father's good pleasure for all the fullness to dwell in Him,"

Colossians 2:9 "For in Him all the fullness of Deity dwells in bodily form,"

Ramsis Ghaly

Www.ghalyneurosurgeon.com

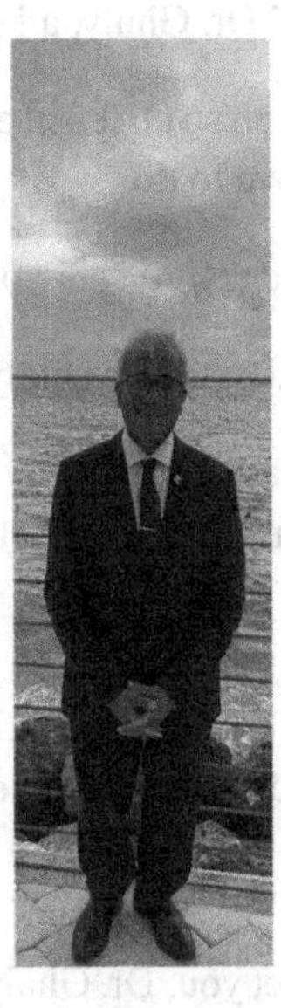

CP, Very nice picture.

MW, What a Beautiful thing to say! Thank you!

ML, Such a sweet photo of you Dr. Ghaly.

DE, U are a true blessing

AK, What a great picture, thank you.

CR, So very well said

DM, Well said Dr. Ghaly you are the Best of the Best

CE, U truly r one of a kind Dr Ghaly. U r the diamond. Unique and beautiful! Keep doing what ur doing.

KO, Your the precious stone that reflects unto others, and the best, great picture God bless you always Dr Ghaly

KL, This is why you are the best!!!

JB, But these traits are what make you one in a million Dr. Ghaly. This is what makes you the consummate professional. Your patients recognize your dedication to the profession as well as each of us individually as patients. We all know how fortunate we are to have you as our physician!!

ML, You're truly "one of a kind" Dr. Ghaly, a !

SM, I never had a doctor that's been so efficient and quick, don't ever change your ways, keep on doing what you love to do.

RF, That's why I love you so much. God sent you to be our healing Angel.

GP, You're a wonderfully blessed man, Dr Ghaly.

JD, We never asked why. You made us ask why all the other doctors don't do it. You are amazing and you are our precious jewel.

MA, You are awesome @

JJ, Your values and trust in God are why you are Dr. Ramsis Ghaly and why we love you. Thank you for all you do for your patients.

I/We hope you are taking good care of yourself, too

LG, Indeed. So blessed to have met you, Dr. Ghaly! An honorable man and blessed steward of the Lord!

KP, You are truly one of a kind as I have never met a more caring doctor let alone do the work that you do! Thank you.

SM, It's because you have your Superman suit on under your other suit and you are a true Superhero!! Best of the best! And thank you for all you've done and continue to do!! We love ya Doc!!

MA, You are wonderful!

KC, You are also just like a diamond one of a kind, wonderful doctor.

NL, Thank you!

JT, amazing doctor...you inspire me

BCD, Great photo, great ethics

DL, The best of all the rest.

LK, Absolutely the best doctor on planet earth! Thank you for all that you do for every one of your patients!!

ET, I love your treatment of patients.

CS, S, You're doin God's work:)

LW, You are simply the best!!

JM, Thank You Dr. Ghaly!!!

SL, I LOVE this response. You truly were the answer to prayer when I had all of my back issues, hurt on the job and they wanted to fire me because they said my condition was minor but yet I couldn't even bend to get dressed. That was 11 years ago now! I I have my full life back, working full time, I swim, garden, mow the grass, power walk and everything. Due to misdiagnosis (for a whopping 6 months) I will always have some numbness (permanent nerve damage) but it is so much better than the alternative - it could have been so much worse had you not taken me in as a patient!!! And you did it without hesitation, telling me to let you worry about them paying that I only needed to focus on myself and healing. You have helped COUNTLESS people with the gifts God has given you and I for one am so very grateful. Thank you Dr Ghaly …

JS, You are the most caring doctorlove you

RM, Hallelujah well said Dr. Ghaly.

JF, Amen. Amen. Amen. Thank you for fulfilling your ministry and cslling. I love Dr. **Ramsis Ghaly**. **#PastorJeff90210**

CN, Love this man. He is a great doctor.

LW, I feel the same way about my patients

SA, The world needs more physicians like you! God Bless you

JP, You are an incredible human being and a wonderful doctor. May God bless you abundantly for your ministry both in medicine and life.

DN, Very nice post and nice picture

LW, God bless you. Wish more doctors had your philosophy.

CG, I love love love that you feel that way about your patients! We all love you because you are such a unique doctor unlike any other

Bless you!

DM, Not just an ordinary doctor.he walks extra miles not only for his pstients but family as well .God bless you always Doc

AP, God bless you if

ONLY WE HAD MORE LIKE YOU

BM, You're a Gem!

JN, I am so lucky to have been one of those patients!

AB, You care about your patients with all of your being!!! I'm living proof! Thank You Dr Ghaly for all you give!

RC, Thank you doctor for Takeshi care all your patients like a real diamond, yóu are a rare gen too

KE, Blessed

TW, I love you and your "helicopter approach" to diagnosing, repairing and healing your patients! I'm LUCKY AND BLESSED to have been one of your success stories!

DL, You amaze me. Where have all the great Doctors gone ? You are one of a kind !

VG, My Dr..... A Godsend. God has blessed this man & his hands...A true genuine person.

RA, If our country had your devotion to seeking God first, our nation would be strong and respected and healed. God bless you Doctor.

JD, Bless you my friend, you are a Godsend to many lucky people.

JD, Excellent

CP, A angel among us. God Bless you my friend.

MB, What an amazing life philosophy to live by!!! Beautiful!!

TC, You are simply the best Dr Ghaly. You make every patient feel equally important and you are such amazing human! Thank you for all you do for so many

Word of Mouth Still Alive in America!

Written by Ramsis Ghaly

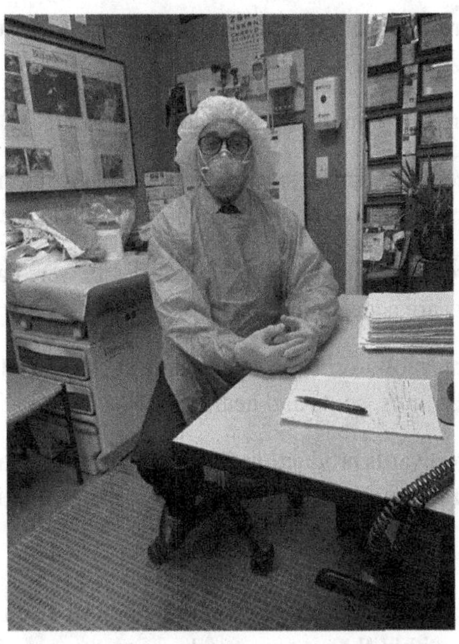

A patient should be able to reach out and to bd cared by a physician and surgeon of his or her choice and the institution of his or her choice —!!

However, the free to choose in healthcare it appears it is gone and America is as follows:

In a time where health insurance plans restrict where to go, health institutions demand where to get for healthcare and to which doctors to receive the care———!

In a time where "Free of Choice" in healthcare is almost gone and the public lost the freedom to choose where it was the norm in the past!!

In a time, healthcare is a mass production and one size fits all where health protocols, policies and pathways must follow with penalties to whoever deviate from!

In a time, where individual care doesn't count as much as group policy and mass production guidelines!

In a time, healthcare is like a Cookbook and the name under which is "Evidence Base Practice" and not individual customized care or hands on individual care!!

In a time, healthcare support institutions and Not Sol practitioners or small medical businesses!

In a time, healthcare support large medical and industrial groups and not limited groups!

In a time, healthcare refers in its own and not to outsiders!

In a time, healthcare is focused on sub-specialization and intermediary healthcare providers and intermediates where the patients as a whole are lost in the middle!

In a time, healthcare is about business and productivity were gaining majority and loosing few patients are acceptable!

In a time, healthcare is follower to computer data and artificial intelligence rather than human brains, minds, souls and hearts!!

In a time, healthcare awards production and profitability and fame in social media and rank in organizations more than individual patients' quality of care!

Yet

The Good News, "Word-of-Mouth", second opinion from "word-of-mouth" referral rather than within the system, reach out to new set of eyes and ears per patient's choice, change health team to another team, search for different opinions are still valid options!

Yet, In America, there is still hope and still room for "freedom of choice"!!

In the meantime, please Don't underestimate patients referred by other patients!!

In my practice, referrals are more than 90% based on "word-of -mouth" since I am not employed by institution or contracted by outside institutions!

What remains consistent that patients know their bodies much more than medical consultants themselves! Many times, I can't believe how smart are patients and highly educated! They diagnose themselves correctly and never settle for less and keep knocking doors until they get the answers that make sense to them and provide the correct answers to their medical and surgical concerns and issues m!

Just in the last few weeks, 10 patients came desperately, and no one could make the correct diagnosis and figure the cause of their health problems! In fact, majority were more than 6months out with day and night suffering despite following their own doctors, ancillary services, reputable medical care facilities! And these patients were following to the medical advice literally! Yet they weren't any better and continued to scream even to the stones of the walls!

And such patients that are lost in the healthcare system are in the rise and those are the ones to seek doctors and neurosurgeons like myself! Physicians that aren't attached to big corporates and follow cookbook medicine!

And the minute they come to be evaluated and in my first phone calls with them, the clock of care including "hands on customized care" starts! The core of MY Care is "Patient-Comes-First", and its highlights are as following:

-Listen, listen and listen then

-Hands on evaluation, then

-Process and come up with differential diagnosis, then start to

-Come up with plan of care

-Recommendations, then

-Follow through and follow up then

-Definitive diagnosis and then

-Definitive Treatment!

-Never give up and always

-Pray for guidance and blessing

-Manage with humble heart and love.

-Keep thinking and thinking until a clear diagnosis and treatment and heart comes to a peace with ongoing plan of care!

- Praying and praying knowing no one is perfect and no textbook available for such a patient until God show the best way for such a patient!

-Be patience and spent as much time until the job well done, and patient is taking care of the best way!

More than forty-five decades ago when I fell in love with the nervous system!

Back in my early years on Medicine after studying all human organs, I knew with certainty Jesus our God gifted treasure and His secret in humanity and in His creation was placed in the human brain and the nervous system!

I also realized that there is no single textbook of computer program or policy, or protocol will ever make the correct diagnosis and decide for each particular patient what is the ideal treatment!!

I asked: If the human brains of doctors couldn't make diagnosis in many medical and surgical conditions, how can artificial intelligence and computer program that feed by human brains be superhuman and make the correct diagnosis!

There is no way that I will ever believe in corporate care or cookbook care! The nervous system is so mysterious and every day even in my stage, I still learn, and I will continue to learn and be open minded!

Therefore, with humble minds, investigative eyes, listening ears and searching engine in a heart full of love and prayers, I approach such patients!!

"Except the Lord build the house, they labour in vain that build it: except the Lord keep the city, the watchman waketh but in vain. [2] It is vain for you to rise up early, to sit up late, to eat the bread of sorrows: for so he giveth his beloved sleep." Psalm 127:1-2 KJV

Amen

Www.ghalyneurosurgeon.com

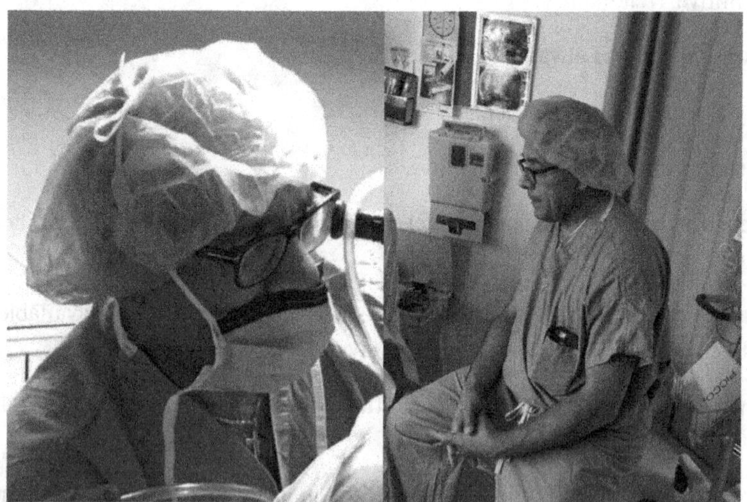

DL, YOU are such a rarity ! Stay Blessed

Charlene Mentzer Glowaty

Everything you said is so true.

You are the epitome of a caring

doctor and surgeon. Many blessings

Jack Jane Cole Duvick

I truly believe everything you said Dr. Ghaly !! Keep up the great work that you do !!!

With My Residents at Post-COVID Time

Thank a Resident Day!

Ramsis Ghaly
Thanks Resident Day 2/25/2022

Today is a special Thank you Day to our Medical snd Surgical Residents nationwide. In 2018, the Gold Humanism Honor Society decided to bring to light the importance of the residence staff and encourage healthcare institutions and medical staff throughout the nation to show their gratitude and appreciation. It also elevate awareness to the public about the great service provided day and night 24/7 of our house staff residents.

As I have been mentioning and working with our residents for 35 years. You aren't forgotten the trainee of the coming generations. Thank you all !!

blob:null/ac2b189c-6ec2-43e8-9fe5-d8ad43052d16

https://lnkd.in/eYA7KuY8

Ramsis F Ghaly, MD

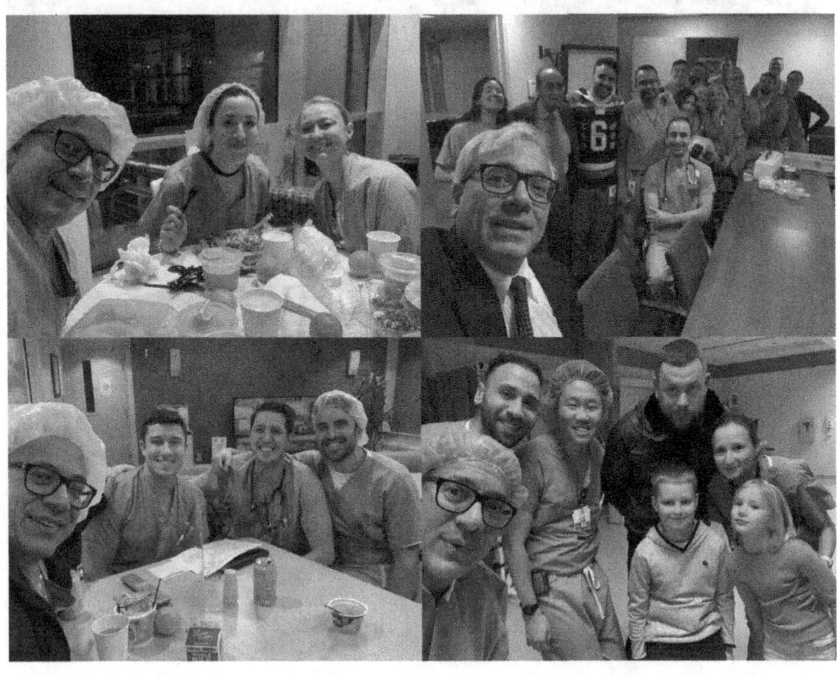

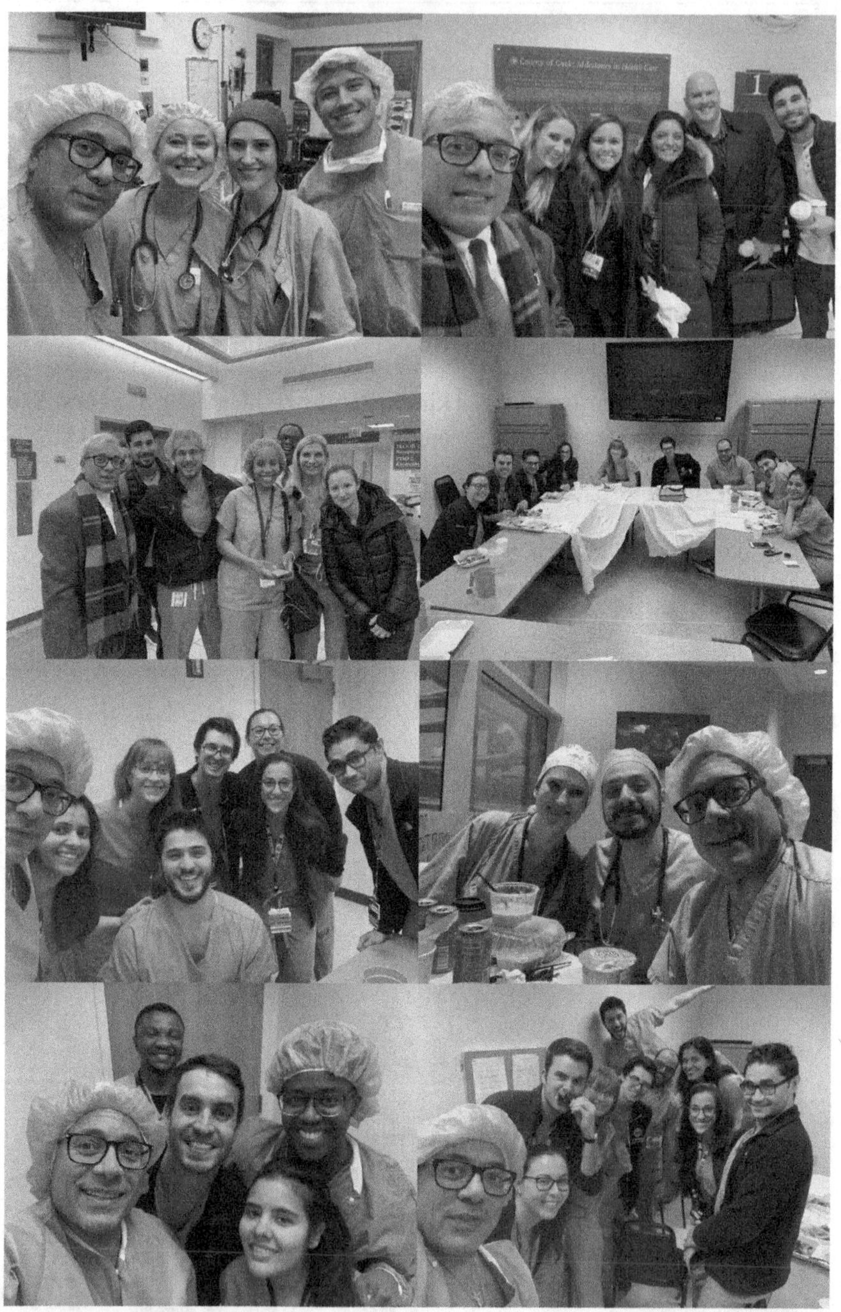

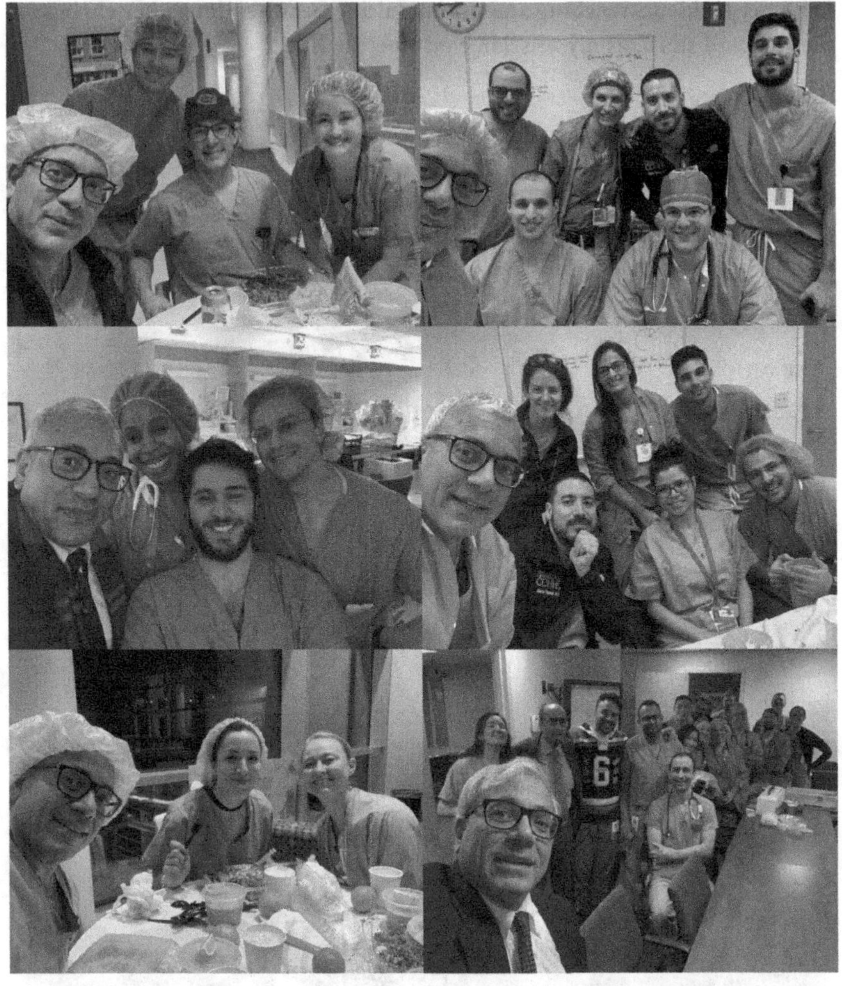

Clinical Professor of Neurosurgery, Anesthesiology, Neurocritical Care and Pain Management

Www.ghalyneurosurgeon.com

AV, Thank you!!

JT, thank you...they are our future healers!

CG, KG, Thank you residents!!!

JM, Thank You All For Your Devotion To Care AMEN

With my residents teaching and dining taking heavy call together caring for the sick and so Ill, as my mission continues in 2022!!

Ramsis Ghaly

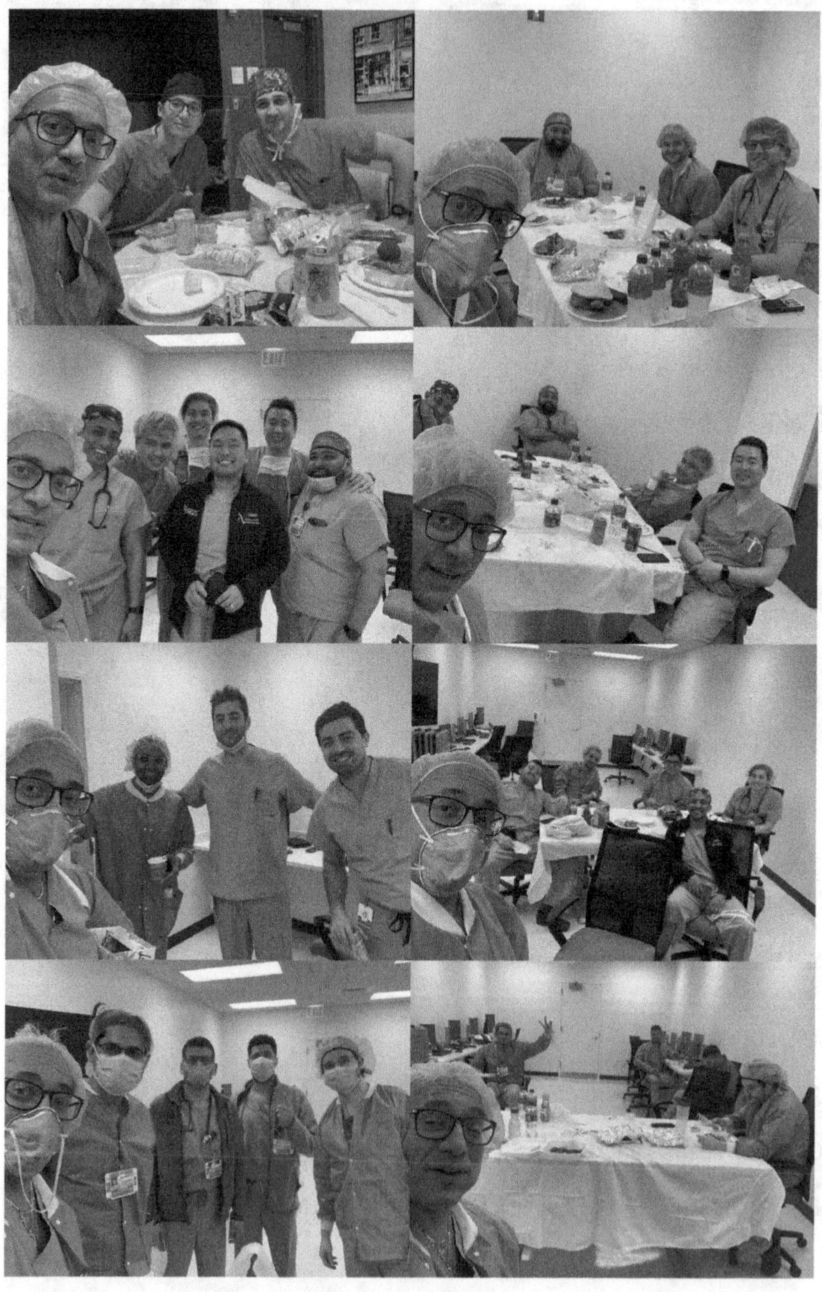

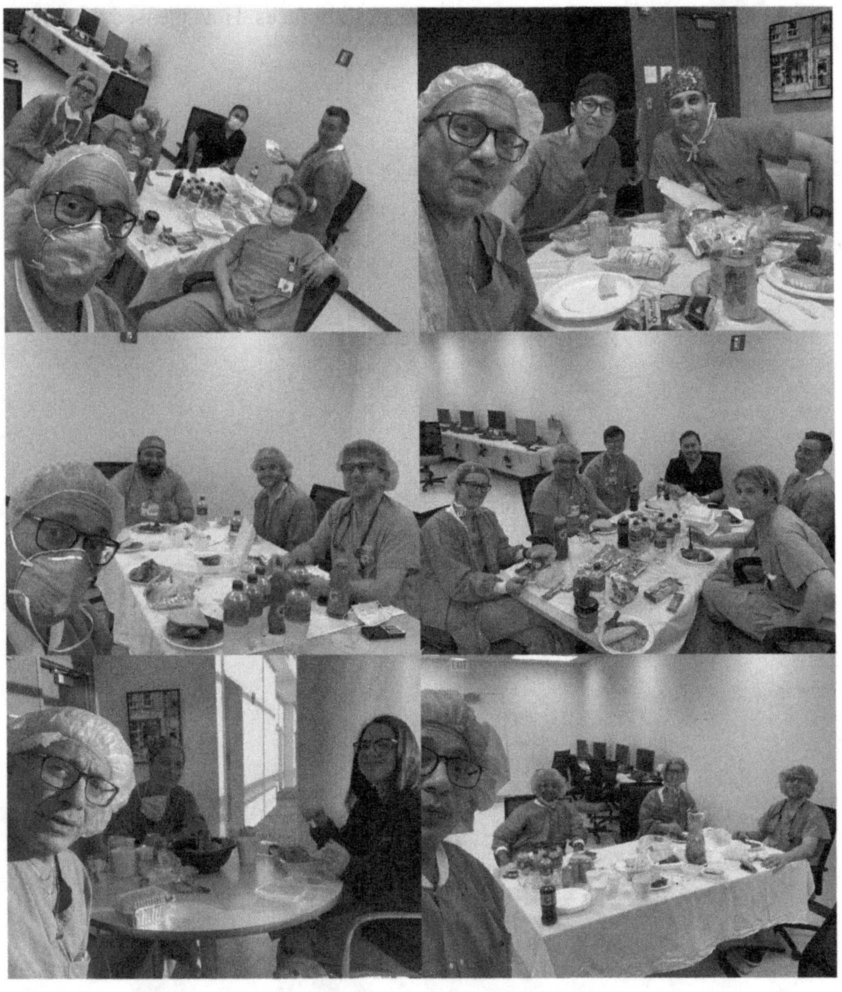

MN. Great looking group, they are lucky to have you sharing your extensive knowledge.

ML. God bless each and everyone of them! God bless you Dr. **Ramsis Ghaly**

JT. i love you all for your dedication and that guy with the camera is the best!!! i think Ramsis Ghaly is a gift from above for all he is doing and continues to do in the name of God...amen

CG. I look at these pictures and see all the smiling faces. How pleased they must be having you teach them all that you know.

Bless you all!

JM, **Congratulations**

"Best To All Of You"

New Class New Academic Year and New Teaching!

Congratulations to the graduate class and welcome to the new class and congratulations to moving to the senior classes!

Comprehensive Didactic Annual Ghaly lecture series and Workshops preparation!!

Ramsis Ghaly

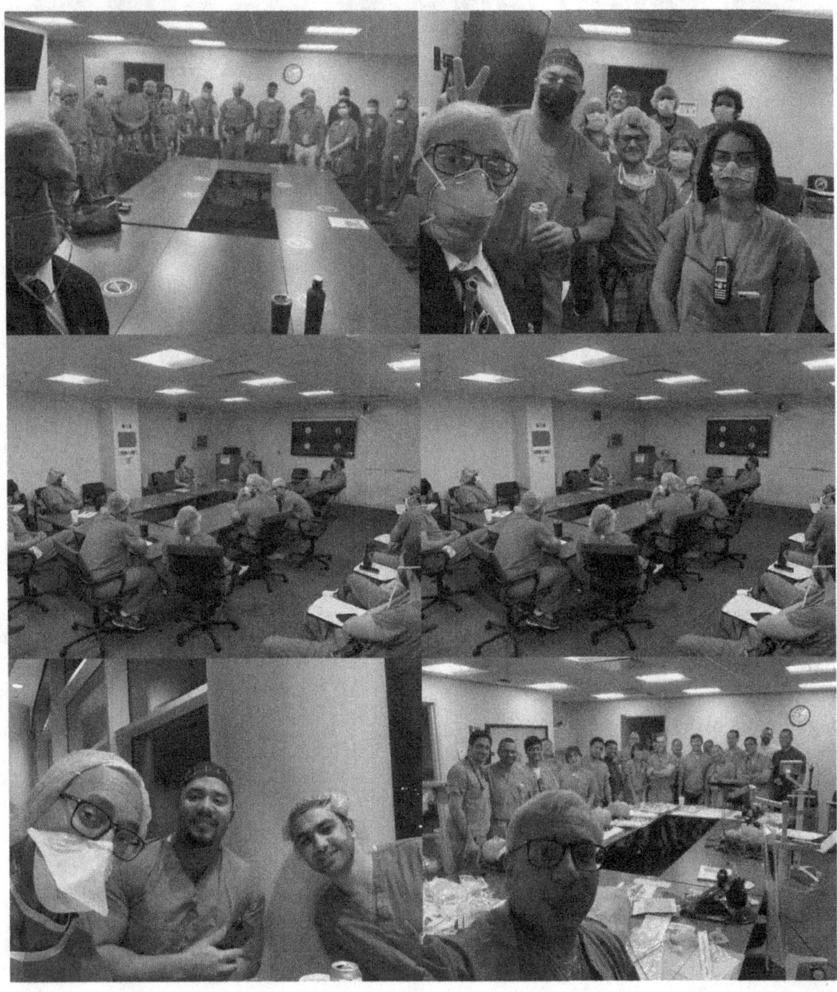

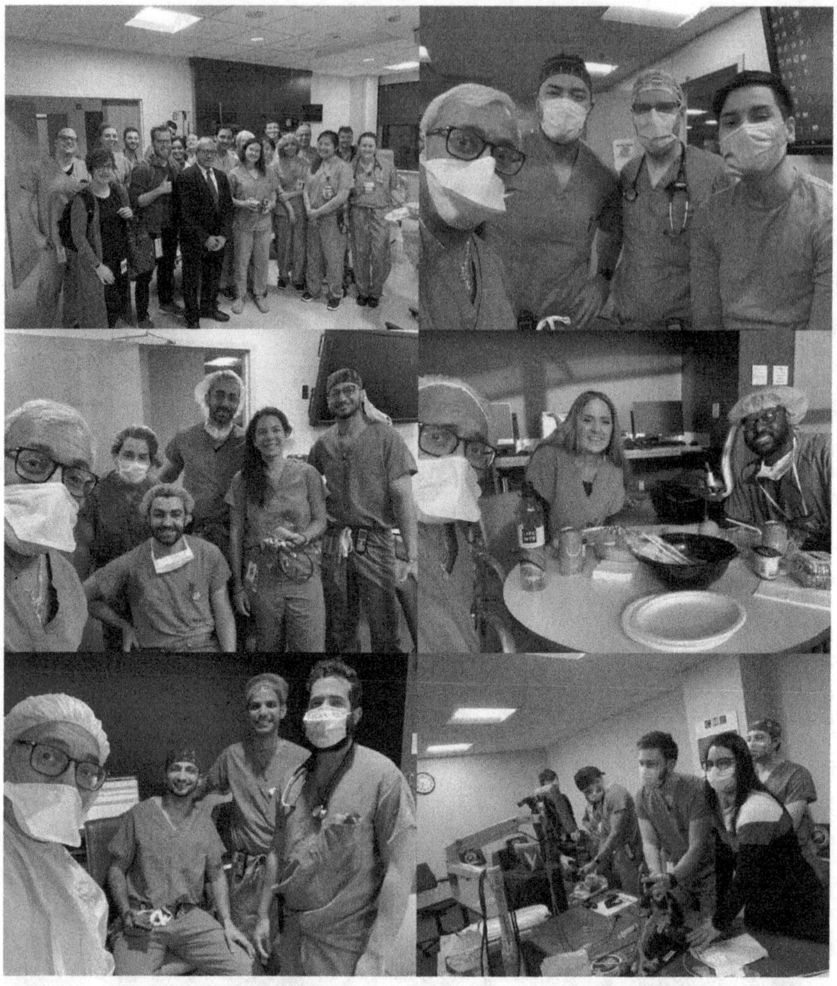

Ma, Em, The world needs more Dr. Ghaly's that take the time, effort and genuine care to improve lives

Cg, That's awesome!

Congratulations

Jd, Great job sir!

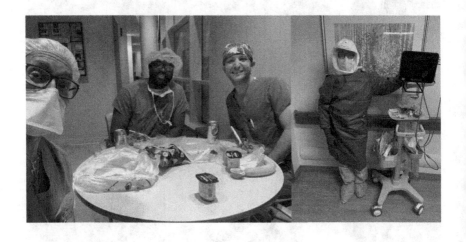

Teaching the Residents!

What a joy to be a teacher to our students and residents!
What an honor to be part of the future!
What a privilege to be a mentor to the coming generations!

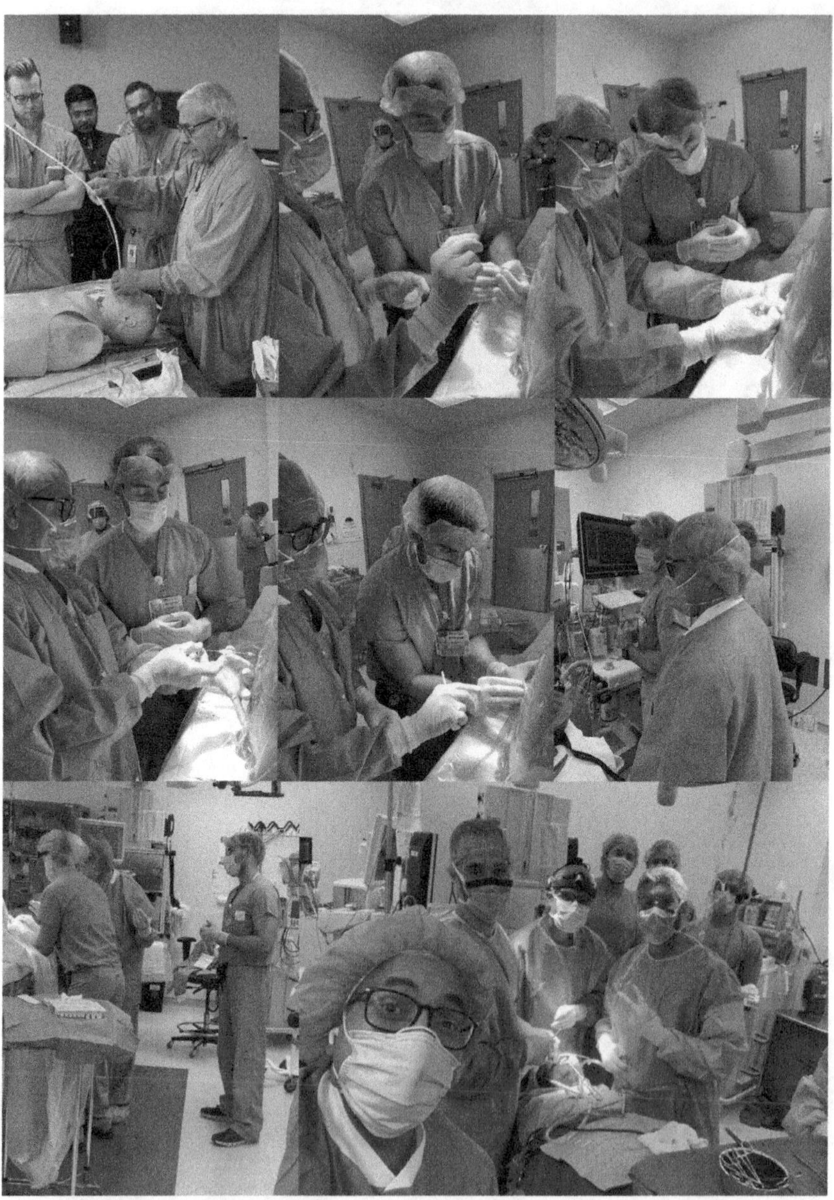

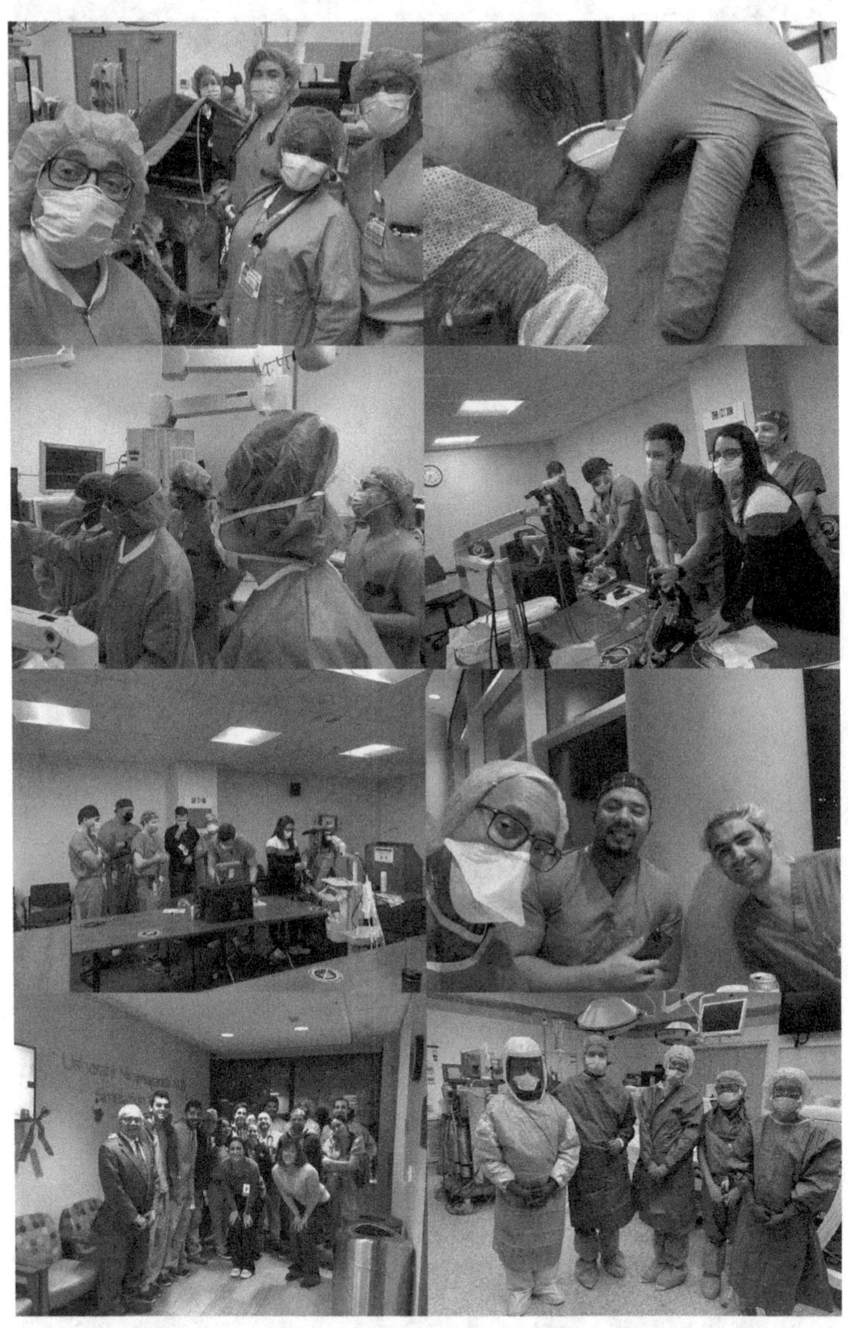

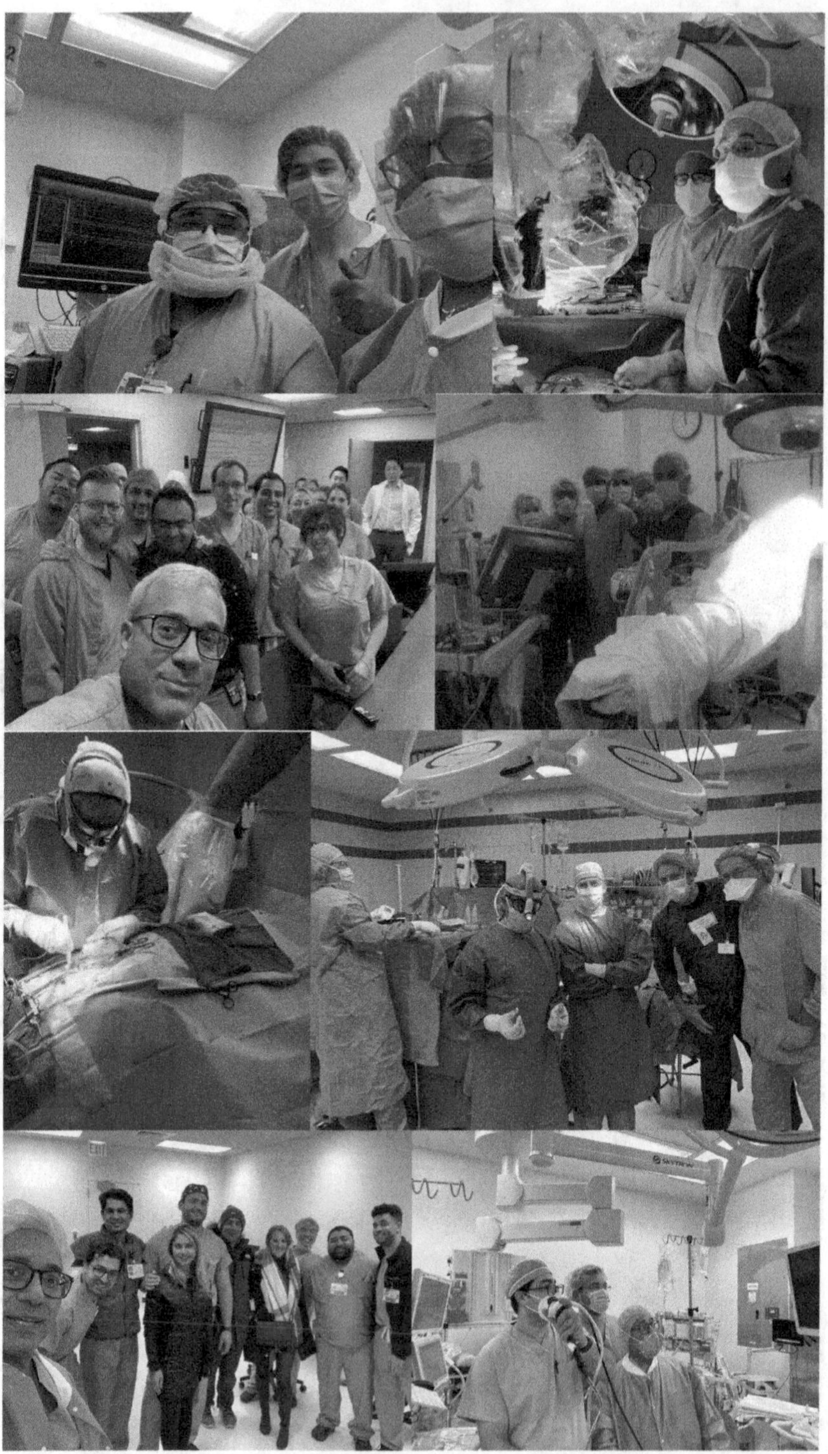

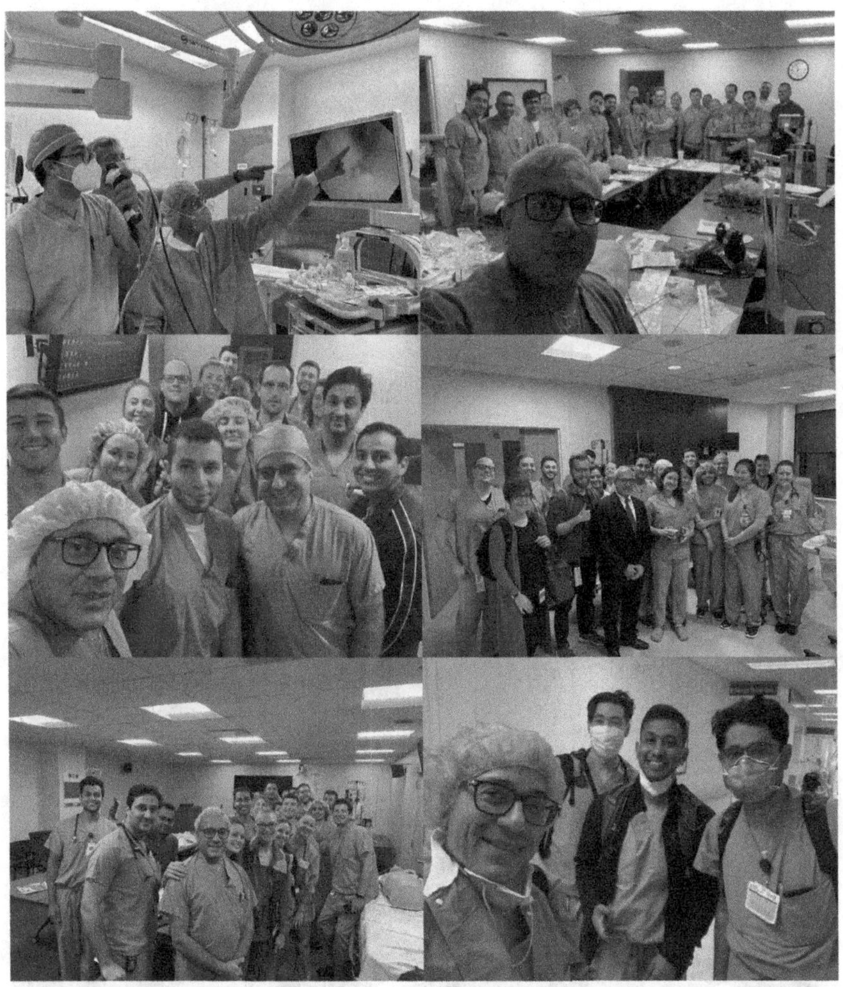

July 6, 2022

Very early morning the Ghaly Annual airway workshop to our residents and students. Thank you for all attendee

Ramsis Ghaly

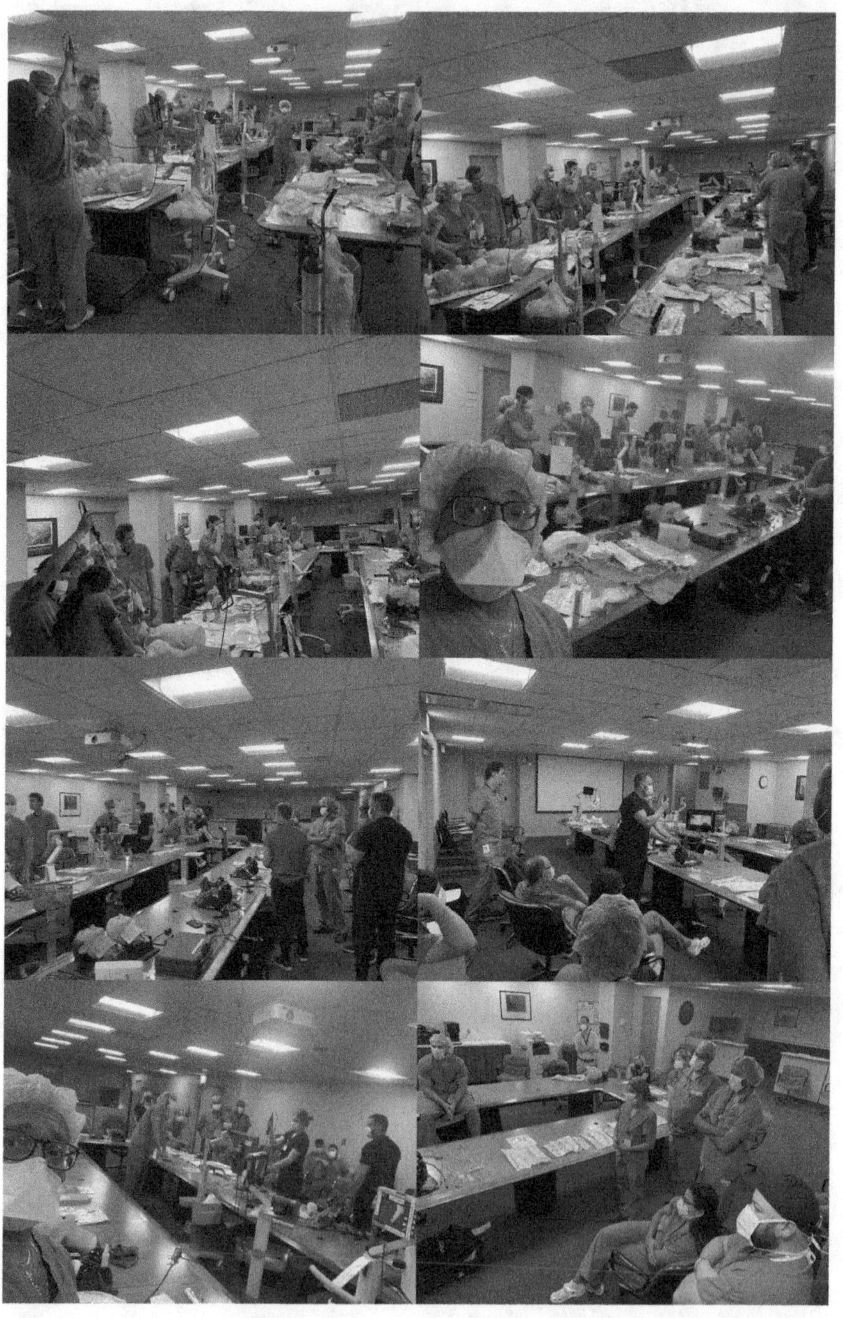

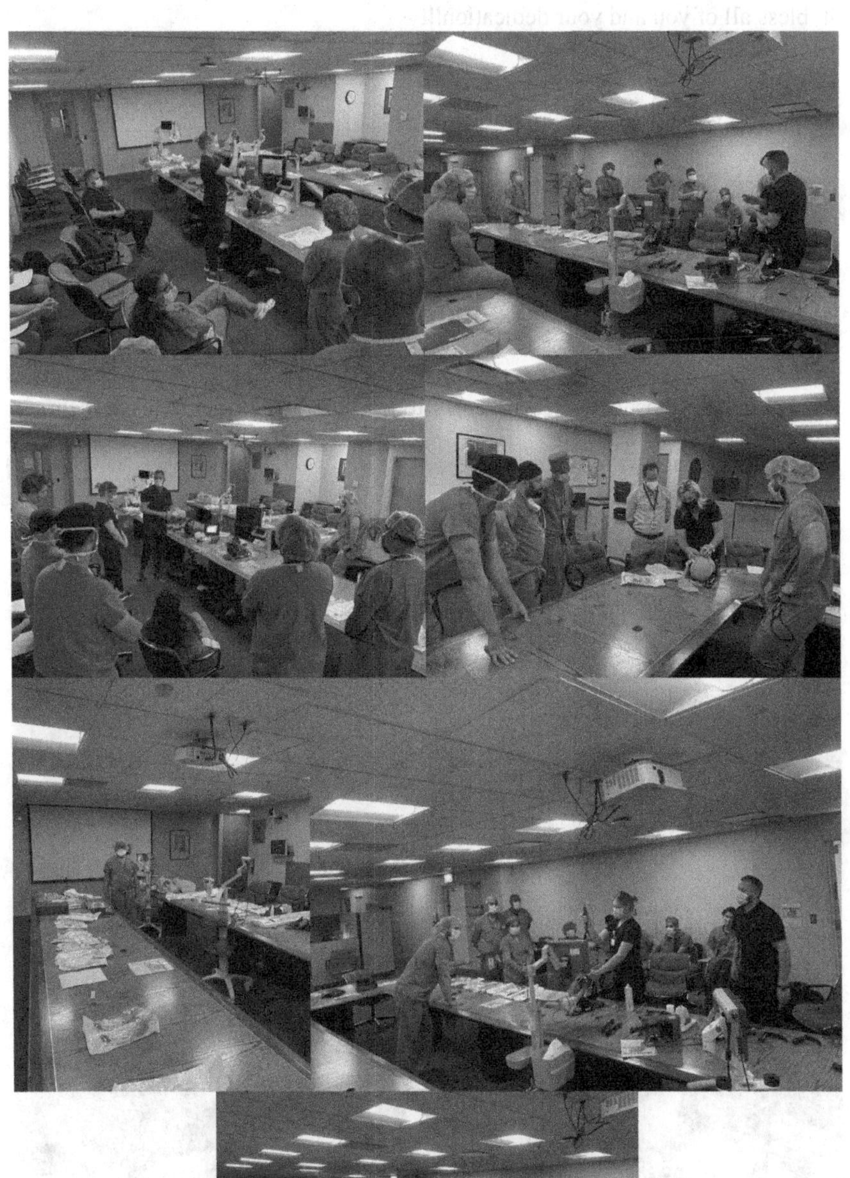

Jt, bless all of you and your dedication!!!

Dd, AbCs!

Jg, Love this

Ed, This is fascinating. God Bless!

Tg, God Bless to all !!

Eo, You have quite the audience. I'm sure they learned a lot. Have a blessed day.

Cb, Visualize the vocal cords

Cg, Look at all those attendees so eager to learn and you eager to teach them.

Rc, **Congratulations** for your work!

Ms, Thank you for showing these inside pictures of learning. Bless you all that will help someone and prevent an heartache of their family.

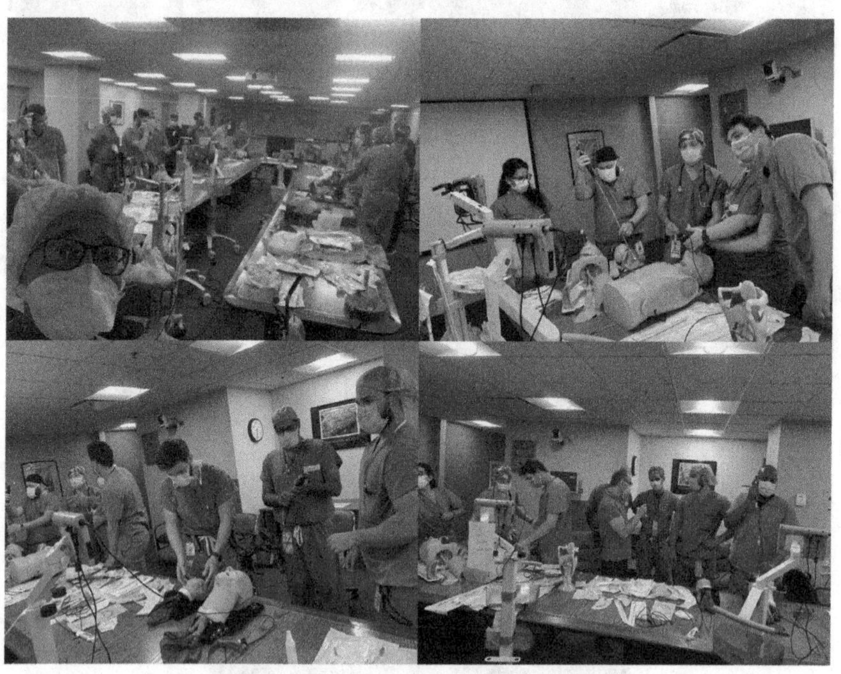

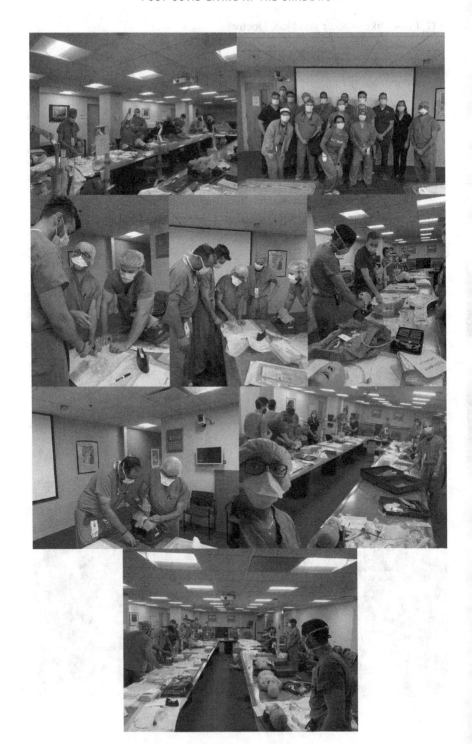

VG, Looks like another good job, Doctor!

SM, They are learning from the BEST!

JT, i am extremely impressed...bless all of you with the healing hands...

KH, Go Dr. Ghaly!

JD, Good for you Ramsis!

Ghaly yearly hands on comprehensive central line and arterial line Workshop! Thank you to all the attendee early the yearly Ghaly central line and arterial line workshop mastering Internal Jugular, Subclavian and femoral central line catheterizations and arterial line insertion. Our next and final this Wednesday 8/24/2022, same time and same place.

Hope you all enjoyed and learned much. It is so important to master these procedures. See you all and thank you simulation lab team!

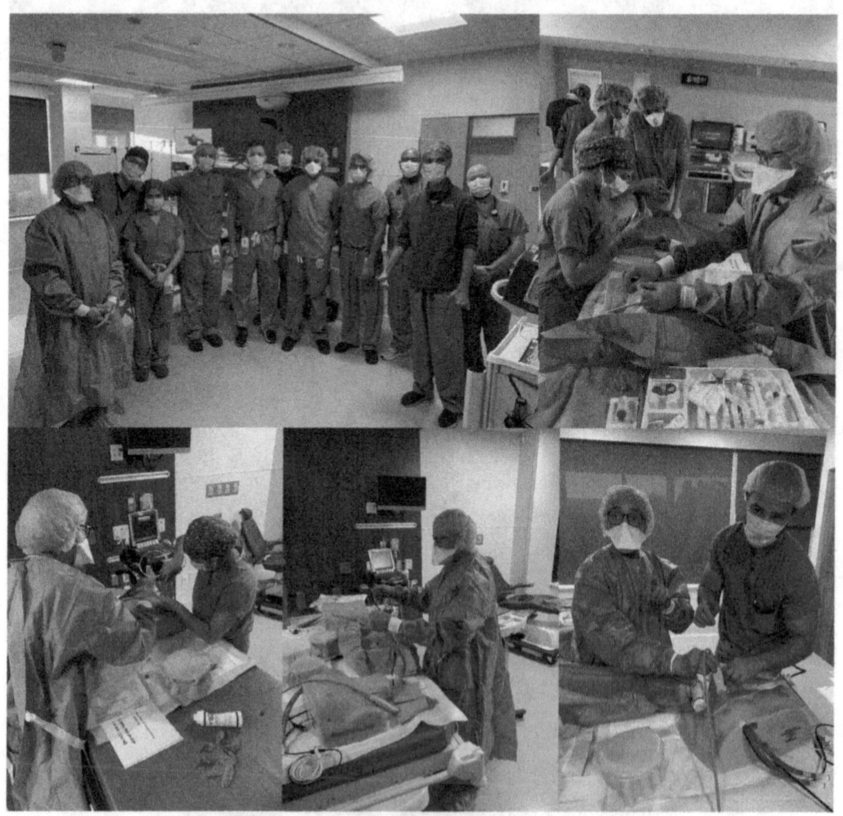

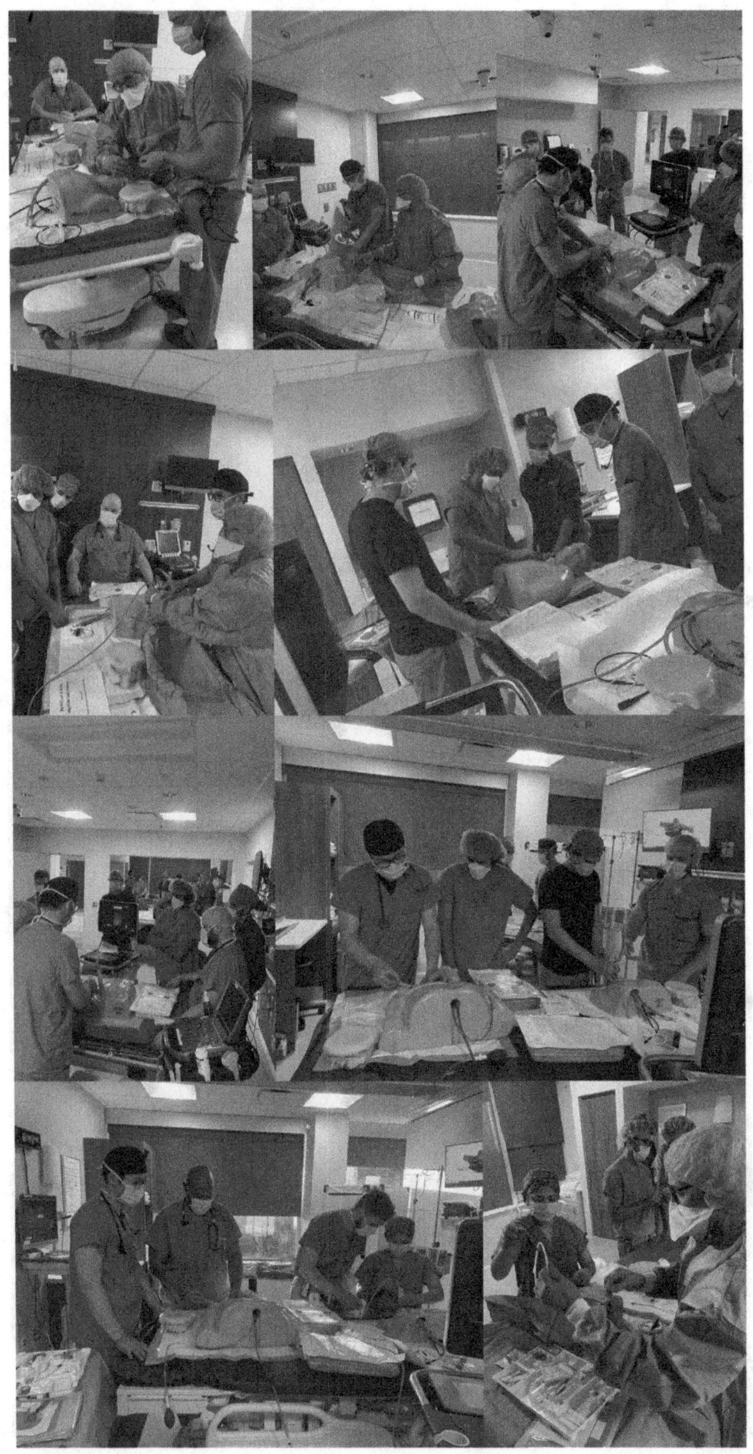

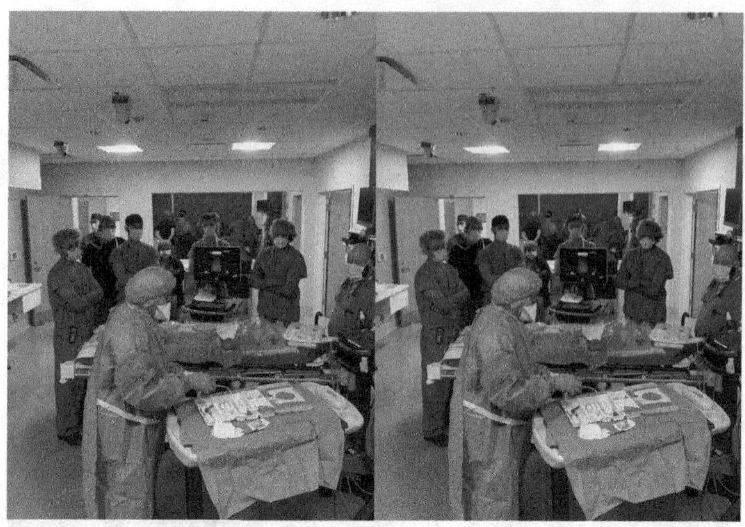

Another day of teaching. Amen to my Lord Jesus, a merciful Healer, our Master and Trach, God Our Lord and Savior

Ramsis Ghaly

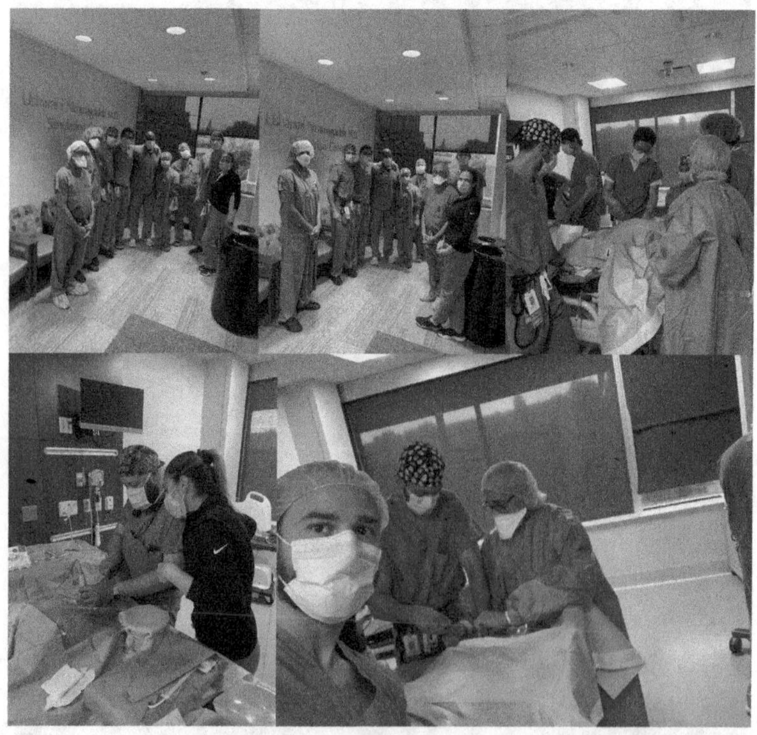

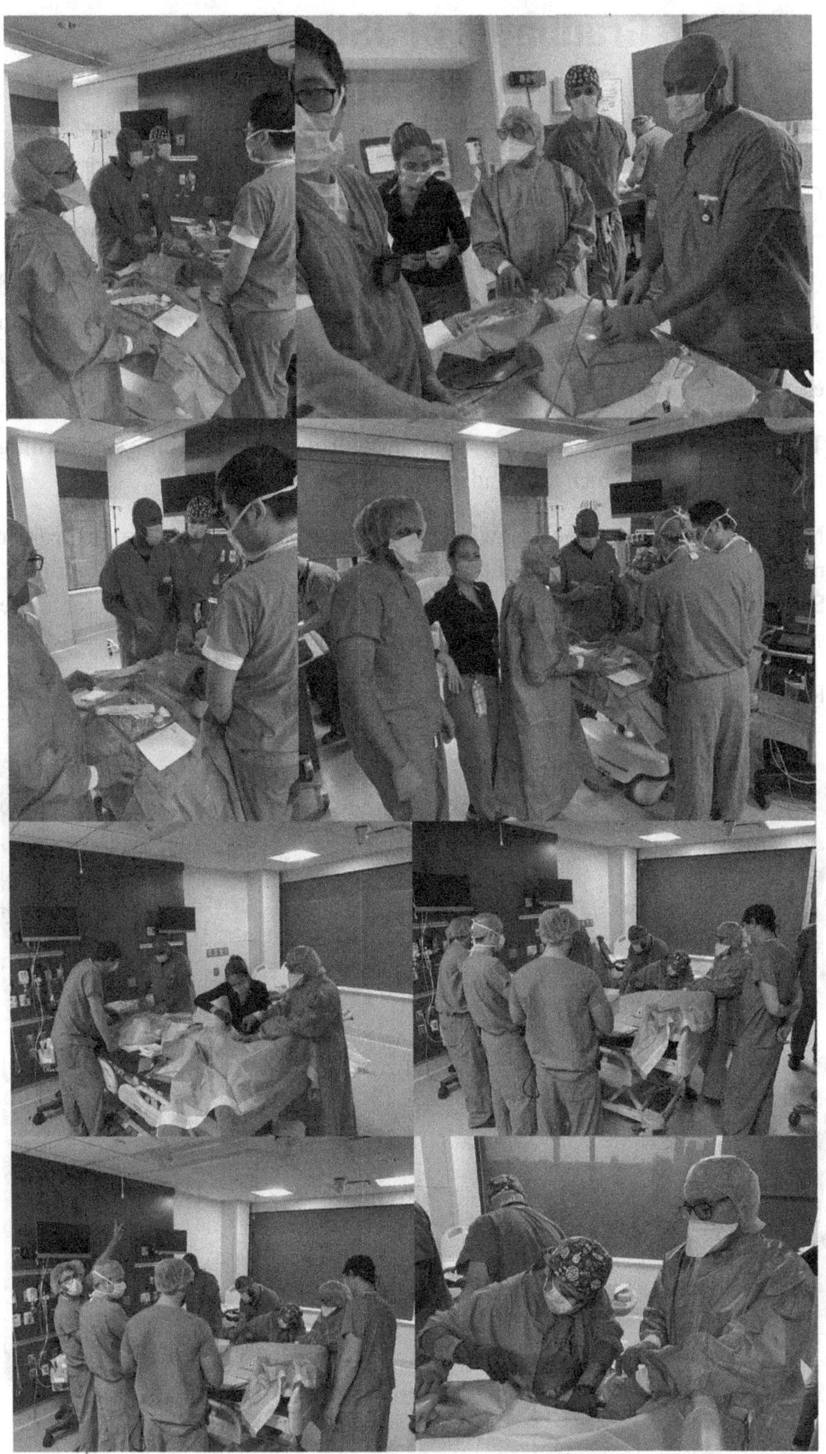

Graduates of JSH of Cook County Hospital 2022!

Congratulations to JSH of Cook County Hospital Anesthesia and pain graduates 2022. Best wishes. Great celebration to outstanding residents and fellows.

Cook County is known to graduate the best as so many very sick patients and various pathological illness are cared for. Four years of handwork going through caring for Chicago trauma victims and COVID patients' day and night weren't easy.

Tonight, the graduating class is celebrating the fruits of their training and earning the certificates for which they had sacrificed their lives.

Now we wish them all the best wishes as they are preparing to their next career nationwide. We are so proud of them, and they are so ready to be in their own. Some are joining practices and others are spending another year for more subspeciality training. ng and saving lives we trust!!

Ramsis Ghaly

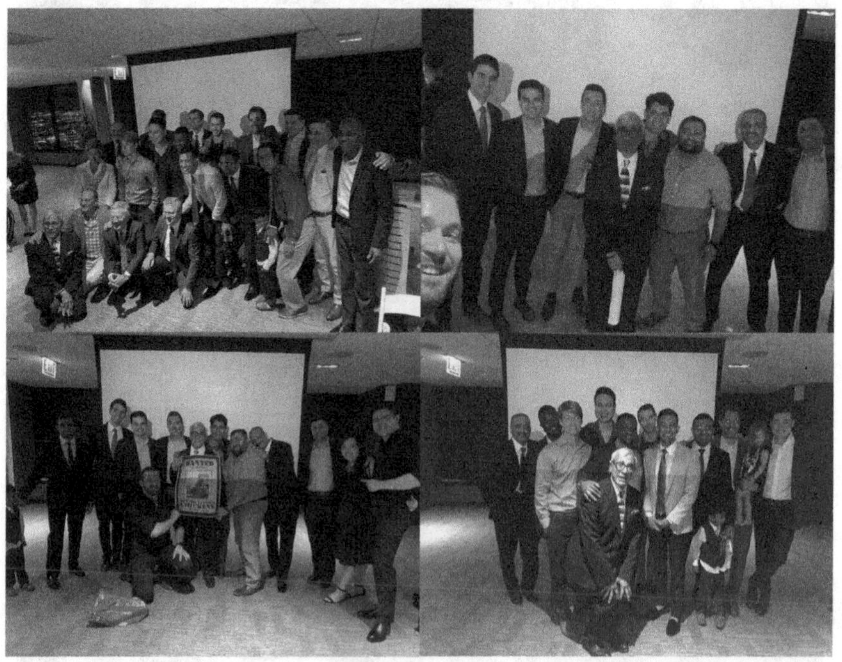

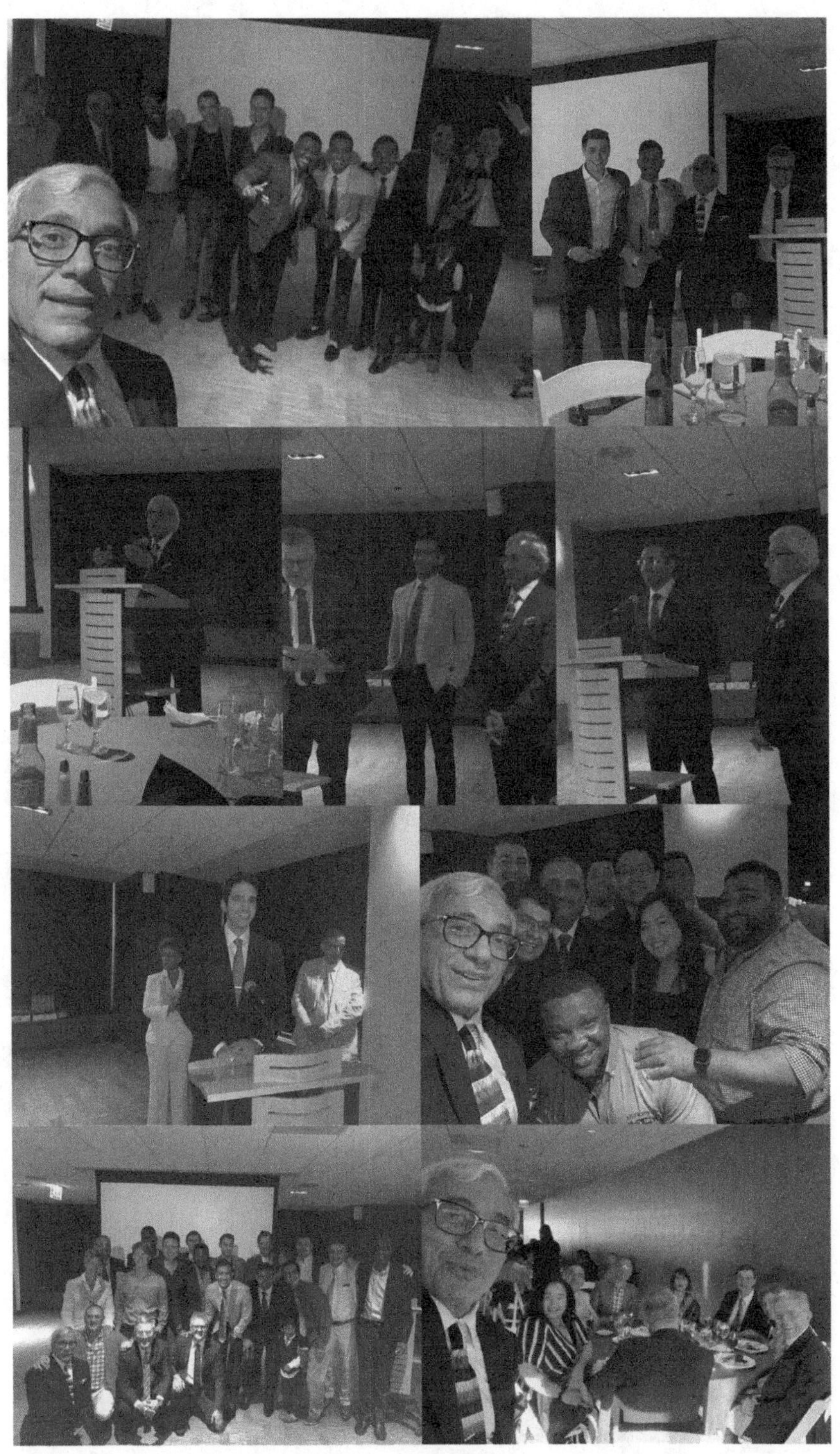

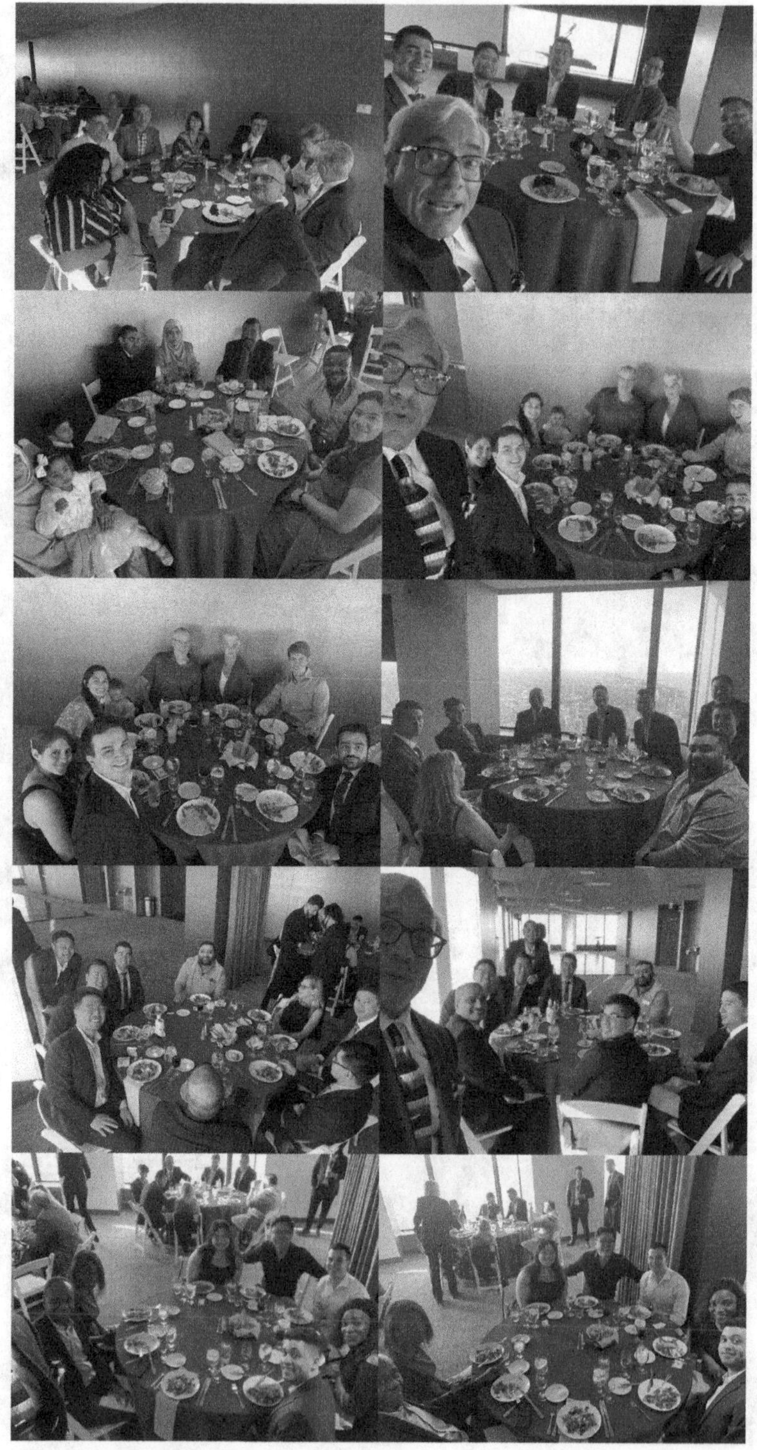

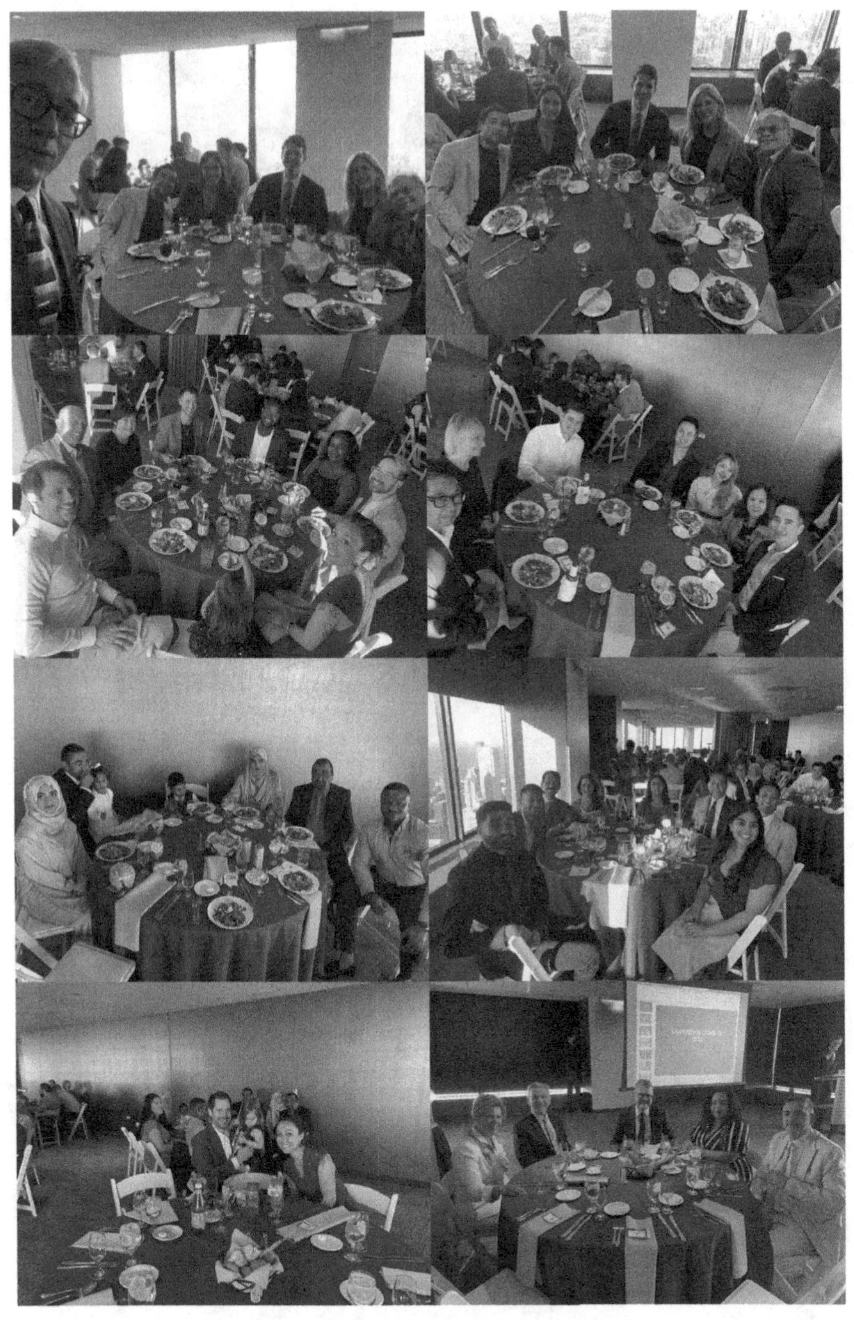

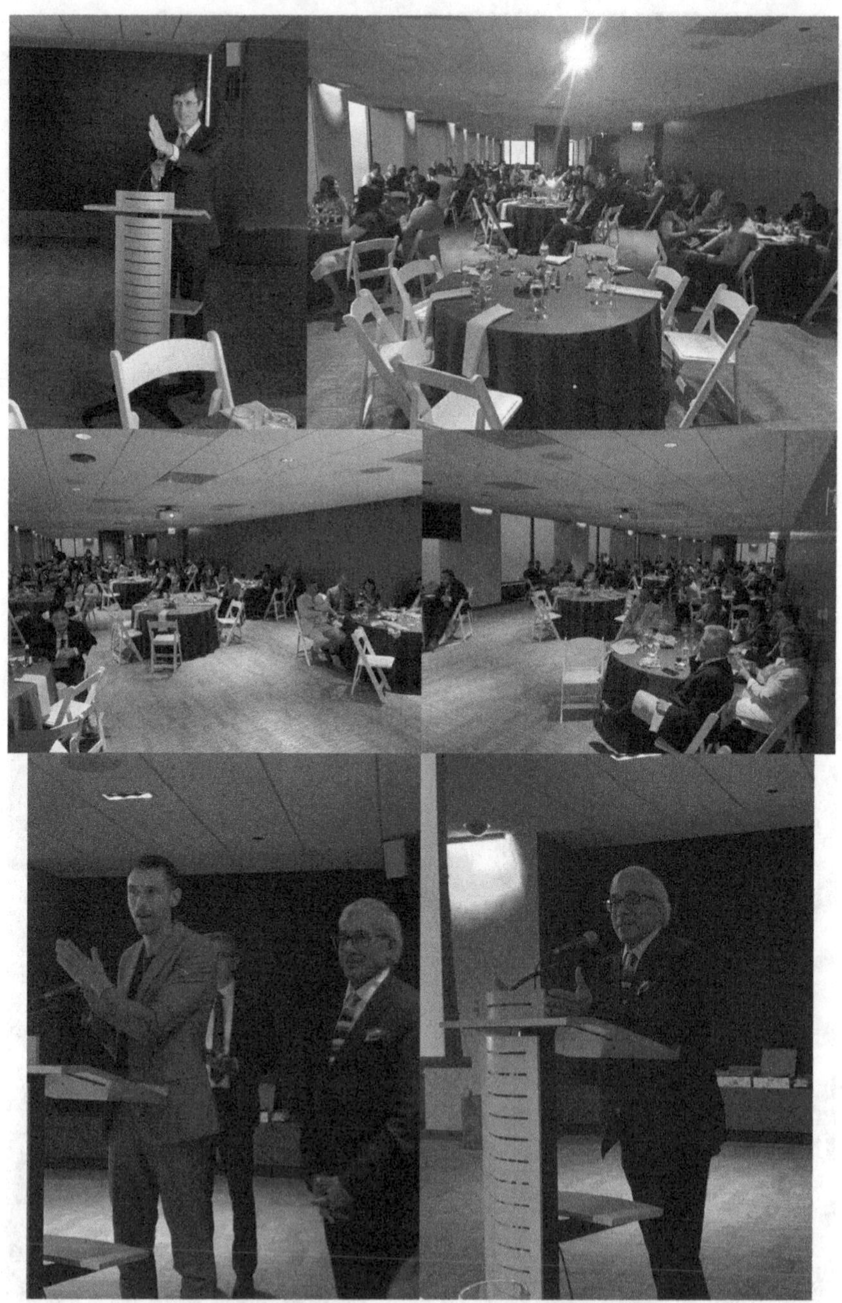

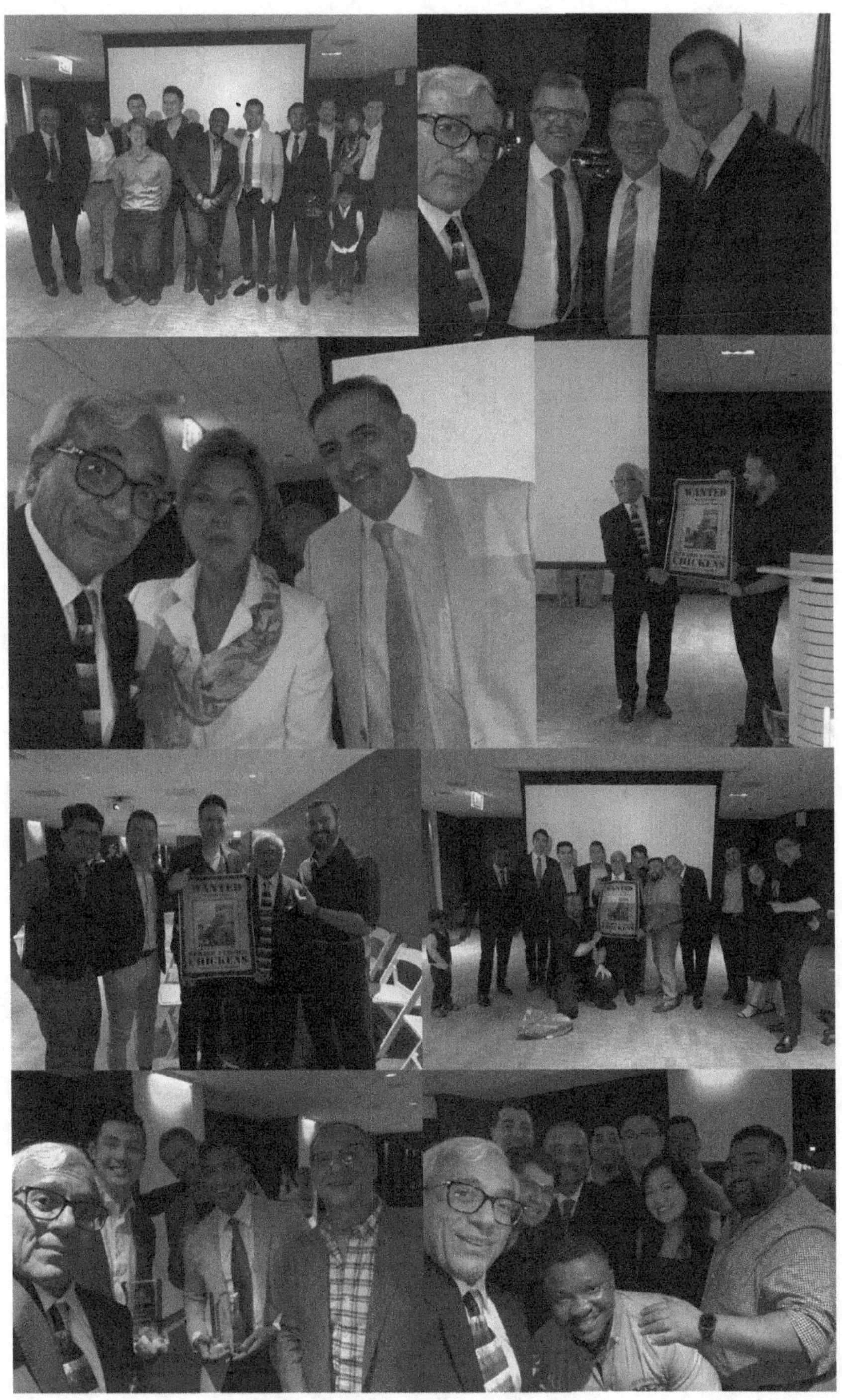
WANTED
CHICKENS

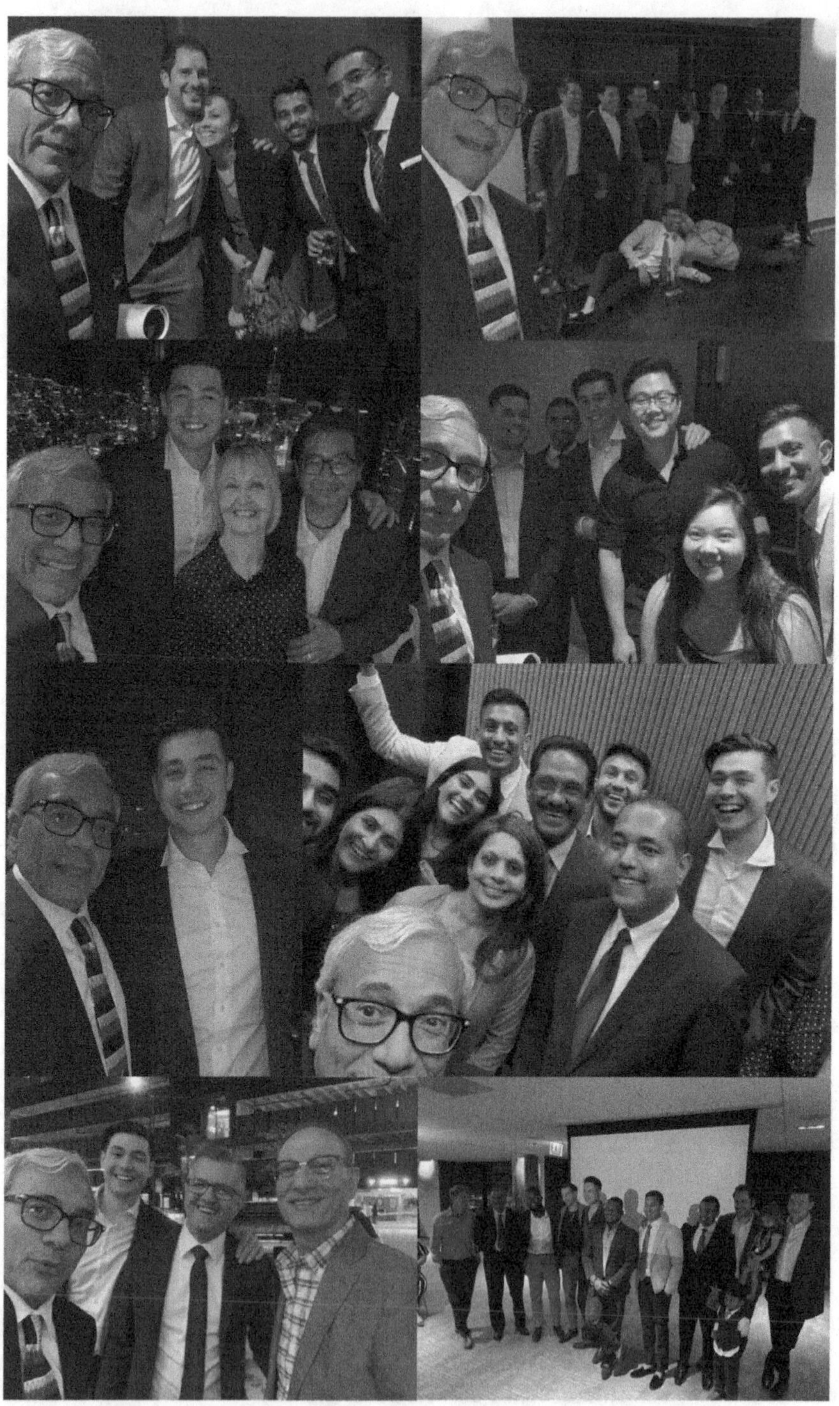

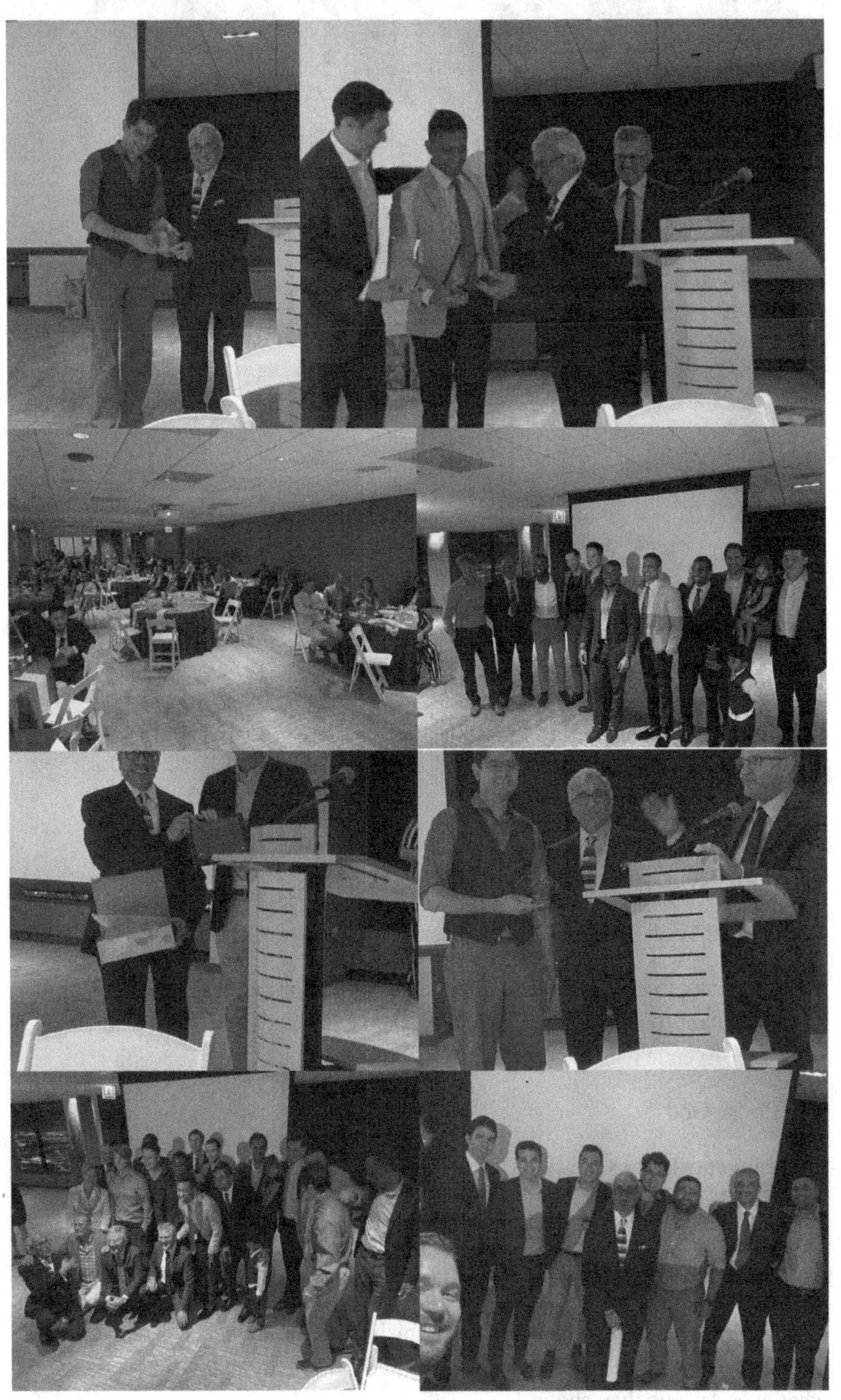

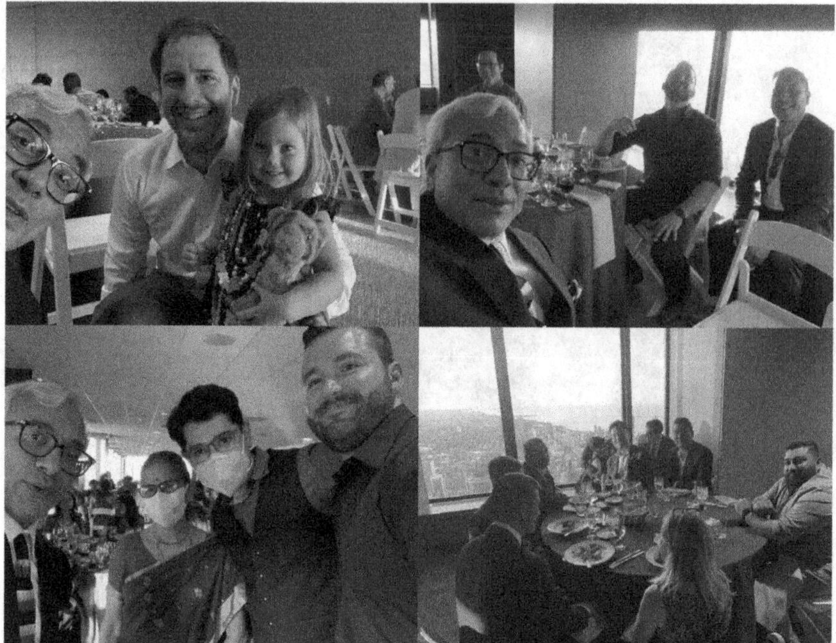

JT, **congrats** to all!!

CG, Congratulations!! May you achieve many more goals in your life and inspire others around you.

JS,Congratulations

CR, Lord, thank you for each one!!!!

BL, I pray they all are blessed in their service for others. **CONGRATULATIONS**

TC, **Congrats** to all! You are such an aspiring doctor and teacher with so much knowledge and I am sure they have benefited from it all and will be amazing in what ever Avenue they choose!

AB, Praise God

ES, Congratulations to all.

DN, My sincere **congratulations** to each and every one

BL, I pray they all are blessed in their service for others. **CONGRATULATIONS**

TC, **Congrats** to all! You are such an aspiring doctor and teacher with so much knowledge and I am sure they have benefited from it all and will be amazing in what ever Avenue they choose!

AB, Praise God

ES, **Congratulations** to all.

DN, My sincere **congratulations** to each and every one

MM, **Congrats**

MG< **ongrats** to all the graduates! My 4 years of county residency were invaluable for the sheer experience!

Dining with My Residents!

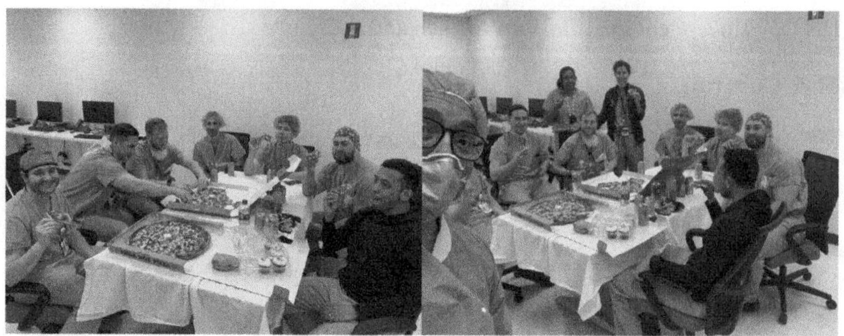

What an honor to dine with our residents on call, they are tired and hungry and appreciate a treat.

It is a golden opportunity to listen to their day events, cases, venting and share with them my personal experiences and feedback.

Theses are the best tines that they will always remember snd appreciate when they graduate and be in their own practices!! Time to Cherish and appreciate!!

Ramsis Ghaly

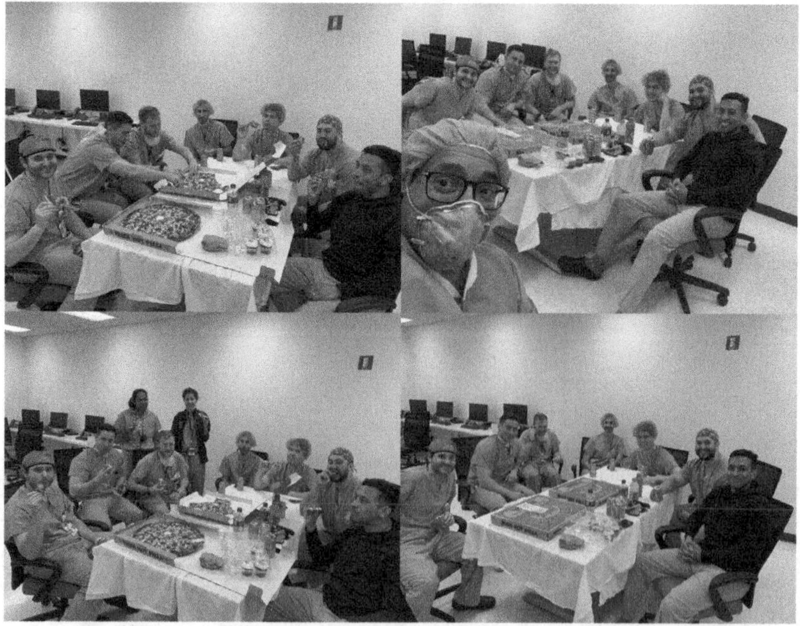

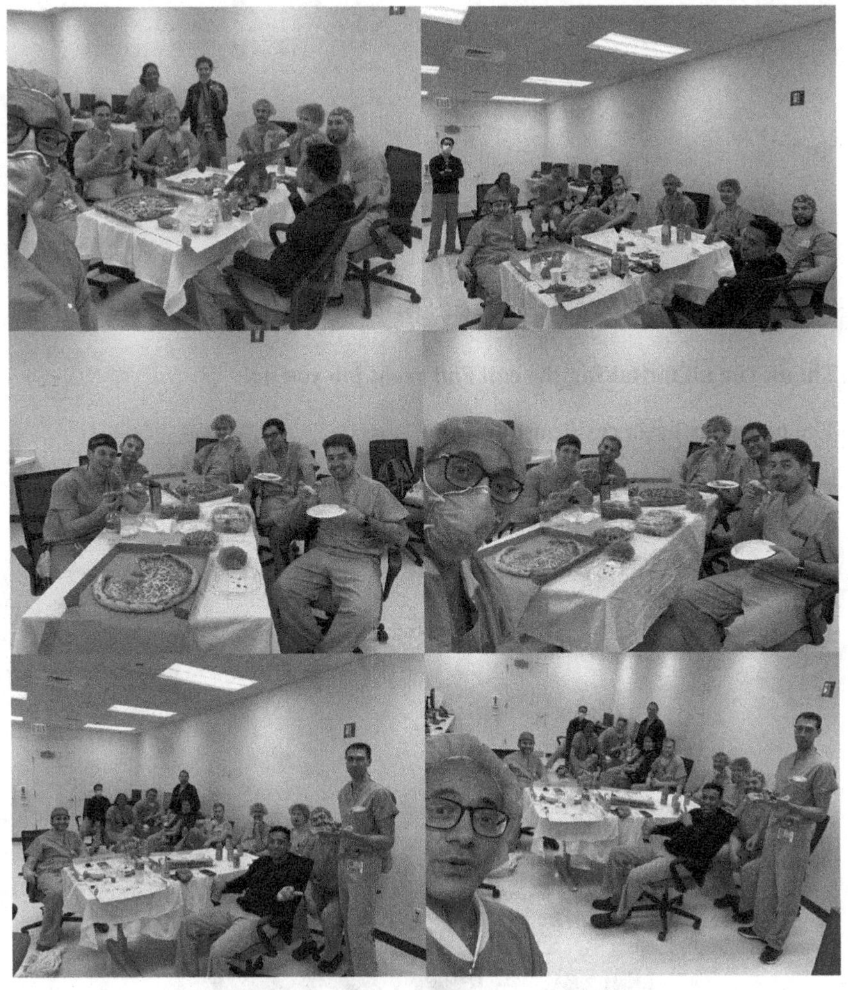

Kg, Keep up the good work!

Ks, That's awesome

Jb. An incredible amount of knowledge in one room!!!

Mh, A "Great!" Way to spend lunch

Jt, this is love for humanity!!

Ed, God bless you Doctor. The faces of hope for our tomorrows. Yes, wonderful memories for all of you

Jm, CONGRATULATIONS TO ALL

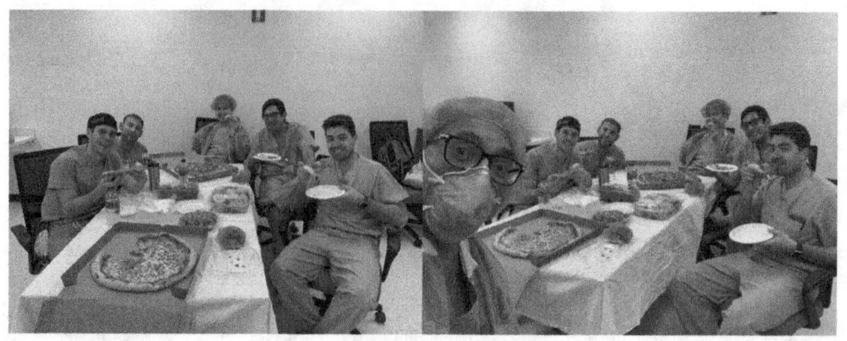

Thank you all for taking the call and great job you do!

The new anesthesia resident dinning

Yesterday we loaded with waters and disposable utensils, coffee, microwave—Always great to dine with our residents after hardworking!

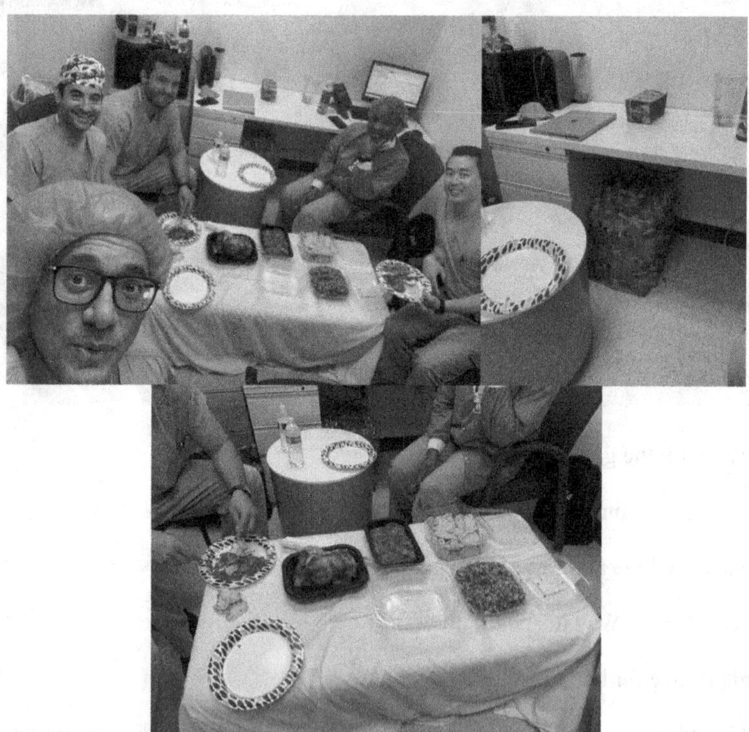

With our residents! So proud of each of them! So fortunate to continue to teach and be part of the future generations!

Ramsis Ghaly

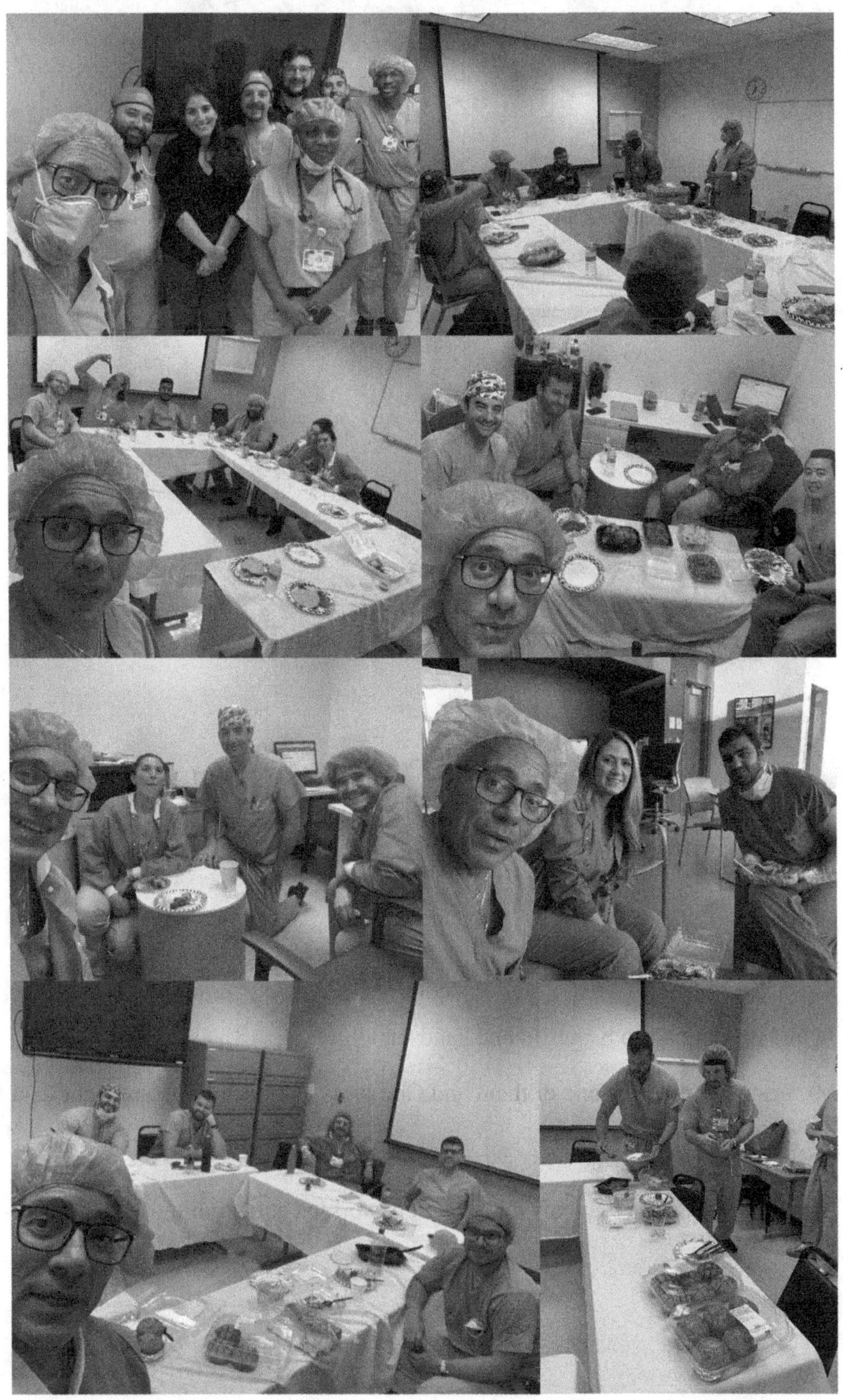

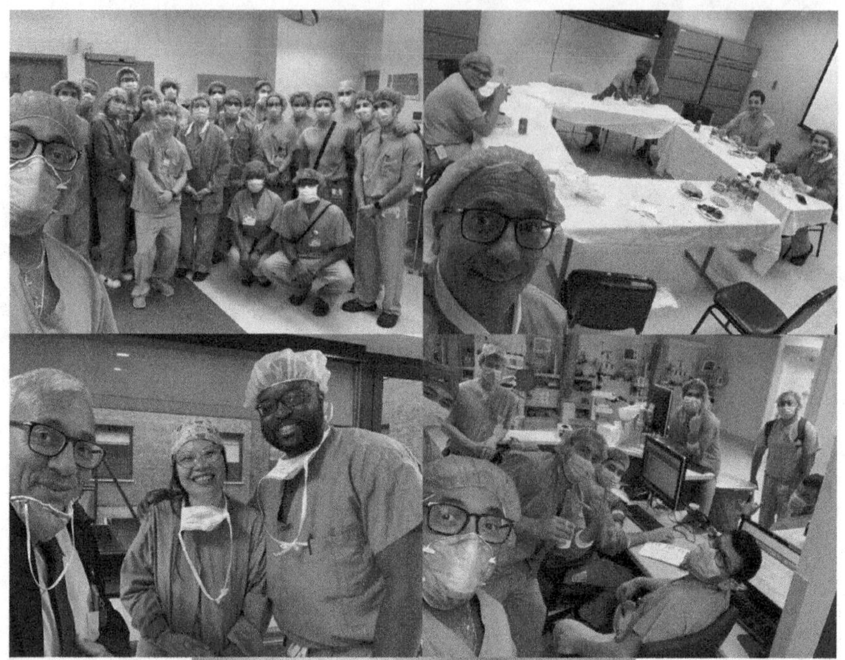

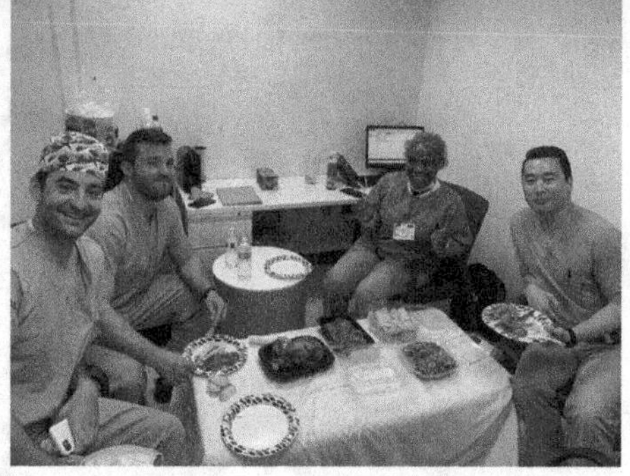

Jt, and they are all so beautiful and handsome!!

Mr, best luck to every one of them and God bless you doctor you are right God bless Dr Ghaly

Blessed to be among them my day and night working and teaching as long as my Lord permit!!!

Ramsis Ghaly

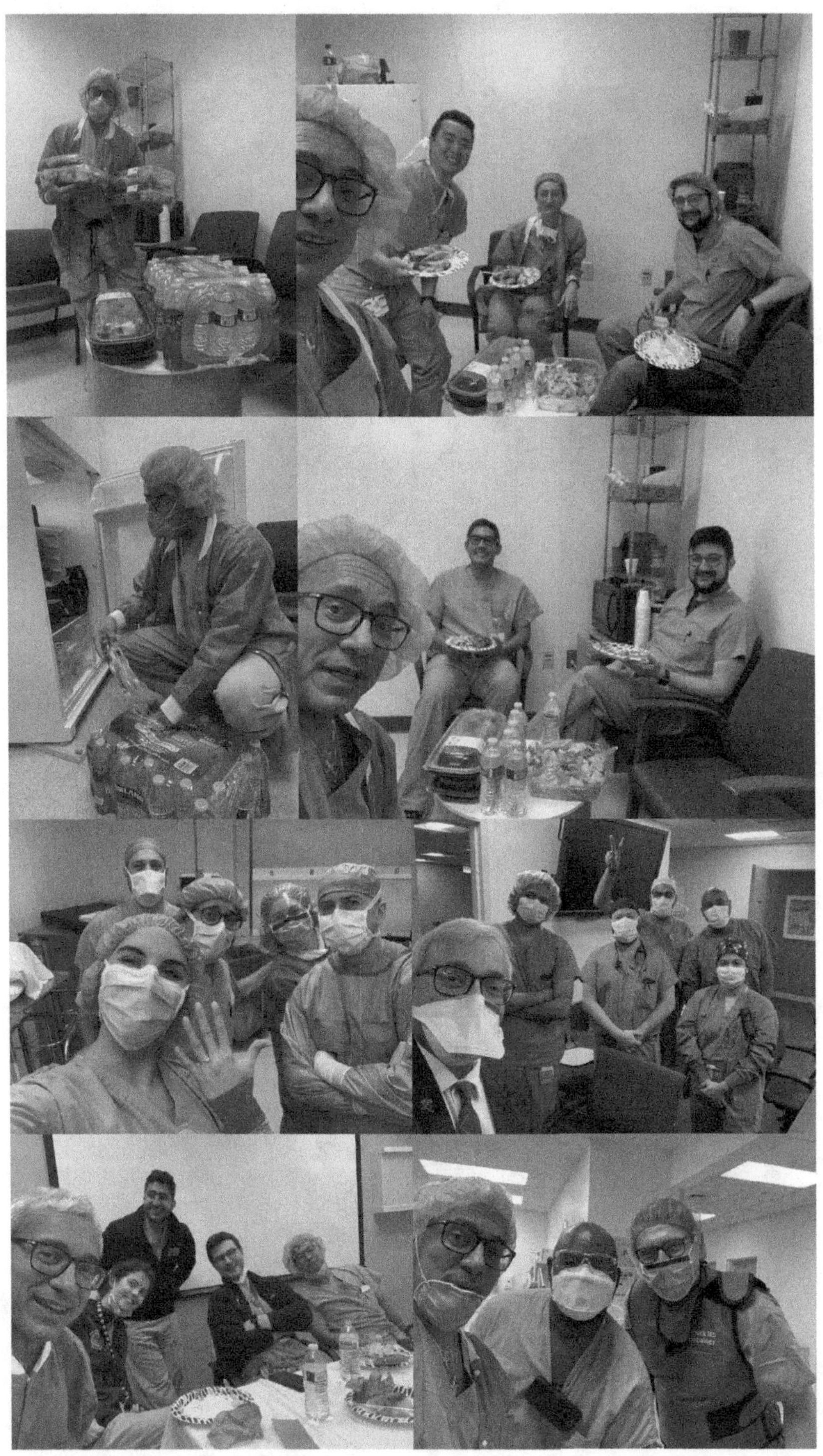

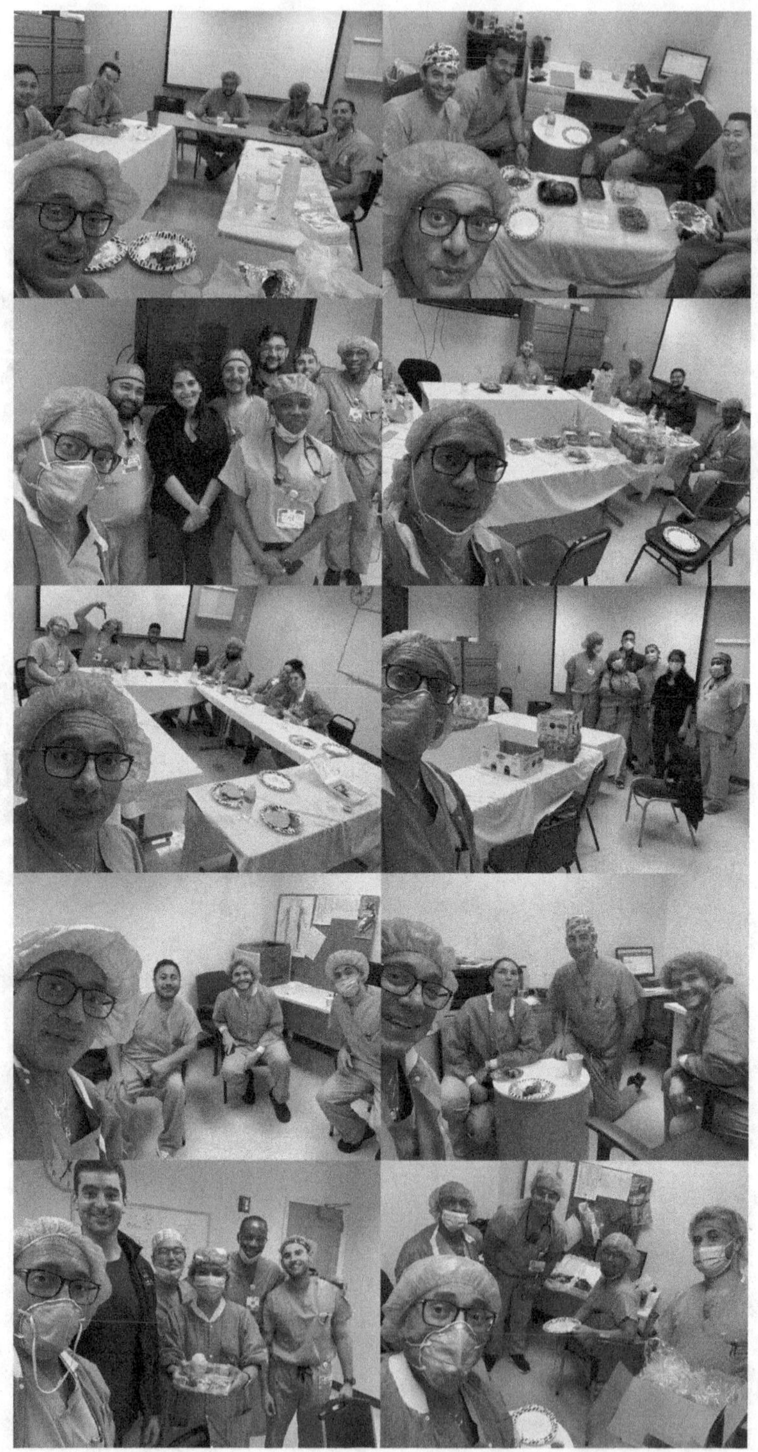

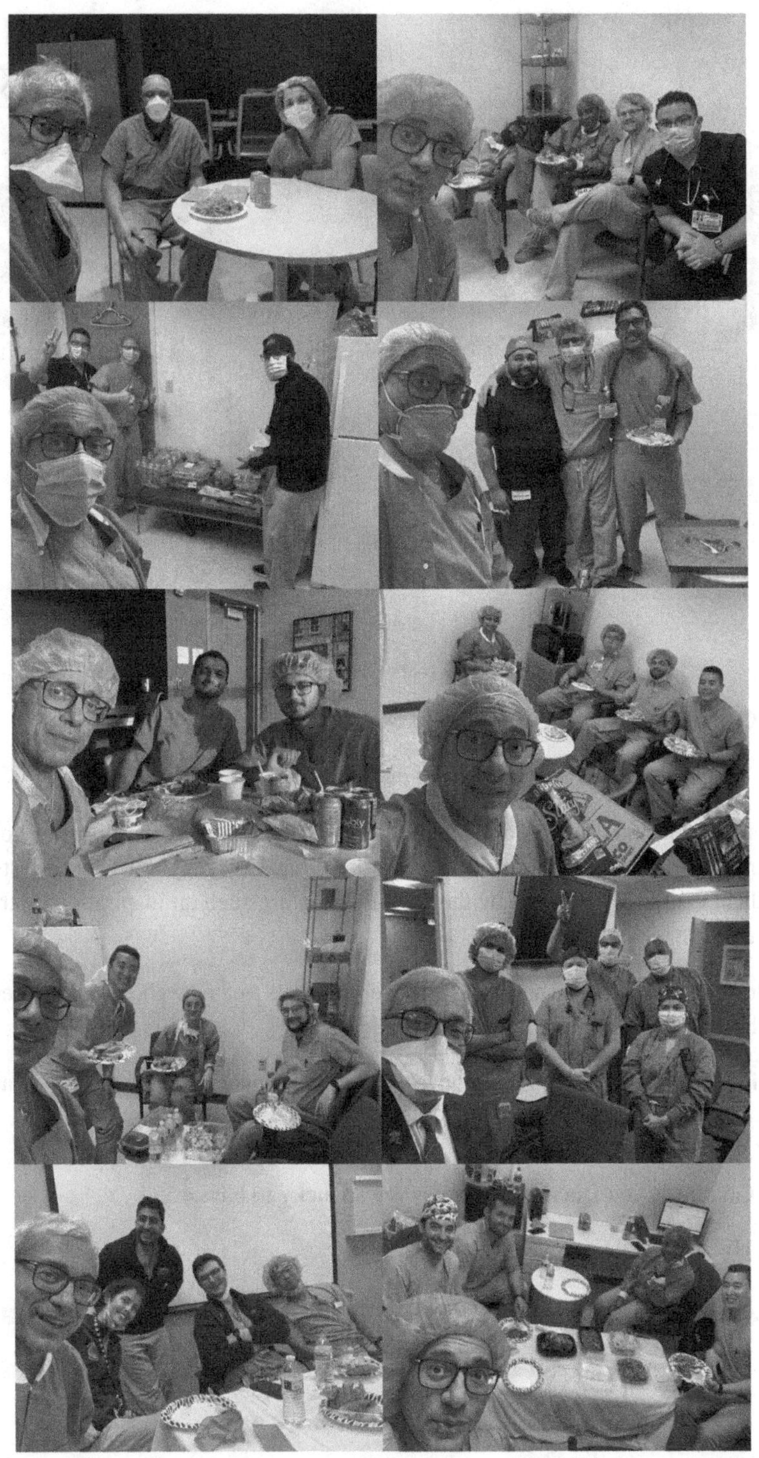

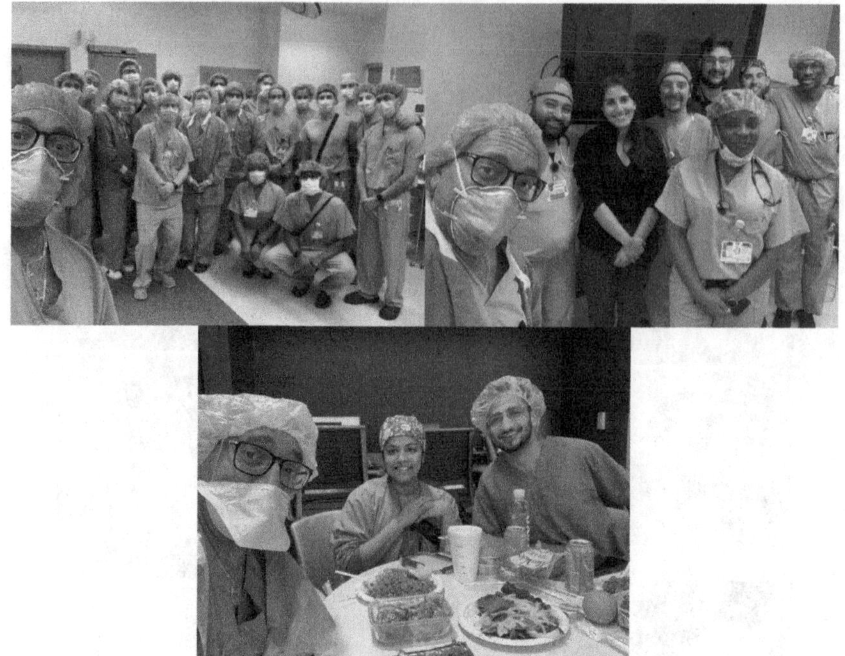

JT, God bless each and every one of you...

Ma, Jc, Clearly I was working late at the wrong hospital tonight!

Rn, Bless you and yours! I post stupid stuff while your out there day after day doing your best and doing gods work too! I work all day everyday at Ut southwestern medical center. Great place by the way. But you are such an inspiration. I strive to be mor…

Jt, love to see such dedication and that everyone gets treated well...they all deserve the best...ty Dr Ghaly for being their leader

cg, I'm sure they feel blessed to have you as their teacher as well. Bless you all.

Lm, Yes, blessed.

Nv, God bless you Doctor Ghaly they are so lucky to have you !

Lk, Hi Dr Ghaly!

Rp, Es, Lucky students. You are the best mentor.

Ss, God bless you Doc ! They are lucky to have you!

Sl, God bless you all! Thank you for your hard work!

Ms, Thank you for showing us, so much to learn from you. God bless you and your students.

Easter 2022 with My Residents!

Happy Easter 04/17/2022

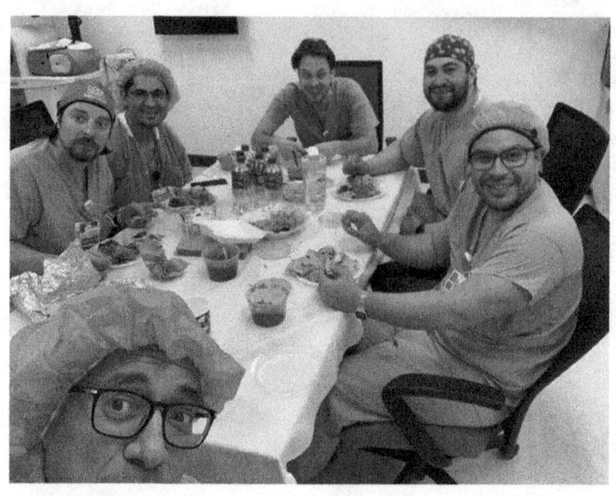

Spending Easter with my residents teaching and caring for patients joining so many faithful servants inspired by the spirit of Easter!

Luke 24:5-7 KJV "And as they were afraid, and bowed down their faces to the earth, they said unto them, Why seek ye the living among the dead? [6] He is not here, but is risen: remember how he spake unto you when he was yet in Galilee, [7] Saying, The Son of man must be delivered into the hands of sinful men, and be crucified, and the third day rise again."

Jesus is Risen Indeed He is Risen!

Happy Resurrection and Easter to you all. Let us pray for the victims of Ukrainian/ Russian conflict and the world!! Amen

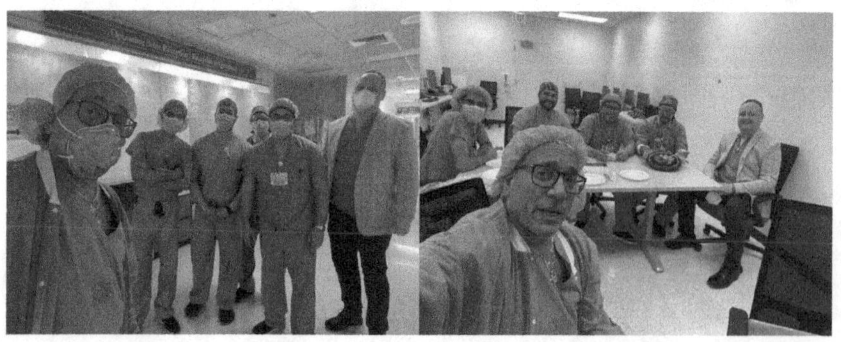

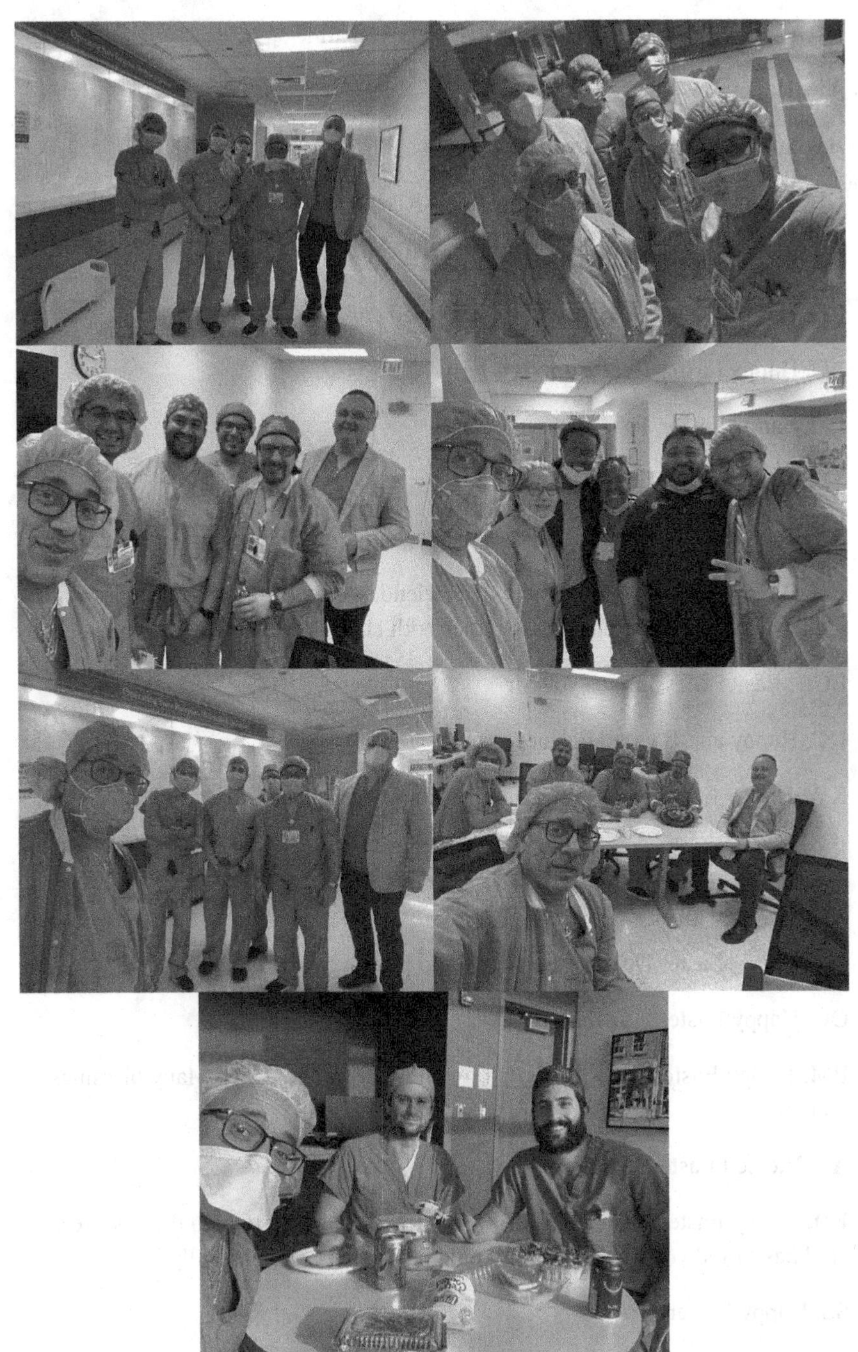

JT, have a blessed and uneventful weekend and enjoy the teachings of our Bible

DL, Happy Easter. He Is Risen ! God Bless you all !

AR, Happy Easter! Dr. Ghaly.

JG, God Bless you for all you do!

DH, Happy Easter to you all! Yes, HE is Risen!

JF, Happy Easter, my precious Dr. **Ghaly**!!! **#PastorJeff90210**

CD, Happy Easter Dr Ghaly. Have a blessed day.

AC, Happy Easter Dear **Ramsis Ghaly**,

LM Happy Easter. Peace be with you.

SM, Good Bless all of you Angels

PR, To everyone, good Easter weekend, sending much love.

EO, Happy Resurrection Day my dear friend. Because of HIS sacrifice, we that are in Him will spend eternity together with HIM. Hallelujah b

BCD, Easter Blessings to you Sir

DC, Happy and Blessed Easter to you!

KW, Happy Easter & Resurrection Day, my friend! Our Christian from Egypt!

Ken & Lena

CB, Thanks and Happy Easter to you!

NV, Happy Easter Doctor Ghaly and God Bless you!

OC, Happy Easter!

BM, Happy Easter Dr. **Ramsis Ghaly** and to your residents. Many blessings to you all

AS, Blessed Easter!

ED, Happy Easter good doctor. Bless you for all you do to help those suffering. God has gifted you to heal those in pain physically and spiritually

SS, Happy Easter

YS, Happy Easter

DK, Happy Easter, Dr. Ghaly!

JC, Happy Easter Dr Ghaly

MB, Happy Easter Dr.Ghaly

LA, Happy Easter!

SK, Happy Easter, Dr. Ghaly

BD, Happy Easter!!

JS, HAPPY RESURRECTION SUNDAY Dr Ghaly, you have a wonderful day. for World Peace but especially for Ukrainian and Russian people. HE IS RISEN,HALLELUJAH

JD, Happy Easter Dr. Ghaly! He has risen! What a glorious day. Jack & Jane

OP, Buona Pasqua!

GH, Happy Easter! God Bless you!

RR, Happy Palm Sunday

KL, Happy Easter!!

KZ, Happy Easter! Christ has risen!

MS, Happy Easter to all of you! May your service to others show His great love for you!

Blessings!!!!

KC, Happy Easter

MS, Happy Easter Dr.G

AV, Happy Easter Dr.Ghaly! God Bless you & your residents!!

LR, Happy Easter. Thank you for your service.

MN, Happy Easter Dr. Ghaly

KH, He Is Risen Indeed! Happy Easter!

DF, Happy Easter Dr Ghaly !!

MW, Happy Easter

NE, Happy Easter !

JC, Happy Easter!

ML, He has risen….

Happy Easter to you and those precious residents.

SF, Happy Easter!!

VA, Happy Easter

MS, A Blessed Easter to you and all your residents.

SK, Happy Easter Dr.

MD, Happy Easter

BN, Happy Easter!

CG, Happy Easter!

RC, Happy Easter.

MD, Happy Easter Dr. Ghaly

D,M, happy Easter

CG, Alleluia He has risen. Happy Easter to you and your residents and all the patients who can't be with families.

VG, Happy Easter

ZS, Happy Easter,Wesołych Świąt

AR, Happy Easter

SS, U r amazing!! Working??

SG, Happy Easter Dr.

DM, Happy Easter to you and your family

RD, Happy Easter Dr **Ramsis Ghaly**.

HH, Happy Easter Pr. Dr. Ramsis Ghaly.!!

RM, Happy Easter Sir

SG, Happy Easter Dr Ghaly!

DB, Happy Easter Ramsis!

My Early Residency Training at JSH of Cook County Hospital University of Illinois at Chicago! !

www.Ghalyneurosurgeon.com

Neurosurgery Residency 1990/1991 at University Of Illinois and Cook County Hospital, Chicago Illinois

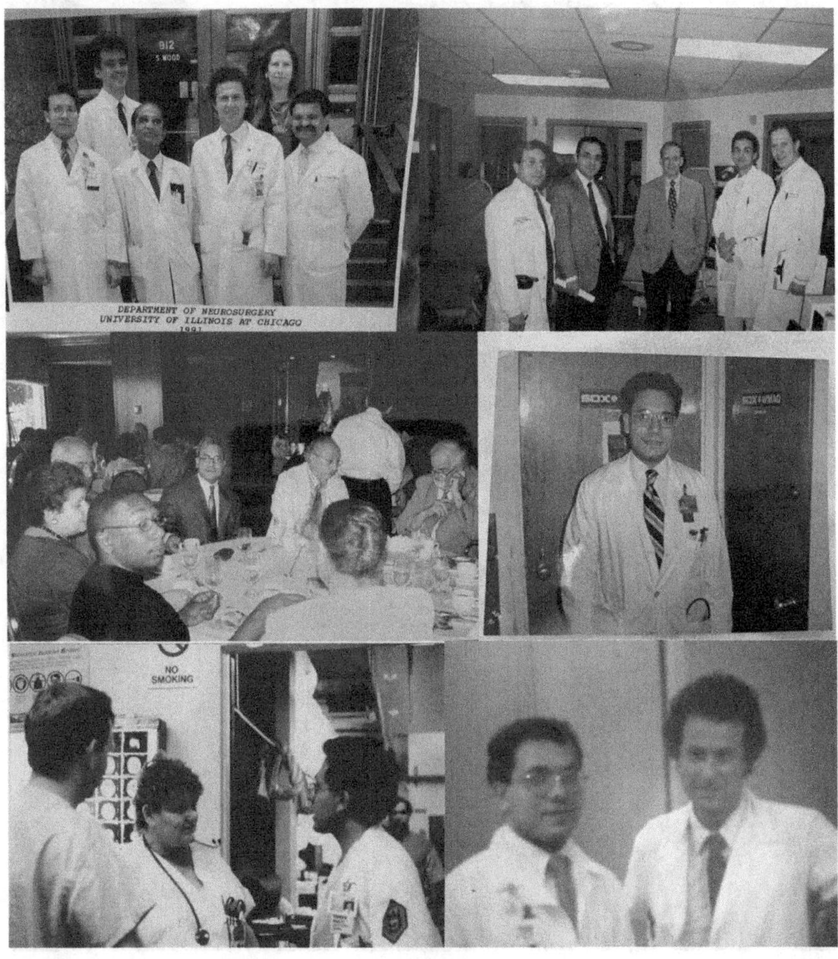

DT, The best neurosurgeon in the state!!!!!

KG, The Best International Neurosurgeon & Doctor of Anesthesiology from the world over! Superman doesn't do him justice. A true Blessing from God! Thank you, Dr **Ramsis Ghaly** for all you do. God Bless you always. Blessings and Love from an American in Egy...

Praise our Lord to who is the glory forever Thank you

KG, Ramsis Ghaly To God be the glory!Amen.

JSH of Cook County Hospital decades ago!

Ramsis Ghaly

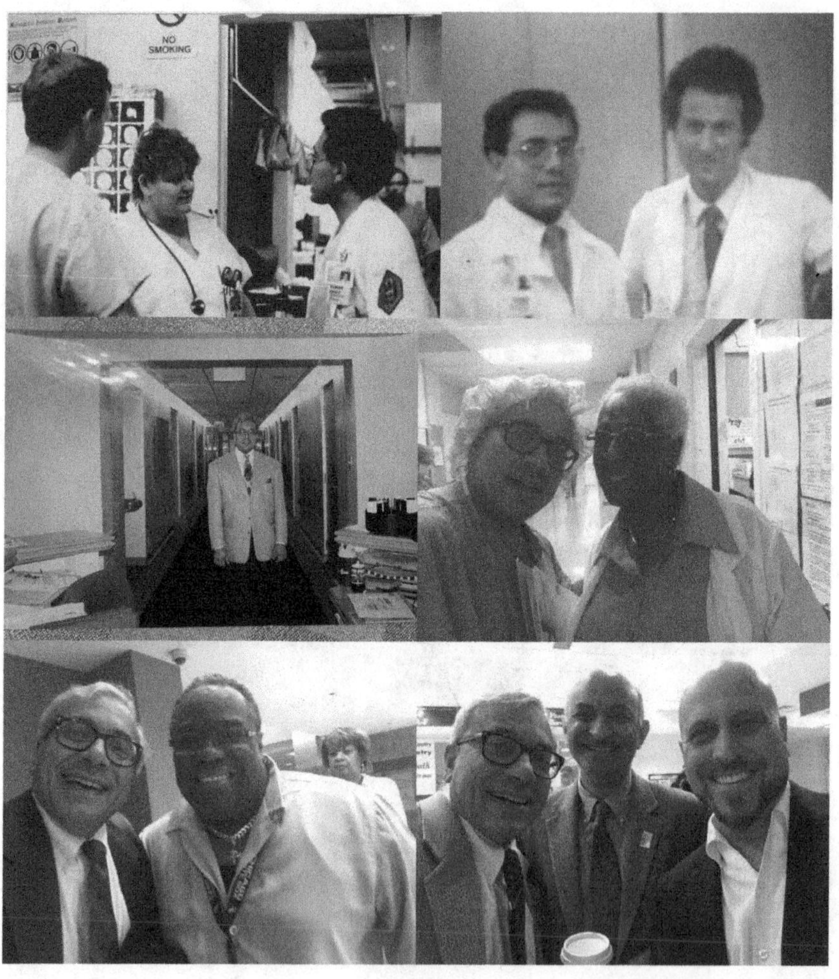

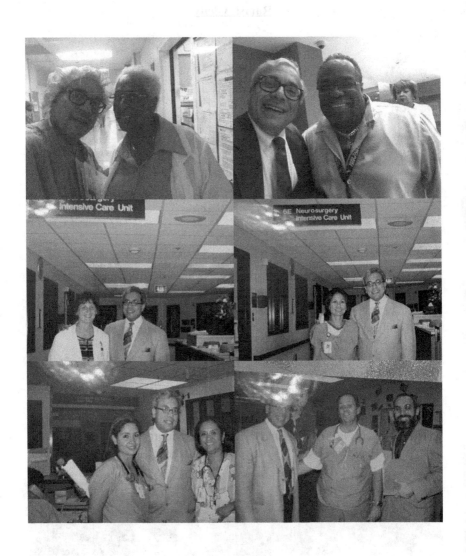
Intensive Care Unit
6E Neurosurgery
Intensive Care Unit

What a Fantastic Surprise Visit by 2018 Pre-COVD Class!

<u>Ramsis Ghaly</u>

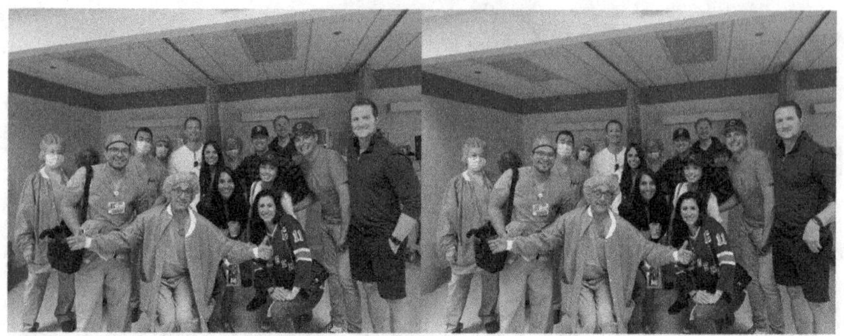

What a Fantastic Surprise!!

<u>Ramsis Ghaly</u>

Our great JSH of Cook County hospital graduate class 2018 kept their tradition as a class of getting together and visit their home where they were trained and spent more than 4 years, Cook County hospital! Each is on a different state and has a family and all made arrangements to unite together in Alumni!! What a lovely surprise!!

They remember their days of training, keep us in the loop of their success and share their experiences with our current residents!

We love you all very much. Very humbling to think of us. So proud of each of you. Your success is incredible and testimony to your greatness. Please stay well and visit us your home again. Thank you and safe travel

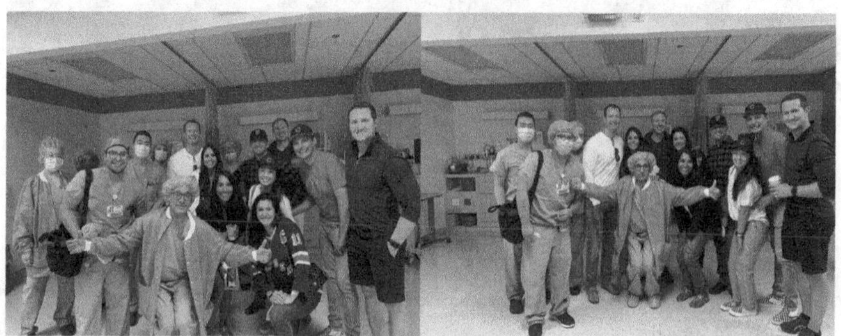

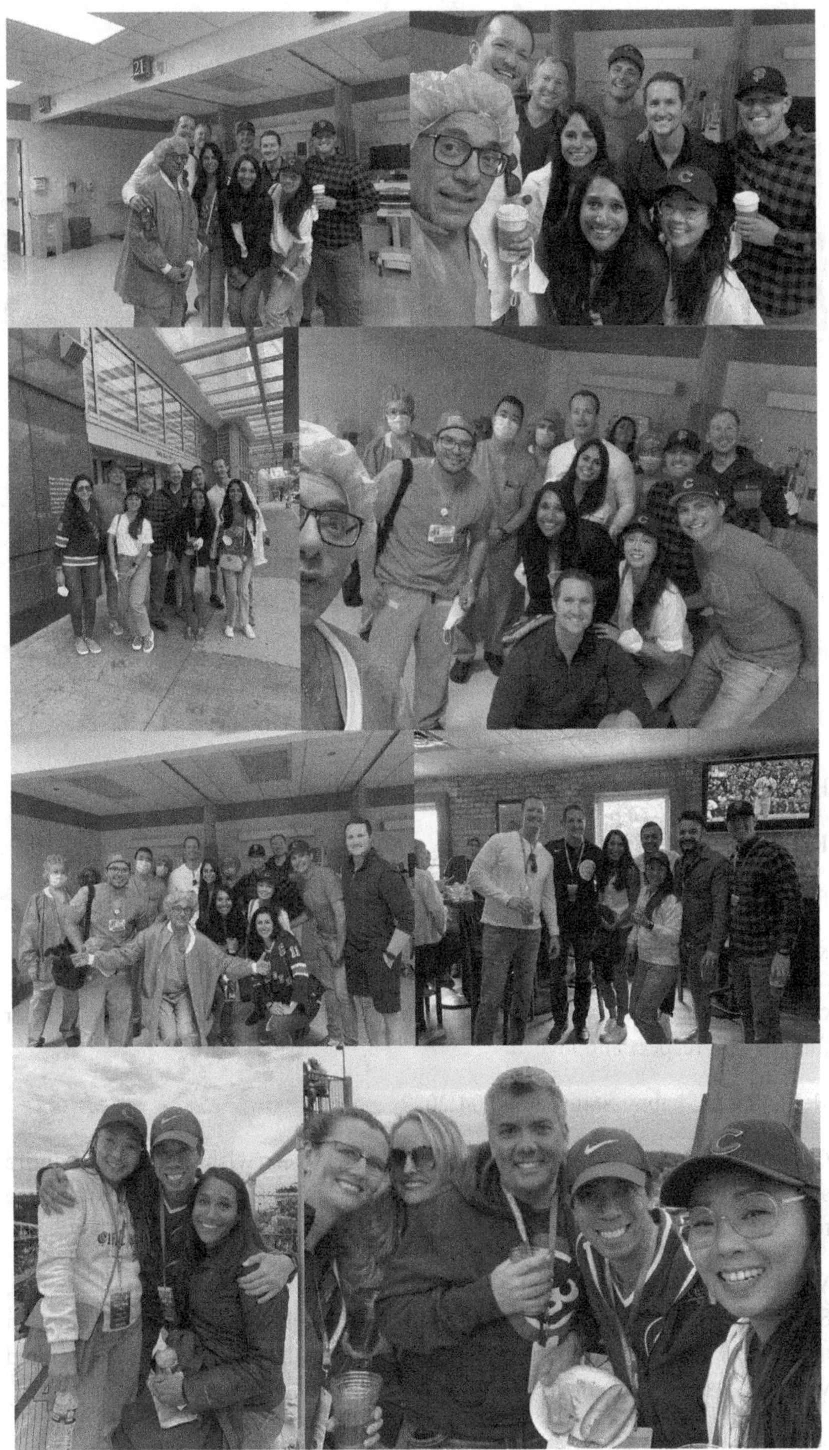

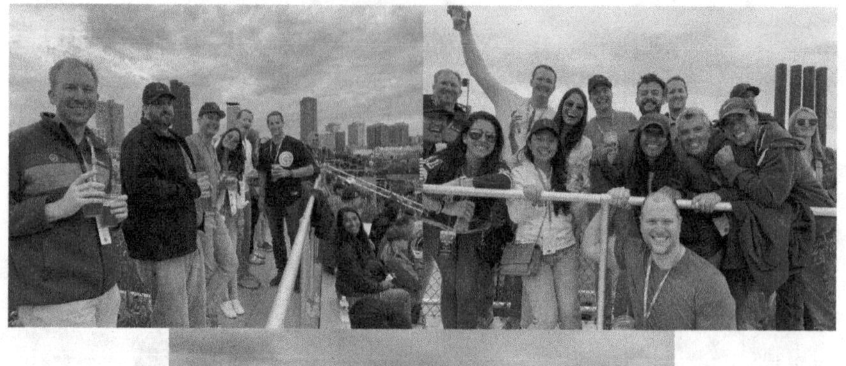

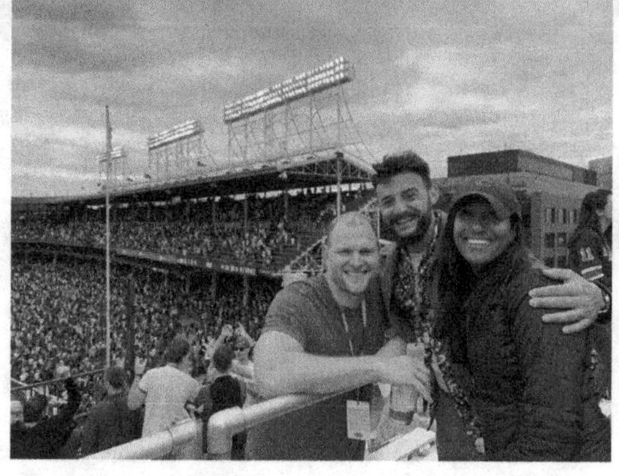

HH, **Congratulations** my Best Dr..!!

KG, Congratulations

from Egypt!

Many Blessings of abundance.

cg, How wonderful that they all come back to where they started and to the teacher that they all respect and love

Hello you all; happy Saturday 06/04/2022

Congratulations to all our graduate class 2022. Best wishes. You all admire success of each of you, your bright future and you all will be missed. We are so touched with celebrating together last night. Thank you all.

What a surprise to see 2018 class came and visit us! Fantastic class Gil, Sheaba, Susan, Kevin snd their partners. Thank you do much. What a heartfelt emotion to see those outstanding anesthesiologists come together from different states and visit with us and share their successes and loyalties!

Today is a fantastic day for our residents especially the new CA Laura and Ainura. Charles is leading the team with Peter, Williams snd San, doing great job. Our CA1 and CA2 are big part of teaching. Thank you to all the seniors fir supporting the new comers.

Saturday is an outstanding day for all new class Please come and learn and enjoy our call and company!

Today both Laura and Ainura mastered the comprehensive pre induction ghaly check list, intubated successfully their cases. We went over the cases including one case high risk aspiration and desaturation and how to prevent complication! Already various cases ortho, general, trauma and pediatric.

Look at all these pictures!!! Please come again and join us for ghaly special and Saturday call and treat of chicken!!!

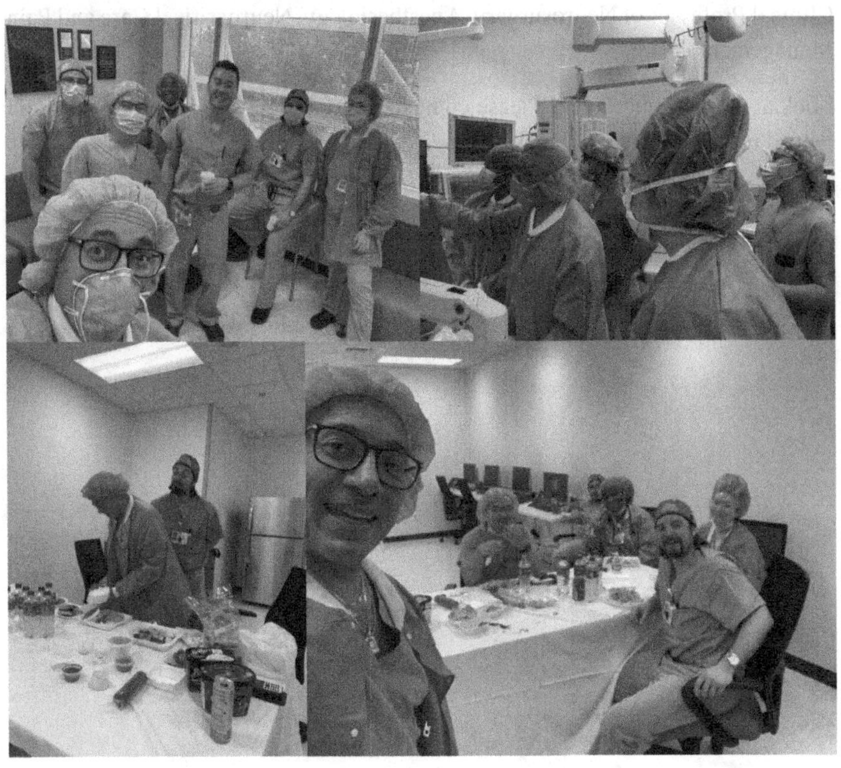

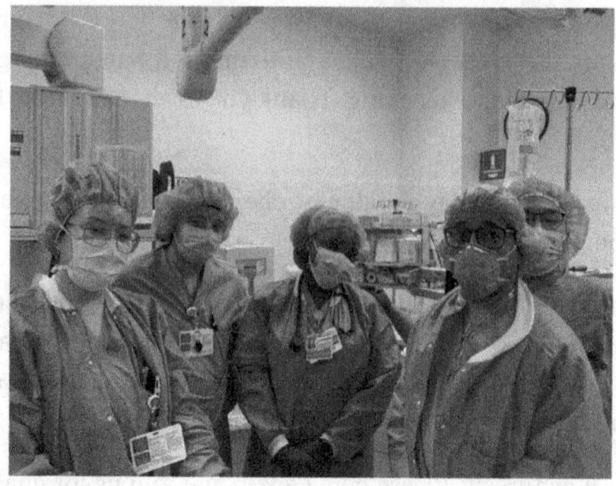

Ramsis F Ghaly, MD

Clinical Professor of Neurosurgery, Anesthesiology, Neurocritical Care and Pain Management

Look at all these pictures!!! Please come again and join us for ghaly special and Saturday call and treat of chicken!!!

You Never Know Who You Might Inspire!

John is a shining star neurosurgeon in virtual reality at Harvard. John's mother was in charge of laundry shop in high rise building where I used to live in early 1990's. Whenever, I left my laundry, she was inquiring about who am I and ask more questions about neurosurgery. Then, the mother asked me if I can talk to her son and try to inspire him.

The mother encouraged her son to be a neurosurgeon like me.

Amazing to see them grown prominent and very successful! At Harvards!

Indeed, You Never Know Who You Might Inspire! Not a trivial to keep inspiring the new generations and be an example and a proof of what your passion and sincere mission in life.

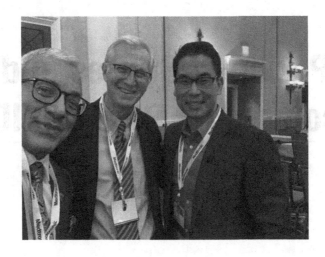

Patients' Stories and comments Post COVID

A Blessing gift for saving My life!

Richard Came Today With His Wife with a Precious Gift!

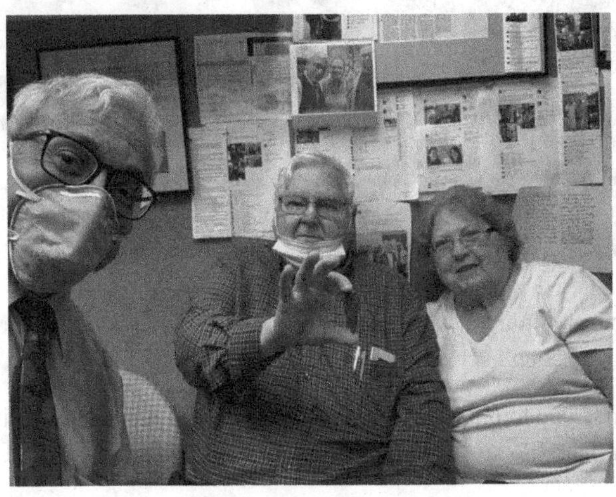

The minute he saw me, he handed me saying: "A Blessing gift for saving My life"

It is from a Native Indian Arrowhead from Stone Bridge tripe used to be in Philadelphia and moved to Ohio where it was settled in Wisconsin!

Actually, we need to thank Lord Jesus, he came to see me to have back Spine surgery and I diagnosed him with compltetely different more urgent problem that was about to burst and die if it continued to be undiscovered!!!

Look how it was all started. I just did his carpal tunnel surgery and as he recovered, and we are about to discuss his back problem that he had for years!!!

This patient was walking with something not neurosurgical that was dangerous to be untreated yet he has not much of complaint. This is to the degrees that With all the care he received everyone missed it. The reason is nothing is perfect and no one test us enough. That is the reason when insurance and those care about cost try to regulate testing and prevent Physician like me from ordering tests and do the right thing for patients!

Bless your heart and speed recovery! Thank you Lord Jesus Amen

Ramsis Ghaly

Www.ghalyneurosurgeon.com

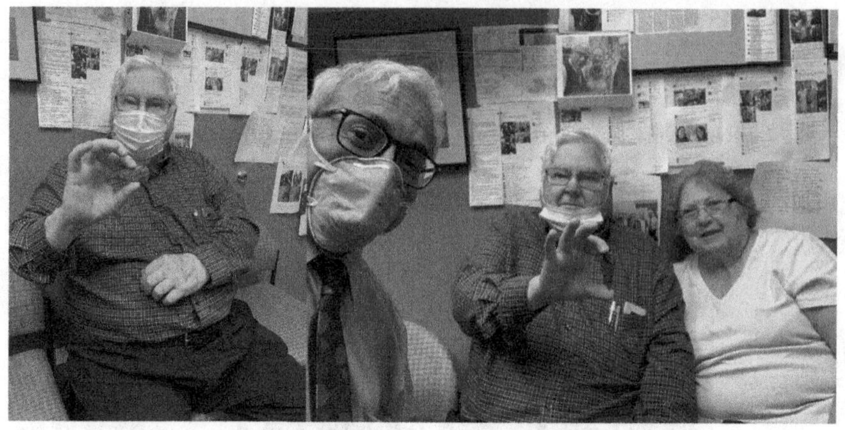

DL, I haven't met you yet, Dr Ghaly, but I sure do love you. You are amazing. Hope to see you soon !

JCB, Of course you found it Dr. G. You actually listen, and take your time treating the whole patient . So so thorough. Bless you as always.

JM, How Wonderful Happy They Are Doing Well

A Miracle Story!

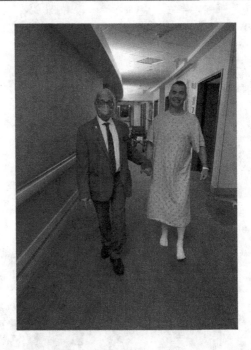

What a story of a rare cause of horrific pain and loss of function put him to tears and suffering for months!!! Early morning, we walked, and we raced, and Jim was granted new lease in life looking forward to hunting and enjoy his grandchildren!!!

Look at Jim early morning after surgery to remove the cause in a very delicate and uncommon location missed by many!!

I told Jim and his wife Lynette a Disclaimer, this is extremely rare and not easy surgery, and both replied in strong faith: "We want you to do the surgery and care for Jim"! And both never questioned their decision or pursued to ask more questions! Much Blessing and love!

We together prayed before direct, during surgery and after surgery giving thanksgiving to our Savior Lord Jesus! Much blessing his recovery!! Praise our Lord Jesus always the Healer!

Ramsis Ghaly

Www.ghalyneurosurgeon.com

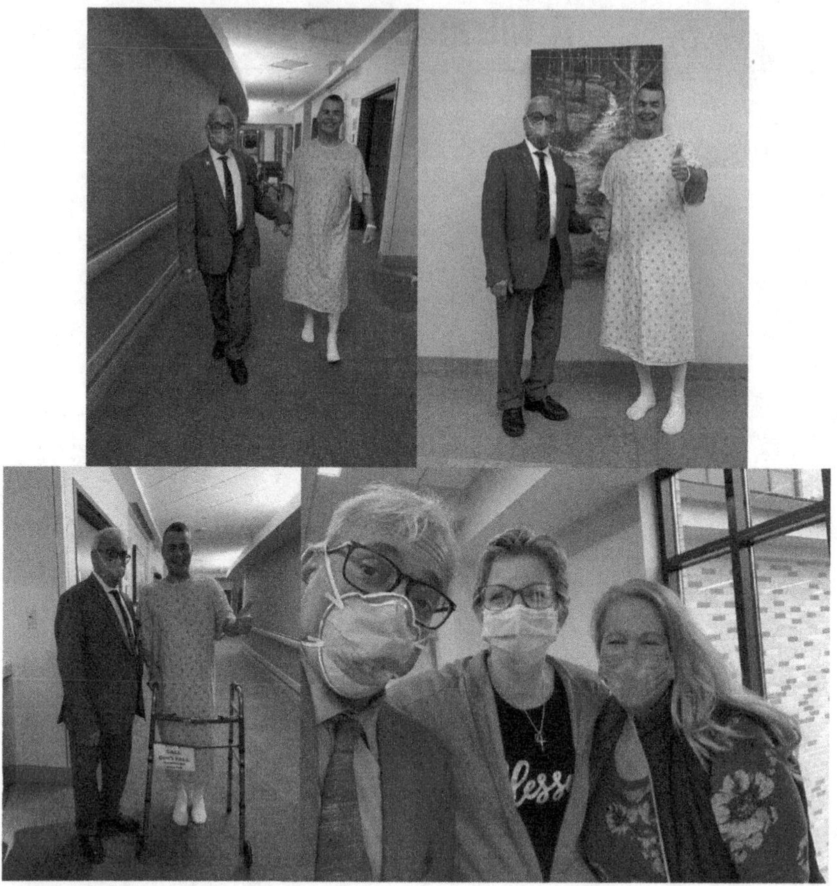

Wife Wrote Next day after Surgery:

Today is day 1 of recovery....Jim's recovery after a 6 month battle with hip pain. Jim is now sleeping after a very long, complicated and significant surgery yesterday at Hospital with an extremely compassionate and kind neurosurgeon, Dr. Ramsis Ghaly. He had been in significant pain for months. He had seen 5 different doctors, had 2 rounds of oral steroids, 2 injections and 5 MRIs to no avail. Then, we found Dr. Ghaly. Without boring everyone with all the details, suffice it to say that God led us to this neurosurgeon! You see, after the 3rd MRI a tumor was discovered in or on Jim's sciatic nerve! We saw Dr. Ghaly last Wednesday (April 27) he saw the significant debilitating pain that Jim was in and he scheduled surgery immediately for May 6th. Yesterday was one of the longest days of my life.

With the delicate nature of this surgery, being at the sciatic nerve, the risks were great. However, Jim and I truly felt God's presence in all of this so we had peace in that

Jim was prepped for surgery at 5:30 am, went under at about 8:30 am and at 10 am, surgery began. Needless to say it was a long day!

When the surgical nurse at CDH texted me at 2 pm that the tumor was out, I lost it! All of the stress of Jim's pain, the difficulty of seeing him suffer and the unknown regarding the location of the tumor was released. I thanked God for 10 minutes.....for everything. Words cannot describe the emotions that I felt at that moment!

At 6pm, Jim finally made it to a room, a little loopy to say the least and now (Saturday) he is home and ready to recover!

Turns out the tumor was IN the sciatic nerve, not next to it! And was the size of my thumb! God surely directed Dr. Ghaly's hands in removing the mass

Thank you to all of our friends and family that have been supportive throughout this process, helpful in helping with ru ning of the business, taking care of our home and dogs, providing food and medical supplies and, of course, prayers! We are grateful for all of you and especially Dr. Ghaly who, in my estimation, performed a miracle!!

Keep praying for both recoveries

AD, Praising God with you! So thankful for **Ramsis Ghaly**!!!

LD, Praise God for all his blessings!!!

CK, Prayers for you both

JZ, Thank God they both came out of surgery ok and Jim has been relieved of the pain!! Now, YOU take care of yourself!!!

MM, Speedy recovery! Prayers for y'all

JE, I will be praying for Jim and your Dad, God is good isn't he!

RL, Thank God for Dr. Ghaly! Praying for an uneventful and complete recovery for Jim. This is what those vows mean Lanette...for better or worse and in sickness and health. You were there for Jim as he would be for you. That strengthens your relationship! Love you

DG, Thank God your Dad & Jim are ok!! Prayers to both for speedy recoveries **Lanette**!!

MM, Just good news for you, Jim and your Dad. God is powerful.

BS, Prayers and thoughts are going your way !!

BL, So glad everything turned out well with Jim he'll feel like a new man!

BB, So happy and thankful that all went well, and praying that Jim comes away pain free!!

DB, Wow! Wishing Jim a speedy recovery.

I can't even imagine that kind of stress Lanette.

LY, I soley rely on God's strength for sure!

DD, Prayers for a speedy recovery for Jim and your Dad!

BO, Praise God, so glad they got it out. Now day to day recouping.

rb, Praise God. Prayers the tumor is benign and true healing begins

Ml, Glad both are doing fine!!

Mb, Will keep a prayer for both of you.

Nm, Healing prayers for Jim

RH, Wishing them both a speedy recovery

OG, Praise the Lord!!!

LJ, Oh my goodness! So grateful Jim's surgery went well. Hopefully removing the tumor and surgery was the hard part!! Now on to recovery and rehabilitation.

TS, Omgoodness….prayers for speedy recovery!

AM, Here for you anytime. You know how to find me. Stay well. Find a smile anywhere you can.

MV, Speedy recovery Jim! So glad surgery went well!

PG, So happy to hear all went well! Prayers for a speedy recovery!

KH, Thankful it all went well…. Hoping the rehab doesn't knock him out… then the drinking can begin!!

CK, Thoughts and prayers to both you and Jim!

RR, What an ordeal, my thoughts and prayers are with Jim and your dad for a speedy recovery🙏

PS, Praying for a speedy and complete recovery

SM, Wonderful

DB, Wow, what a great outcome!

RS, Praise God! So happy to hear that great news.

JS, You tell Dr Ghaly that you know me. I worked with him long time ago. Very compassionate man. I'm glad you have answers and are on the mend.

JS, how are you Jaime. All the best

MP, Dr **Ramsis Ghaly** is one incredible human! I've never experienced anyone else like him and I only know him through rehabbing some of his patients!

JT, your prayers for healing have been answered

JS, Oh WOWWW praising God and praying for Jim's recovery!

SK, Sending prayers for a quick recovery for your special guys!

MA, Here's hoping for a speedy recovery

FC, God is Great!

DN, Thanks so much for the update! Prayers for a speedy recovery for jim & for God to give you strength as you care for both Jim & your dad!

MT, God is good !!!

JN, Dr Ghaly is the best. Love him. He actually cares about and loves his patients. He did my first surgery in 1996. He was at Silver Cross Hospital in Joliet at that time.

JM, What a story with a happy ending!!!

LJ, Glad it went well! Praying for a speedy recovery

LS, Happy to hear all went well with the surgery.

JD, Thinking of you guys !!!

SF, Continuing prayers! So happy to hear the good news!

EW, Wishing Jim a speedy recovery. Sciatica is very scary and takes time to heal. More than most. Keep his mind busy take it easy ?!!

AV, Praise God all went well!

PG, You have both been through so much. I pray Jim has a complete and comfortable recovery.

LL, What a journey for you both, so thankful that God guided every step of the way. "Come and listen, all who honor God, and I will tell you what he has done for me. I cried to him for help; I praised him with songs."

Psalm 6:16-17 GNT

LS, Does he do cervical spine surgeries?

LY, yes! He is amazing!

DW, Glad all came out on the good side. for Speedy recovery for both

MP, Prayers he's feeling better soon.

JP, Sending prayers for your husbands recovery. . Dr. **Ramsis Ghaly** is truly the best and you are all in the best hands.

MN, Omgwow, that is just amazing. And yes Dr. **Ramsis Ghaly** Is an amazing surgeon, he did my back surgery, in 2008 and it's been amazing what a difference it is to not be in pain anymore..he is a miracle worker, and we love him..when you see him for fol…

BC, God is so good! Happy Mothers' Day weekend!

Great news. Hoping for a speedy recovery!!

AB, Oh Lanette!! I'm so happy to hear this good news. Praying for you and Jim both in his recovery.

SL, Dr. Ghaly is the most skilled doctor! He performed back surgery on my dad years ago. I truly believe he was sent here from God almighty to be a healer for his people.

KC, Oh wow! I hope Jim has a speedy recovery!

JJ, SO SORRY TO HEAR THIS. JIM IS AN AMAZING GUY AND HE HAS AN AMAZING AND BEAUTIFUL WIFE BY HIS SIDE. LOVE YOU GUYS. JOYCE AND DENNY.

Praise God for a successful surgery!!

CW, So glad jims on road to recovery and surgery went well

JZ, Wow, prayers for Jim!

AS, for a fast recovery

PS, What a testimony! Yes, God sent you to the best doctor. Dr. Ghaly was the instrument for my nephew and a dear friend. Both needed a miracle. Thank you God for your intervention and the talents and compassionate Dr. Gahly possesses. Praying for healing and comfort.

SP, Another amazing outcome

SS, Looking good Jim!! **Lanette Sellers Yingling** prayed for a successful surgery and grateful prayers were answered

JD, Wonderful

CG, Prayers are being sent your way with the hopes that you will feel better soon.

AB, Praise God

LG, Praise God!

JY, Thank you Dr. **Ramsis Ghaly** for removing the tumor from Jim with an amazing surgical procedure....done with precision, accuracy and God-given wisdom!! You are a blessing

SS, **Jim Yingling**God has certainly blessed Dr Gahly with amazing talent and skills.

RM. Great job Sir

GC, Dr **Ramsis Ghaly** #1!

NG, Amazing!

RN, Thank you for helping so many people. Amen.

DN, You have a wonderful talent Dr.

RB, Praise God for a fantastic team to help heal him!

DH, Great news Dr Ghaly! Great news for patient

CB, You are the best.

Jim Yingling

Thank you Dr. **Ramsis Ghaly** for removing the tumor from Jim with an amazing surgical procedure....done with precision, accuracy and God-given wisdom!! You are a blessing

Susan Smith Jim Yingling God has certainly blessed Dr Gahly with amazing talent and skills.

Diane Nelson You have a wonderful talent Dr.

Cristina Batelli You are the best.

Amy Merkel Daly Praising God with you! So thankful for **Ramsis Ghaly**!!!

Gary Chandler GC, Dr **Ramsis Ghaly** #1!

Jamie Riffell Schultz

You tell Dr Ghaly that you know me. I worked with him long time ago. Very compassionate man. I'm glad you have answers and are on the mend.

Rhea Hagar Lumsden

Thank God for Dr. Ghaly! Praying for an uneventful and complete recovery for Jim. This is what those vows mean Lanette...for better or worse and in sickness and health. You were there for Jim as he would be for you. That strengthens your relationship! Love you

Mandy Phillips

Dr **Ramsis Ghaly** is one incredible human! I've never experienced anyone else like him and I only know him through rehabbing some of his patients!

Mary Nixon

Omgwow, that is just amazing. And yes Dr. **Ramsis Ghaly** Is an amazing surgeon, he did my back surgery, in 2008 and it's been amazing what a difference it is to not be in pain anymore..he is a miracle worker, and we love him..when you see him for follow up please tell him mark and Mary Nixon said hi!! So glad Jim is doing well

Jennifer Daly Petrucci

Sending prayers for your husbands recovery. . Dr. **Ramsis Ghaly** is truly the best and you are all in the best hands.

Carol Nelson

Dr Ghaly is the best. Love him. He actually cares about and loves his patients. He did my first surgery in 1996. He was at Silver Cross Hospital in Joliet at that time.

Stacia Robinson Little Dr. Ghaly is the most skilled doctor! He performed back surgery on my dad years ago. I truly believe he was sent here from God almighty to be a healer for his people.

Patti Stiegleiter

What a testimony! Yes, God sent you to the best doctor. Dr. Ghaly was the instrument for my nephew and a dear friend. Both needed a miracle. Thank you God for your intervention and the talents and compassionate Dr. Gahly possesses. Praying for healing and comfort.

Lanette Sellers Yingling Dr. Ghaly's post this morning! I swear this man doesn't sleep!!

Ll, Wow. I'm amazed at the surgeons words. Just how rare this was and how he not only relied on his own skill but also prayed for the surgery. you Jesus!

Lk, Dr. Ghaly did my surgery 2 years ago. I would go back to him in a heartbeat. He is truly a miracle doctor!

kw, Blessings to the max! Keep working miracles, Dr Ramsis!

First clinic visit of our angel Jim after 6 months of suffering and misdiagnosis. Look at him now few days after his rare surgery. Praise our Lord Jesus. Speed recovery. Excellent loving couple!!

Ramsis Ghaly

www.ghalyneurosurgeon.com

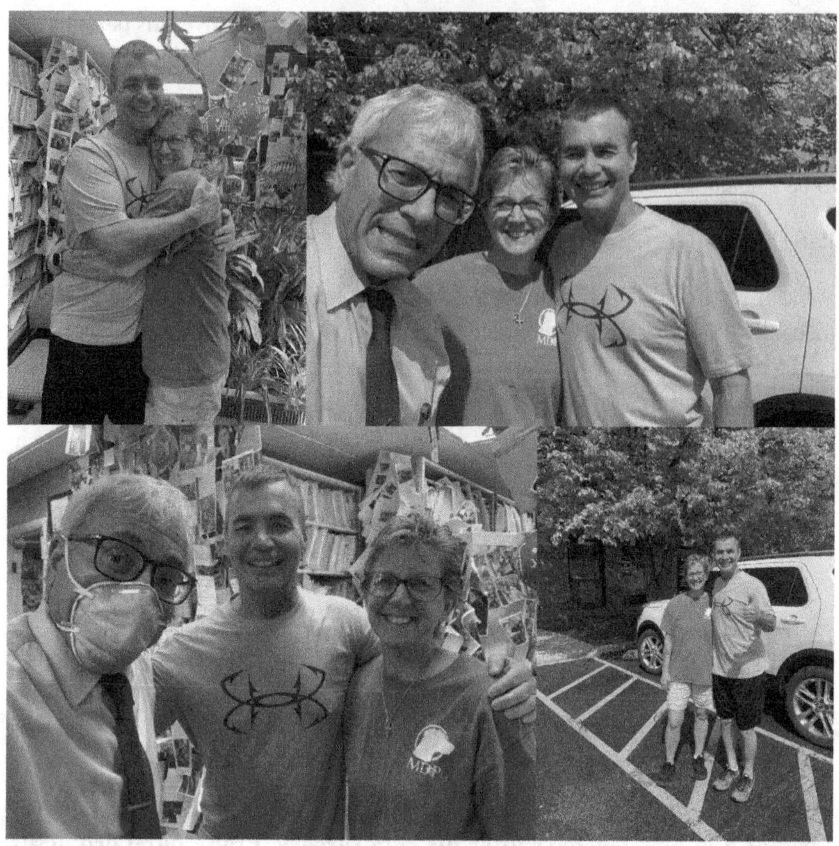

LY, Day 6 of recovery and all is well!! I wish that I could describe how grateful we are, specifically Jim, to have had Dr. Ramsis Ghaly be the one to have performed surgery! He is truly a gifted surgeon that has dedicated his life to helping people. He has not only given Jim hope that his pain has an end, but he has also shown us....again....that God is in control. You see, just 24 days ago, we had no hope for an end to Jim's pain....we were getting nowhere with the doctors that we had been seeing....then we saw Dr. Ghaly. That same day, he scheduled surgery after seeing the MRI reports of a tumor in his sciatic nerve and saw the pain that Jim was in! Thank you so much for your love for people, your love for Jesus and your love the the gift that God has given you! Praise the Lord that the tumor is benign!

CC You're wonderful! You give healing to the hopeless.

DN, So wonderfl

BO, Dr Ramsis Ghaly, you are our friend Jims Guardian Angel. Thank you sir, for your expertise and skills.

CS, Praise God!

AV, Praise God for you Dr Ghaly!

LG, That is so awesome! God is good.

yes he is Sis!!

CG, Sending happy thoughts, good wishes and prayers your way so that you continue feel good.

PM, Amazing!!!

DH, You are Awesom Dr. GHALEY!

JY, Words cannot express the gratitude that Lanette and I have for you. Not only your professionalism as an amazing doctor, but also your compassion as a friend. God Bless you Dr **Ramsis Ghaly**!!

RC, Amazing! Is so nice to have healt feelings. Speed recovery and good tougths.

PS, Wonderful news! Dr. Ghaly used by God to bring healing again. Amazing servant of God.

MN, Yes Dr. **Ramsis Ghaly** Is amazing.

I tell people all the time how great he is and so glad that you are doing well jim... God is good.

S, DM That's so awesome!

JE, Praise God, I'm so glad the tumor is out and benign!

AG, This is incredible! I'm so happy he got the help he needed.

DG, So glad for the good news! And wishing Jim a speedy recovery!

OZ, Praise the Lord!

mo, Good news on Jim's health Prayers answered.

Mm, Praise god! So happy for you both!!

Js, May GOD bless Dr Ramsis Ghaly. He sounds like a man of GOD. So thankful he helped Jim.

MS, Wonderful news! Dr. Ghaly used by God to bring healing again. Amazing servant of God.

MO, Thank you for sharing the good news Prayers answered

RP, So happy for you Jim!!

Six weeks later back to work:::

Update from wife Lanette 6/9/2022

Update on : after just 4 weeks of recovery post surgery, Jim is back to work! Dr. Ramsis Ghaly is a miracle worker!

Ramsis Ghaly

Amen Praise our Lord. much love and blessing

Ramsis Ghaly we owe it all to you!!

rl, That is so awesome and we're so happy for Jim and thankful to God for Dr. Ghaly.

Pc, Wonderful news!

Jl, Awesome, great news!!

Sf, So good to hear!

Mb, So glad to hear.

Me, Wonderful news!!

ms, I'm not sure what happened, but so glad he's on the mend. he had a tumor in his sciatic nerve that got so bad that he couldn't stand

lj, He is pretty amazing! He goes above and beyond any doctor I have been too. He truly cares about his patients!

A Smile Pain Free after Fourth Month of Suffering!!

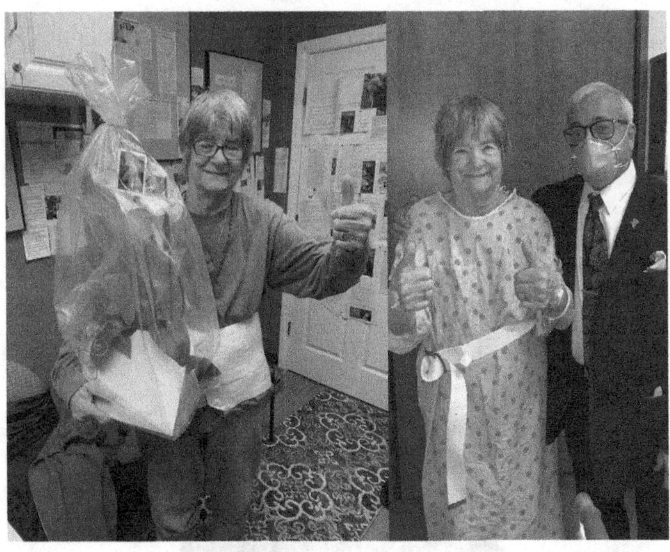

Four months of sever pains and unable to walk straight. Nothing could help her offered by pain clinic and therapy.

An 85 years old determined to live in good health. She never agreed to be dependent in injections and pain meds whatever years remained for her to live.

She is a very active lady, and her life was miserable with suffering. She prayed day and night to God. Out of desperation she reached out to her friends. She was directed to see me.

I took my time, listen carefully and hands on care reviewing images, getting the records, working her up, review all thoroughly and put all these data together in God's hand and pray to God to do what is not written in textbooks for all but what is good for her! We found the exact problem and discussed the curative surgery option. Nothing to replace hands on care and thoroughly and have the Patient and God in center!

Her senior age didn't stop her from seeking the correct curative surgery! Always strive whenever possible to do curative treatment and not palliative treatment getting you addicted and dependent in pain meds even if you 85 years old!! Step in and reach out your comfort zone perhaps you find better options!!

Surgery was done and next day she is at home pain free walking upright praising Lord Jesus our Savior and Healer. Hallelujah home sweet home with no much of suffering as her prayers heard!!

Speed recovery our angel! Amen

Ramsis Ghaly

Www.ghalyneurosurgeon.com

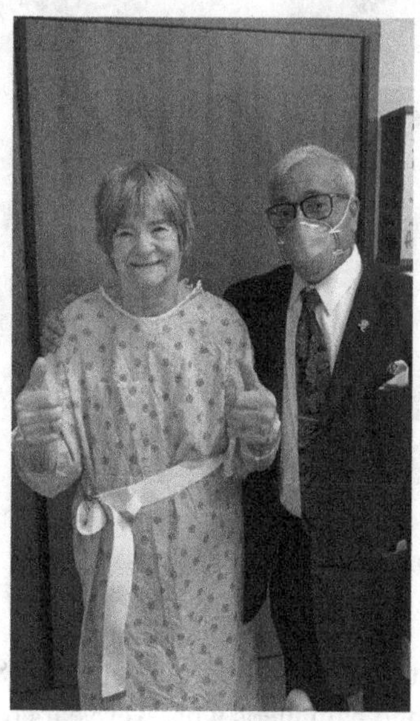

Ten days later after surgery, Dorothy the 85 years old, doing well and brought beautiful Hawaiian 🌱 Orchid flowers and plant for my indoor garden.

After four months of being drugged with medications and horrific nerve pains, simple surgery resulted lifetime cure and now free of all suffering praise our Lord Jesus. Age is not a contraindication to do the corrective surgery!! Surgery is also cost effective and avoids the costly pain injections and meds and disabled individuals!!

She has a new lease in life being normal and independent again without the need for future meds or injections!

As the patient leaving the office she kept saying "you are a great doctor I love you ——I am going tell the world about you". Yet I only did small surgery snd Judy her care giver asked her to come and see me. God world in a mysterious way!!

My practice garden increased by the patients blessing and green blossoming for ever through their blessing and prayers!!

Ramsis Ghaly

www.ghalyNeurosurgeon.com

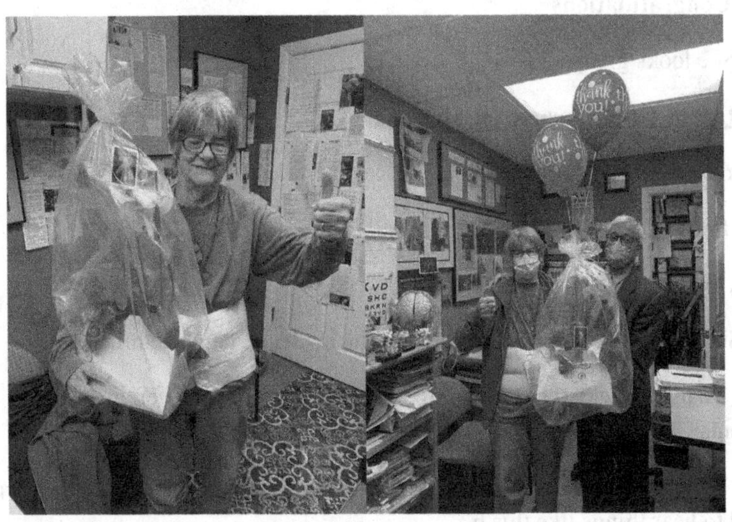

DL, That's such wonderful news !

ED, It's wonderful to hear that this beautiful woman was able to find relief after years of suffering. You continue to do good works through the Grace of God dear Doctor. Bless you.

MA, **JT,** ou need a green house Ramsis...i have an indoor jungle as well

CG, That is such good news. She can live without pain.

You're the best

.

That is a wonderful thank you gift.

DH, That's AWESOME

MN, Speedy recovery!

AV, Praise God!

ML, She is amazing… and so are you.

RC, Both, she and you are a warriors. A lot of blessings!

JN, You are a wonderful dr.

ES, She was and is in the hands of an amazing doctor. Thank you Dr G for helping so many. The Lord has given you a great gift.

JK, Congratulations

JK, She looks great.

dr. **Ramsis Ghaly** you are walking angel.

I could used your blessings....

AB, Praise God

MG, God bless you Doc abundantly!

PI, She was a pleasure to care care of. She made me laugh so much

RG, Thank you doctor for helping so much. Blessings to you always and your patients!

MS, What an inspiration to all of us. Thank you for the beautiful words. It's really good to hear things like this.b

JS, God Bless Her & you also

JC, You're a champion Ramsis Ghaly

MP, Praise the Lord, Dr Ghaly works through Jesus, Amen.

"Age Is Just A Number"!

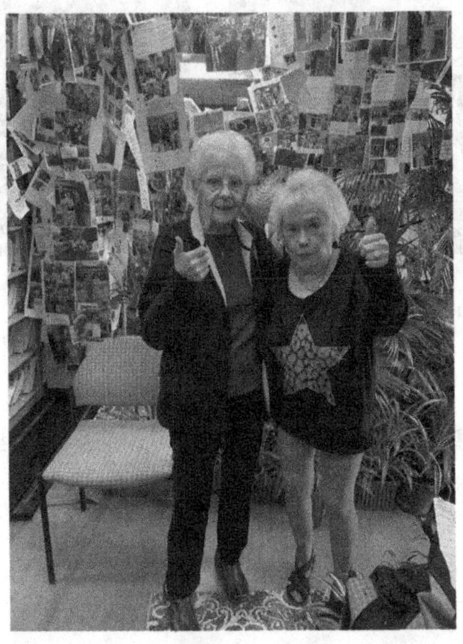

My patient today Diane taught me a lesson with her friend Marianne!!

How lovely and gorgeous both of young ladies; Marianne and Diane, their message to the world is "Age is just a Number"

No masks -well dressed - stylish-very active -and still working —. Her hobby is dancing all her life and she is proud to be in the show in those days with Jim Lounsberry record hob, Dick Clark Show —-

Let us learn from Diane and Marianne. Stay active, dance, work and know "age is just a number".

Praise our Lord Jesus for His creation and Beauty!!

Psalm 103:5 KJV "Who satisfieth thy mouth with good things; so that thy youth is renewed like the eagle's."

Bless you both!!!

<u>Ramsis Ghaly</u>

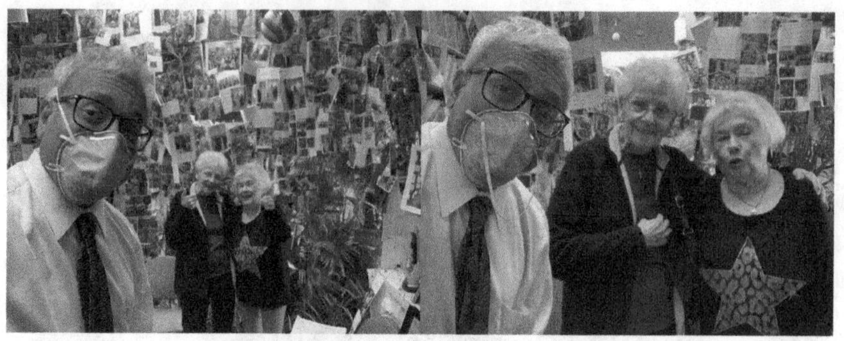

Ec, Beautiful Dr. Ghaly! I agree

Rc, Lovely ladies!

Cg, Bless them. There are so cute and absolutely correct "Age is just a number"

Fifty Years In Suffering, A Story to Tell!

Our shining star Brad recovering well praise our Lord Jesus after long brain surgery yesterday.

You can't beat this beautiful angelic smile full of hope, faith and energy with much gratitude. A smile with thumb up says it all!! And all family are around him!

Speed recovery and thank you all for your prayers

Ramsis Ghaly

Www.ghalyneurosurgeon.com

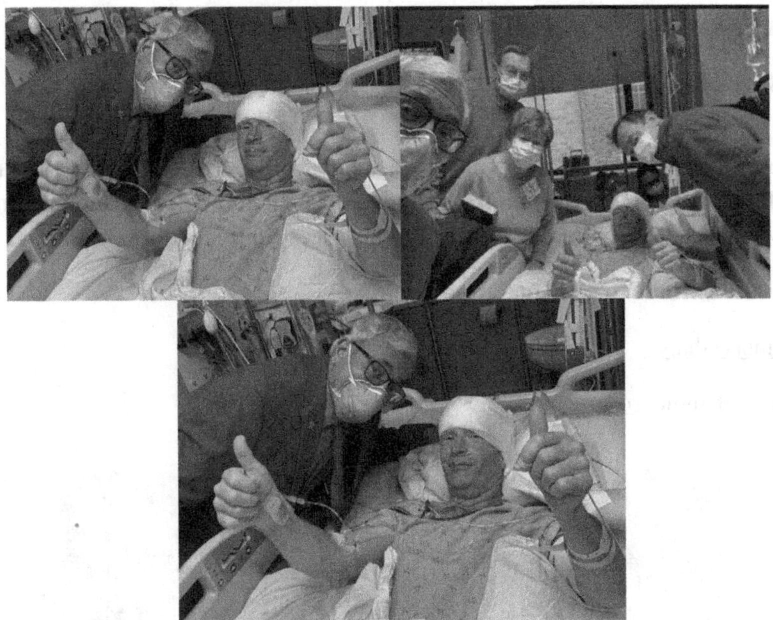

KL, Thank you Dr. Ghaly!!! We love you and are so grateful for all you do for our family and these special guys of ours

SB, Praise Jesus!! Thank you Dr. Ghaly, you are such a wonderful doctor. Our family is so lucky to have you.

CS, There aren't enough words to express our deep gratitude!! We love you!

AC, The best doctor!

DM, Thank you Dr. Ghaly for all you have done for Brad and for Stephen!!! You have touched our family in the best of ways!

LM, Dr.Ghaly **you're the Best**!!!

RM, Speedy recovery Brad I've been here No worries your in good hands with Dr Ghaly and our Lord

DN, So wonderful

TC, Thank you Dr. **Ramsis Ghaly** for being a faithful servant and using your talents as a blessing for those in need. Our family has been blessed twice and we are so grateful!

KS, Fantastic news!

MS, So glad all is well.

JM, "Awesome" Dr. Ghaly

DS, You have the best Doctor ever Brad. Sending healing prayers.

Going home today sweet home!! Praise our Lord. Walked around the unit hallway flattering the unit nurses and tell them all about his fog and farming! Everyone loves him and his smile and his exceedingly love and kindness!

Let us continue to pray for speed recovery

Ramsis Ghaly

Www.ghalyneurosurgeon.com

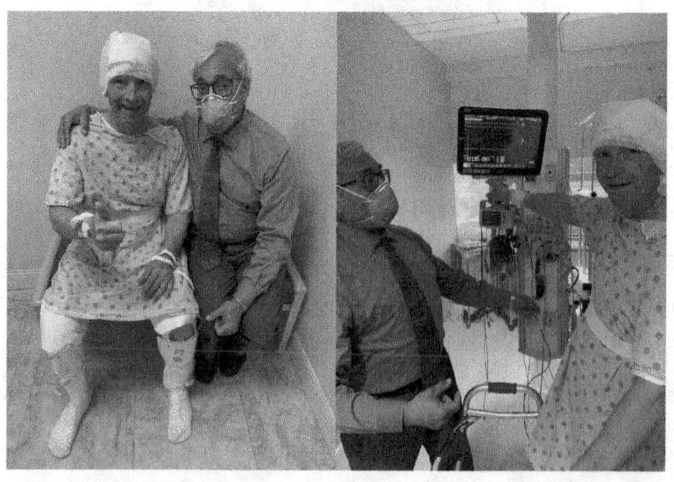

DH, You are an amazing talented surgeon Dr Ghaly. You have a gift from our high God

4KL, He looks great!

PD, Great to hear! for continued healing.

TC, Hooray Brad!!! And thank you again, **Ramsis Ghaly**!!!

KO, Have a good fast recovery sir you were in the best hands w Dr Ghaly

DM, Brad you are looking great and hope you will feel better every day!! Love your smile. And thank you Dr Ghaly for your skill and knowledge as you care for Brad!

CS, Praise the Lord!!!! So happy!!

AC, The best doctor in the world

RS, Wonderful news!

TB, Look at that! So awesome!

JD, Wonderful news!

JS, Thanking GOD and for a safe recovery

SB, So elated for Brad and family. Dr. Ghaly **you're the best**

and know how much our family appreciates you for helping Brad. God bless you!!

JA, to you all and keep up the good work Brad!!

DC, Way to go Brad! Thank you so much Dr Ghaly! You are the best

RD, This makes us so happy!

SP, Dr Ghaly you are amazing! God Blesses you to heal others

MO, That's so wonderful!

JB, Yeah Brad. So happy you are doing well! Looking good.

MS, Thank God!!

SP, Sending healing prayers.

JK, Great job. Ramsis Ghaly

Look at the most elegant man with a surgery white hate!! Handsome with great smile!!

Brad came today for his first visit a week after crucial surgery!

A fantastic different person looking good and recovering well. Praise our Lord!!!

Much love and blessing

Ramsis Ghaly

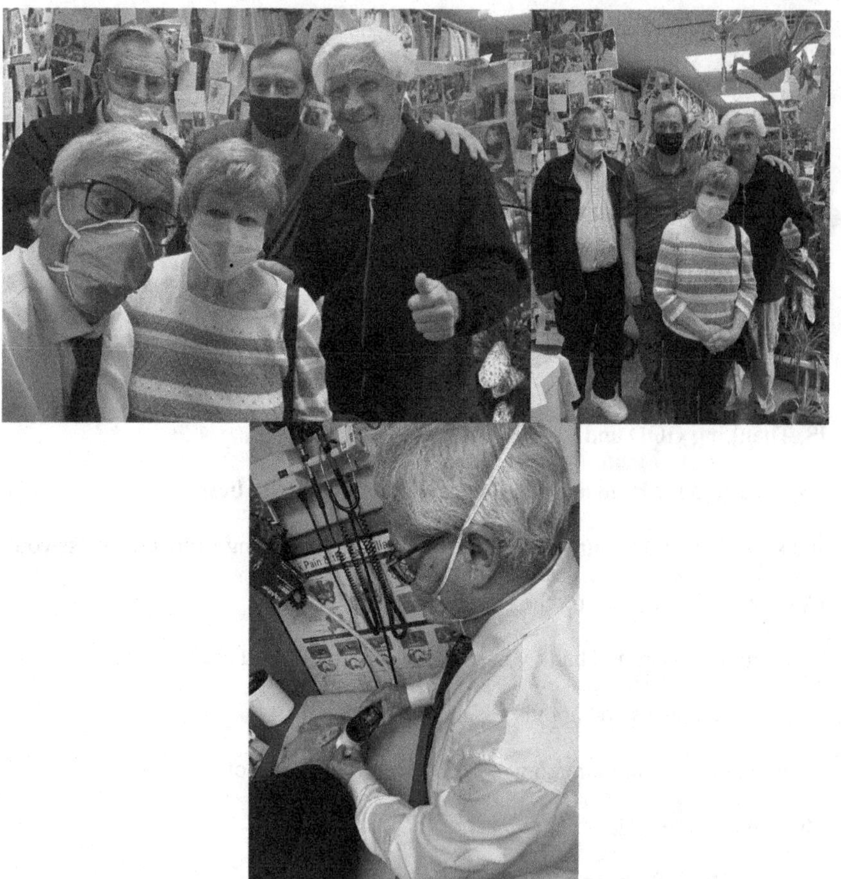

Rd, This is so wonderful!

Vg, Another great job, Doctor!

Ms, Thank you Lord for Doctor and God bless you all.

Dh, Praise you Dr Ghaly! Praise God, All the Glory to God

Jam, reat news!!!

Bs, Awesome news!! One day at a time.

CS, Continued prayers of thanksgiving!!! One week post op and doing amazing!!! We're blessed to have you Dr Ghaly as Brad doctor-

LL, Love this!

TA, He looks good

Todd Appleman yes. Getting a little bit better every day. Like Mrs G said. 1 day at a time. We've seen a great improvement already in just 1 week.

A week later after Brain Surgery

What a joy to see my two miracles' patients Stephen and Bradley.

What a miracle after delicate brain surgery!

They continue to beat all the odds performing spectacularly full of love, joy, kindness and blessing!

He is shopping, conversing, watching news and rendering opinions while maintaining his kind manners and politeness!! So honored to see the Conderman's and Schott's families all together today! What a great surprise!

Much love and blessing and Ed co to help to pray for speed recovery!!!

Ramsis Ghaly

Www.Ghalyneurosurgeon.com

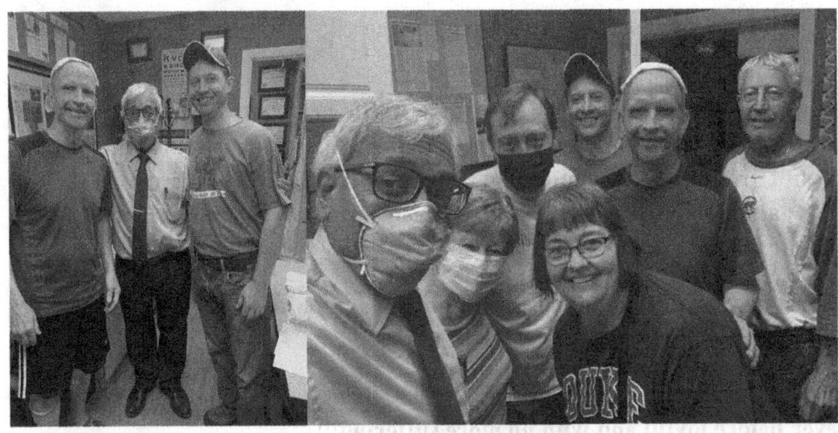

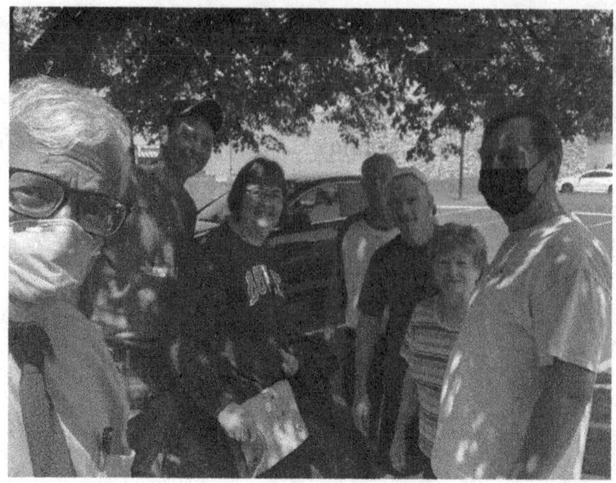

Cg, Caring thoughts and prayers are with you as you get better.Bless you both.

Ja, Keep fighting the good fight men!!!

Kg, God Bless you both on your healing journey. And God Bless Dr Ghaly Always for guiding his hands to perform the most delicate of miracles. Much continued success. Blessings from Egypt

xoxo

ms, Love that you show your precious families. God bless you and all you care for.

Rc, Blessings for all, and you dr. Ghaly

Cl, HIS Blessings to all!

Dn, They are miracles and thank god you had a miracle worker Doctor good luck with your recoveries, god is with you

Cs Brads doing great!! So thankful to Dr Ghaly!!!

What a joy to be part of a New lease in life occurred by surgery through which Brad was granted a life worth living while so many major institutions didn't grant him that chance for 50 years! Miracle to see in two weeks, Brad has gained so much that he and his family have never seen in decades! Glory to our Savior!

Surgery was done and God was so gracious to do so for Brad!!! Amen!! We all so proud of you Brad.

Praise our lord as we all witness everyday Brad is doing more and more than ever before joyful and with no more suffering!!!

We pray for more blessings!!

Ramsis Ghaly

Www.ghalyneurosurgeon.com

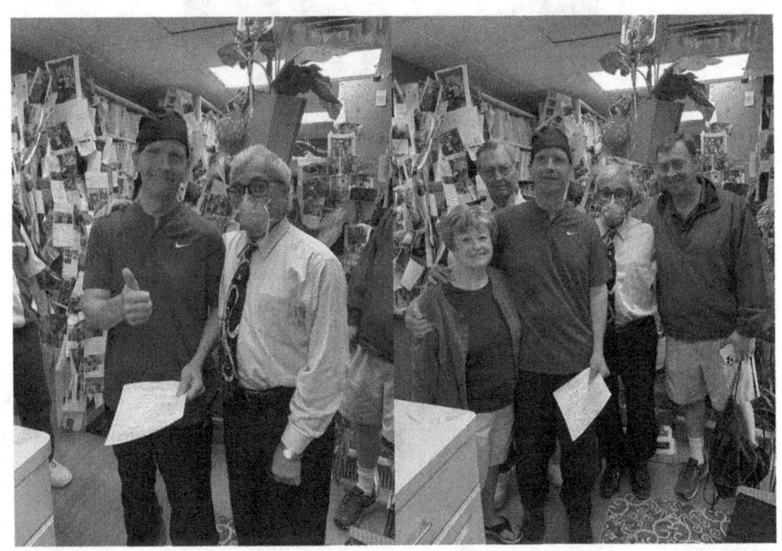

DM, Brad we are so excited for you!! Sending you much love and hugs!!!

TR, I truly believe God sees your heart and uses your hands to do HIS work

TB, Truly an Angel on earth.... what a gift!

JA, Great news Brad!! Can't wait to see you!!

TA, Awesome news! Get well Brad!

BG, Awesome

TH,amazing

AV, Praise God!! Blessings to all of you!!

Joshua Story!

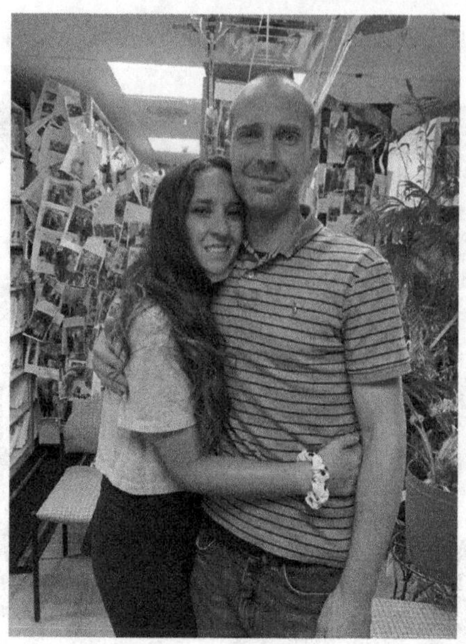

06/09/2022

I saw this wonderful couple and Joshua has been miserable since 2017 with no hope or help devastated. He had five years of horrific illness journey suffering miserably beyond imagination and many procedures, meds,—— no help

I pray his visit with me today is the beginning of new lease in life to regain his self back to himself, to his wife, to his kids and to the world . He was a genius engineer and lively hardworking man!!

Let us pray in Jesus name for Joshua. Amen we pray!!

Ramsis Ghaly

Www.ghaly Neurosurgeon.com

Ke, Prayers for you Joshua! U r in the best hands ever with Dr Ghaly! I'm living proof twice.

Av,Praying for all of you!!

Kg, Praying for Joshua! You're in the Best of Care with Dr Ghaly. My family is proof and I'm almost 7000 miles away. A minor medical procedure left me NOT really walking right...more like a wet noodle and NOT able to really feel my legs. HUGE Thanks to Dr Ghaly for correcting the issue. And my husband having a rather hard fall that Dr Ghaly was consulted on, correctly handling. Huge prayers and Blessings for you that God sent you a very special Angel to us all! God Bless you and rest easy now. God Bless, Dr Ghaly,an Angel disguised as friend.

Xoxo

Dn, Praying with you for Joshua

Se, Prayers

Jh, Praying for you Joshua!

Jk, Prayers

DC, Praying for you Joshua! May the Lord Jesus use Dr Ghaly's hands and God given skills to fix whatever is wrong. Amen!

CG, Prayers for you Josh. You have the best doctor taking care of you.

JG, Prayers for Joshua!!!

JY, Prayers!

RC, Let's pray for him, for his recovery in order to have a new life in good hands

ML, Amen

JG, Prayers for Joshua!!!

JY, Prayers!

RC, Let's pray for him, for his recovery in order to have a new life in good hands

ML, Amen

ED, Prayers sent to this wonderful man. Amen

AP, Wishing you a speedy recovery

DH, Prayers for Joshua ...May God shine his Grace upon him and his family, and if you are doing surgery, May God Bless and guide your hands for a new look at life, thank you Dr. GHALY

ALL THE GLORY TO GOD

BM, Praying for healing

jb, Sending healing prayers

Rs, Ma, Prayers for all

Ko, Prayers are on going

Dg, Praying for you Joshua! May the Lord Jesus use Dr Ghaly's hands and God given skills to fix whatever is wrong. Amen!

Cg, Prayers for you Josh. You have the best doctor taking care of you.

Jg, Prayers for Joshua!!!

Jy, Prayers!

Rc, Let's pray for him, for his recovery in order to have a new life in good hands

Ml, Amen

Prayers sent to this wonderful man. Amen

Ap, Wishing you a speedy recovery

Dh, Prayers for Joshua ...May God shine his Grace upon him and his family, and if you are doing surgery, May God Bless and guide your hands for a new look at life, thank you Dr. GHALY

ALL THE GLORY TO GOD

Bm, Praying for healing

Au, Prayers your way Josh for recovery in Jesus' name

Bk, Amen

Dm, Praying god will guide you in giving him a new and wonderful future

Jp, He's in great hands with you.

Jj, Amen!

Mc, Praying for his well being may Jesus Christ help him regain his health back. May He lay hands on him and heal him, for his loved ones. Our Father in heaven hear our prayers. We trust in you and pray thy will be done. Amen

06/10/2022

Look at Joshua and Natasha smile for a new lease in life in just few hours!!! Hallelujah

Ramsis Ghaly

Look at Joshua and Natasha smile for a new lease in life in just few hours!!! Hallelujah

In less than few hours, the correct diagnosis and simple treatment started, the man is cured and in less than 24 hrs a huge smile and big relief. No more terrors, pains, fear of pains, cries, headaches and misery day and nights—-! Praise our Lord Jesus. Thank you praising His Name always.

It was a persistent phone calls from wife and patient and Facebook message if can cut a nerve or redo brain surgery? I did not know if I can help since he already had the brain surgery. The cries and tears were pouring for help!! I prayed to try to listen and see if I can help and to be a vessel!

After I saw him and spent three hours, I wrote this post asking for prayers: "I saw this wonderful couple and Joshua has been miserable since 2017 with no hope or help devastated. He had five years of horrific illness journey suffering miserably beyond imagination and many procedures, many teeth pulled, injections, surgeries, meds,—— no help. I pray his visit with me today is the beginning of new lease in life to regain his self back to himself, to his wife, to his kids and to the world . He was a genius engineer and lively hardworking man!! Let us pray in Jesus name for Joshua. Amen we pray!!

https://www.facebook.com/1150861349/posts/10228723793656978/?d=n

As soon as he left yesterday night my clinic, had a severe attack, immediately he applied the treatment I recommended and Within 20 minutes the attack ceased. This morning after long night sleep uninterrupted he never experienced such a good straight night sleep as he did last night in 5 years, Joshua and his wife came today absolutely phenomena, joyful, regaining his life back and family back. Joshua back to himself and his wife and his children and to the world with hope and appreciation for a new lease in life after five years of hell from intractable pains and headaches——-and so many procedures and meds—-

Amen to Lord Jesus and his gracious unlimited mercy and love to His children, the only One and by His word!

Let us pray for Joshua and family for healing from the past and speed recovery

Ramsis Ghaly

Www.ghalyNeurosurgeon.com"

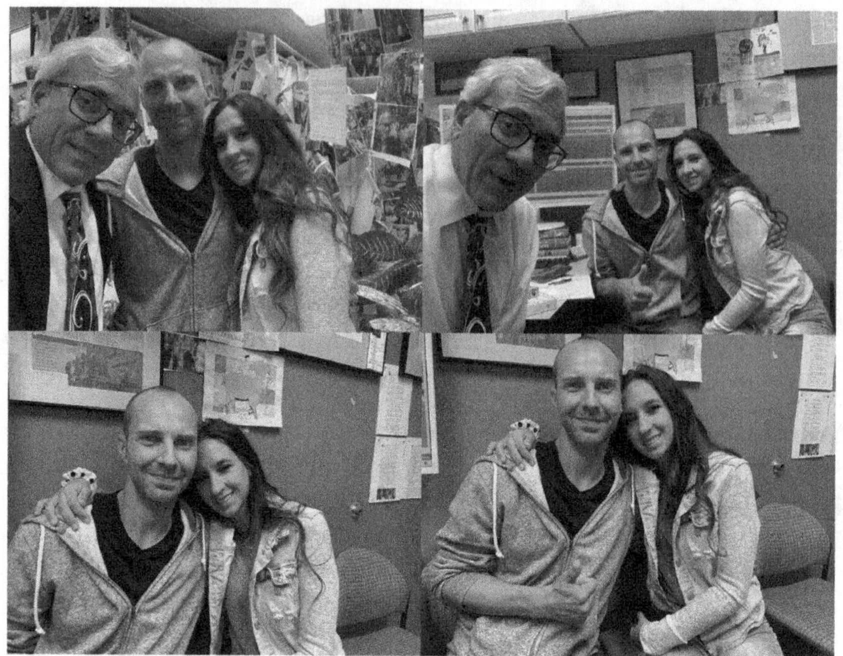

SC, your amazing dr Ghaly

KG, Speedy Healing and Complete Recovery to Joshua and Family.

God Bless you all.

Thank God for Dr Ghaly!

BO, Your the best Dr Ghaly, God sent for sure,

BD, You will not find a more honest Dr. and one who cares more for his patients than Dr. Ghaly!!

CG, So happy for him. Wishing him continued healing. God bless and watch over you both.

SC, Oh my...I could cry for him. He must be so happy to have found you and to have new hope!

RC, Amazing healing, amazng doctor¡£

NM, Amazing Dr. G!!!!!!

VW, Healing Hand

NM, Amazing Dr. G!!!!!!

VW, Healing Hand

DB, God's Dr. Ghaly! We are so blessed to have Dr. Ghaly in our lives!! Thank you, Father!!

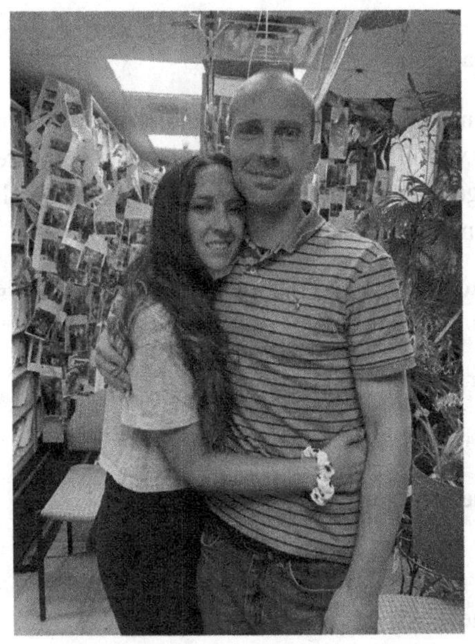

06/20/2022

It was the best ever Father gift to Joshua and to myself!!

I just heard from our Joshua that: "Joshua is doing miraculously and he has his life back again. He is alive again after 5 years of dying everyday. Joshua is back to himself, to his kids, to his wife, to his family, to his friends, to his work and to the world with tremendous excitement and hope for the future"

"Jesus said unto her, I am the resurrection, and the life: he that believeth in me, though he were dead, yet shall he live: [26] And whosoever liveth and believeth in me shall never die. Believest thou this?"

John 11:25-26 KJV

Jesus said to old son, the earth and heaven are so happy because the younger son was dead and alive again:, "And he said unto him, Son, thou art ever with me, and all that I have is thine. [32] It was meet that we should make merry, and be glad: for this thy brother was dead, and is alive again; and was lost, and is found."Luke 15:31-32 KJV

"And he said, The things which are impossible with men are possible with God."Luke 18:27 KJV

Amen Lord Jesus thank you and thank you all to your prayers !!

Ramsis Ghaly

Joshua and Natasha Prim

Thank you very much. We are so grateful and always thinking of you. 48 hours no pain!!!! 5 years waiting. I can't thank you enough. We are on the right track and you have changed my life in the best way ever. We will call you soon and give you an update. From all of us and especially me .

All of our prayers were answered thank God and thank You! **sy,** Praise the Lord!

Charlene Mentzer Glowaty

Just amazing what a caring doctor can do .

Wishes for continued recovery for Joshua.

Rita Castillo

Awsone! Best wishes

Sandi Benedict Crites

your the best dr ghaly

Joan McGrath Pocius

Answered prayers

Kathy Hogan

You are a gift from God. Thank you Jesus!

For five years he was miserable incapacitated and look at him now. Back to himself, his life, his family and to the world. Praise Lord Jesus. Amen Hallelujah

This is today his words to me: "I no longer have bad days. I never had as such good days in the last five years as now in the last two months. I feel awesome. I have been damaged and hurt fur the last five years. I lost do much money

and years were taken away from me and my family. I learned much. I think about you every day and my family appreciate you!!"

To Lord Jesus is the glory forever and ever Amen!

I wrote his story in June 20, 2022: https://www.facebook.com/1150861349/posts/10228783514189954/?d=n

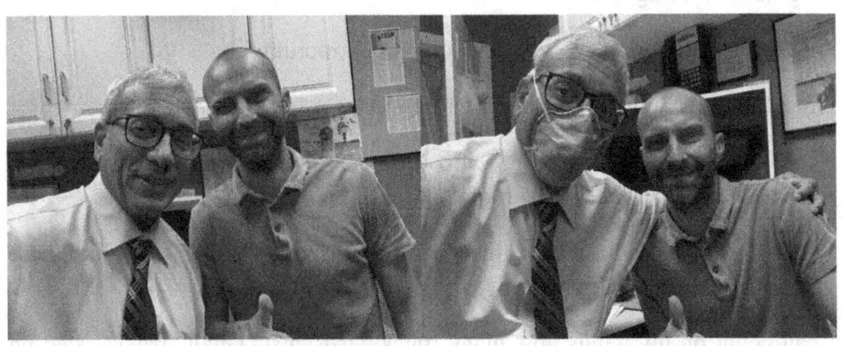

Eo, The Lord is wonderful. Blessings to you my dear brother in Christ

Dh, Hallelujah! Thanks be to God

Rn, Your an Angel from heaven to work everyday to improve people's lives. I pray for you. You had to be sent from God. You're a remarkable human being!

Ko, That's so awesome Dr Ghaly is certainly a life safer for all his pts, God bless

Sy, Praise God!

Dm, When jesus is the center of life miracles happen

Jp, Thanks be to God

Sometimes God Send Us Angels!

Sometimes God sends us Angel's disguised as friends.....

So Blessed and Thankful for this Doctor.

Originally from Egypt.

America's, Chicago, IL, Best Neurosurgeon Extraordinaire.

One Man CAN and DOES make a Difference!

The BEST American Doctor, a Neurosurgeon, who took time to assist us when Basha had a sudden fall on the roof, 27 May 2022.

I am so very Thankful to have this Doctor as my friend and brother all of these years even BEFORE I came to live in Egypt.

I can count on my hands how many times, Dr Ramsis Ghaly, has assisted on Consultations when things just didn't seem right.

When sudden surgery left me unable to feel my own legs, here, in a foreign land and

NOW

Basha having a sudden fall that left him in terrible pain with bruises and tears to the Gluteal muscles on one hip. Very Thankful the leg, Mansour's hip, was not broken.

Very VERY THANKFUL FOR

DR. RAMSIS GHALY.

Shokran Khteer

Thank you

Thank you

Thank you

God Bless You Always

Dr Ramsis Ghaly

Mansour Khalil

June 5 at 7:05 AM ·

Thanks and appreciation

For Professor Dr. Ramses Ghali residing in Chicago, USA ... Brother and dear friend

For your precious time . And your daily prayers and follow up of the blisters and bruises I suffered while I was on the roof. Thank God, the first and the last, for not having a break. Now I'm fine, thank God, thanks to Dr. Ramses Ghali and Dr. Andrew.

Also I thank everyone who asked about me by all means

.... Thanks to all of you

Kg,

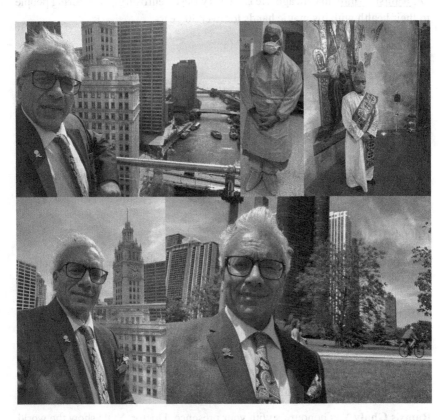

Bp, Not many Doctors are like that nowadays. Glad you and your family have a wonderful and trustworthy doctor!

Kathleen MacGregor Grace

Bp, I am so Blessed and Honoured to have this Doctor in a world that often devalues and negates people as they step on each other to get ahead instead of helping one another as we should.

I can't even imagine where I would be without THIS Doctor as so many times he has guided me here and even when I had a iffy unneccessary procedure that left me unable to walk properly, just to "Keep the peace" and "Fit In." I've since remembered MY Worth and will NEVER do such again or ever allow another to denegrate or devalue me again.

This Doctor is Amazing and I am so grateful to call him my friend and brother.

If you know anyone who needs a wonder Doctor with outstanding skills and chair side manner for even the most delicate brain or spine issues, please send them to Dr. **Ramsis Ghaly** in Chicago. He is the very Best Neurosurgeon restoring people to their health with his magic hands for over 30 years.

We Love Doctor Ghaly

Thank you, Sis!

Blessings

Kathleen MacGregor Grace

Merci! Shokran Khteer, Dr Ramsis Ghaly! Thank God for you. Basha is healing well and we are staying the Protocol you prescribed. Thank you so very very much!

Ramsis Ghaly

Very touched **Kathleen MacGregor Grace** and unworthy. we all servants helping each other as our Lord Jesus taught us and He blessing all of us. Please send my love and regards to my homeland Egypt where the very ancient Coptic orthodox Christianity was born and alive to the end of ages despite the persecution in the Middle East. So happy you all stand strong. Speed recovery much love and blessing!!!

Kathleen MacGregor Grace

Ramsis Ghaly You honour us with your presence, Doctor. YOU show the world that YES! 1 Man CAN and WILL make a difference. YOU ARE the TRUE

ANGEL among us all, teaching and sharing your craft with the next generations as we all should. NOT keeping all a secret to be envied and fought over.

WE are so Blessed and Honoured to call you our friend and brother.

I can still remember returning from my own time in a hospital and unable to move my legs properly leaving me to wonder what I could do and afraid again when Basha had his fall 27May 2022.

And GOD answered those prayers as there you were to guide us on these adventures to restored mobility. A True Angel disguised as friend.

I truly cannot ever Thank you enough for the purest heart of Gold and gifted as you are helping from so far away.

I am deeply deeply honored.

Shokran khteer,.Doctor!

Thank you so very very much, Dr Ramsis Ghaly.

Gs, Great man a real hero

Kathleen MacGregor Grace

Gs, Yes, He is!

The very Best! I'm so glad he has helped Basha. You don't know how awful it looks. Very Thankful it's Not broken and just needs some time to heal which it is just nicely. Thank you, George!

Kathleen MacGregor Grace

I'm glad he's doing okay hope things will heal faster just a matter of time and everything will be back to normal thank God again he is doing wonderful and Hope that he will take care of himself

Kathleen MacGregor Grace

Gs, ou KNOW he is chomping at the bit being down and out!

He has the VERY BEST DOCTOR/Neurologist from Egypt, too, George, so he can speak quite nicely with him AND the proper care, treatment and medicines to American Standard, George. THANK GOD!

Just need to keep him home..no stairs for awhile yet.

Very Thankful for Dr Ramsis Ghaly in Chicago.

Kathleen MacGregor Grace

I'm totally agree with you but the most important thing is he's in good hands with you and I have to give you all the credit for the hard working and the excellent care you provide for him anyway thank you for taking care of my buddy

Kathleen MacGregor Grace

Thank you so much!

I have to Thank God for giving me Dr **Ramsis Ghaly**, George. Because I could never see me dragging him back down any stairs for more tests and unnecessary things.

We have All we need when we believe. Thank GOD!

Dr Ghaly is an Angel

A true miracle of all the people.

Thank you so much, Dr Ghaly.

Kathleen MacGregor Grace

George Salib Thank You so much! IF you saw it, you wouldnt believe it was a sudden fall on a piece of irregular concrete slab.Noone would believe it. More Like a Car crash or worse.

You would never ever believe that was a fall. I promise! I'm still s…

Kathleen MacGregor GraceMansour Khalil

June 5 at 6:54 AM ·

Thank you for helping Mansour and I when we needed you.

Merci, Dr Ramsis Ghaly.

God only gives the Best

When we believe.…

See more

— with **Mansour Khalil** and **Ramsis Ghaly**.

www.ghalyneurosurgeon.com

One of the Best Ever Blessing Award I have received as an unworthy servant is from Pope of Vatican his holiness Benedict XVI in 2006!!

Ramsis Ghaly

www.ghalyneurosurgeon.com

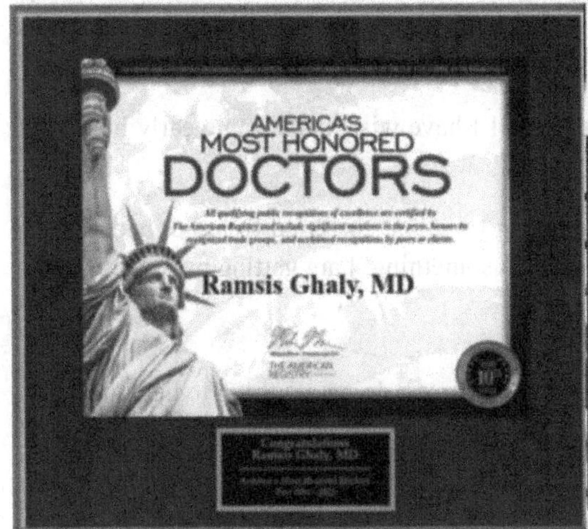

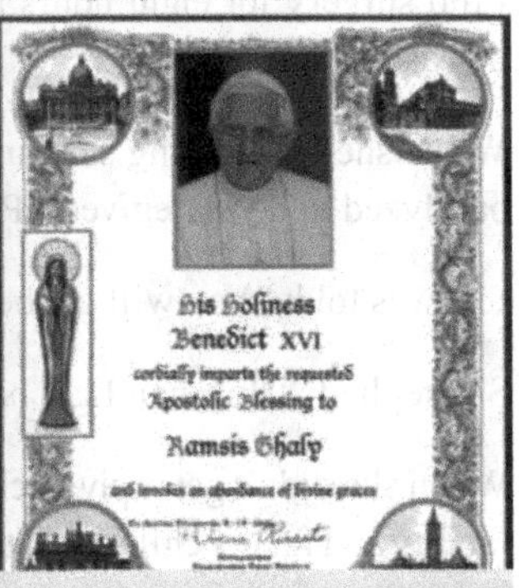

The Story of Virginia No Other Name But His Name! Please Pray!

I did surgery in an unfortunate patient already paralyzed and the disease is far advanced and are her bones at two different locations. There is No way that the patient will ever walk again even after my surgery and extensive rehabilitation. It is already too too late. The spinal cord is already damaged!

She is a beautiful angel with a glorious soul like a diamond, looked at me today laying in her bed saying: “Please let me walk again! You are a miracle worker”. I cried as she was talking to me shedding my tears couldn’t open my mouth to dare to say a word. I am who I am with broken heart for her!!

I said:” Lady there is No other Name that can do the impossible than His Name!! No other Name but Jesus our Lord!! Absolutely No other Name in the entire universe and in heaven but His Holy Name that can let you walk again”

I did surgery for eight hours all night! I have wished she came early before the disease took over!!

While she was getting sick and losing function, she cried from her bed helpless paralyzed to her caregiver: “Please do something. I am getting paralyzed”

She was told: “You will get better”

She replied: “How can I get better if you aren’t doing anything to help me??”

When she didn’t get reply back and all around left her, she demanded to leave the facility and for her children to take her home paralyzed and helpless. Heartbreaking indeed!!

She reached out to me and her son late in Friday evening asking for a miracle!! My heart is heavy aching for her! Indeed, there is No other Name but Jesus Christ the True Healer Above all!!

She looked at me and said: “In the meantime, if my heart stops, please let me go to be with Jesus my God!””

It reminded me with our Lord words to His Heavenly Father: “And he said, Abba, Father, all things are possible unto thee; take away this cup from me: nevertheless, not what I will, but what thou wilt.” Mark 14:36 KJV

We pray and you all let us join to pray for this angel that served our Lord tirelessly as nurse for 60 years since 1961 and raised her children the best they can be!!

St Peter said: "Neither is there salvation in any other: for there is none other name under heaven given among men, whereby we must be saved." Acts 4:12 KJV

For nothing is impossible with God as it is written: "For with God nothing shall be impossible." Luke 1:37

"And he said, the things which are impossible with men are possible with God." Luke 18:27

"But Jesus beheld them, and said unto them, with men this is impossible; but with God all things are possible." Matthew 19:26

"And Jesus looking upon them saith, With men it is impossible, but not with God: for with God all things are possible." Mark 10:27

"But without faith it is impossible to please him: for he that cometh to God must believe that he is, and that he is a rewarder of them that diligently seek him." Hebrews 11:6

"And Jesus said unto them, Because of your unbelief: for verily I say unto you, If ye have faith as a grain of mustard seed, ye shall say unto this mountain, Remove hence to yonder place; and it shall remove; and nothing shall be impossible unto you." Matthew 17:20

John 14:13-14 "Whatever you ask in My name, that will I do, so that the Father may be glorified in the Son. If you ask Me anything in My name, I will do it."

Philippians 2:9-10 "For this reason also, God highly exalted Him, and bestowed on Him the name which is above every name, so that at the name of Jesus every knee will bow, of those who are in heaven and on earth and under the earth,"

John 1:12 "But as many as received Him, to them He gave the right to become children of God, even to those who believe in His name,"

Colossians 3:17 "Whatever you do in word or deed, do all in the name of the Lord Jesus, giving thanks through Him to God the Father."

Acts 3:16 "And on the basis of faith in His name, it is the name of Jesus which has strengthened this man whom you see and know; and the faith which comes through Him has given him this perfect health in the presence of you all."

Psalm 148:13 "Let them praise the name of the Lord, For His name alone is exalted; His glory is above earth and heaven."

Psalm 99:3 "Let them praise Your great and awesome name; Holy is He."

Matthew 18:20 "For where two or three have gathered together in My name, I am there in their midst."

Ramsis Ghaly

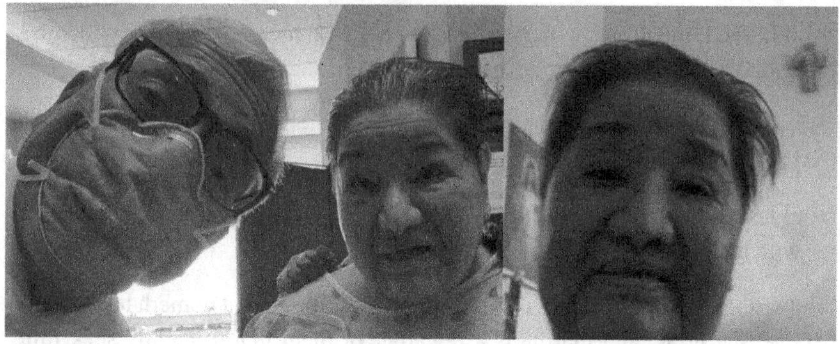

BC, God bless

JG, Praying for this sweet lady! We know the Lord is still doing miracles! Blessings

KE, All things are possible with God. Praying she be miraculously healed by our Lord Jesus Christ! Amen!!!

RM, Praying

DL, Praying for a miracle for this sweet angel, Dr Ghaly. You did your best, let God do the rest ! prayer warriors do your thing !

Heavy is your heart and your gift through God to heal It is Gods destiny of the outcome You are a vessel of his miracles What will be will be. God bless you for your faith, gift and strength May the lord bless you as your heart is truly compassionate

DS, Heavy is your heart and your gift through God to heal It is Gods destiny of the outcome You are a vessel of his miracles What will be will be. God bless you for your faith, gift and strength May the lord bless you as your heart is truly compassionate

DB, Praying for her!

LM, Sending prayers

JT, Breaks my heart! Nothing is impossible with Jesus! I speak life and health and mobility over her! Do a miracle Lord!

AMEN! ALL THINGS ARE POSSIBLE WITH GOD, IN HIS NAME, GREAT ARE PRAYERS ANSWERED WHEN 2 OR MORE GATHER TOGETHER,, LORD GOD PLEASE HEAL THIS WOMAN OF FAITH AND DR. GHALY, SAY IT, BELIEVE IT, HIS WILL BE DONE! Those of the Faith of...

VG, Prayers

CR, This breaks my heart

JM, Our Lord is able, nothing is to hard for Him.

ED, You did your very best Doctor. Prayers for you and this Angel.

LSA, Everything is still possible to God, when we are praying

MD, Prayers

RL, Prayers for your sweet patient and her family. I pray for her comfort of mind and body.

And prayers for you and your comfort in knowing God is in control.and His will be done. May He bring you insight and comfort.

RC, Matthew 18:19 ASV

Again I say unto you, that if two of you shall agree on earth as touching anything that they shall ask, it shall be done for them of my Father who is in heaven.

CR, Only Jesus

DW, Prayers for your patient and for you.

MB, Praying, thank you for posting the powerful scriptures.

LK, Let's pray for a miracle!

MM, Amen to the word of God prayers for God will to be done in her life.

LB, You have our Fathers Eyes"!

GM, Heart breaking so sad

SM, Praying hard.

JP, Sending healing prayers

KO, Prayers ongoing

KM, Praying for complete healing in Jesus name. Amen.

RC, Praying for her tonight!

TA, Prayers

DM, Prayers going up blessings coming down

MJ, You're in our prayers. May

DG, Prayers for your dear patient to be miraculously healed by one touch or one word from Jesus. May His will be done on earth as it is in Heaven. Also prayers for your tender heart Dr.Ghaly. May you feel the peace of God. All prayers said in the name of Jesus!

DM, My prayers for you and your patients i know you always do your best.but ItsGod only God,like what you said can make it happen

GH, Prayers said for this dear patient and you Dr Ghaly. Thank you for the scriptures. Some of my favorites and my deceased moms favorite verses. Have a blessed day.

DU, Praying...

RC, Pray for she first and for all who need all the lord's blessings

LM, Prayers. Thy will be done.

CC, Please dear God hear our prayers and bless her with a miracle

BM, Praying for a Super Natural Miracle, in Jesus name

GV, Ow almighty Lord Jesus heal my friend Virginia bless her, gave more years to live, gave her a miracle to walk again, amen .

JH, Prayers

JK, Prayers..

AN, In the precious, Holy Name of Jesus, I pray for complete healing!!!

MM, Praying for her healing,Almighty God I trust in you,I hope she will get her miracle just like I did.Dr. Ghaly you **you're the best** GodBless

CR, You are doing your best my dear doctor. Praying for her.

BD, OMG,. So beautiful, this made me cry too

DK, Praying in agreement with other believers for her full miraculous healing in the name of my precious Lord and Savior,Jesus.

She's a beautiful soul. She has the best, you Doctor and our almighty God. I will be praying for both of you. God's miracles happen everyday. I will be praying for this one to happen.

CL, Thank you for your continued dedication Doctor. You have surely earned your wings.

KG, Prayers and Healing in Jesus Name. Lord, we say to you, from the Holy Land in Egypt, we beseech Saint Spyridon, Miracle Worker from God, Please Intercede and bring healing to our sister in Christ. And it is done. God Bless you. **Xoxo**

MS, Thank you for explaining so much. Yes, I will pray for this dear lady.

TM Both of you are in my prayers, dear Ramsis. Heartbreaking

DH, Sarah Cooper-Young AMEN! ALL THINGS ARE POSSIBLE WITH GOD, IN HIS NAME, GREAT ARE PRAYERS ANSWERED WHEN 2 OR MORE GATHER TOGETHER,, LORD GOD PLEASE HEAL THIS WOMAN OF FAITH AND DR. GHALY, SAY IT, BELIEVE IT, HIS WILL BE DONE! Those of the Faith of...

FA, Prayers sent

AP, So heart breaking to hear this I will pray for this dear lady

CR, Would it be possible to have her first name so we can pray for her by name? I understand if you can't. I put it up on my Prayer Warrior list. Jehovah Raffah, The God who Heals.

KP, Prayers

In her way to Renown Rehabilitation Center!!

Our Miracle Angel is getting slowly better!! Hallelujah! She showing the world a miracle. Praise our Lord Jesus and you all you prayers and support.

I am Much blessed to care for an American hero as her served as a dedicated phenomenal nurse to care for the indigenous of Chicago at cook county hospital in 1970's and 80's and American warriors and causalities at VA Veterans hospitals all her life!!

Look at her smile and hope and extreme faith in our Lord Jesus! Amen in His Name, any little progress and little recovery is a great deal when you talk about complete paralysis in a patient in dire need of any neurological recovery even if it appears too late or impossible!

She is in her way to a renowned Rehabilitation Center!! Best of wishes.

https://www.facebook.com/1150861349/posts/10228975759435965/?d=n

Ramsis Ghaly

Www.ghalyneurosurgeon.comRamsis Ghaly

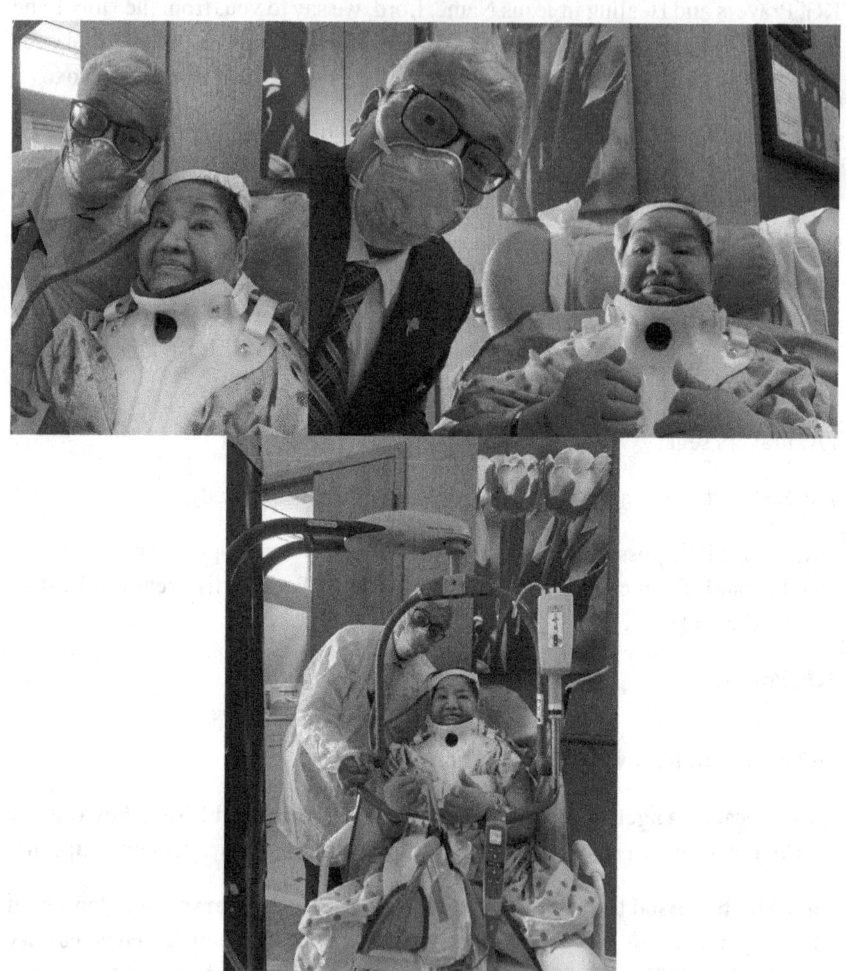

SY, Praise the Lord!

JT, our prayers are being heard!

PH, Thank you Dr. Ghaly, and thank you to her for her service also. And great thanks to our Lord!!

SJ, Praise God

KO, Ongoing prayers fantastic Dr Ghaly thank you Lord

SL, Still praying for this angel

JG, Amen! Prayers for healing!!!

KE, Hallelujah JESUS IS OUR HEALER!

KC, Great news!

JS, GOD BLESS HER in her recovery

AU, Praise in the name of Jesus!

AV Praise God! & Thank you Dr Ghaly!!

DH, Prayers for this Angel for overwhelming healing. Glory to God, Thanks be to Dr. Ghaly

GE, KP, Praying

LA, Thank you Lord, you hear our prayers

KP, Prayers for a speedy recovery

RM, God bless you

AL, Amén

AB, Praise God

DL, The best Doctor ever. I would fly across the world for you. May God continue to bless her and you Dr. **Ramsis Ghaly**.

JS, This is great news!

AN, I knew it!

MD, Prayers

BM, Thank for your Service! Praying for a speedy recovery

DL, Jesus hears our prayers for this Angel ! Godspeed !

JD, Glory be to God! Thank you Jesus!

CL, God bless you. Praying for a speedy recovery.

DN, Thank you Jesus

MS, You bring me closer to Our Lord Jesus with your faith. Thank you.

Jp, Sending healing prayers

Afte long journey to death 💀, Virginia life was restored after my surgery on July!!

Ramsis Ghaly

She made it with grace of Lord Jesus not only new lease on life but also going home sweet home after almost 5 months away!

What so strange but common in my practice, she referred herself as a word of mouth otherwise she was two weeks maximum to die the severe death!!

Virginia and her fantastic children by her side fought the good fight despite all the odds even in her age above 80's!!

Lord Jesus always looks after her children even if we all failed her!!! Amen praise Lord Jesus.

Look at her smile and appreciation!! She was so kind to bring me a bottle of wine!!! Thank you . Much love and blessing!!

Speed recovery and congratulations!!

Www.ghalyneurosurgeon.com

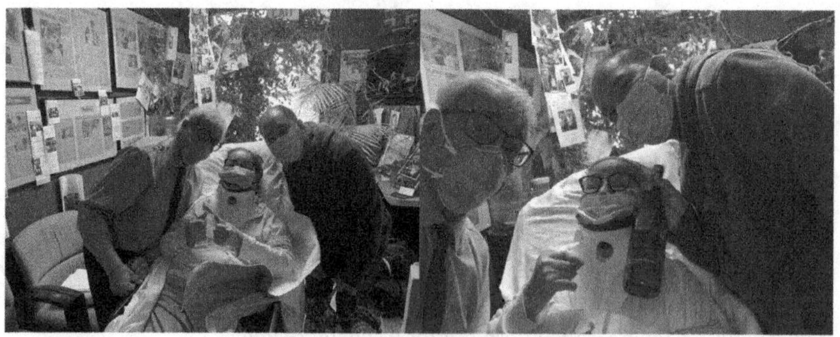

DE, What a true blessing

CR, So so beautiful Dr **Ramsis Ghaly**

JK, Dr. Your hands & mind is threw are lords guidance's, your a great dr. Bless you & all you help heal threw there healing journey!!

P.S: am i still on your wall of gods grace?? In your office??

MA, I remember you also had the newspaper clippings of when you take took care of my brother, Jorge Salas Sr. He passed now, but at that time we owed you his life. Forever grateful to you and God's hands that guided yours.

TF, Awesome

DH, Praise God and your healing thru Jesus Christ Dr Ghaly

DK, God given talent,skill and compassion!! May God bless you as you bless others!

RM, Outstanding Dr Ghaly

EL, Dr. Ghaly - you are an amazing man. God gave you a wonderful gift!! He is working through you!!

RC, God is manifesting thougt you. Blessings of gif!

Td,God Bless you Dr. Ghaly!

Jm, God Bless "**CONGRATULATIONS**"

Kb, God bless congratulations.

SJ, Praise God for working through you, Dr. Ghaly

JS, GOD bless her with a healthy recovery

CG, How wonderful! What a blessing. Wishing her a continued success in her recovery.

DL, You are AMAZING !

AV, Praise God!! Thank you Dr Ghaly!!

HG, You and Jesus are the most amazing team Dr Ghaly!!

Our Miracle Patient from complete paralysis four months ago due to advanced spinal cord injury and look at her today how much she had gained and recovered. We pray for more recovery!

Look and see how Our Lord Jesus healing three months after surgery. Virginia has been recovering at home with her dedicated family! Her two sons are always at her bedside full service! What a dedicated children giving the difficult times our children going through!

Let us continue to pray for Virginia recovery!

Virginia is our Thanksgiving and our joy!

Ramsis Ghaly

Www.ghalyneurosurgeon.com

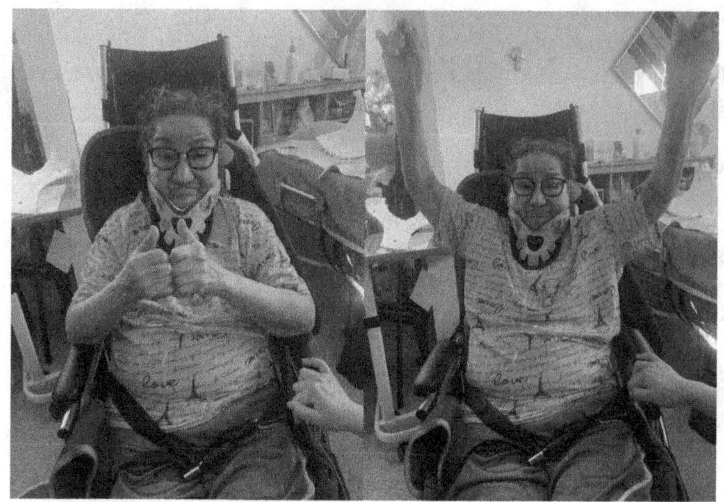

JS, Congratulations. May ur body heal by leaps & bounds

CG, My thoughts and prayers are with you as you continue on your road to recovery.

CC, A miracle. Thank you Jesus!

We Need You! A Real Story, a Mother Saving her Paralyzed Daughter!

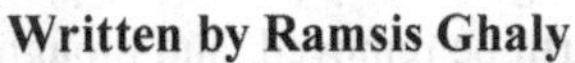

Written by Ramsis Ghaly

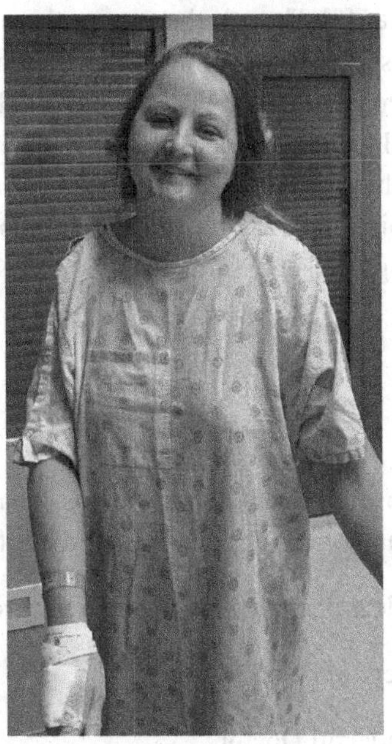

A mother called yesterday and demanded for me to see her disabled daughter suffering for two month unable to walk. I called back, she couldn't talk in church and send me a text "we need you". They couldn't find help heads hitting the walls but their visit to church open the eyes!!

I called and said why should I see a patient that has no neurosurgery problem!! The mom cried and was persistent! My heart moved and my spirit ached!

It was touching. The story was painful and the fries were so loud! The daughter was in and out the hospital losing her legs in horrific pains and unable to walk screams day and night, yet the hospital discharged a crippled patient with no diagnosis and no help——.

I saw her today! I was in tears just looking at this young lady! No one to go to but my God to open my eyes! And her prayers to find the diagnosis was revealed!! And she is in her way to downtown for further care she urgently needed for two months!!!

Let start a chain of prayers!!! Please pray for the special daughter speed recovery and next steps of the care she deserved! We pray isn't late!!!

Lord Jesus in control and us our Refuge when in trouble!!

"God is our refuge and strength, a very present help in trouble. [2] Therefore will not we fear, though the earth be removed, and though the mountains be carried into the midst of the sea; [3] Though the waters thereof roar and be troubled, though the mountains shake with the swelling thereof. Selah. [4] There is a river, the streams whereof shall make glad the city of God, the holy place of the tabernacles of the most High. [5] God is in the midst of her; she shall not be moved: God shall help her, and that right early. [6] The heathen raged, the kingdoms were moved: he uttered his voice, the earth melted. [7] The Lord of hosts is with us; the God of Jacob is our refuge. Selah."Psalm 46

We pray in Jesus Name! Amen

Ramsis Ghaly

jd, Shame on the bad hospitals and bad physicians. Thank you Heavenly Father for giving us Ramsis Ghaly! praying for Gwen and her family.

GM, This is my sissy, please help her we are all heartbroken!!!

KO, Many prayers for her are being said

MK, God bless this wonderful Doctor.

Believing your treatment and Jesus for a complete healing. Thank you for helping Gwen and this wonderful post.

CG, God bless you, thank God you are able to help!

JS, Praying for Gwen

MA, prayers for Gwen

KK, Kristen Robert Kirkland

DF, Prayers

KG, In Jesus Name we Pray. Thank you, Dr Ramsis Ghaly for all you do. You are a wondrous inspiration to the whole world and a Beautiful Gift from God to All. GOD BLESS YOU ALWAYS. Love from Egypt

RC, Pray for speed recovery. You are a magnificent doctor!

MS, Praying.

CR, Very touching you are in gods hands Dr Ghaly is a true Angel on this earth!

BM, So glad you were able to help her! Praise God and God Bless you always

CF, Well Judy you took her to the right Dr. Prayers for a speedy recovery

CB, Praying

DL, God bless you

CG, Praying for her to get the care she needs.

You are a true blessing

EH, Praying in Jesus name for her

DL, Amen

LW, Dear Ramsis, You are a miracle worker!!

LA, Joining all others in praying for Gwen's speedy recovery and continued success in her rehab.

DH, Praying for Gwen and her family. God is Powerful, Asking for God's healing Love and you Dr Ghaly. to help her!

TG, Thank Gd for you dear doctor!

LF. Father you lead. You already have the answer. Touch everyone here we pray in Jesus's Name.

JI, Amen

DE, Amen

AV, Thank you Dr Ghaly for seeing this patient!!GBYD and I will pray for this sweet young girl!!

WP, Yes we do!

JK, Prayers for fast recovery...

What are diagnosis doctor Ramsis Ghaly?

The reason l am asking, bc l have similar problem now....

YH, Prayers

RFFAMILY UPDATES PRIOR TO SURGERY

Update on Gwen.

First off, Gwen isn't doing so well. However, she does have a team of specialists working with her. She is in a lot of pain, has a hard time breathing and can't walk without assistance. Due to all the meds she's on, she sleeps very little and has a hard time reading and remembering things. So, she hasn't been able to read and reply to all her messages. She's asked me to tell everyone that she appreciates all the texts, messages and well wishes and that she loves all of you. It's going to be a long journey before she is herself again, therefore she won't be on Facebook and the such often. Just please continue to pray for her and keep her in your thoughts.

I will periodically post on Facebook to try and keep everyone informed on her fight with all these symptoms which thus far includes;

Osteoporosis, hashimotos thyroiditis, pulmonary fibrosis, pulmonary sarcoidosis, interstitial lung disease (with 51% lung capacity), scoliosis,

peripheral neuropathy, peripheral disc bulges L1-L5, with encroachment at right L4 nerve root.

It's a lot to take in, and very overwhelming for her, but she's fighting a good fight and trying to be positive and placing all this in Gods hands. Thankfully she also has a loving family that she can depend on to be with her when I can't be.

I also want to thank everyone for all the support that you've given her through this difficult time. It raises her spirits and gives her something to look forward to.

Thanks again and have a good day

Back here to see Gwen

She is STILL in pain all over. She says it feels like the pain is coming from all her bones.

Getting a bone scan in a couple hours, and her white blood cell count is elevated.

I still think half of all this is from the prednisone. Nasty steroid.

Back up here, hoping SOMETHING is going to get done for Gwen today. So far it's just been hurry up and wait. She still can't walk on her own and and isn't feeling very well. Not even sure if they're going to look into her back, which obviously needs to be addressed.

Not impressed by this place so far.

After being in a hospital, 11? days in about 3 weeks, Gwen is finally getting surgery this Friday morning at North Western Central DuPage hospital. Apparently the tumor is pressing against her spinal cord and needs to be removed. How the others missed it is beyond me. It is a risky procedure as you can imagine, and will take several hours along with weeks of therapy. Hopefully she'll be back home by Monday. She is in a lot of pain at times and most of the time unable to walk on her own even with a walker. Sleep also is quite a challenge with the pain and stiffness.

Please continue to keep her in your thoughts and prayers. I'll keep everyone posted.

Thanks.

CG:

Update on my mom… (long post below)

After being in and out of the hospital the last couple weeks and progressively getting worse without many answers. A surgeon hopefully has found the reason why she's been in excruciating pain and why she can hardly walk with a Walker and some days not able to walk at all… He found a mass that's pressing on her spinal cord and causing her to become potentially paralyzed so he will be performing surgery tomorrow morning to remove it. With that being said this surgery is dangerous not only because it could also paralyze her but as well with the state of her lungs it makes going under anesthesia dangerous. We're all hoping and praying that is what my mom needs and that the surgery will be successful without complications. Its hard for us to not have so many mixed emotions and worry about our mom when all of this happened so quickly. On my birthday last month my mom took me shopping and to dinner as if everything was normal besides her having shortness of breath, getting around a little slower than normal and experiencing pain in her legs. To the next day being admitted into the hospital getting released 4 days later then ending right back into the hospital 10 times worse… One minute things seem okay and like she's getting better then the next she can't talk because she's in so much pain. It's hard to understand why all of this is happening to her when she's the most caring and loving person I know but my mom is so strong, she will get through this and come out on top!

All of us girls (her daughters) have been with her as much as we can be with all of us having kids we can't be there as much as we'd like to be. Thankfully my grandma has been by her side every single day doing all that she can to help my mom from taking her to all of her appointments (sometimes multiple in one day) to sitting in the hospital waiting for a room for 10+ hours all 3 of the times she went, to cooking/cleaning and overall just going above and beyond for her daughter while also having her own health struggles and being worn out. Judy Johnson Kladis we can't thank you enough for all that you do for ALL of us, your amazing and we love you more than you'll ever know

Gwen L Favero even though I can't physically be at your surgery just know I'm there with you and im thinking of you wishing I was there! You have a mom, 4 girls and 10 grand babies that all love you most

Prayers for surgery to go as planned and for a good recovery would be greatly appreciated! Also to any of my moms friends that want updates on my mom feel free to message us.

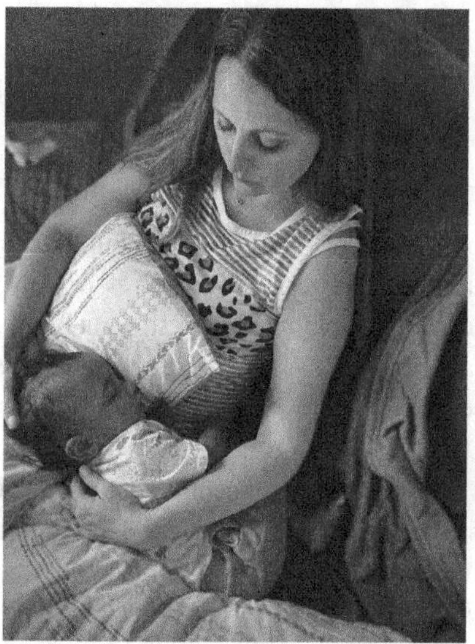

Well. It's surgery day for Gwen.

Please keep her in your prayers. She'll be in surgery for several hours and staying here for a few days. Step one to getting her better

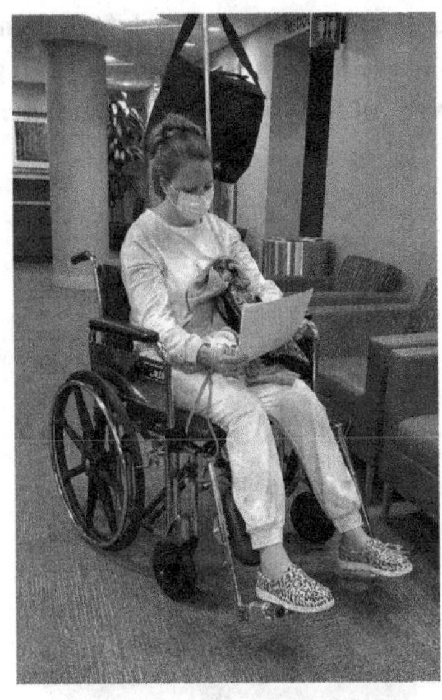

Thank you everyone

Rob will update on here as he hears from Dr. Should have updates every 2 hours

Should be going in to surgery soon

God has Me, and I know He has a Plan For Me!

Love you All More!!!!

everyone please pray for my mom as she goes under a very risky surgery today I love you momma, and I know you'll be just fine Gwen L Favero

RF: The doctor successfully removed the mass from Gwens **back!**

CF: I just spoke to my mom on the phone and she is doing much better! When she first got out of surgery she was in a ton of pain and the drs had to sedate her to ease her pain. She has to stay in the ICU tonight but hearing her voice and hearing her excitement when she told me that for the first time in awhile she was able to feel her feet was exactly what I needed to hear! I've been all over the place today with my emotions but now I finally feel at peace🩶 I will give another update when I go see her tomorrow. Thank you all for your thoughts and prayers, it means a lot to all of us!

My mom was just moved into a regular room! She was able to take 9 steps this morning but dr wants her to stay flat in her bed today and rest before they

push her hard tomorrow so that she's on track to go home Monday with home health. As hard as it is to see her in pain I know it's all going to be worth it in the end. Again thank you all for your thoughts and prayers!

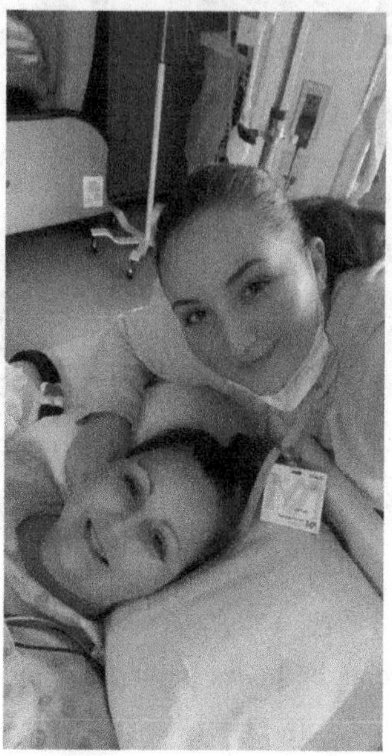

Gwen is Cured and Healed! Hallelujah!

Written by Ramsis Ghaly

Gwen is Cured and Healed! Hallelujah! Mom is back in her feet and God heard her crying and all your prayers!! We aren't worthy of our Lord love and mercy. Our Savior is gracious!

"This I recall to my mind, therefore I have hope. The Lord's lovingkindnesses indeed never cease, for His compassions never fail. They are new every morning; great is Your faithfulness."

Lamentations 3:21-23

What a true miracle, our Lord Jesus heal our angel from the keg paralysis and horrific pains, tears and cries fir three month. Just hours after the surgery, here is our miracle Gwen L Favero**! Gwen has her life back!! Her smile and joy forever!!!**

Many institutions and doctors have failed her and some thoughts weird diagnosis, yet Gwen believed in herself together with her family. Going in and out hospitals with no answer.

And in faith, she is healed with new lease in life. The surgery was so delicate and risky but His hands had made it easy!!!

Gwen is Cured and Healed! Hallelujah! Mom is back in her feet and God heard her crying and all your prayers!!

Medicine without Faith is empty and limited. In faith in our Lord, all things are possible as He said: Matthew 19:26 KJV "But Jesus beheld them, and said unto them, With men this is impossible; but with God all things are possible."

No computerized textbook available for each patient, but only through HANDS ON, caring thoughtful humble sincere patience and perseverance with skill, experience and knowledge in faith provide the best living textbook for that patient!

Thank you all for your prayers and trust and praise our true Healer, always Lord Jesus!

Psalm 124 "If it had not been the Lord who was on our side, now may Israel say; [2] If it had not been the Lord who was on our side, when men rose up against us: [3] Then they had swallowed us up quick, when their wrath was kindled against us: [4] Then the waters had overwhelmed us, the stream had gone over our soul: [5] Then the proud waters had gone over our soul. [6] Blessed be the Lord, who hath not given us as a prey to their teeth. [7] Our soul is escaped as a bird out of the snare of the fowlers: the snare is broken, and we are escaped. [8] Our help is in the name of the Lord, who made heaven and earth."

Ramsis Ghaly

Www.ghalyneurosurgeon.com

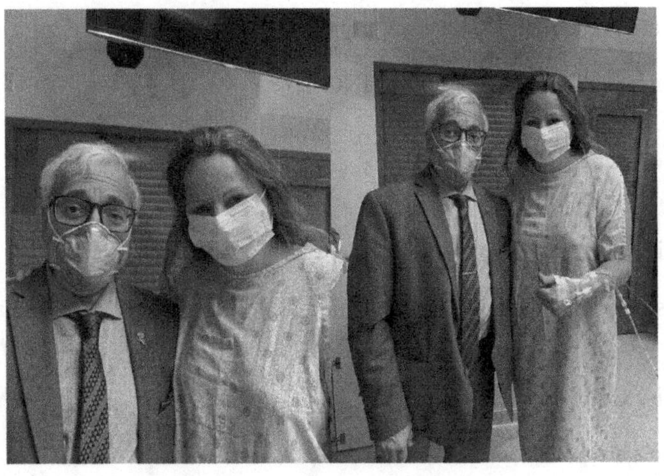

JK, Praise God !!!

CK, God be all the Glory, thank you Dr. Ghaly for your faith and skill in Jesus name

What a great, Dr. Ramsis Ghaly . Thank you from the bottom of my heart I'm so glad to have you as Gwen's Dr.

CK, This was our song of hope throughout this time and yes He heard our cry! AMEN

BN, Amen. Thank you for all you do Dr. Ramsis Ghaly . Thank you for taking such humble pride in healing others. It's people like you that make the difference. You're a blessing.

AS, Praise God now praying for you complete healing.

WJ, Great news

DC, Thank you my friend, God gave you the ability to help other and you are every patient's blessing.

LC, This post certainly made my day. Thank you Dr. Ghaly for helping my friend. Thank you God for guiding Dr. Ghaly's hands.

MS, Hallelujah! God is good.

PB, Praise You Lord, thank you Jesus!!!

MK, Thank you Jesus! God is so good. All the time.

VW, GOD IS GOOD! So happy for you Gwen and your loved ones

SE, We are rejoicing!!! Praise almighty God!!!

CL, Praise the Lord! This is AMAZING news!

EH, Praise the Lord

TD, Yes!!!!!!!

KT, Praise The Lord!!

TJ, Praise God! Hallelujah! Only By God's Grace, Love, and Mercy! Thank You God!

ER, Praise God!!

We serve a awesome God

Amen and Amen

RC, With faith everything is posible!

LB, Thank you Lord for the healing of Gwen through lord Gwen's dr were able to heal her aling body. You are the Lord jesus through all things are possible

ES, God-bless you Doctor Ghaly for all you do. The Lord has given you a wonderful gift.

CT, Thank you god and thank you dr Ramsis Ghaly

LP, Praise The Lord!! God Is Faithful!! Thank you Dr Ghaly for allowing God to use you!!

PP, Praise the Lord! God bless you Dr. Ghaly for all you do and allowing God to work thru you.

CR, You are an amazing physician! Thank you for healing my dear friend Gwen!

CO, What great news!!!

DL, All Glory be to God ! Amen

DH, Amen! Praise God!

HM, Praise God for His goodness

DN, Thank you Dr. Ghaly and thank you God for healing Gwen

GK, Glad you're feeling better and everything went well

JS, Thank You Lord

LJ, Miracles STILL HAPPEN!

Prayers STILL WORK!

DR, Thank you God

CL, God bless her. She's so blessed to have you as a Surgeon.

What a Touching Story and a Living Testimony of Our Savior Continue to Do Miracles on Earth for Those Who Believe in Him!

Ramsis Ghaly

He came at night while all were sleep and touched her and she was healed!!

Isn't our Lord Jesus Gracious, merciful and full of love and kindness??

Isn't our Lord Jesus is the Living Almighty the Savior of the world and the Only capable to raise those crippled in wheelchair and let them back in their feet healed wholeheartedly??

Early morning after major delicate surgery, Gwen standing and looking for the breakfast menu, it is her very first time to feel normal and hungry. She hadn't have any appetite for months and has Berlin in horrific pains drugged up and sick to her stomach!

As expected with all the useless dangerous medications and wrong diagnoses, she was lost miserable ready to kiss the death bed!!! Never she had such a smile for a year!

Yet with the grace of God, she is full of hope, looking for life worth living rejoicing with the Lord of hosts that because of his kindness extended His holy hand and healed from wheelchair to run!!

Gwen is singing to Lord saying; Psalm 23 "The Lord is my shepherd; I shall not want. [2] He maketh me to lie down in green pastures: he leadeth me beside the still waters. [3] He restoreth my soul: he leadeth me in the paths of righteousness for his name's sake. [4] Yea, though I walk through the valley of the shadow of death, I will fear no evil: for thou art with me; thy rod and thy staff they comfort me. [5] Thou preparest a table before me in the presence of mine enemies: thou anointest my head with oil; my cup runneth over. [6] Surely goodness and mercy shall follow me all the days of my life: and I will dwell in the house of the Lord for ever."

Www.ghalyneurosurgeon.com

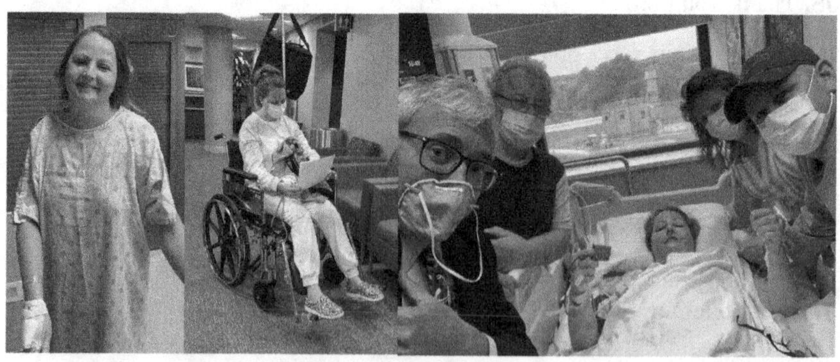

JK, That's what my God can do,just believe.

GM, Praise God. So happy for you all.

DC, Amazing!

MA, Praise God! Dr. Ghaly is his hands!

JD, We ask in faith for nothing less than this Praise God

MK, So excited for you Gwen. Thank you Jesus. Love you

WJ, That smile says it all

AV, Praise God for His Blessings!!

DK, Love this so happy all went well!!!! Our lord is a great lord

BC, Great to see that smile!!

RJ, PTL!!! Isn't He Wonderful!!

Love you Qwen !!!

MS, Praise God!!

MB, Praise the Lord

DL Amen !

DS, Praise God!!

JT, amen...

LP, Awesome awesome!!

NH, Amen thank you lord

TJ, Continued prayers!

KH, Amen. God is good. Love you.

MJ, Thank the Lord

JV, Continued prayers

LB, Congratulations

all the prayers is healing God was listening

JP, Praise God

GS, Amen thank you Lord!

CK, Dr. Ghaly thank you again for your servant attitude. You are an inspiration to us all..God has blessed you and will continue as you partner with the Devine Healer...Jesus!

KB, Thank you Lord.

DK, Praise God and I thank him for the healing gift and talents he has given you!!

LW, Thank God…and you!

RH, Miracles every Day in so many ways praise God

LJ, Thanks be to Our Lord and Savior for putting His People in place to serve Him.

Ramsis Ghaly is one of those servants that through Jesus is performing miracles that no one thinks are possible, but God knows they are. I stand in awe of God's will and know that He does hear the prayers of His People. I will forever praise Him for his good works unto us.

Glory be to God in the highest.

LM, This makes my heart so happy!!! Love you all! Paise the Lord

DF, Praise the Lord

MK, I'm doing a happy dance.

GV, Makes me so happy

BB, **CONGRATULATIONS**

GWEN keep it up prayers for you and family and friends

TJ, God is good!

LO, Awesome

SK, I am so happy for Gwen and all her beautiful girl!!! This is awesome news!!!!

BP, Praise the Lord!

NH, Great, prayers for a speedy recovery.

VJ, Thank the Lord!!

AG, Yay! What a relief! Was thinking about her all day! Lit my candle

And it burned all day

PH, This is Amazing!!!! So glad to see she is up and moving. Gwen here is to many years of happiness your way.

DA, Wonderful ⚘. Prayers for a speedy recovery.

AM, That is awesome!

TM, She has a great doctor. Glad Gwen doing better.

JM, Awesome news!!!

TG, Great news!! Praying for continued healing!

RC, Thank you Lord Jesus! So happy to see this! Big ((Hugs))

LR, God is so good !!!! Continue praying for complete healing ! Hugs !!!! God we thank you and praise You ! Use this for your glory

RS, Wonderful news!! Glad to hear

AM, Just amazing praying for a speedy recovery.

TM, This is the best news!

JD, We have been praying for nothing less than this fantastic to hear

BH, **Jeffrey DeBoard** praise God!

MG, Good to see her on her feet. Glad the surgery was a success!

TL, Thomas Lepper

Great news still praying for a speedy successful recovery

JS, Amazing!!

LJ, Great news, prayers for speedy recovery

RR, So glad for you God is the greatest

LP, Praise Jesus for answered prayers Will continue to pray for her whole body to be healed

TZ, Roman's 8:18.....For I consider the suffering of this present time is not worth comparing to the glory about to be revealed to us. Amen. We're continuing to pray for you **Gwen**

JW, Awesome news

TN, Great news

LK, So, so happy for you. The greatest thing news Ive heard today.

AK, Great news! Rock that recovery.

BA, Great news

SC, I'm so happy she's better now!!

Thank you a lord Jesus? Who will dare to deny that Gwen is a true 2022 Miracle ftom GOD!

In two days after major complex surgery, Gwen is going home with no assisted device, no pain, able to walk with good strength in no major medications.

And soon Gwen is going back to work and absolutely turning her back from the past and she shall be even more angelic and wonderful than ever before after the horrific illness journey!!

Thank you all for you prayers and speed recovery. Home sweet home ! Praise our Lord! Amen

Ramsis Ghaly

Www.ghalyneurosurgeon.com

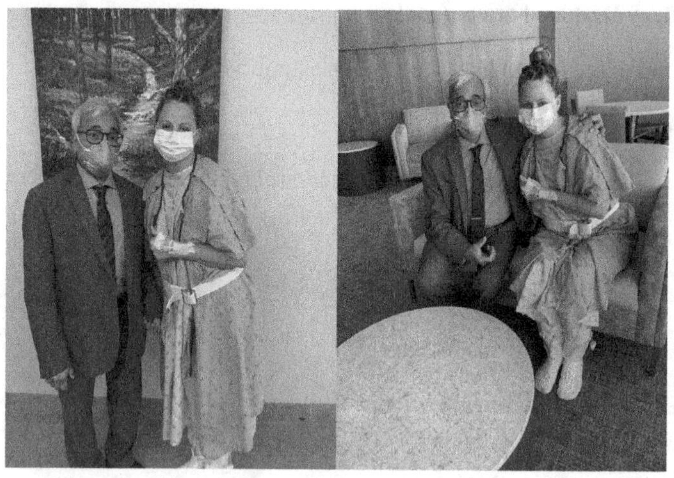

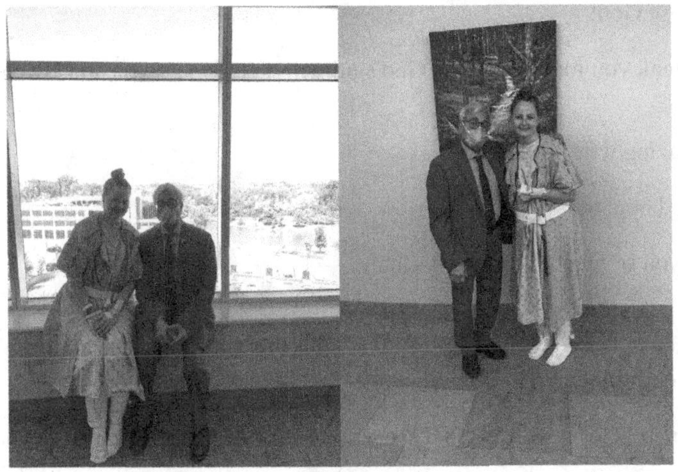

GF, There are no words to thank you enough for saving me from becoming crippled Dr. Ramsis Ghaly I'm so thankful for you and that you allow God to use you to save people's lives!!! You will forever have a special place in my heart!!! God bless you!!!!

DC, Gwen L Favero he truly has been a Miracle Worker to so many.

KK, That is awesome news. Awesome

NH, God's love is endless.

AO, Amazing!!! This is the best news ever!

ML, So happy to see this.

L, Praise The Lord

DF, He's the best !!

CT, Praise Jesus and Dr. Ramsis Ghaly

JS, PRAISE GOD for giving you the knowledge to work the unthinkable. Dr Ghaly, your mind and KG, Speedy recovery to Gwen and God's Blessings. Thank God for Dr Ghaly.

CK, PRAISE THE LORD

CM, This makes me beyond happy !

DK, thank you Jesus and Dr Ghaly!!

DN, Thank you god and Dr. For healing Gwen

TJ, Praise God!

MS, Thank you for showing us God's miracles. God bless you and Gwen.

My amazing wife, Gwen.

Coming home today

Thank you so much Dr. Ramsis Ghaly.

TZ Amen. Glad you guys will be home, together, this has been a huge blessing. We're continuing to pray for you guys.

KN, Amen!! God is good!! Glad everything is going so well!! Loves to you both!!

JW, Glad to hear this wonderful news

TJ, Awesome news!!!!!!

AH, Incredible new, **congrats**

JC, That is wonderful news!!

RP, That's just wonderful!!

LH, Yay!!!!

AH, WTG Gwen.

LP, Answered prayers there's no place like home

LR, God is so good !!!! Sending big hugs !!!!!!!

RR, Amen!!

LH, That is awesome.

JG, Wonderful news!!

DG, Thats AWESOME...

DS, Glad to hear that there's no place like home!!

JD, Outstanding

AM, Great news that's Awesome.

AB, What wonderful news!

MR, Good to hear!

AK, Take great care of her **Robert**! Wonderful news for all.

SH, Amen

LP, Speedy recovery Gwen!!!

MR, Such wonderful news! God answers!

PJ, awesome!!

PZ, So happy for you both speedy recovery prayers

RAMSIS GHALY: THANK YOU Much much blessing. Speed recovery. So touched with your humility endurance and strength. We pray

Gwen L Favero is feeling thankful.

I just wanted to give an update about the tumor I don't think anyone had updated about it. Dr. Ghaly said if you have a tumor this the kind you would want to have, because it's benign...thank God!!! It's called a Schwannoma tumor of the spine. Before surgery we weren't sure if the tumor was related to my Sarcoidosis or if it was something else now we know. I somehow had two unrelated rare issues going on in my body at the same time. I will not sit around and say why me... because you know what....why not me?! I'm just like everyone else, and anything can happen at anytime to any of us! As I sit here and think of it all I'm just so very thankful to Dr. Ramsis Ghaly before he did surgery I didn't know if I would ever walk or walk normal again or even feel my feet or legs!!! He listened to me, did the correct testing, and allowed God to use his hands to fix me, and I'll forever be so grateful!!!! I'm praising God that the surgery went as perfect as it possibly could have went, and believing that my recovery will go just as well!!!! Thank you Everyone for everything I cannot say enough about how much love I have felt through all of this

SD, So happy you're home and on the mend! Love you!

AS, I'm so happy you went to Dr Ghaly. He is such a special gift from God who takes the best care of his patients. So glad you are feeling better! me too Allie!! You are one of the reasons I trusted him so much!!! Thank you!!!

GF, that makes my heart so happy. You have had a hell of a year but have approached it with such grace. You are a fighter who will get thru!

KR, So glad you are home now and praying for speedy recovery

GF, Thanks Uncle Keith I love you bunches!!!

RB, Best news ever!! So very happy for you!!

SW, So happy for you Gwen!!

EM, So happy you're healed! Thank God! Stay blessed beautiful lady

KM, So happy to hear!! I hope you're recovering quickly and well!

MG, So happy that this tumor was benign. Glad you are on the road to recovery.

CK, Well spoken, I'm so proud of you for the Woman you've become. I love you and am so proud you call me Dad! thanks Dad!!! Have a great time in your trip you deserve it!!! I love you!!!!

CP, Glad to hear your home and everything went well many prayers to you

CO, Great news and so happy you're on the mend!!

AM. Good news glad your home.

SH, So so happy for you and more prayers and hugs for a speedy recovery and enjoy the summer…

TZ, God is everything every day. We'll continue praying for your recovery.

LC, That news really made my day. If anyone could remove that tumor with no other problems, it's Dr. Ghaly. Continuing prayers, because you are certainly proof the power of prayer works.

TD, So glad you found Dr Ghaly

TJ, So Thankful for God to use you to show your Faith, Strength, Love, Compassion. Also thankful you got a Doctor who believes in God and that God is using him to fix and heal people thru his hands. Love you **Gwen L Favero** and I'm truly happy for you. God …

CT, God bless you my friend love you and miss you!

VW, That is the bestest new Gwen!!! So happy for you!

EL, am glad to here your surgery went well. Hope you are feeling better each day.

CP, Thank God. Praying for your ongoing recovery

TJ, I'm so glad to hear the great news! Love you and may. You have a speedy recovery!

BH, You are amazing. Keep healing sister!! Love ya. YAY!!!! That will make my day

At the miracle workers office

0:04 / 1:51

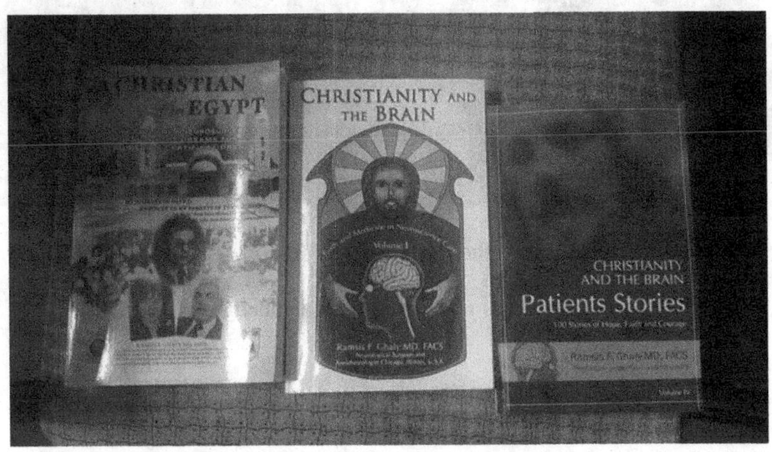

Lynda Welch Christensen

He certainly is. All of the articles are so fascinating.

Ramsis Ghaly

What an honor to be your neurosurgeon. Amen to the grace of our Lord and His healing hand to His children. Through our Lord Jesus all are possible. Thank you

Gwen L Favero

Ramsis Ghaly I'll never be able to thank you enough much love Dr. ! All honor and Glory to God for using your hands to do such an incredibly delicate surgery!!!

Sh, Awesome

First clinic visit three weeks later

Our shining star Gwen L Favero visit after the surgery with her husband Robert W Favero. Hallelujah praise our lord Jesus.

Lovely couple. We pray for Speed recovery

Ramsis Ghaly

Www.ghalyneurosurgeon.com

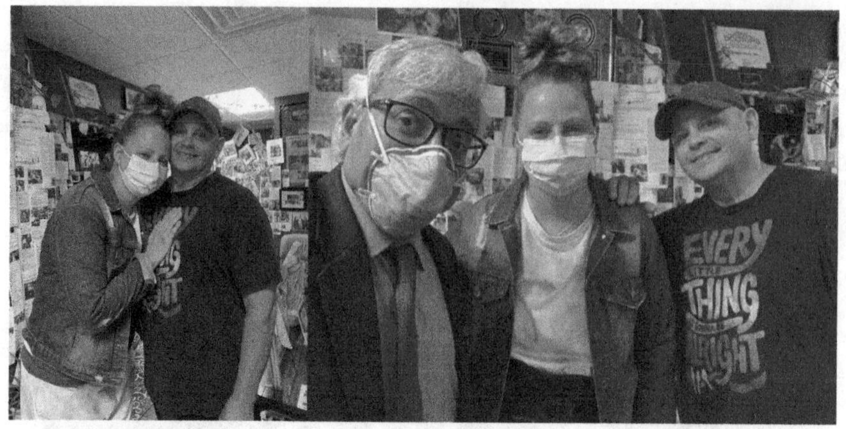

Kg, Hallelujah, Gwen! Praise the Lord. Speedy Recovery and Blessings.

Pp, Praise the Lord! God Bless you Gwen with a speedy recovery!

Jm, AMEN !

Cr, My beautiful friend! My favorite doctor! What a blessing!

Am, Amen life is good.

Up, Praise The Lord!

Kr, My Prayers are always with you sweetie

Av, Amen! Praise God & Thank you Dr.Ghaly!

Mj, What a wonderful Doctor.

Rc, Blesdings for the recovery of surgery!

Some hot chick and some bum...

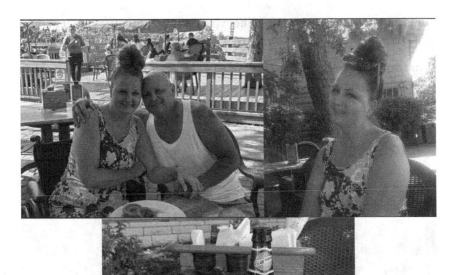

BC, Great pictures

RG, Y'all are so sweet

JA, It is so good to see you both out together having fun! God is good!

L, So sweet! Glad you got out of the house for your Anniversary!

JC, Glad to see her out and about! You look wonderful Gwen!!

Ramsis Ghaly

O thank you Lord Jesus. You both gorgeous

Ramsis Ghaly

Happy anniversary. So happy for you both Excellent

SZ, So happy for you two. Glad to see your wife back on her feet and looking wonderful!

Our angel Gwen L Favero came for her visit three months after surgery ready to go back to work after a long journey!

What a miracle from intractable day and night suffering to a new lease in life with a bright future full of joy! Throughout she has never lost her faith and continued her utmost determination. What an angel with a smile!!

Much love and blessing and more and more recovery. We all are blessed by you! Praise our Lord Jesus!

Ramsis Ghaly

Www.ghalyneurosurgeon.com

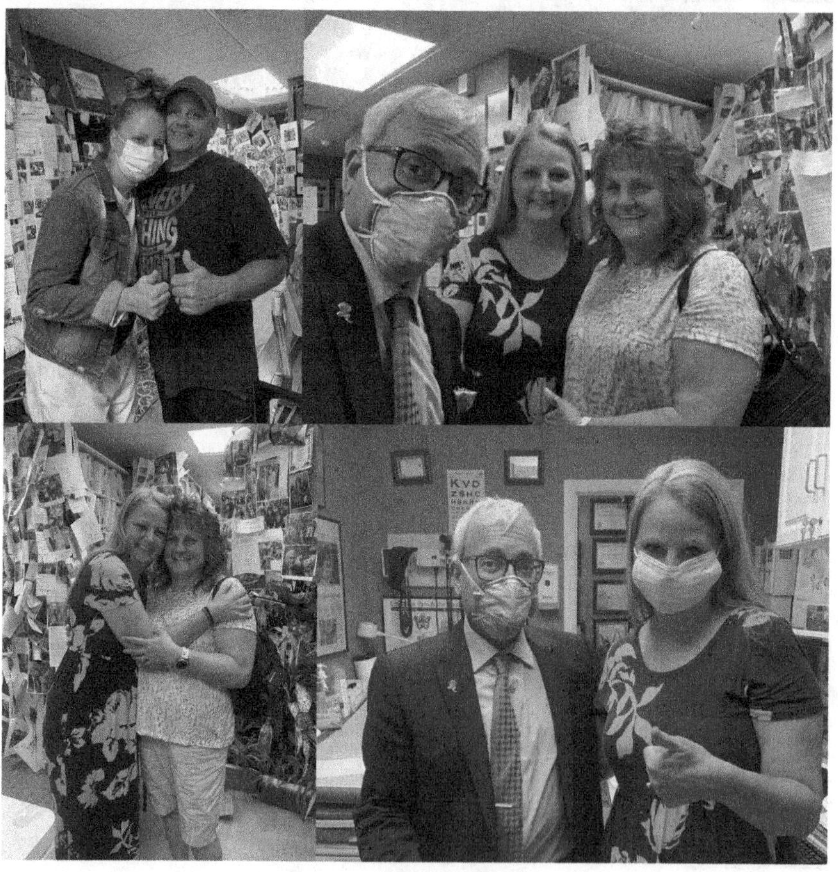

Dh,Praise the lord sister

Lr, God is so good !!!!! Hugs

Jd, God is good

Kw, Wish you All the best!

RV, My warrior

What A Miracle!

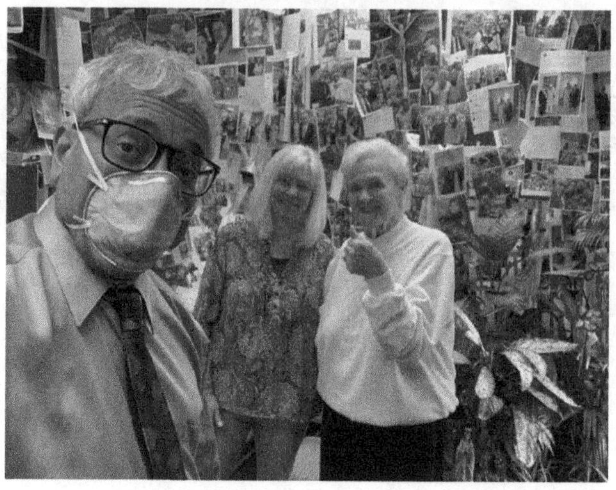

What a miracle praise our Lord Jesus from paralysis bedridden to upright walking with no device. It took 6 months since the surgery.

Majority with this type of condition won't have walked or regained ambulation!

Prayers, Faith, Endurance and Skilled Surgery bring Healing and Grace!! Only Glory to Our Lord the Healer!!

She is enjoying new house and driving!! Much much blessing to you and much glory to our Lord Jesus!!

Ramsis Ghaly

Www.ghalyneurosurgeon.com

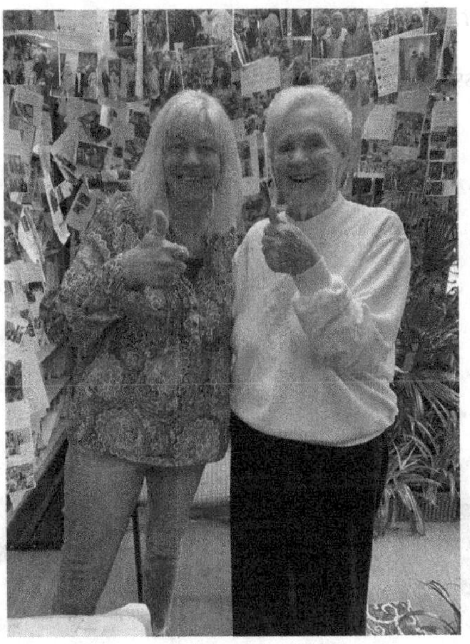

MP, Praise the Lord! Awesome Dr. Ghaly

DL, Wow ! Miracles still happen !

CG, How wonderful! She is so blessed you were there to do her sugery. Wishing her continued healing.

KM, How Beautiful! Wishing all the best.

RC, It's increíble wha can we do with blessings, falta and love!

JM, Wonderful Dr. Ghaly

JK, Most definitely Dr Ramsis Ghaly you are a Miracle Worker.

God Sent to you Special Blessings on your hands, mind and your body...

May Our Loving God always Bless you...

BM, Praise God

What a miracle less than a year, my patient is a 79 years old, look and do as an 18 years old preparing for her grand daughter wedding!!

Her big 80 birthday at the door and feel young! God blessed her with great recovery ftom major surgery!

Bless your heart. So proud of you!

Congratulations for the wedding of your granddaughter!!! Bless you all.

Much love and blessing. Praise our Lord Jesus!!

Ramsis Ghaly

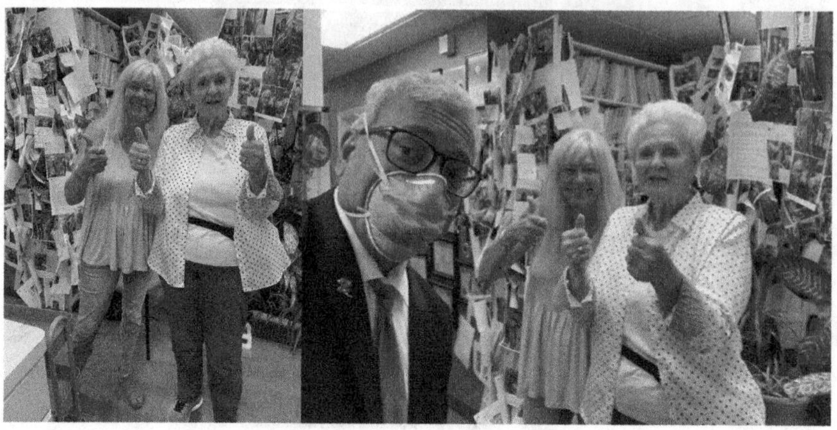

JM, Wonderful Dr. Ghaly

Look how miracles occur when you listen to the Holy Spirit and ask Lord Jesus to intervene?

Written by Ramsis Ghaly

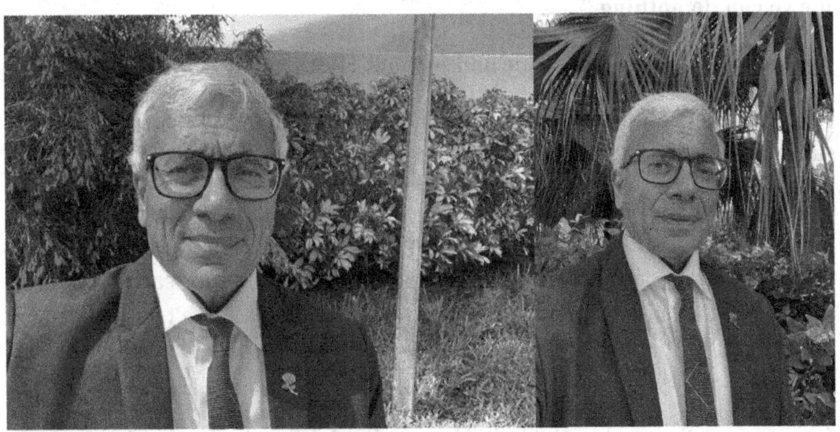

Patient was so ready for surgery and cleared from all his physicians to go for surgery. The surgery is scheduled, and the date already booked. The patient and family all signed the necessary papers and already to go sealed well by science and medicine!!

I usually like to see the patient and family several times prior I commit to do surgery. And this what I did for this patient!!

In my patient last visit toward the end, it was exhausting day and somehow, a thought came to my mind to order a test (Doppler) for the legs for no good reason just to make sure, a suspicion!! There was no good scientific reason or medical reason, the patient already cleared by his physicians and had necessary testing and already! But God Almighty said no he isn't ready for surgery My son!! It was only a divine intervention!

O my God, the test came so positive, and the patient's leg was loaded with clots and venous thrombosis ready to go to heart and brain to kill him immediately!!

Imagine I took him for surgery with clots in the legs laying down during surgery for hours with messaging boats during surgery and after surgery!!

These clots in the legs will have gone to the heart and the brain and killed him 100% with absolutely no doubt! His heart will have arrested and never survived or walked out of the hospital!

Despite he was cleared for surgery from his physicians and all set for surgery, the Holy Spirit comes at the last minute and save lives. The voice rings in my ears all the time: John 15:5 KJV "I am the vine, ye are the branches: He that abideth in me, and I in him, the same bringeth forth much fruit: for without me ye can do nothing."

Indeed, Jesus is my True Vine and without Him I can do nothing!!

If I can tell you all, I can't count How many times I have lived seen innumerable times of my Lord intervention!! Countless miracles over my career!

Although I am a Neurosurgeon, but I look at the patient as one and care for the person as a whole. I also put my nose into my patients care, I get involved and review and provide comprehensive care surgical and kind surgical, I work them you before the surgery because of my extensive training. I don't hesitate to step on the toes for the sake of patients. I always strive to prepare the patient the best shape for surgery!

Let us never forget everyday miracles our Lord Jesus do for us with the Holy Spirit. Our God is a Living God!

A man is a man and not a perfect man, a physician is not a perfect physician and science is not perfect science either! Be humble and reach out to our Lord, our perfect Healer!!

Some said, "It is gut feeling" and I reply "No! It is Lord Jesus Blessing and the Voice of Holy Spirit". God so loved all His children in the world and care so much as it is written: John 3:16 KJV "For God so loved the world, that he gave his only begotten Son, that whosoever believeth in him should not perish, but have everlasting life."

To my patient, I always say: "God loves you! He wants you to live and He grant you a new lease in life. What happen is a miracle and wasn't out of science or my skills. There is a reason God wanted you to live and so find His calling and purpose He wish for you to do!!"

To my Lord Jesus and Holy Spirit, I always say: "I worship You and Thank you for making me a vessel for Your Divine Glory and a living testimony to Your Glory O my God Lord our Savior and Heavenly Father! I am not worthy by all means!"

Amen

Www.ghalyNeurosurgeon.com

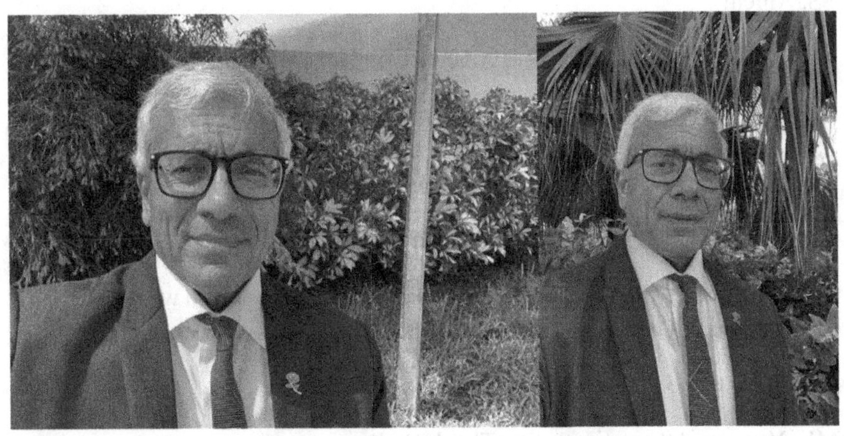

SH, You are amazing! So glad you pray and wait on God's guidance

KR, Love your words—-

As a nurse I love hearing your thankfulness for your patients relief of pain and wonderful outcomes-your not just a surgeon, but a God send to your patients. What a miracle this story is—Thanks so much for sharing!

CR, Beautiful

LK, Amazing!!

KG, **Ramsis Ghaly** Our God is an Awesome and Amazing GOD to bring such miracles for the world to witness through your devoted care, expertise and unfailing faith. Thank you,Dr Ghaly, for all that you do helping all of the world through HIS glorious interventION. and Wisdom! Amen Amen Amen

God Bless you in HIS mighty name forever and ever.

We all love you, Dr Ghaly.

Blessings from Egyp

BC, I feel like God helps us every day. You are a true blessing!

MI, God bless you! and Wisdom! Amen Amen Amen

God Bless you in HIS mighty name forever and ever.

We all love you, Dr Ghaly.

Blessings from Egyp

SS, Amen!

MP, Always listen to the voice, Amen ! God works through your hands I have no doubt.

PS, God is awesome. From everything I have read in the past 2 years, blood clots seem to be a much more common problem these days.

CR,That's a Holy Spirit Wow! Only God.

SY, Wow! Praise the Lord! It's because of your obedience to do what Holy Spirit says! Amazing Dr. Ghaly!

CY, Glory to God for divine intervention

ML, You saved the patient's life. Thank God!

JD, Bless you my friend!

SJ, What a wonderful diagnostician and Servant of God you are, Dr. Ghaly.

EM, God bless you Dr. Ghaly for all you do for others

JT, such a good man here...

TF, Prayers of guidance, knowledge, divine surgical skills, strength, comfort and Godspeed on the healing.

KE, Grèat Man and very gallant,*

SM, Amazing!

KL, What a blessing!!

CK, Yes, you are used of God and stepping on toes is a part of that. I firmly believe as it is written in the infallible Word of God

"obedience is better than sacrifice " God bless you Dr. Ghaly and yes listen to that still small voice!

MS, Thanks be to God for this Divine Intervention!

JK, You are a great Dr. For you care about the person.

KH, God uses you in a powerful way! Blessings!

HD, I love that you honor the Lord & listen to the Holy Spirit! You are blessed & continue to bless those around you!

ES, God has given you a special gift. With that gift you have saved and enriched many lives of people. You hold a special place in the hearts of your patients and their families.

LY, What an incredible testimony to the power of the Holy Spirit guiding you Dr. **Ramsis Ghaly** !!

I am trusting you implicitly with my surgery on Friday

RC, Thank you for miracles!

MJ, Yes. A doctor is a great profession as sacred as an angel. You should be a gentleman.

Yes. A doctor is a great profession as sacred as an angel. You should be a gentleman.

LM, Amazing.

AK, Prayers, Brother.

OB, Dr Ghaly did my back surgery 4 years ago. I was released from hospital the very next morning. This Dr. is a genius.

Cristina Gift of Superhero!

My patient Cristina Rojas-Rutkowski gift!
Thank you so much
Ramsis Ghaly
Www.ghalyneurosurgeon.com

SM, Best pic ever!!!

CR, You are! You are our hero and best doctor ever!!!!

JG, So accurate

SR, Love it!!!

CG, You are my super hero and also that of every patient you ever had and every student you ever taught.

JD, That's great super doc!

NV, Doctor Ghaly the Super neurosurgeon hero

BJ, Love it

MP, That's worth framing, because you are Superman in so many ways.

JB, Love this!!! WTG Dr. G!!!

DL, You are Superman. Lol.

CR, Perfect!

MB, Awesome !

CP, Yes you are.

KG, You're our Beloved Super Hero, no doubt! Best ever! God Bless you, Dr **Ramsis Ghaly**

KC, You are!!!!!

SM, Love this

RC, I say so!

DK, Perfect except you need a Bible under one arm!!!

CG, You are a SUPER DOCTOR.

AR, Love it

SJ, Love it

JC, Everyone's superman

TG, Love it

KN, This REALLY " suits YOU"

LW, Love it!

RM, Very fitting, You wear it well Sir

SB, So fitting. He is definitely a Super-Hero.

My Patients Getting Married and Celebrating Happy Anniversary!!

Let us congratulate Tricia and Dan getting married soon.

Congratulations

Tricia came today to her anniversary surgery clinic visit doing fantastic after years of suffering

Back then Dan would have walked in aisle pushing her in the wheelchair !

Instead after the surgery praise our Lord Jesus will walk and race in the aisle!! What a gorgeous emotional moment and tribute to our Lord and for His children!

Let us glorify Lord Jesus and congratulate Tricia and Dan, the first and life time marriage forever!!!

Ramsis Ghaly

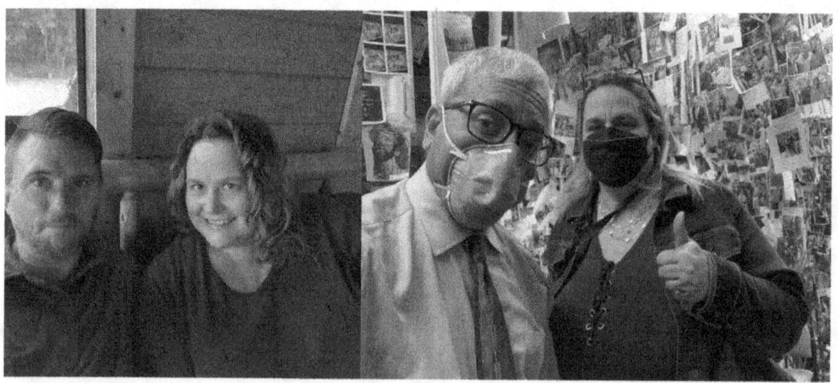

JP, Kudos to you Dr Ghaly

DF, **Congratulations** May God keep blessing you

KO, **Congratulations** to this couple

Dr Ghaly, you are remarkable surgeon God bless you always

WW, **Congratulations**

MS, **Congratulations** to you All!

DA, Dr. Ghaly is a fantastic dr! He took care of my son many years ago when he was suffering with a spine problem. No one else did what he did! So thankful for him! So happy you found him, too!

MR, Very nice couple **congratulations**

BF, **Congratulations** to you all.

SB, **Congrats** Beautiful people.

CT, **Congratulations**

JT, such good news...have a beautiful wedding and remember love is a gift from God

RE, **Congratulations**

Dan & Tricia!

MQ, When's the date?!

Congrats

LS, Love them both! Praise God for Tricia's healing!

BS, **Congratulations**

KL, So excited!! For healing and the upcoming wedding!!!

TT, **Congratulations**

RC, Paise Jesús.

CG, How wonderful for them and thanks to you she will be able to walk to her husband to be.

PA, **Congratulations**!

ES, **Congratulations** on the upcoming marriage.

KG, Mabrouk from Egypt!

BL, Dr **Ramsis Ghaly** you are a life changer and loved so much!

VW, Dr Ghaly, God sure gave us "ALL" a blessing when you came into this world. You are not only the best neurosurgeon but you are the best a person can be. You care. You laugh with your patients. You remember us all. My eyes water up how great and amazing you are. I don't with this type of surgery on anyone but if you do please and I mean please on see Dr Ghaly. You mean the world to me and I appreciate you for everything you have done for me and my husband. I thank you for everything. You made my burdens lighter

Rg. your words brought tears to my eyes. Praise our Lord for His works. Much blessing and grace. Thank you

Jb, Well said Valerie. You express the sentiments of many of us!! Thank him for you Dr. G.

Cp. **Congratulations**

It was her dream to walk down the aisle in her wedding! She underwent surgery and God granted her to walk not the aisles only but mountains. We all so proud of you and your husband to be soon!!

Let us congratulate Tricia for her coming wedding!

Best wishes and full of prosperity and joy to Tricia and her fantastic husband Dan!

In our Lord Jesus Name Amen

Ramsis Ghaly

Www.ghalyneurosurgeon.com

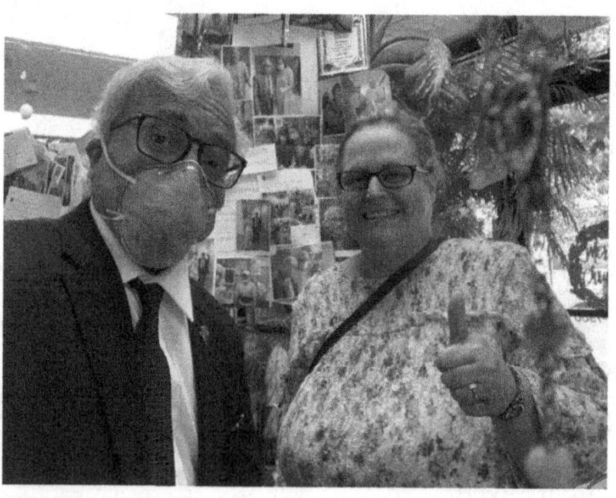

40Dianna Lynn, Kathleen MacGregor Grace and 38 others

Ls, Praise God!

Ko, Congratulations to you mam

Mp, **Congratulations** Trisha!!!

Kg, Praise God and

Congratulations

Kw, Congratulations so happy for you .

Nw, **Congratulations**

,Tricia! I am so happy for you.

Pg, **Congratulations** Tricia!!

Cg, How wonderful, that because of you she gets to fulfill her dream of walking down the aisle to the man she loves. **Congratulations**

Bm, I am so happy for you Tricia.

Congratulations

Cheryl and her husband are celebrating tomorrow the Sixtieth (60) anniversary.

I have done her surgery 6 years ago. Tomorrow is her 60th year anniversary. What a blessing! Praise our Lord. Happy anniversary you both and many more years in joy and health!

Ramsis Ghaly

Www,ghalyneurosurgeon.com

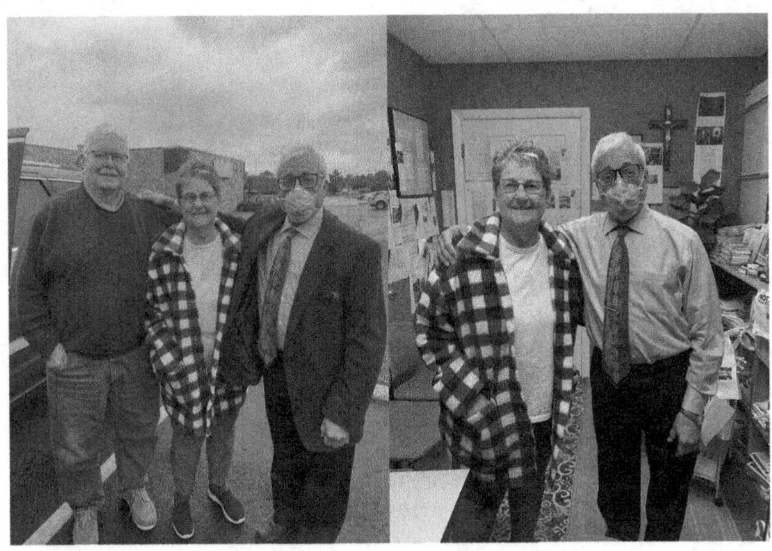

CG. Happy 60th anniversary!

MH. Happy 60th Anniversary!

Yesterday these two celebrated 55 years of marriage. They have been through a lot and keep making great strides. Thank you for showing us what true commitment means. Love you both with all my heart.

Photo credit: Ramsis Ghaly

Our Easter gift!!

A week later after anniversary Cheryl underwent surgery. Look at our angel had a major surgery two days ago and look at her. Fantastic recovery snd going home sweet home today.

Praise our Lord Jesus. She celebrated the 60th anniversary last week and much blessing.

Just remember never too old to have the correct surgery and stay away from meds and palliative pain clinic treatment.

Speed recovery. Hallelujahs Hallelujah

Ramsis Ghaly

Www.ghalyneurosurgeon.com

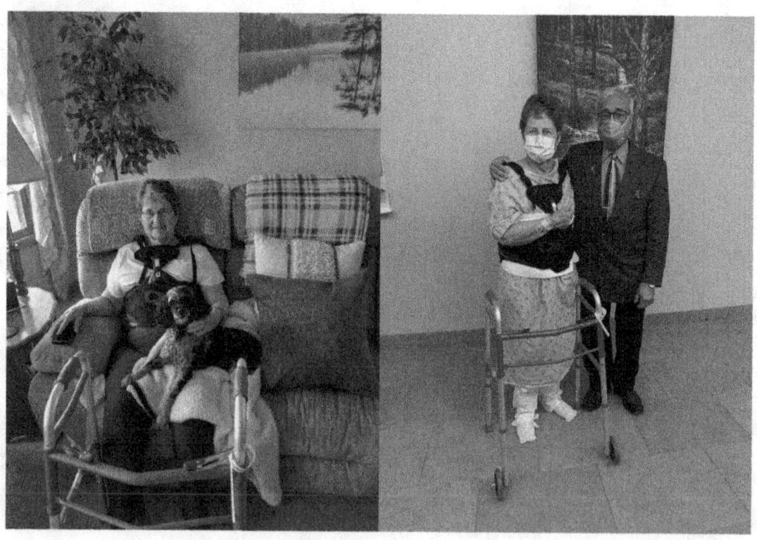

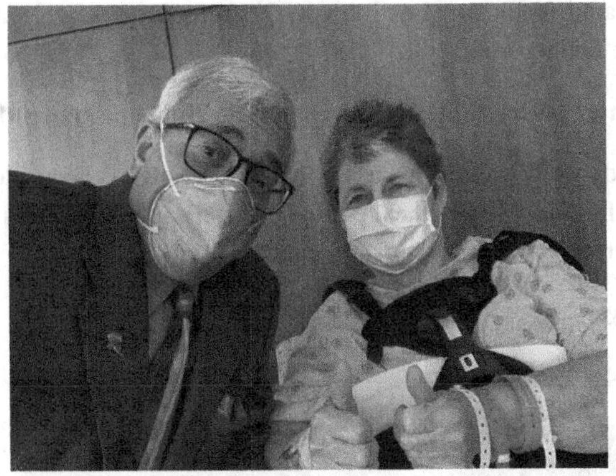

LT, So happy to see you're doing good Cheryl! Happy 60th Anniversary to you and Dick

CS, So happy to see your up and going Cheryl

HM, So glad to hear this !!!

JD, **Congratulations** Cheryl! Great job Dr. Ghaly. You are an amazing doctor! Jane.

CB, Way to go Cheryl!

WA, Looking good, way to go! Wishing you a speedy & full recovery .

NW, Sending prayers and healing thoughts your

JF, Can't keep a good girl down for long!!

CS, You look great! Hoping for a speedy recovery!

MS, Glad to see you are on the mend.

CG, Wishing you a speedy and full recovery.

LP, Good to see you are home and looking good!

BK, Wishing you a speedy recovery

CK, Cheryl, good to see you are on the mend!

JK, Glad you are doing well! I know the dog missed you. Looking great!

What a miracle from our Lord Jesus, 3 weeks later after major surgery, Cheryl came for her visit!

She is all healed, skin stables removed and no single pain or suffering.

Cheryl already went to church and her husband Dick has been a loyal husband flourishing the floor with red carpet for his lifetime pride. Bless you both; 60 years anniversary and sixty more to come. Amen

Ramsis Ghaly

Www.ghalyneurosurgeon.com

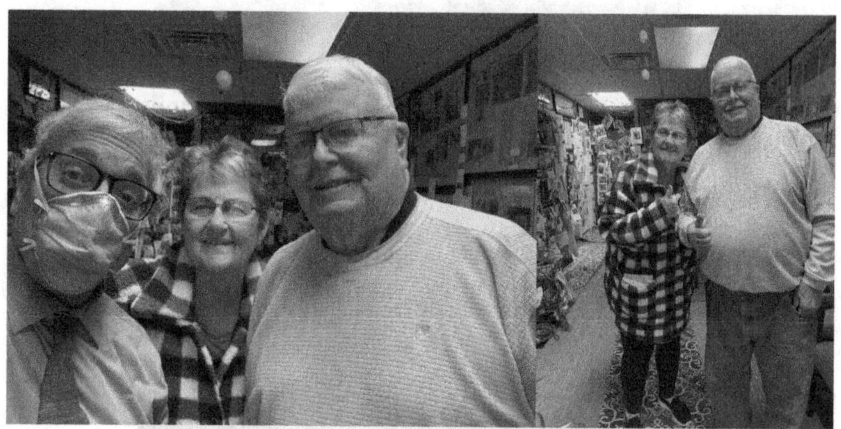

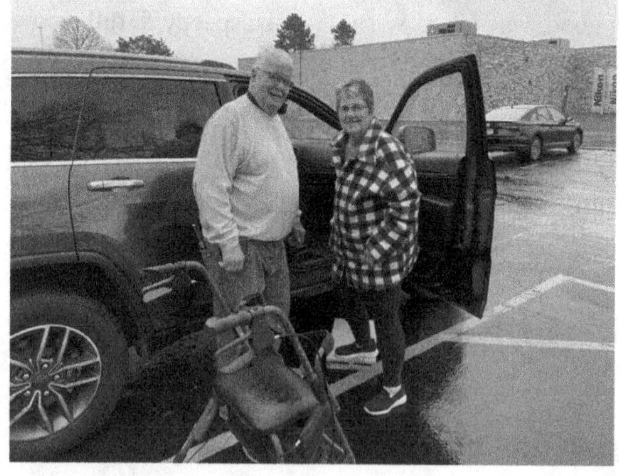

Great news! Glad you are doing so well!

NJ, Cheryl is a miracle and a great friend!

NJ, I'm glad there is a doctor she trusts to take care of her. Thank you.

AS, You two look Great! Prayers for continued healing, the Esgar men are wonderful care givers

RS, With LOVE

SW, Awesome news

CS, Glad you are doing so well and it sounds like Dick is taking good care of you

LK, That's great!

KJ, This is great!! Great news.

NW, Wonderful news! Continued prayers and healing thoughts

WA, Great news

E,Lookin' good Cheryl!!

LT, Glad you're doing good Cheryl! You and Dick look great

DH, "Happy 60th Anniversary"**Congrats** dr **Ramsis Ghaly**! You're awesome! Just one day I may make it up to see if you could help me... All the Glory to God

JT, amazing!!!!

LC, Glad you are doing so great!

LW, Way to go Cheryl. Glad you are doing well.

RS, Good news Cheryl! Good picture of you folks—except Dick are you getting old?

JF, Great news Cheryl!!

KW, Good to see you up and about.

KV, Happy to see you doing great! Happy Anniversary!

TV, So glad to hear you're doing great! Also Happy Anniversary!

CW, Praising the Lord for good news! I had no idea, Cheryl. Sixty years! It's a good match! Love you both.

PE, You look wonderful Cheryl! Have a Happy Mothers Day!

AV, Praise God!!

CM, That's great Cheryl!

JD, Another miracle my friend

JM, A Very Happy Ending Dr. Ghaly

My patient Cheryl and her husband Dick made me a home-made hand-made acrylic comfort Pen and executive Pen made of Purple Heart wood!!

What a privilege!! What a talent!! So much appreciative. Praise our Lord!

Cheryl doing terrific after surgery a month ago walking and dancing!!! Hallelujah

Ramsis Ghaly

Www.ghalyNeurosurgeon.com

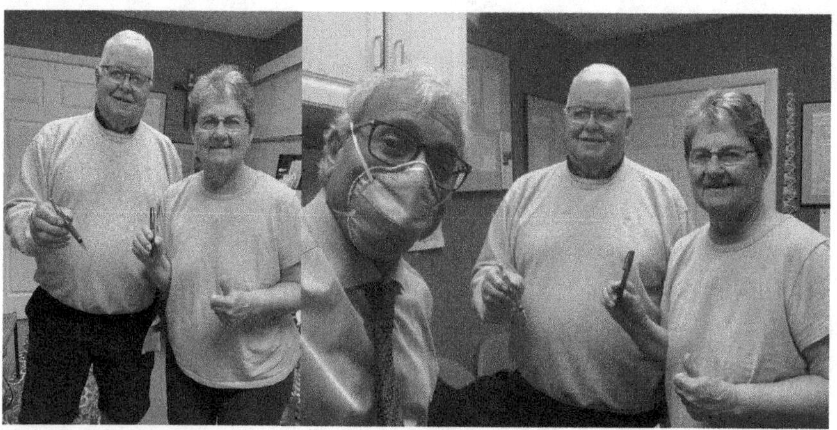

NG, Such a sweet Doctor! Apparently very caring.

KO, S0 awesome, gifts from the heart your truly appreciated Dr Ghaly and loved

RS, Wow! Great job folks. Love those projects—need to visit your workshop!

DC, Amazing

NJ, Great people, I've known them all my life!

NW, What a talent and good news that Cheryl is doing so well

AV, Fantastic! PRAISE God for His healing upon her! And so thankful for you Dr Ghaly!! I know Jesus guides your hands!!

LW, **Congratulations**

Cheryl glad you are doing well,

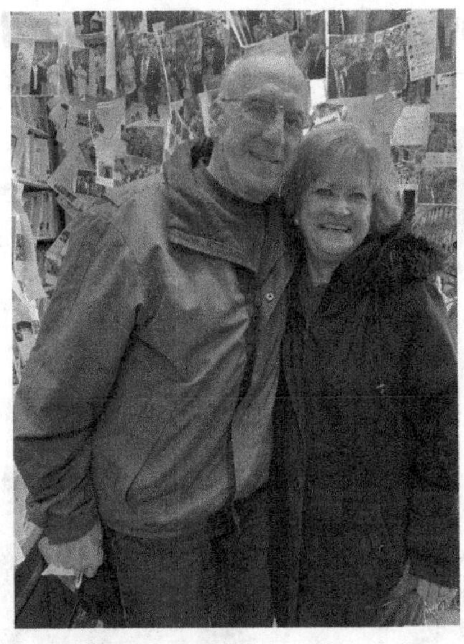

cc. You were our angel. Don't know how we would have made it without you

In memory of my patient Sandy Smith!

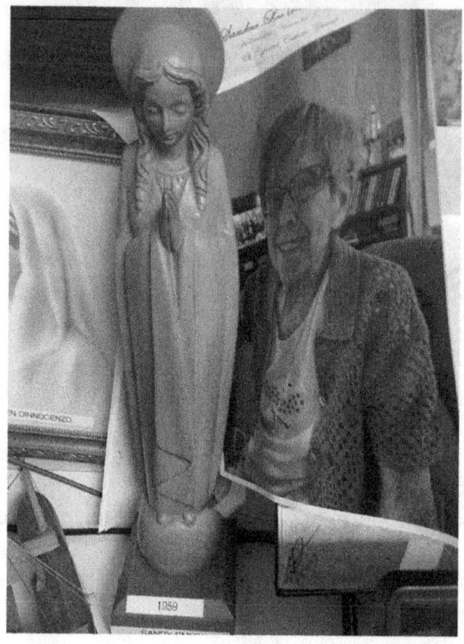

Less than two decades ago after surgery in a wonderful mother, Sandy brought me this Gorgeous historic statue of St Mary as a gift. Since then, I kept it by my working desk.

The surgery and recovery were remarkable, and she had new lease in life. Since then, she hasn't forgotten the blessing and so her family!

Sandy told me this previous gift no other place to keep except by you. Back 1959, she was praying hard with tears interceding to the mother of God to have a child and she did.

Now Sandy our angel is at heaven, blessed her soul in the bison of St Mary and her Son Jesus! Amen!

Ramsis Ghaly

DW, Amen

CR, Rest on peace

KS, Amen

MH, Beautiful Amen

MC, Amen

KB, Beautiful

RC, Peace for the woman she was with your help

CG, What a lovely angel she was. Bless her.

JZ, Beautiful statue and gift!

BS, Thank you Dr Ghaly … she so appreciated and admired you not just as an incredible doctor but also as a friend. God bless you as you continue your amazing work with peers, students and patients.

My Patient Gifts They are in my Heart Never Forgotten!

Ramsis Ghaly

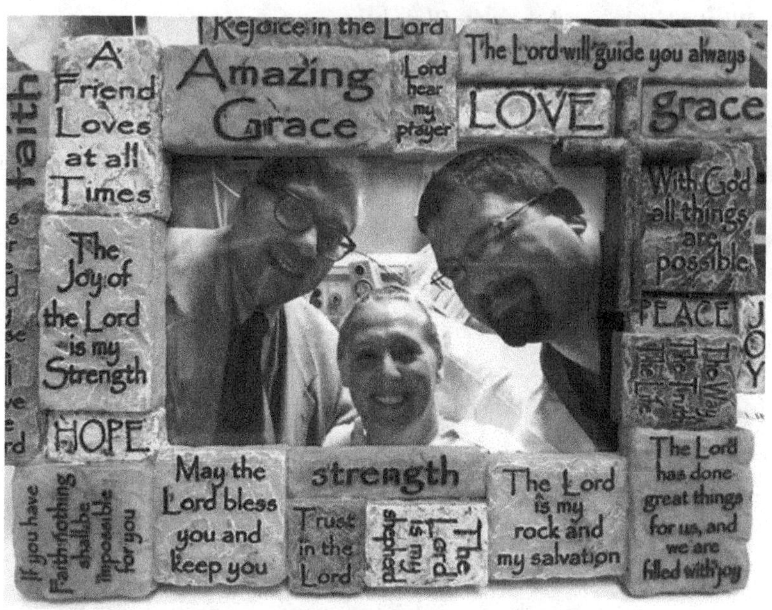
Rejoice in the Lord
A Friend Loves at all Times
Amazing Grace
Lord hear my prayer
The Lord will guide you always
LOVE
grace
faith
With God all things are possible
The Joy of the Lord is my Strength
PEACE
JOY
HOPE
If you have Faith nothing shall be impossible for you
May the Lord bless you and keep you
strength
Trust in the Lord
The Lord is my shepherd
The Lord is my rock and my salvation
The Lord has done great things for us, and we are filled with joy

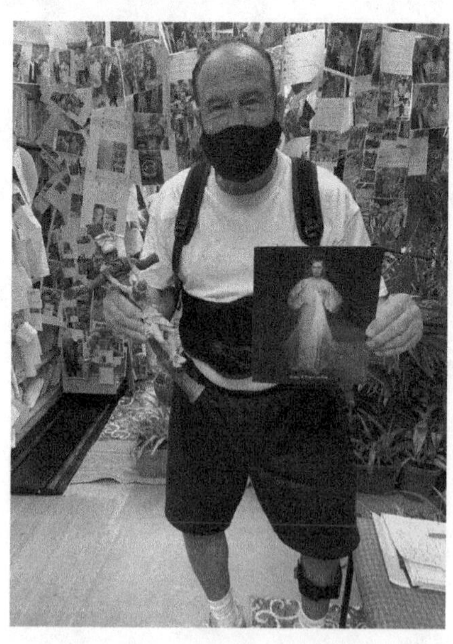

Patient to Get Know Each Other at Their Clinic Visit!

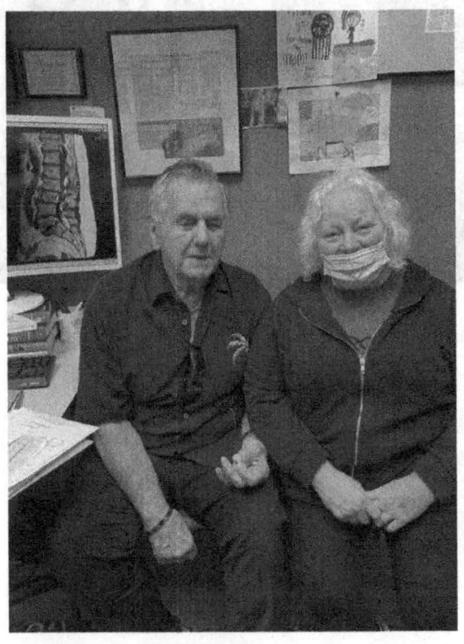

Patients don't know each other! They meet in my office during their clinic visit.

They be one close friend and support each other.

They become close each other and reach out to help out, talk about their experiences through surgeries, what work and what didn't work and lessons learned!!

Let us pray to our patients!! They are our love and comfort to know we are for them!

Amen to patient's love !!

Ramsis Ghaly

www.ghalyneurosurgeon.com

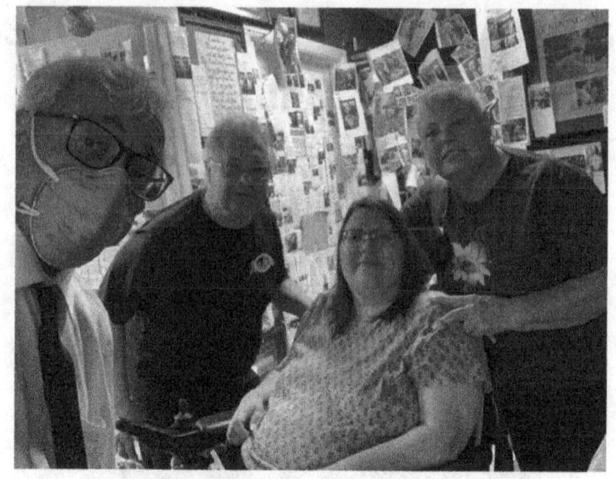

18Dianna Lynn, Margaret Agamy and 16 others

4 Comments

1 Share

Like

Comment

Share

4 Comments

Janice Moss

Wonderful Amen!!!!

Kristine Nelson Collins

You are great at putting people in contact with each other and helping. I know my mom was happy to share her experience with trigeminal nueralgia with other patiences. People who dont even know what they have or anyone who has been through some of these strange issues are really lucky to have you as their Doctor.

- **Love**
- **Reply**
- 6h

Sarah Cooper-Young

This is true!

- o **Love**
- o **Reply**
- o 5h

Charlene Mentzer Glowaty

That is one of the things I like about your office. You come out and introduce us to each other.

- o **Love**
- o **Reply**
- o 3h

My Patients are the Angels And I Pray for Lord Guidance!

Ramsis Ghaly

Real today's story!!

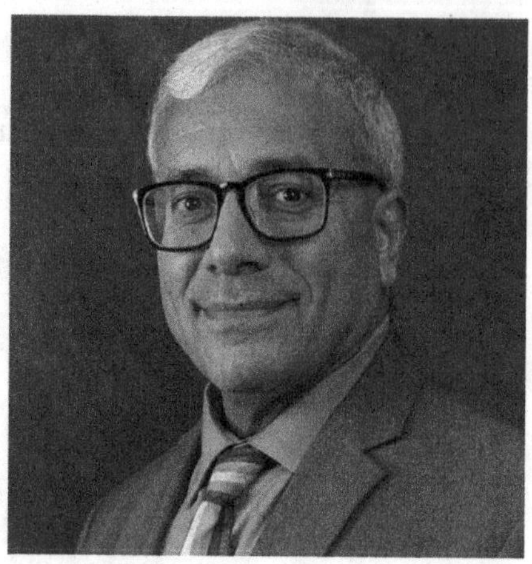

I called my patient to check on him after my treatment! He is in his seventy and has suffered so much!

He replied: "I feel much better, and I am driving now picking up pumpkins for the church for the first time after three months of horrific pains and numbness in my legs!!"

I replied: "Hallelujah praise our Lord."

He replied: "I have been in suffering trying to get help since July and although my daughter is a nurse Practitioner trying to get me an appointment!!"

I replied: "Thank God you feel better! God guided you to my way."

He replied: "Two weeks ago, I was talking with my wife about angels and last night I dreamed that you are an angel. So who are you?

I replied: "By no means I am one, but a servant and I pray to my Lord Jesus that have given me the gifts so to use them for His glory and heal His children. But you are the angel"

Then I called another patient to check on him after my treatment. This patient is in his twenties and has suffered so much with horrific pains and immobility for ten months!

He replied: "I am doing terrific the first time in ten months and giant part of my pains are gone!

At this time, I merged phone calls with both patients! O my gosh both were in the waiting area yesterday complaining to each other of miserable pains and both were praying for each other. One in his seventy sitting with wife and another in his twenty with his three-week newlywed wife!

Both were so excited and so happy to be free if pains and suffering g after king time!

Now, I told my two patients: Who is the angel among us?? I replied to you both are definitely. You both were suffering so much and praying, and God answered your prayers. Therefore, you both are angels!!

Indeed, there is no specific medical book for each patient? Each patient is different from another!

So, I see, hear, examine, evaluate and processing all together! With deep thoughts and prayers, I proceed!

So isn't Paul and isn't Apollos but God: 1 Corinthians 3:6-7 KJV "I have planted, Apollos watered; but God gave the increase. [7] So then neither is he that planteth any thing, neither he that watereth; but God that giveth the increase."

Proverbs 20:24: "The Lord directs our steps, so why try to understand everything along the way?"

Psalm 119:105: "Your word is a lamp to guide My feet and a light for my path."

Proverbs 19:21: "Many are the plans in a person's heart, but it is the Lord's purpose that prevails."

Isaiah 58:11 KJV "And the Lord shall guide thee continually, and satisfy thy soul in drought, and make fat thy bones: and thou shalt be like a watered garden, and like a spring of water, whose waters fail not."

Thank you, Lord Jesus!

Www.ghalyneurosurgeon.com

SC, Nice

CG, That is such wonderful news that he is pain free. You may not be an angel but you are close to being one.

KB, So glad he pain free because you,and God.

DM, You are a chosen angel of God

CS, U r such an amazing person!! U call your patients & make sure u c them again!!! U r definitely a Godsend!

MH, I'm so amazed at just how many people you do heal. Also just how much your your patience really do appreciate just how much you do for them. You have a good relationship with them and they have a good relationship with you. The Lord gave you the gift of healing his people & you make him proud each & everyday your parents are looking down from heaven and are very proud of you also. You are definitely The Lord's servant by healing his people may the Lord continue to bless you each & everyday. Sincerely Margaret

DH, You are truly Amazing Dr. Ghaly

May God continue to Bless you

CR, You are my angel my dear doctor and I will always be grateful for your great help and time.

Patients Stories!

My loyal patient is every anniversary of the surgery that changed her life to be more active with no more nerve pains of back pain, send me a wonderful memoir gift. This time is a terrific holiday classy tie!

Thank you so much. Thanks go to our Lord Jesus

Much blessing!

Ramsis Ghaly

www.ghalyneurosurgeon.com

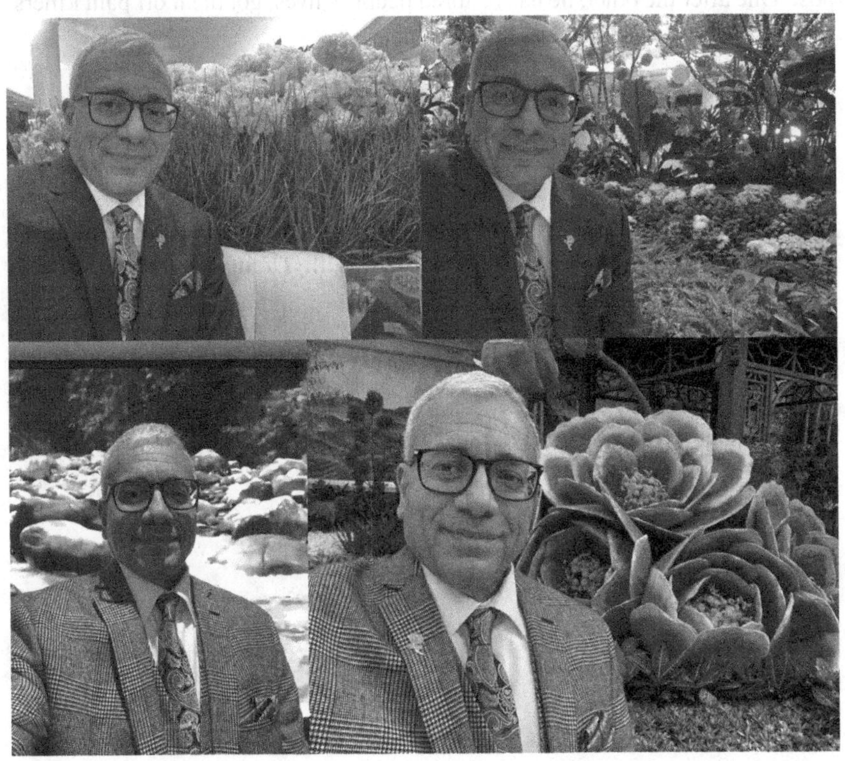

ED, Very handsome

CP, Very nice pictures.

KG, God bless you Dr.Ramsis

KC, Looks very nice!! You wear it well

JC, Looks great on you

MS, Goes with all the excitement you are and around you.

CL, Wow... so beautiful! God bless her soul.

MP, This is Dr. Ghaly, chief neurologist surgeon, and medical teacher to the interns. This Dr. Is a special God's healer. Amazing story here about removing nerve pain. I have witnessed many patients cured with life debilitating problems, some unable to walk or stand or sit. I wish there was some way you could see Dr. Ghaly. He is not in Florida, he is licensed as a Dr. In several States. He is an author of many books too.

I do believe he has a connection through Jesus. Follow him and see what he post. One after the other, he has restored people's lives, got them off pain killers, changed their worlds. Removed their pain.

NV, Nice tie! It looks good on you !

AS, Thank you

Our patient is at home with his beloved sisters and mom recovering after long surgery. What a great and loving family!!!! Their love and tenderness are very touching!

Praise our Lord Jesus getting better day by day. Much blessing and speed recovery.

Ramsis Ghaly

Www.ghaly neurosurgeon.com

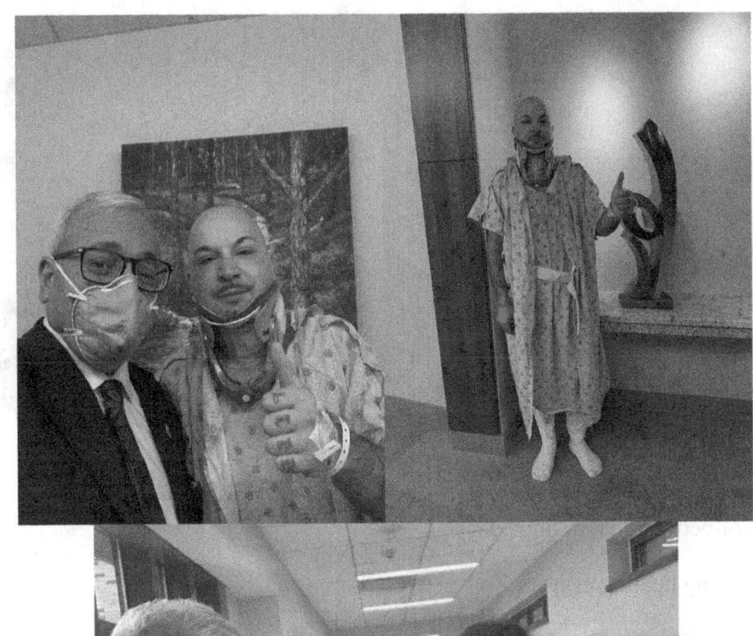

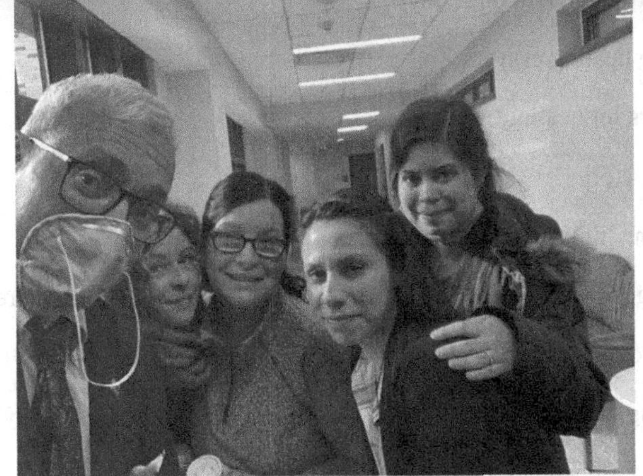

Our angel Baltzar came for an offic visit. Doing well two weeks after surgery. So happy for both.

Praise our Lord and Healer. Speed recovery

Ramsis Ghaly

Www.ghalyneurosurgeon.com

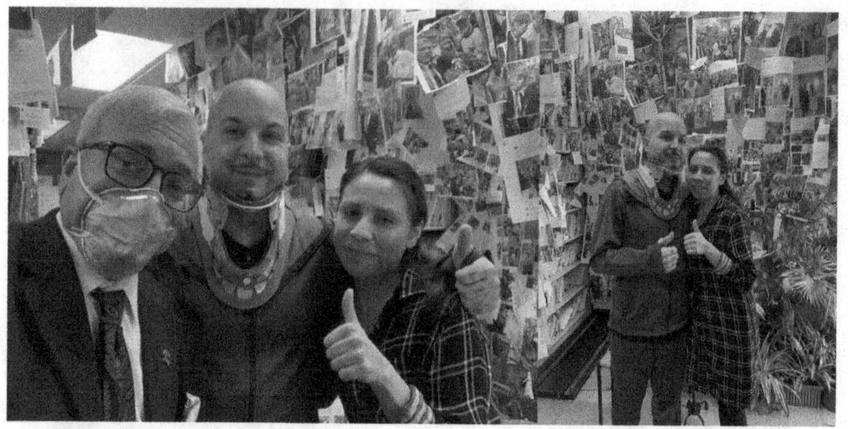

Cg, Another happy patient. Wonderful!

RC, For better and blessings days

JT, sending healing prayers

MS, Prayers for healing!

Thanks, Doctor!

CG, Wishing him well and a speedy recovery.

JG. Praying for a speedy recovery! Dr. **Ramsis Ghaly** is the best there is

JD, Bless you my friend

GK, sending prayers for healing. God bless you Doctor Ramsis Ghaly

JP. Prayers for healing **Congratulations** On Your Recovery

AP. Wishing you a speedy recovery

What about our miracle man Richard! In less than a year, had two major surgeries and look at him! A strong and blessed man. St Michael is his Saint. Praise our lord standing in his two feet

Speed recovery Richard. Praise our Lord Jesus.

Ramsis Ghaly

Www.ghalyneurosurgeon.com

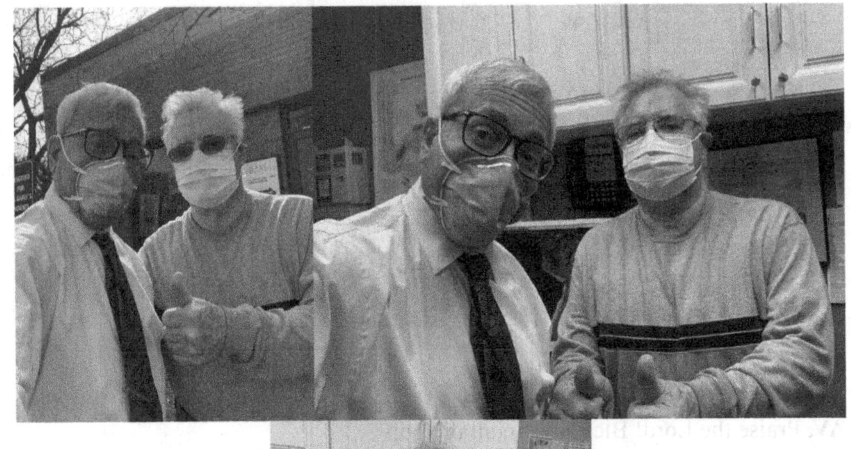

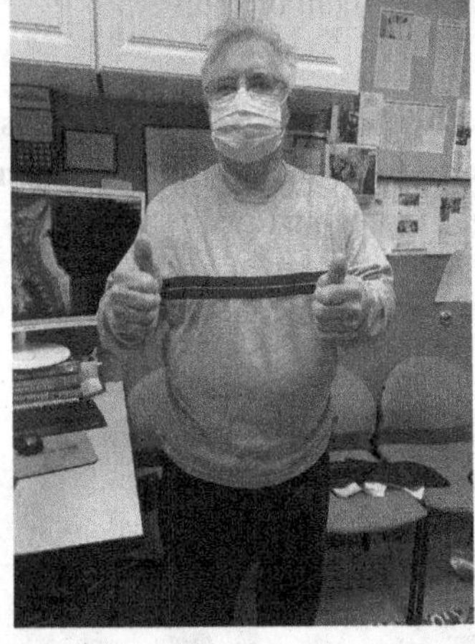

Cg, Another thumbs up! Good for him. He is fortunate to have had you as his surgeon.

Our angel Richard came today to visit full of blessing walking after two major Surgeries!! Looking forward to go home and do some traveling.

Archangel Michael is our saint!

It was a long journey and look at him now!!

Praise our Lord Jesus. Amen

Ramsis Ghaly

Www.ghalyneurosurgeon.com

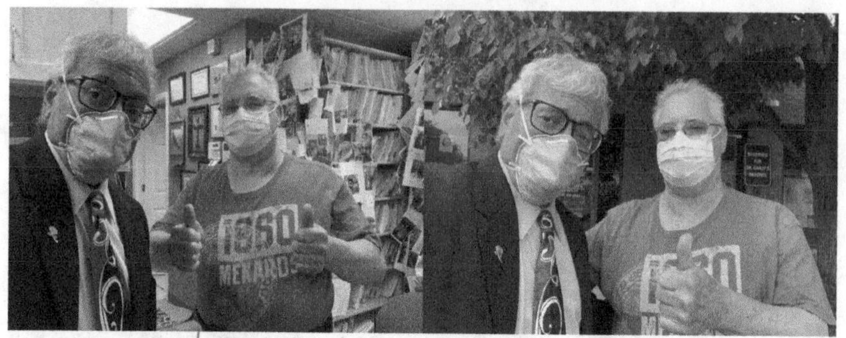

DN, Praise the lord amen

AV, Praise the Lord! Blessings to all of you!!

Our commander and father of Danny Candy store is doing well week after surgery and both came to bless me and clinic. Thank you speed recovery. Much love and blessing. Praise our Lord

Ramsis Ghaly

Www.ghalyneurosurgeon.com

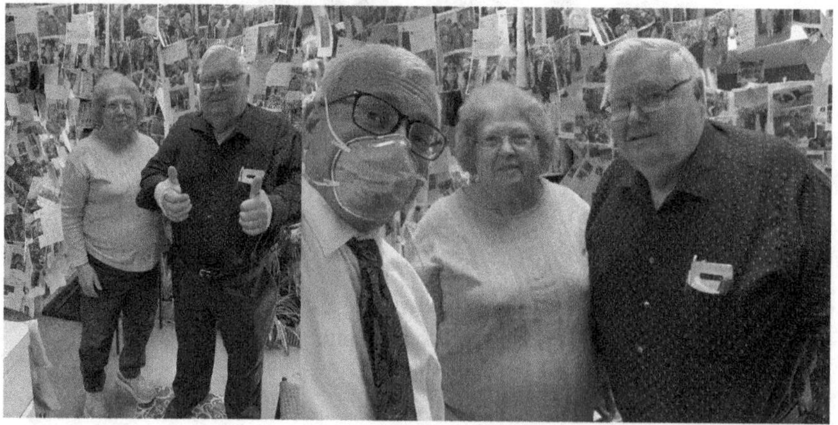

33Sandi Benedict Crites, Charlene Mentzer Glowaty and 31 others

4 Comments

Kc, I knew he would be in great hands.

Jg, They are such a sweet couple I'm so glad we were able to meet them

Cg, Wishes for a quick recovery recovery.

Ms, It's nice you said, they came to bless you, I like to remember that when people come to visit. God bless them and you.

Our Saint servant Donald came today ten months ago he was miserable of pains and had long big surgery! look at him now!! Back to work and helping many others. Praise our Lord Jesus.

Ramsis Ghaly

www.ghalyneurosurgeon.com

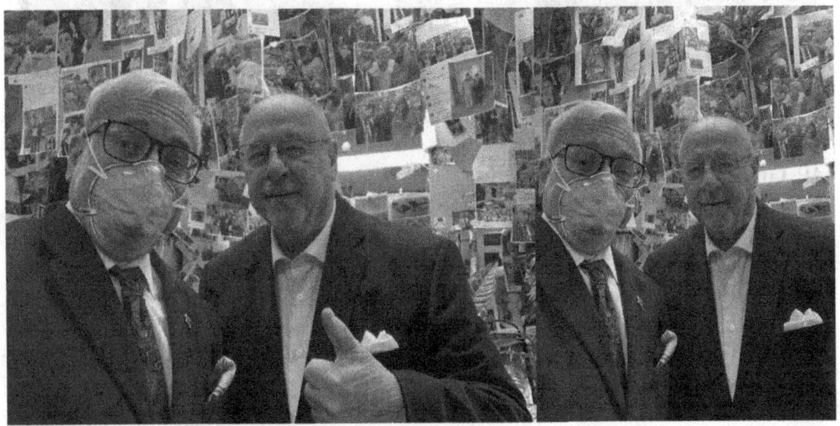

Cg, The smile on his face says it all.

Ws, Lookin' good, dad! Thank you so much, Dr. **Ramsis Ghaly**!

Rc, That makes all worth!

Our wonderful angels Carolyn and Jim survived the most life scary event and now look at them, smiling in faith and love.

My long life time patients. Much Bless and love. Praise our Lord Jesus and pray to keep you in good health

Ramsis Ghaly

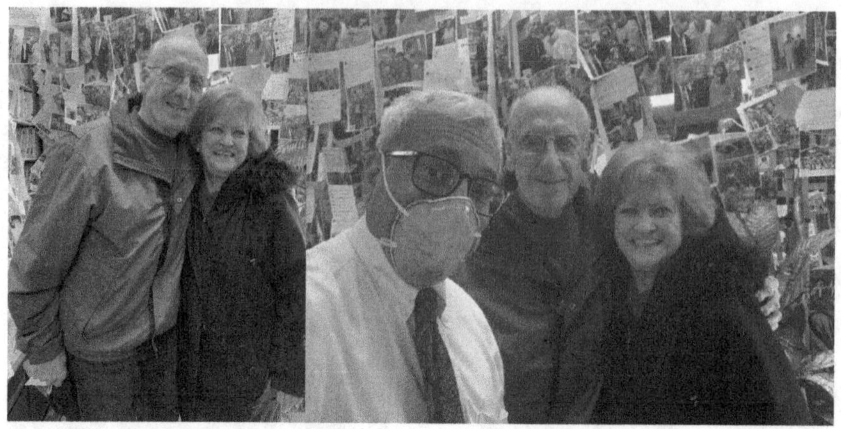

JT, beautiful smiles!

MP, Great picture!!!Love you guys!!!

Our wonderful angels Carolyn and Jim survived the most life scary event and now look at them, smiling in faith and love.

My long life time patients. Much Bless and love. Praise our Lord Jesus and pray to keep you in good health

Ramsis Ghaly

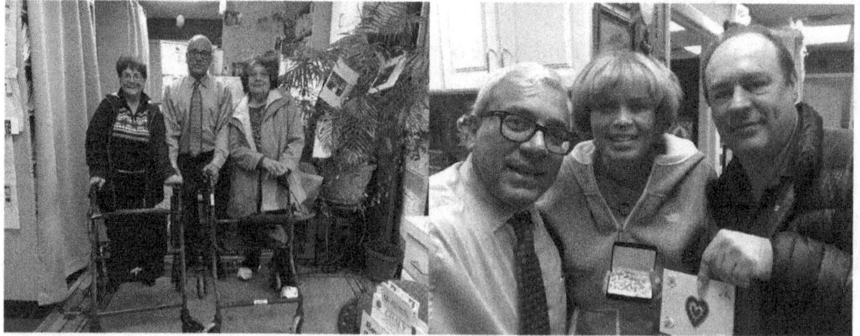

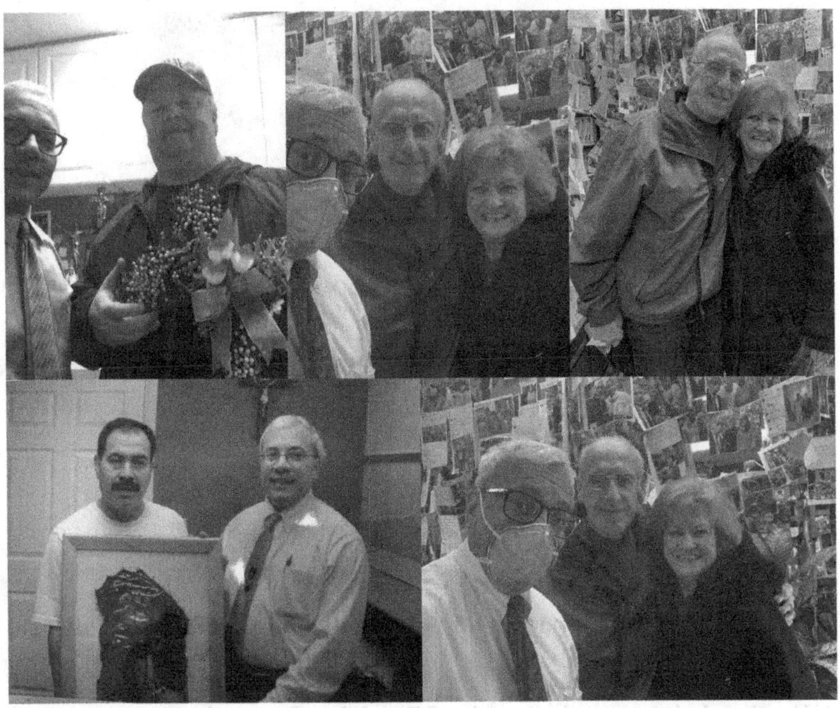

Jt, beautiful smiles!

Mp, Great picture!!!Love you guys!!!

Cc, Thank you Dr. Ghaly. It was so good see you

Sc, Thank you for the kind words Dr Ghaly!!! They have come a long way. I kept telling them to keep the faith and they will get through this. They look amazing. Love you mom & dad

Sm, Looking great! Thanking the Lord for your recovery!

La, So glad they both made it through that tough time

Look at this beautiful Easter card by Char. Happy Easter. Thank you and much blessing!

<u>Ramsis Ghaly</u>

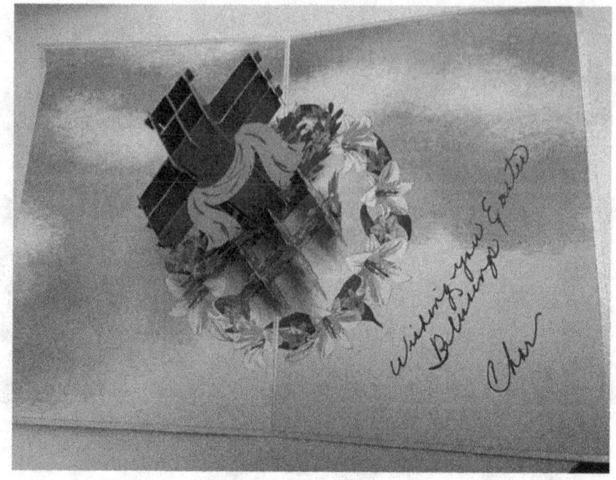

KO, Beautiful card

AV, Beautiful

A gorgeous gift from my patient his wife just did his surgery two month ago. He was suffering of paralysis.

A Handmade by my patient made of Revolving Carousel of verses wooden with a beautiful verse selected by my patient Balazar and his wife Estela.

What a great gift!!! Thank you so much. Glory to our Lord Jesus

Ramsis Ghaly

Www.ghalyneurosurgeon.com

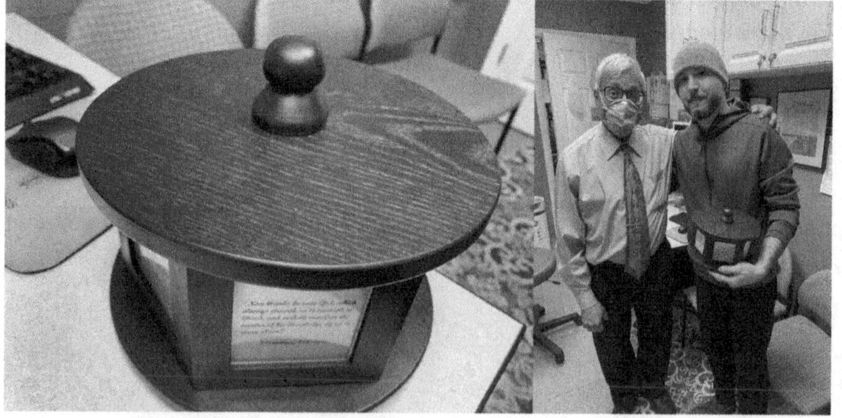

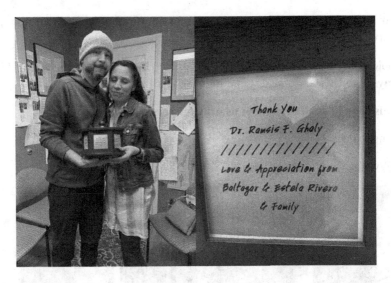

Bk, Beautiful.

Jh, Beautiful

Mp, What a wonderful gift. Handmade with hands you gave ability to use legs and arms, and that gift was made with Love.

Av, Wonderful gift with great Bible verses!!

Bl, You are loved so much and your patients want to share their talents with you in love and appreciation. Blessings You have changed their quality of life!

Cp, Beautiful

Ds, Just beautiful!!

Personal request for all my Prayer Warriors, family and friends of my brother Brad.

. Brad is going to have a shunt revision Monday at 9 am cst. Praying for God to work through Dr Ramsis Ghaly and all medical team assisting and caring for Brad . Prayers for successful uncomplicated procedure and a speedy healing and recovery. Asking for a peace and complete trust as we place our dear brother in our Lord's hands. Mother Mary watch over Brad, guard and protect him

God bless you all!

Cindy

Our angel Emily going home with smile and joy and brightness after major neurosurgery two days ago.

Look at her smile and incision covered. Her husband at bedside and kids praying for her at home day snd night with all her friends.

Praise our Lord Jesus and let us pray for her speed recovery

Ramsis Ghaly

WWw.ghalyneurosurgeon.com

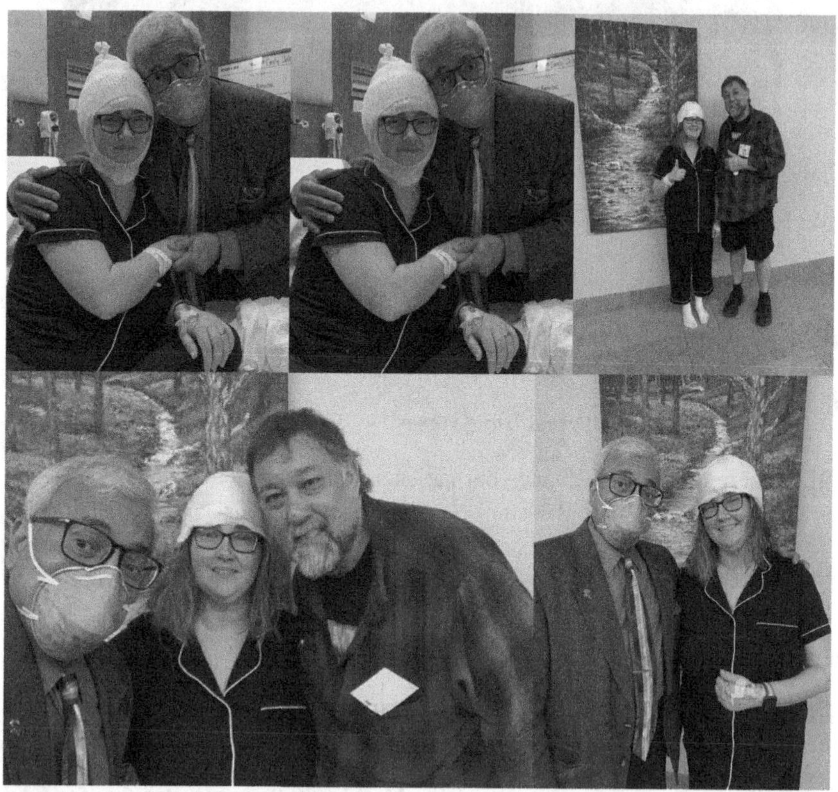

KM, God bless you Dr Ghaly!

CP, Wishing you a speedy recovery

JD, Bless you both

SC, your in good hands

EO, Blessings. You don't waste any time getting your patients back on their feet.

JK, Dr.Ramsis Ghaly,

I need your miraculous hands to heal my feet, so I can go home and walk safely again.

Your patients they are so blessed to be under your care...

JM, Prayer's and A Speedy Recovery

AP, Wishing her a speedy recovery

AT, our Lord sent you Ramsis to help and heal...

AC, The best doctor

RC, Both are great!

JJ, Healing prayers are sent for Emily, God Bless You !

MA, Dr Ramsis Best doctor

GB, You got this, Muffin

MH, She is a warrior!

TW, You look Fantastic **Emily**!!! You've sooo got this

JG, This makes me so happy! Love you Em!

SG, You look fantastic, Em! Heal quickly!

TC, We love you **Emily**! We are grateful for your Doctor too!!!!

TM, Many prayers for you Emily!

JB, Sending healing prayers

NG, DL, God bless you both.

TT, You got a tough girl mike. Good luck to you too. Never give up

LC, Love u Em and God bless Dr **Ramsis Ghaly**

AB, Praise God

JU, Get well soon!

NH, So happy to see these pics

KD, Continued prayers for you Emily!!

KC, Your have God's hands when your healing others

MB, You look amazing and strong!!! Thankful for your doctor for getting you through this!

RM, God bless you Sir ! The Great Dr Ghaly does it again

EP, God is good all the time wish a speedy and full recovery ! Wonderful doctor

CB, Sending you prayers for a speedy recovery

JM, Wonderful that All is Well.

XS, Sounds like an amazing doctor you look great Emily.

God

RH, God works amazingly stay strong and praise God AMEN

TN, A beautiful story about the gift of God and the hands of surgeons.

WO, so happy to hear you are doing well, Emily!

Our angel Emily Linn first visit after major surgery. Look at her full of joy and blessing praising our Lord Jesus for new lease in life.

What a journey and today she received the best news of her life!! Glory to our Lord! Amen

Ramsis Ghaly

Www.ghalyneurosurgeon.com

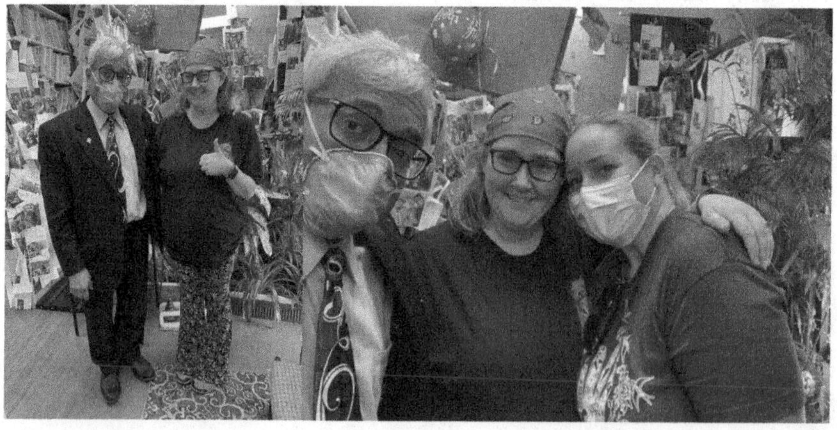

LC, U look amazing Em!!

Had my appt with the amazing Dr Ramsis Ghaly yesterday with my amazing husband Michael. Going back to work soon. Let's be honest, no one ever really wants to go back to work after being off for 3 mos right? But I'm happy that I'm ABLE to return to work. And it'll back to my old routine in no time.

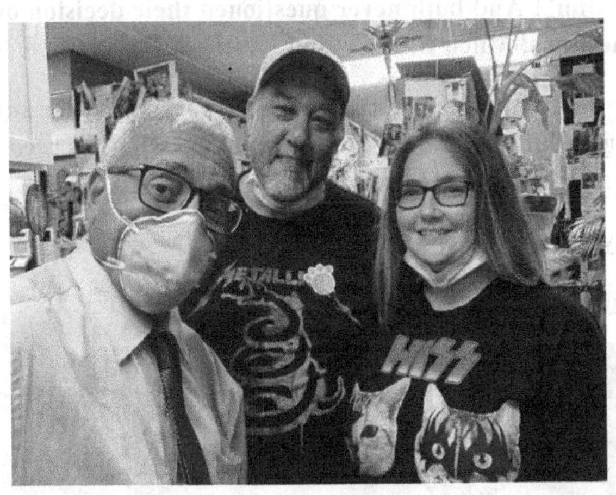

Jp, GREAT NEWS!!!

Nh, Can't wait to see that beautiful face!

Jl, I'm so glad

Sj, Emily! You look amazing and I'm so excited you get to go back to work!

Jl, Good news

Jm, Yes

Mh, Wonderful new Emily! Enjoy your time and continue to rest- see you soon!

What a story of a rare cause of horrific pain and loss of function put him to tears and suffering for months!!! Early morning, we walked, and we raced, and Jim was granted new lease in life looking forward to hunting and enjoy his grandchildren!!! For the first time looking up and taking steps with confidence with no tears and screams and crying from the severity of the shooting pains and agony of electric jolts and hypersensitivity to touch and falling from heaviness of the legs, not for a month or two but for a year. After being exhausted and no one to help, God had a good plan to remedy his illness.

Look at Jim early morning after surgery to remove the cause in a very delicate and uncommon location missed by many!!

I told Jim and his wife Lynette a Disclaimer, this is extremely rare and not easy surgery, and both replied in strong faith: "We want you to do the surgery and care for Jim"! And both never questioned their decision or pursued to ask more questions! Much Blessing and love!

We together prayed before direct, during surgery and after surgery giving thanksgiving to our Savior Lord Jesus! Much blessing his recovery!! Praise our Lord Jesus always the Healer!

Ramsis Ghaly

Www.ghalyneurosurgeon.com

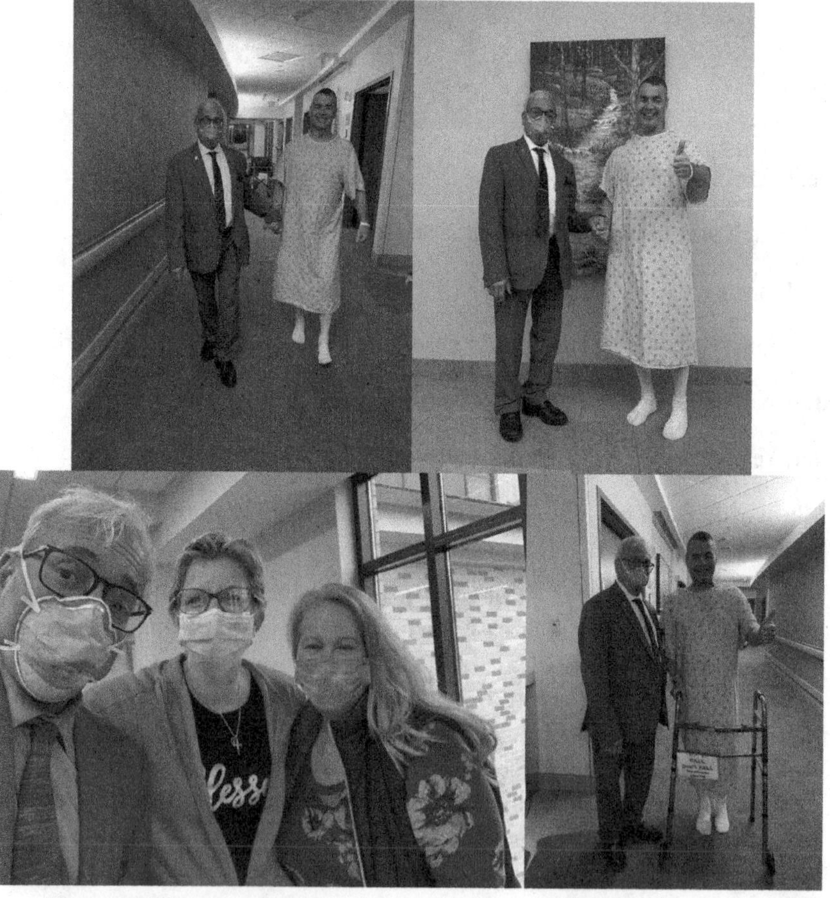

SP, Another amazing outcome

SS, Looking good Jim!! **Lanette Sellers Yingling** prayed for a successful surgery and grateful prayers were answered

JD, Wonderful

CG, Prayers are being sent your way with the hopes that you will feel better soon.

AB, Praise God

LG, Praise God!

JY, Thank you Dr. **Ramsis Ghaly** for removing the tumor from Jim with an amazing surgical procedure....done with precision, accuracy and God-given wisdom!! You are a blessing

RM, Great job Sir

GC, Dr **Ramsis Ghaly** #1!

NG, Amazing!

What about Karen, pain free after surgery 10 days ago.

A new beautiful life ready to go away for vacation for her anniversary and her children stepping up caring for mommy. So proud of you all

Praise our lord Jesus Amen

Ramsis Ghaly

Www.ghalyneurosurgeon.com

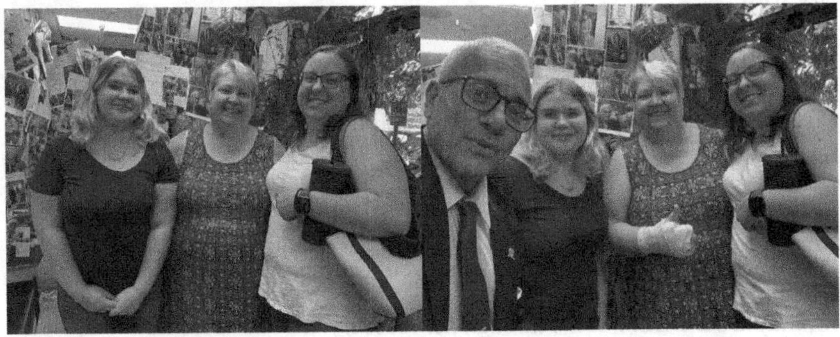

kg, God Bless you all!

Cg, Just wonderful. Wishes for a happy vacation. Bless you!

cn, Best doctor ever

DK, Thanks for helping them!! Hi Carol and Karen!!

Our shining star going home today! Praise our Lord for your speed recovery ! We pray for full recovery in our Lord Jesus. Amen

So proud of you! Much love and blessing!

Ramsis Ghaly

Www.ghalyneurosurgeon.com

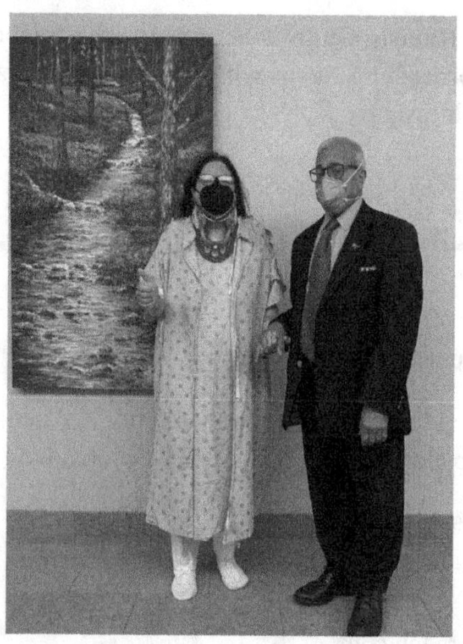

CG, Wishing you a speedy recovery.

KO, Health fast,You had the best surgeon

MN, DRGHALY as always another job well done your the best. Pray for a fast recovery.

RM, God bless

DN, Wonderful doctor gods speed with you recovery

JS, May GOD BLESS HER through her recovery

LS, Thank you for everything Dr. Ghaly!

JK, You are so fortunate having the best from the best

dr. **Ramsis Ghaly** ...

We need you in Las Vegas

Praise our Lord for our angel. Surgery 10 days ago and regained back her life. Hallelujah. Praise our Lord Jesus. Speed recovery

Ramsis Ghaly

www.ghalyneurosurgeon.com

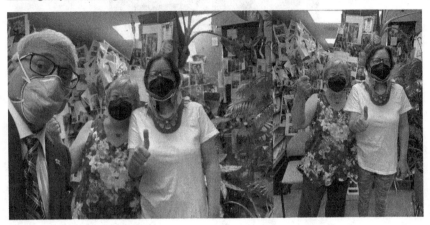

DM, God is with yoi always

JH, Praise God

Early Morning Ready to walk after hours of surgery with No pains! He has suffered for years.

Let us pray for speed recovery. He came all from the great State of California. I pray to our Lord Jesus all the time to hear our prayers and heal our sick! Amen

Ramsis Ghaly

Www.ghalyneurosurgeon.com

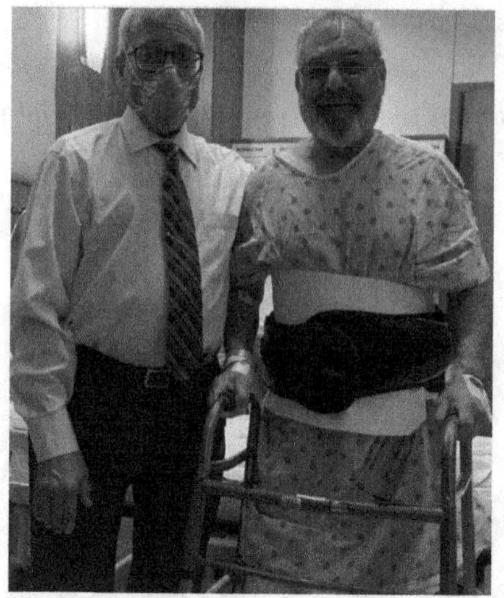

BN, God bless you! Such a beautiful soul. You live and love to help people.

EG, Dr Ghaly, you are an amazing physician!

JT, blessed hands...

JS, I pray JESUS gives you a complete recovery

DH, Thank you Lord. Thank you Dr. Ghaly..

DM, Praying for your early recovery and continuous strength and health for our Dr Ghaly that He continue to help more people

AB, Amen praise God

DL, How wonderful !

Home sweet home with No pains and regaining all function back!!!

Much live and blessing

Hallelujah praise our Good Lord. Amen !!

Ramsis Ghaly

Www.ghalyneurosurgeon.com

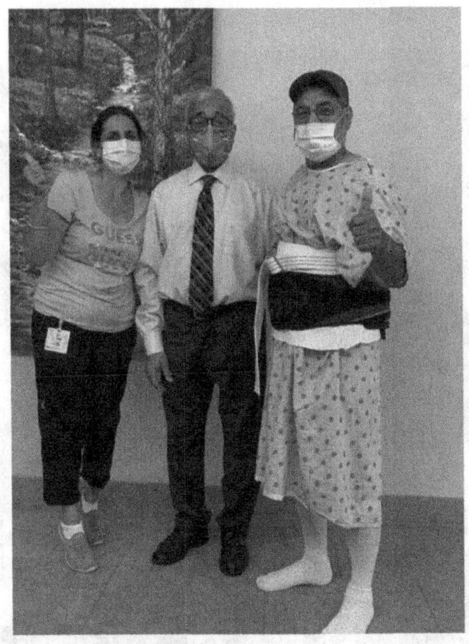

AV, Praise God!! Thank you Dr Ghaly!!

KO, PrYers and God's blessing Dr Ghaly your the best

JS, Praying for a smooth recovery

MA, You are a miracle worker

JS, Amazing!

MS, Praise God for your love of helping us all.

Delicious Indian gifts and famous indian teas, my wonderful patient showed up for her clinic visit three weeks after surgery with these generous treats. Thank you so much.

Bless our Lord. He is doing fantastic healing fast ahead of many. Regaining strength and no pains or taking pain meds

Much love and blessing and continue healing.

Ramsis Ghaly

Www.ghalyneurosurgeon.com

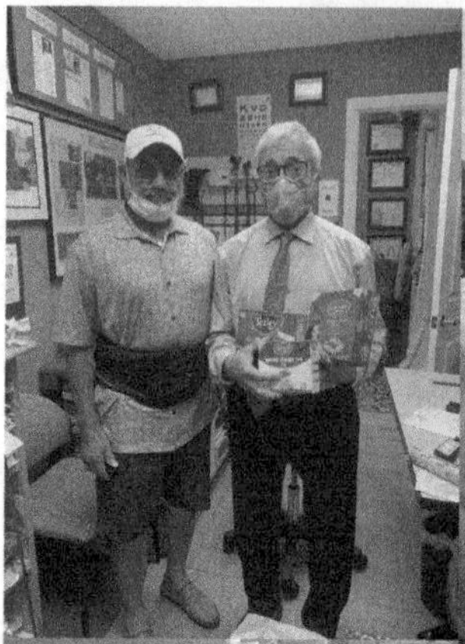

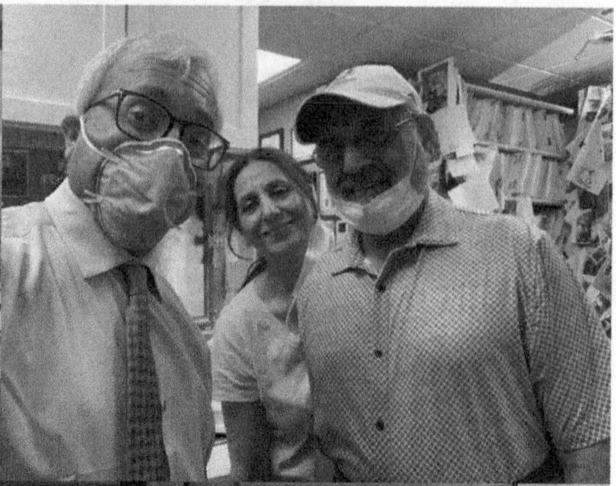

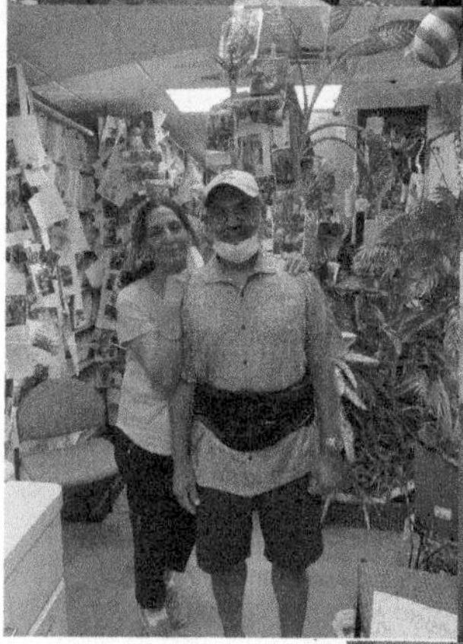

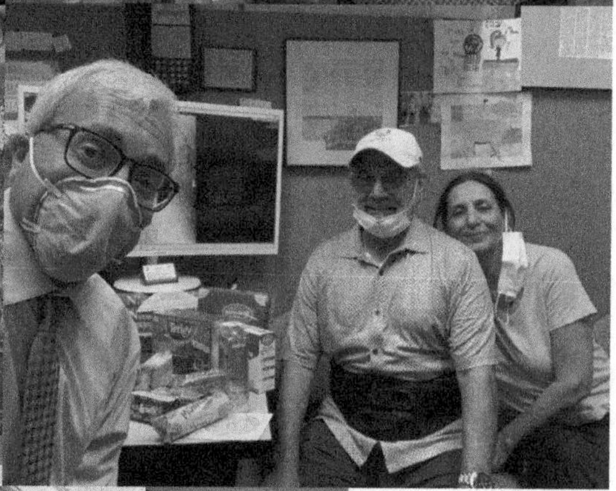

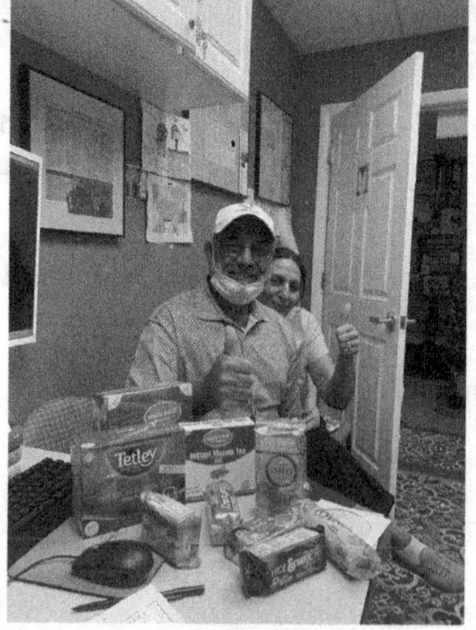
Tetley

KG, Blessings and Continued healing! Awesome treats. God Bless you. Xoxi

CG, Aren't you the lucky one. Prayers for continued healing.

KG, You were meant to be a doctor !!!

LG, Continue to be a blessing, Dr. Ghaly! Lifting you up as the Lord God continues to use you as an extension of His healing hands.

MA, Dr Ghaly is a miracal worker

My patient for 25 years ago came with his partner Margret to visit. A great man. A fantastic couple. A father of grant great children. Much love and blessing

Ramsis Ghaly

Wwwghalyneurosurgeon.com

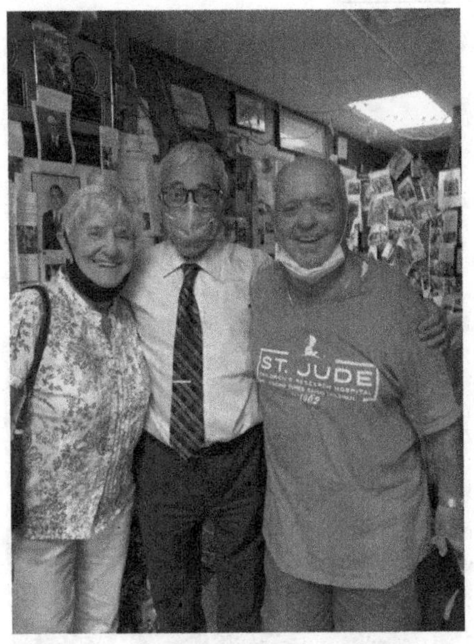

BM, Dr. Ghaly did my back surgery 20 years ago!

DAM, ooking fantastic Peggy and R J

GL, Looking good Rich and Peggy We miss yours

KD, Yes, he's quite a guy!!! God threw away the mold after making my big brother.......

MS, Great picture

KH, Nice Picture, Looking good Peg!

JC, How nice.

JV, Ole RJD looking goo

Early morning walk day after surgery feeling great and ready to go home Home Sweet Home !

It is indeed a new beginning for our angel!! We pray for speed recovery!

Praise our Lord Jesus for His Hesling endures and do His Mercy!! Amen

Ramsis Ghaly

Www.ghalyneurosurgeon.com

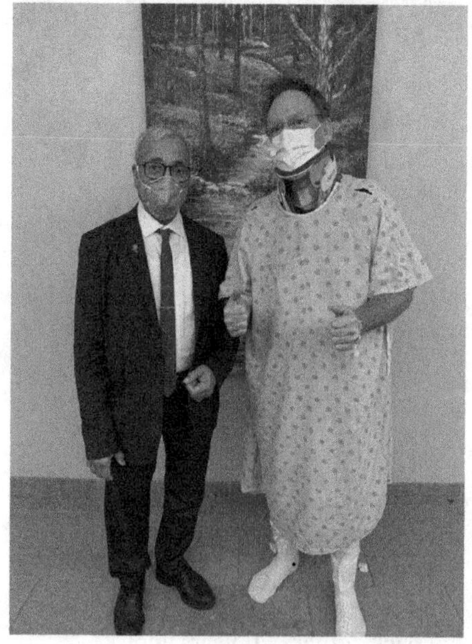

KG, God Bless you and all that you do! Speedy recovery to your patient. Blessings from Egypt

AB, Praise God

Home with no more pinched nerve pains or aches or tingling after surgery!! Praise our Lord Jesus!! Honored to be the Neurosurgeon for my patient

Jeff. Going home today after surgery, sweet home . A special family with spectacular back yard Farm 45. All organic and vegan with no insecticides of fertilizers all Natural—- "Organic gardening with Tomato, peppers, Brussels, onions, garlic, chives, tri-color beans, herbs, summer squash, ground cherries, strawberries, asparagus, raspberries, blackberry, elderberry, popcorn, and 23 chickens. Adding bees next spring!!"

Humbling to learn about our Angelic family Jeff and Katie. We pray for speed recovery Amen

Ramsis Ghaly

Www.ghalyneurosurgeon.com

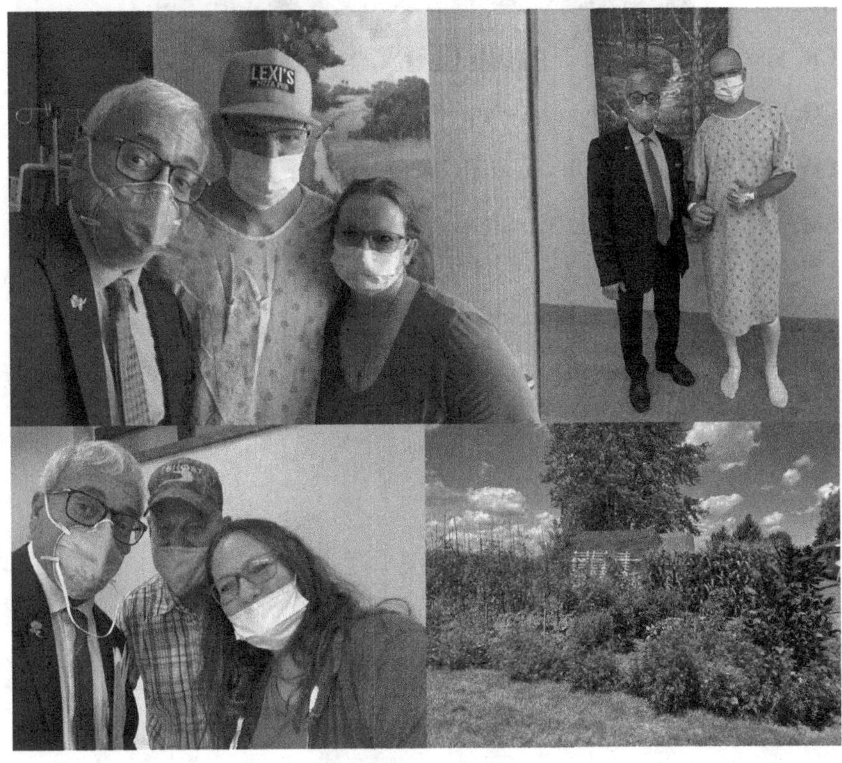

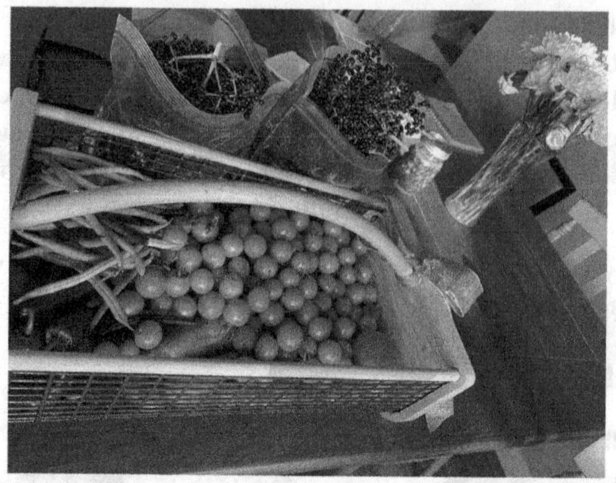

CR, You are an amazing dr **Ramsis Ghaly**

CG, Prayers for a speedy recovery!

LW, God blessed Jeff with you as his doctor.

SM, You are amazing Dr. GHALY and so dedicated. I have so much respect for you.

Kg You were meant to be a doctor !!!

Lg, Continue to be a blessing, Dr. Ghaly! Lifting you up as the Lord God continues to use you as an extension of His healing hands.

Patients Stories 2!

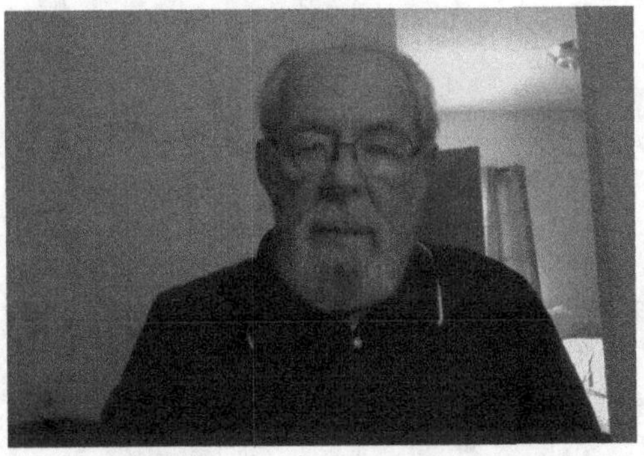

Norman W ParksRamsis Ghaly

What a accomplished Handsome Man. Anyone that knows him and has him fix you up will love him. That includes me. Dr Ghaly is the best of the best.

What a wonderful man and great couple Lance and Maren. Surgery only two weeks ago and ready to work and celebrate.

What a joy!! He also brought The DASH and wrote a touching note thank you. Praise our Lord Jesus.

Much blessing and love

Ramsis Ghaly

Www.ghalyneurosurgeon.com

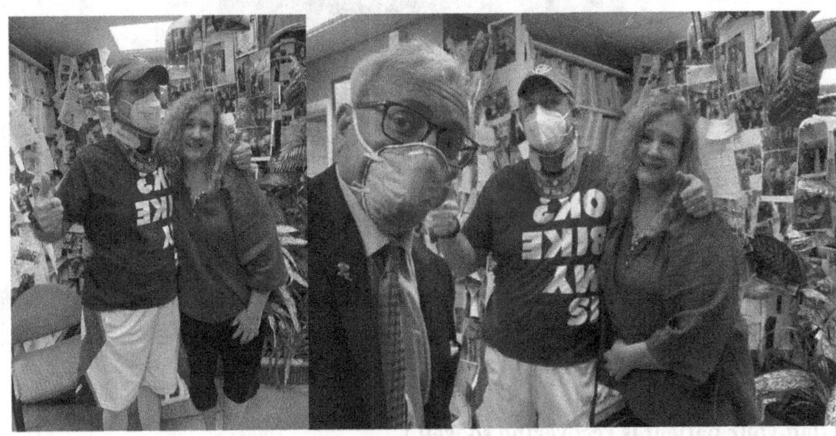

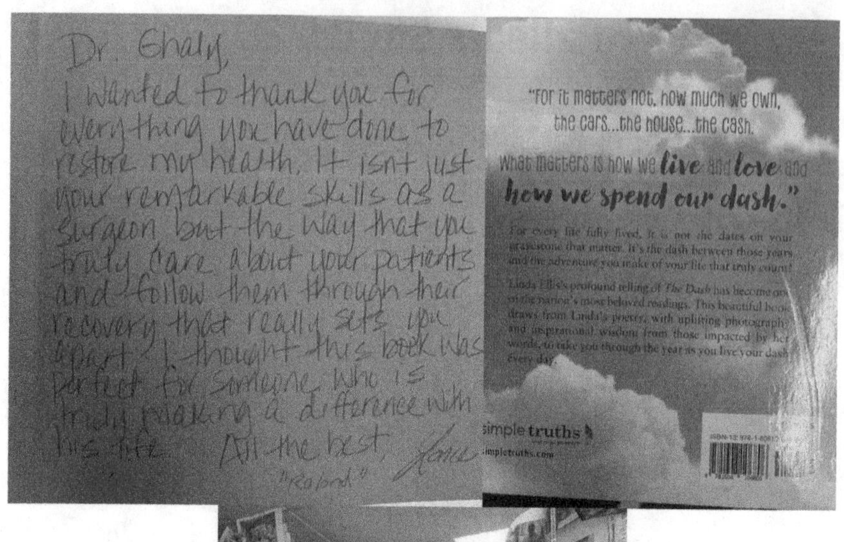
Dr. Ghaly,
I wanted to thank you for everything you have done to restore my health. It isn't just your remarkable skills as a surgeon but the way that you truly care about your patients and follow them through their recovery that really sets you apart. I thought this book was perfect for someone who is truly making a difference with his life.
All the best,

"For it matters not, how much we own, the cars...the house...the cash.
What matters is how we live and love and how we spend our dash."
simple truths
simpletruths.com

4Sandi Benedict Crites, Kathleen MacGregor Grace and 22 others

2 Comments

Like

JP, Glad to hear you're doing well

dl, We read "The Dash" at my daughter's wake in 2009

Glad your patient is recovering so well !

Out angel is so happy done with surgery and neck collar.

Congratulations

. Lance did terrific.

Look at maren and Lance smiles. So proud and happy fur you both. Much blessing to you both praising our Lord Jesus

Ramsis Ghaly

Www.ghalyneurosurgeon.com

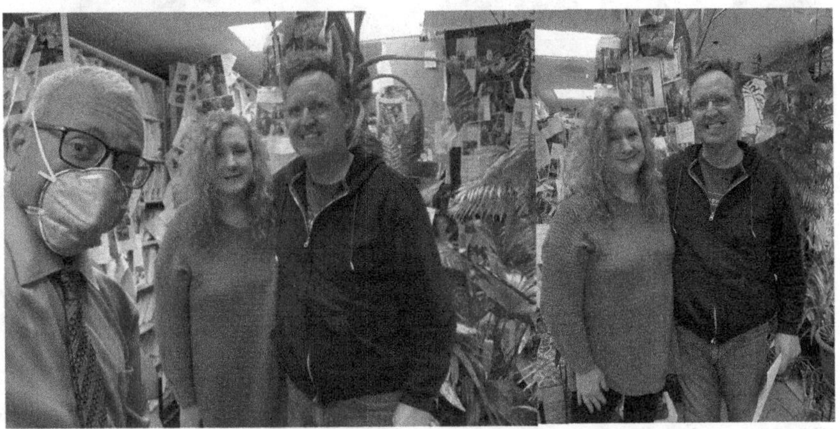

LH, Good for you Lance!!! Must feel great to have that off!

LW, They are so lucky to have had you there for them.

JV, Great news

LK, Some people they don't even realize, how lucky they are to have a doctor with blessed hands by Our Loving God...

Doctor you are the World Savior of many complicated cases.

We need you in Las Vegas...

Why don't saved us suffering here...

May God keep sending blessings on you...

KG, Speedy recovery

LD, Yay!!!!!!!

SH, Time to shotgun a beer.

Home sweet home . What a miracle recovering well after major surgery. Praise our Lord Jesus. Thank you Jim and Deanna

Speed recovery we pray

Ramsis Ghaly

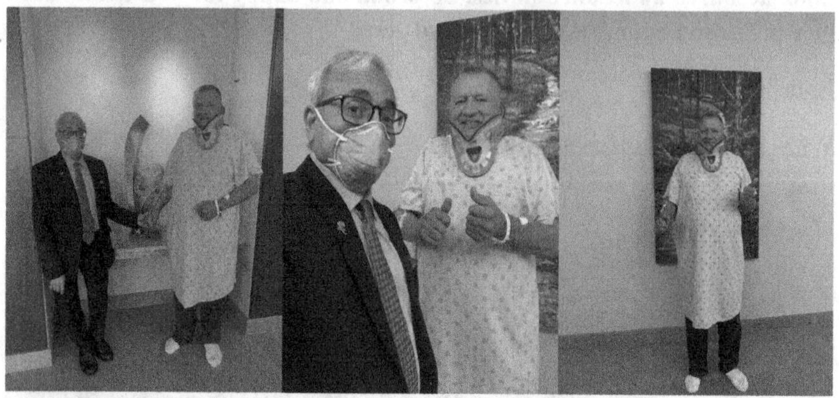

KB, Wait what I just seen Jim Tuesday a picture of heath,hope for speedy recovery

MP, Oh my gosh! That's amazing!!

KG, Speedy recovery and Blessings

TN, Great to hear!!

ES, Best wishes for a speedy recovery Jim!

DH, Best wishes and playing for speedy recovery.

CY,Oh wow! Praying for a full recovery.

CC, Happy Healing!!

KA, Sending healing prayers!

KL, Oh no! Best wishes for a speedy, full recovery Jim.

SP, Wishing you a speedy recovery Jim

LS, Get well soon

CB, Heal well!!!

BC, Get Better soon

Jim and Deanna came to our office as a follow up from Jim surgery! What a blessing to be his neurosurgeon. Much love and blessing always. Praise our Lord for your recovery and healing. Amen

Ramsis Ghaly

Www.ghalyneurosurgeon.com

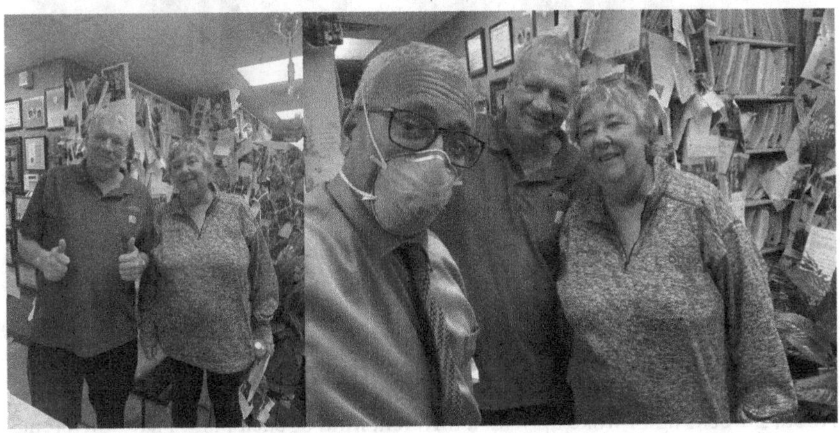

KO, God speed to them

TS, Thankful his surgery was a success.

DD, You are a hero Rhamsis!

CB, So happy for you Jim

CG, Wishing him continued healing.

What a spectacular miracle to see our angel pain free, walking with full strength, going home sweet home after surgery! Lanette and Jim are full of love and blessing with strong faith and positive energy. Praise our Lord Jesus and all the prayers. Much blessing and speed recovery we pray

Ramsis Ghaly

Www.ghalyneurosurgeon.com

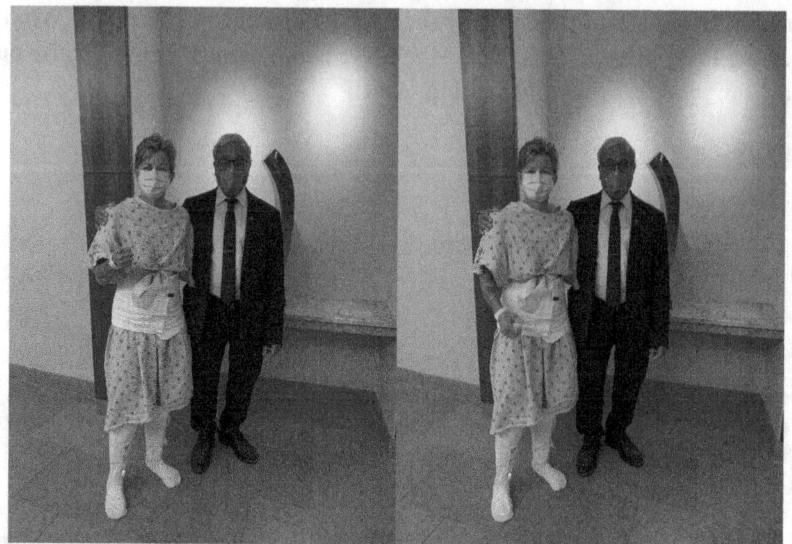

Lanette Yingling

About 2 weeks ago I woke up with a different kind of back pain. I say "different" because I am no stranger to back pain....have had problems since my early teens. This was very different and continued to worsen to the point of numbness and weakness in my leg! I texted Dr. Ramsis Ghaly the next day when I realized that this was more serious than a pulled muscle. He had me come in 3 days later, ordered an MRI immediately and found a badly herniated disc at L3/4. He talked surgery but tried oral steroids for a week and then injection the following Monday.

However, with my symptoms, Dr. G scheduled surgery for that Friday (yesterday)! He did say it was up to me if I wanted to do it, but had the room scheduled anyway. Boy, am I glad he did!! My pain and weakness continued to worsen this past week and by the time I got to the hospital yesterday at 5:30 am I was miserable!!

Surgery was a success and God was with the doctor. This pain AND strength in my leg is back....praise the Lord.

Dr. Ghaly has been such a blessing for Jim and I this year! Two surgeries in 4 months!! Oy...pretty sure we are done for now!

MS, To God be the glory on this healing ministry!

MV, Great news **Lanette**! Take it easy at home!

JS, Oh good Lanette, I was thinking about you last night. So worried after our dog tripped you . Thanks again for the meal!

SY, Oh yay!!!! So good to see her picture up and moving. Praise God! Thanks for helping a great person Dr. Ghaly! I'm so happy she will be out of pain!

RC, Praise our god. Thanks for you great help dr. Ghaly

AV, Praise God for His healing! And for you Dr Ghaly! You truly are a blessing!

AD, Praise God! Thank you for helping my friend, Dr. Ghaly!

CL, God Bless you for all your miracles you perform.

KJ, So glad you're feeling better!

PI, Yes they are, I took care of them both

LG, Bless you.

MA, You are the best Dr

BM, Praise God!

ED, Many blessings to this beautiful lady. She had the best doctor

LK, **Elle DeLacy**Dr Ghaly is the best doctor and surgeon!!! I would go back to Dr Ghaly in a heartbeat

DB, **Lanette Sellers Yingling** sporting that patient gown very well.

Going back to work soon

Jeff and his wife Kati came for clinic visit and brought delicious and healthy goodies from their own garden. So much appreciate their love and blessing!

Fresh goodies from Farm 45. Tomatoes, eggs green beans, garden salsa, peppers and blueberry jam! Home raised chickens and organic garden. Given to our favorite doctor so he can live long and prosper.

Praise our Lord and thankful to Jeff recovery

Ramsis Ghaly

Www.ghalyneurosurgeon.com

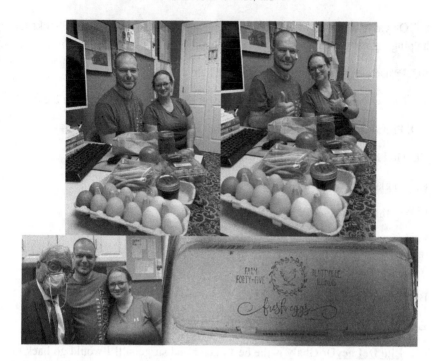

KG, Speedy Recovery

SW, Super nice family. We love them.

MS, Love this

KM, So happy for you guys!!

EM, Amazing

AU, Love dr g! You deserve it! Where is this farm?

RM, Yummm

Thank you Lord Jesus! After more than three months with horrific pains and Inability to sleep bouncing from one doctor to another and one injection to another, taking a huge Toll in himself and family, I did his surgery and immediately pain free slept like a baby with much joy. A new lease in life a new person!!! Amen !

Praise our Lord Jesus who dues wonders!

We pray for speed recovery

<u>Ramsis Ghaly</u>

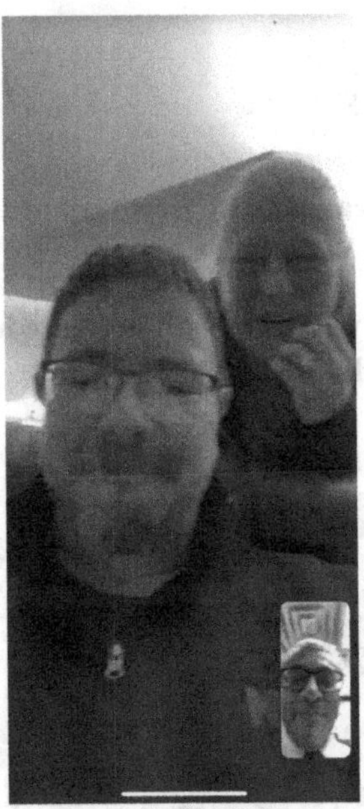

Rv, Amen

Jv, Thank you Dr Ghaly! You have been such a blessing to us. We are so glad that you were able to help us and get Jonny out of pain. You have a true gift from God. You're caring and dedication to your patients is unprecedented. God be with you!

Sn, God Bless you Dr. Ghaly

Cd, Amazing!!!

Tf, Awesome my friend. God driven hands with lots of soul.

Km, You are the best Dr in the US!

Cg, Wishing you a guick recovery! Dr Ghaly is a gift from above.

Sa, Amen

Lw, He was so lucky to find you. God does his work through you.

Jk, Dr. **Ramsis Ghaly**

You are very special to all.

No doubts about, that your hands and you are received special Blessing from God...

I wish you come to Las Vegas, and help us here...

God bless you ways.

Fa, God bless you Dr Ghaly

Our angel and his great caring wife first visit after surgery. He did it. Two in the same time. What a Warrior!

Praise our Lord. recovery terrific with no more horrific pains. Thank you all for your prayers. Much love and blessing

Ramsis Ghaly

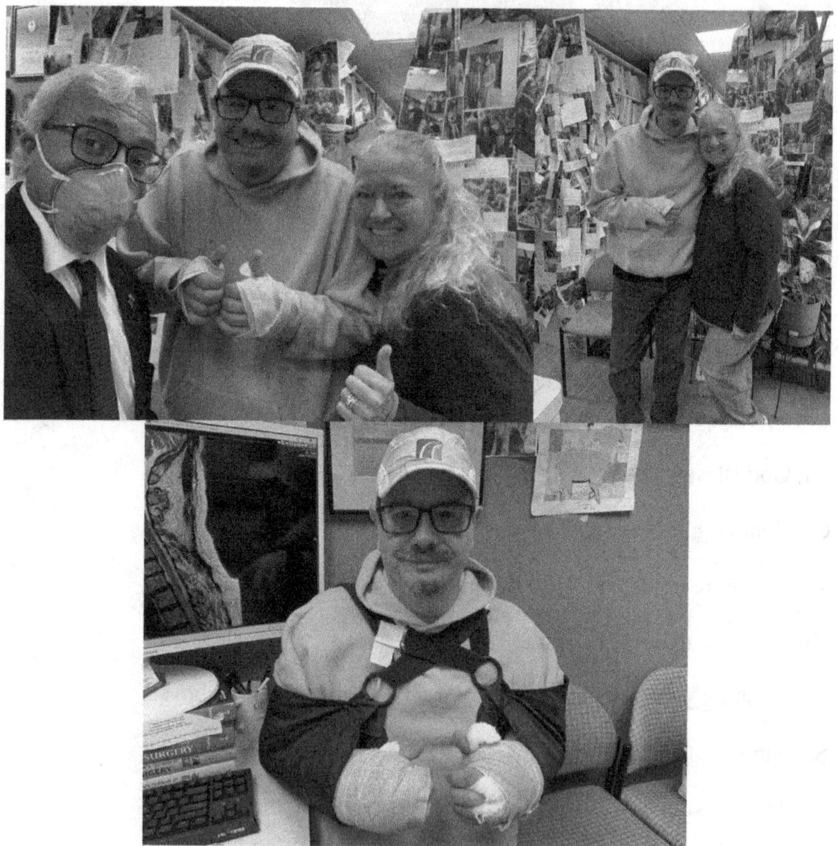

Ko, You had the best dr to care for you sir

av, Praise God! Thank you Dr Ghaly!!

Cg, Wishing him a quick recovery and bless his wife for taking care of him.

jv, Thank you Dr Ghaly. This was not possible without you. His pain was terrible and the recovery has been very easy because of your amazing surgical skills. You have a true gift. Thank you!!

Home sweet home!! Walking early morning with my patient after surgery, Full of energy and joy. Thank you Lord Jesus

We pray for speedy recovery!

Ramsis Ghaly

www.ghalyneurosurgeon.com

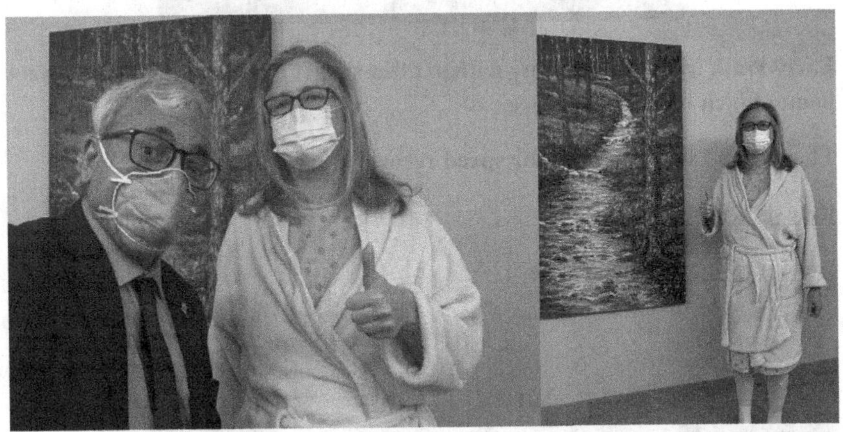

Here is another happy patient two weeks after surgery. These patients come to the office before the surgery almost crawling in the floor from the severe pains and horrific achness.

To see how the Lord help them is just an honor and humble experience. Glory to our Lord God our Savior! Congratulations Connie much more blessing

Ramsis Ghaly

Www.ghalyneurosurgeon.com

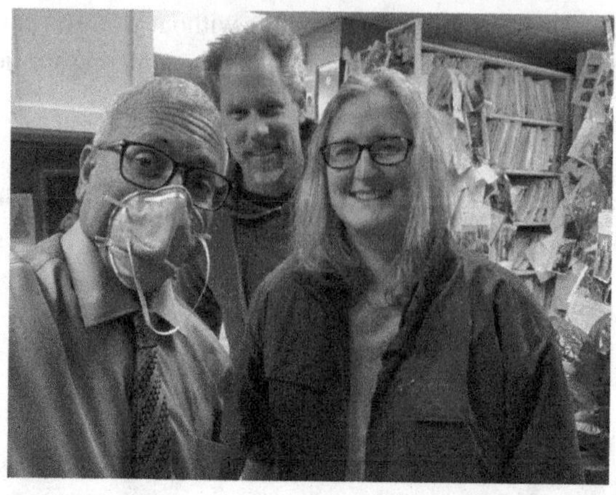

Early Walk in Round with my patient after surgery before going home sweet home. Much blessing and love.

Thank you Lord. We pray for speed recovery!

Ramsis Ghaly

Www.ghalyneurosurgeon.com

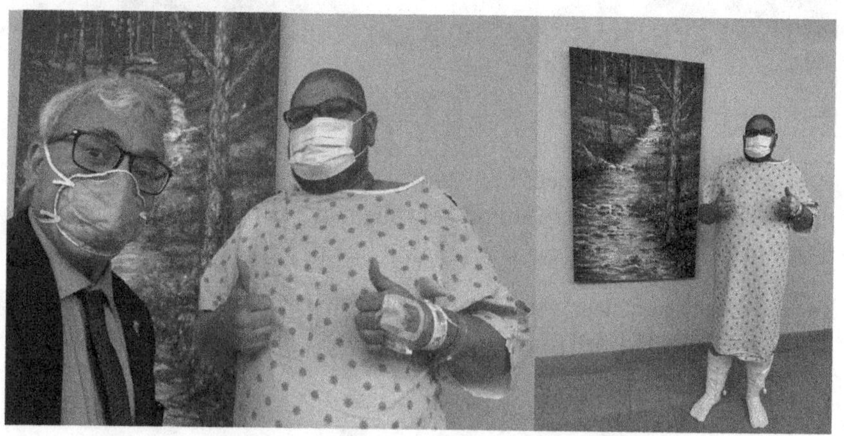

KB, I wish I could have that.So happy for your patient.

MH, Awesome job you did,

congratulations

on healing her so fast.

JS, GOD bless her recovery

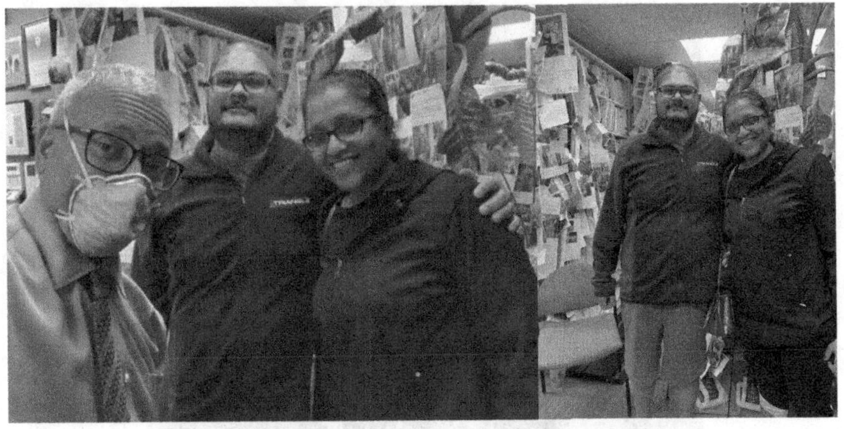

Two angels came from downtown Chicago. Much blessing and speed recovery !! Both love the angels displayed in my clinic!! Thank you!!

Ramsis Ghaly

Www.ghalyneurosurgeon.com

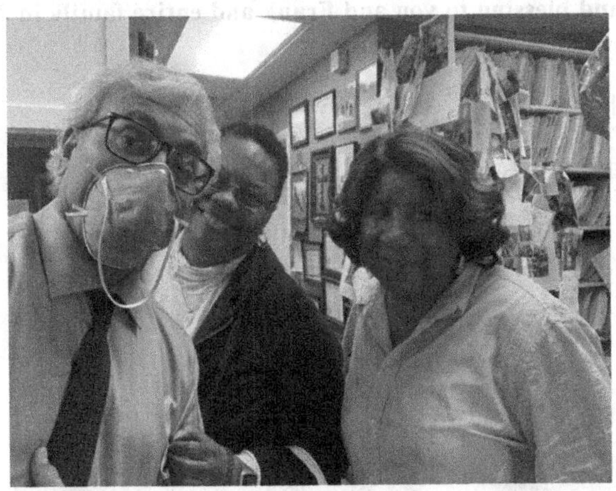

What about these gorgeous smiles in our patients Roger and his wife Imelda

Much Love and blessing Speed recovery

Ramsis Ghaly

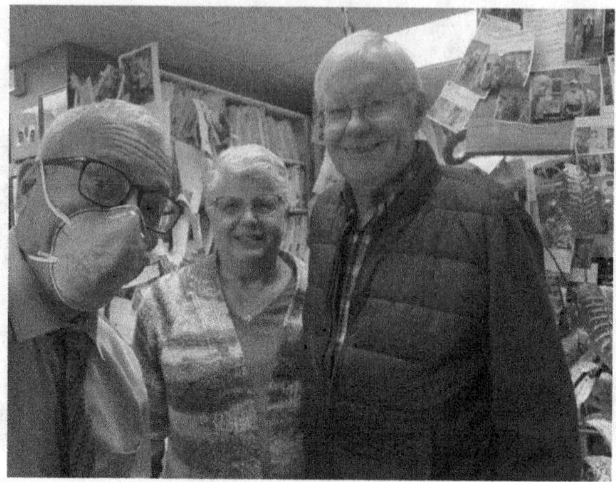

Our angel Charlene Mentzer Glowaty came today to visit and brought a gorgeous plant to add to my office garden. Her surgery was 2017 and God has blessed her, and she is blessing her entire family and the world! We all are fortunate to have Charlene in our life.

Much love and blessing to you and Frank and entire family in Jesus Name, Amen

Ramsis Ghaly

Www.ghalyneurosurgeon.com

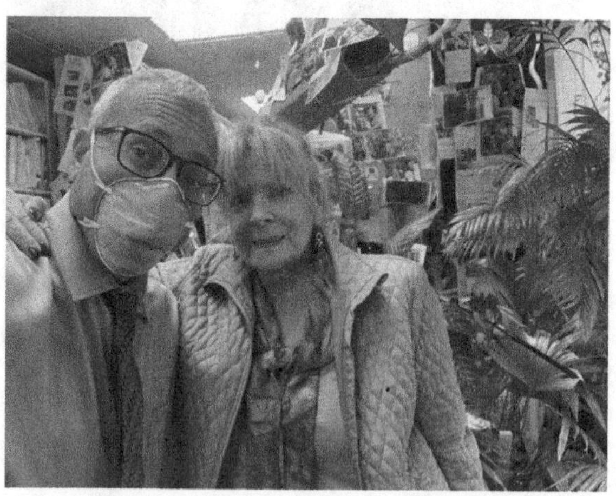

Jb, And thank you for helping Char

Sa, Char is such a beautiful human being.

Ko, Amen blessing to you dr and all of the Glowatys, prayers ongoing

Today was last visit of Our beloved patient Mary Smith Rehm. What an honor. Her back healed and she brought my a treasured gift: St Theresa the little flower from France. There is an Article about lady making glass statue in her shop and the blessing of a nun.

What an honor! Thank you so much to you and all your family. May our Lord Jesus bless you all more and more.

Ramsis Ghaly www.ghalyneurosurgeon.com.

Our angel going home I sweet home after surgery! He has been through so much of pains and suffering! Let us pray for speed recovery !

Ramsis Ghaly

Www.ghalyneurosurgeon.com

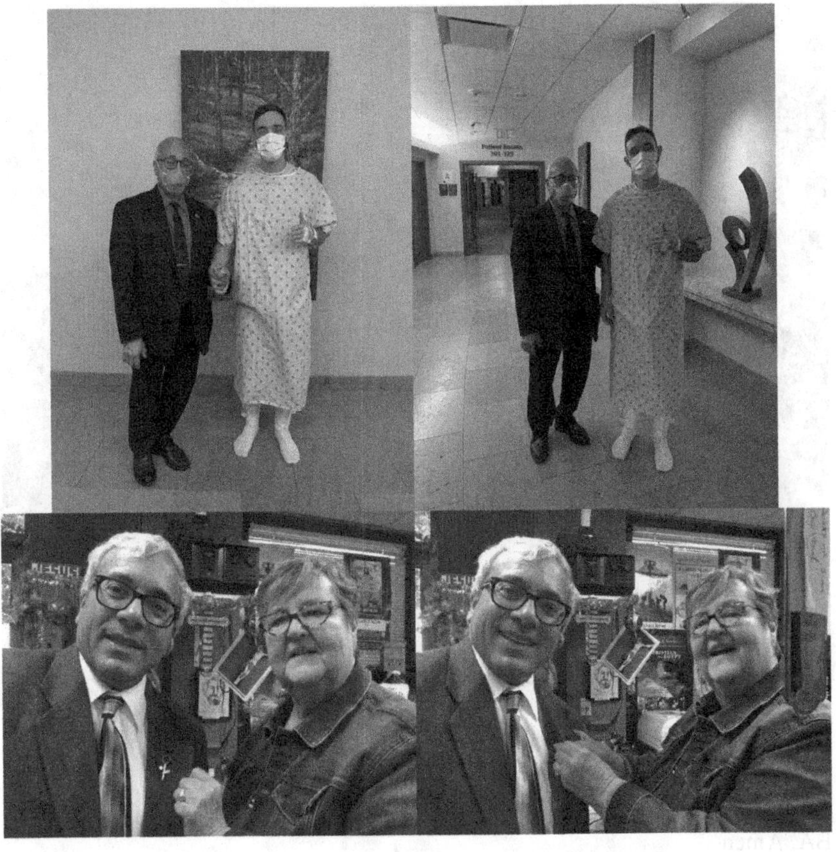

My patient, Lonny, told me before going to undergo major surgery: "I pray that God getting me through surgery and the first thing I see when I wake up in Recovery Unit will, be you and I see your face!"

I did his surgery and our heavenly Savior blessed him and Our Lord granted him what he prayed for: "to see my face in recovery care unit PACU!"

Next morning Lonny is walking, thankful and praising our Lord! And even ahead of many other patients!

Thank you Lord Jesus and thank you Lonny for faith and trust! Speed recovery. And now we all praying for speed recovery in Jesus Name. Amen

Ramsis Ghaly

Www.ghalyNeurosurgeon.com

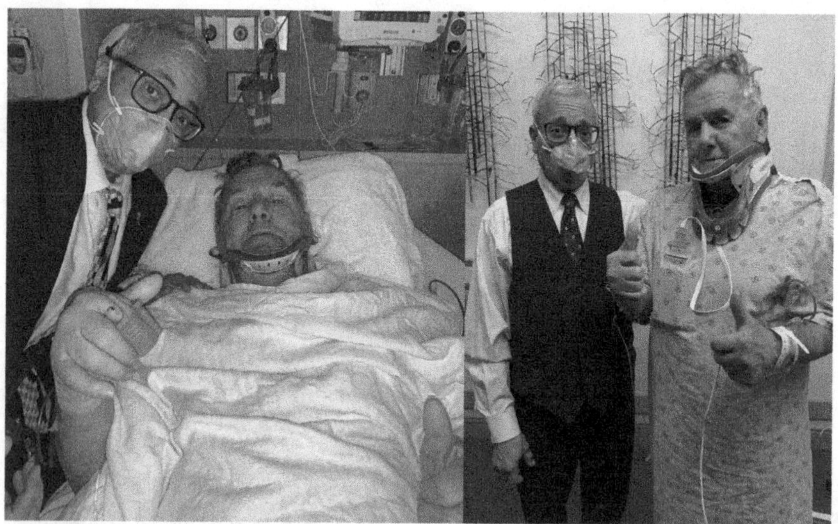

EL, Speedy recovery!!

ED, Amen

BL, Amen. Lonnie has the best surgical care anyone could pray for.

LM, Praying for a speedy recovery

BV, Amen

BA, Amen

CG, Sending warm wishes of healing as you recover from surgery.

DE, Speedy recovery!

SJ, You are an Angel doctor! I wish there were more Drs. Like you

JS, Amazing!

Patients and Colleagues Comments!

<u>Sherry Lee</u>

I'm so glad she found you as her Doctor!! I understand, I was one of those patients.... just about crawling in, couldn't hardly walk upright. I'm so happy that you are there to help so many!! When the other doctors tell you that it must be just "you" and make you feel terrible, then you look and see the real problem and you - with Gods help - fix the problem, and life is normal again, it's the best thing in the world! The world needs more like you. May God continue to bless you and your healing hands

<u>Jolanta Krol</u>

Some people they don't even realize, how lucky they are to have a doctor with blessed hands by Our Loving God...

Doctor you are the World Savior of many complicated cases.

We need you in Las Vegas...

Why don't saved us suffering here...

May God keep sending blessings on you...

Val Aldret

Ramsis, what a great news that you and Cook County are welcoming, and that you will be teaching Navy Lt. Henderson DNP, CRNA. He is an American hero. <u>But you are a hero as well !</u> You have been serving our country by saving lives of American Citizens; every day for the last 36 years. I am proud of your service to USA,

Charlene Glowaty

You have so many achievements to be proud of through the years. The Lord has been by your side the whole time. Blessings!

Becky Neitzke

I remember when Mary Daniels called me about Sue Ann. You performed a miracle! Mary always spoke of you with the highest regards!

You're the best

Dr. Ghaly!

Dawn Smothers Morrison

Sir there is no question that God has given you surgical abilities that are stellar and a faith in him that is unwavering!! You have given life to two of my family members and we are so blessed by your hands!! Stephen Schott and Brad Conderman

Milena Paunovic

Your life story impresses and inspires. Nothing happens without a clear goal, without faith in yourself, and without faith in God. Your life and dedication to your profession and to the Lord is admirable.

Happy Birthday! Happy birthday!

Val Aldrete

You are an incredible blessing to these patients after all doctors failed them, hurt them, abandon them and left them to suffer and die. You are amazing surgeon!!! I am so proud to be your friend. Val

Linda Reeves

I enjoyed meeting you today! Your medical office is like a shrine to God. Thank you for helping my cousin! Gratefully yours, Linda Reeves

Cristina Rojas-Rutkowski

You are my angel my dear doctor and I will always be grateful for your great help and time.

Heather Stonehill-Garcia

You and Jesus are the most amazing team Dr Ghaly!!

Jack Jane Cole Duvick

I truly believe everything you said Dr. Ghaly !! Keep up the great work that you do !!!

James King S

Dr. Your hands & mind is threw are lords guidance, your a great dr. Bless you & all you help heal threw there healing journey!!

P.S: am i still on your wall of gods grace?? In your office??

Martha Lorena Aranda

I remember you also had the newspaper clippings of when you take took care of my brother, Jorge Salas Sr. He passed now, but at that time we owed you his life. Forever grateful to you and God's hands that guided yours.

Elizabeth Landes

Dr. Ghaly - you are an amazing man. God gave you a wonderful gift!! He is working through you!!

Dianna Kay

God given talent,skill and compassion!! May God bless you as you bless others!

Donna Hentsch

Praise God and your healing thru Jesus Christ Dr Ghaly

Diana Lynn

So handsome & professional looking...as always Dr !

Charlene Glowaty

God is the true King and we are all his children and so therefore we are all Royals. You are a special Royal because you spread the word of God.

Julie Volk

Thank you Dr Ghaly! You have been such a blessing to us. We are so glad that you were able to help us and get Jonny out of pain. You have a true gift from God. You're caring and dedication to your patients is unprecedented. God be with you!

Linda Williamson

He was so lucky to find you. God does his work through you.

Charlene Glowaty

Wishing you a guick recovery! Dr Ghaly is a gift from above.

Katia Moura

You are the best Dr in the US!

Jolanta Krol

Dr. Ramsis Ghaly

You are very special to all.

No doubts about, that your hands and you are received special Blessing from God...

I wish you come to Las Vegas, and help us here...

God bless you ways.

Holly Brockman

Blessings for a complete healing and recovery. I know that you got the best talented doctor. Fantastic!

Lanette Yingling

You are such a blessing Dr. Ghaly

Sandra Crites

I dont know doctor i dont think me personally would have liked robotic hands in my glad you had the skillful hands that you did thank all mighty jesus!

Josh Prime

Good morning, I wanted to thank you for all these amazing days I get to have because of you. I miss, think about you and love you so much. Have a wonderful weekend

Kristina Collins

You are great at putting people in contact with each other and helping. I know my mom was happy to share her experience with trigeminal nueralgia with other patiences. People who dont even know what they have or anyone who has been through some of these strange issues are really lucky to have you as their Doctor.

Kathy O'Brien

You had the best dr to care for you sir

Julie Volk

Thank you Dr Ghaly. This was not possible without you. His pain was terrible and the recovery has been very easy because of your amazing surgical skills. You have a true gift. Thank you!!

Diana Martin

Thank God for Dr. Ramsis Ghaly.

Gina Svara

We just met with Dr. Ramsis Ghaly and were given amazing news. After a very long day he was able to make her spine look beautiful! He spent countless hours cleaning up the mess from her failed surgery 10 years ago. She will be moved to a room soon and the recovery begins. I do not know of any other surgeon in this world who would dedicate his life to patients and spend countless hours viewing scans and preparing the best plan. I am forever grateful! He believes God moves his hands and Cheri is one lucky patient to have his skilled hands fix her!

Charlene Glowaty

How wonderful, that because of you she gets to fulfill her dream of walking down the aisle to the man she loves.

Congratulations

!

That is one of the things I like about your office. You come out and introduce us to each other.

Lanette Yingling

We always love to give our testimony at the amazing work you have done in our lives to the people in your waiting room!

Heidi Walker

Happy Birthday Dr. Ghaly! God Bless you and all you do for others

Shelley Peyton Alexander

Happy Birthday Dr. Ghaly! Thank you for all you do for your patients, including me! I hope you had a wonderful day today!

Cheri Polich

May God continue to bless you in all your work & for a healthy & happy future. You are a miracle worker and have helped so many people. I am grateful to all you have done for me. Happiest of Birthdays to you Dr. Ghaly!

Kathy Manthei Sitar

Happy Birthday, Dr. Ghaly. I remember when you were in Joliet and the Herald News had a great article on you. You saved a classmate of mine by removing a tumor from her brain and she made a magnificent recovery . May God bless you today and every day.

Annette Cozzi

A Blessed & Happy Birthday to you Dr Ghaly. We who have been blessed by your gift in this lifetime are eternally thankful for the day you were born. God had such a beautiful plan for your life. We are grateful to be part of it.

Karen Boland Geheber

Happy happy Birthday Dr. Ghaly Your story is an inspiration to all of us to never give up, pray hard, and always believe that God hears us and answers our prayers

Deanna Brockman Johnson

Happy Birthday Dr Ghaly, you have been a gift of healing to so many, your compassion and care of your patients and their families is very rare indeed God bless you always

Tanya Rand

Dr. **Ramsis Ghaly**, you are not only a healer, you are an inspiration, reminding us that God will always show us the way if we allow it. Happy birthday

Darrius Washington

Happy birthday Dr. Ghaly God bless I know your parents are watching over you from Heaven with so much joy, you are their gift to the world and you help heal the world and we are so grateful for you. Hope you enjoy your birthday

Giza Salas

Happy birthday to a great man! May God bless you today on your special day and always..

I will forever be thankful for everything you did for my father. You rock!

Terry Lee Ebert Mendozza

Happy birthday to my special friend, Healer and Anointed of Christ our Lord, to whom I am so grateful for your caring friendship. I cry when I read your stories, but I am always inspired by them. May the Lord's blessings always fall upon you, Ramsis. Happy birthday to you, my dear friend

Gabriela Miller

Have a blessed birthday, you are a living inspiration and your words… full of wisdom for those who (including myself) at times, forget God and all his call and love every day

Angel Schultz

Happy happy birthday you are a wonderful person . Everyone in my son-in-law's family told me what a wonderful doctor you are . I hope you have a beautiful birthday enjoy

Michael Plunkett

May you always have God's Blessings. You are a faithful one, Amen . You are the special healer. I see you everyday enjoying the Present, life offers. You share and help others enjoy their present 's too. You are a special human. Enjoy the Present !

SA, Dr. Ramsis may God bless you and be with you all the time & to help you continue your great work which you do with so much love and care, may this year be filled with love & joy and all God's blessings showers you

Sally Brady

Happy Birthday, Dr. . Ghaly. Thank the Lord you never gave up. Your Faith kept you going and He never lets us down so long as we focus on Him and thank him continually for all our blessings. You are one fantastic doctor and our family loves you. Thanks for being there for us when we were so in need for you. May our Heavenly Father continue to bless you.

Bretonya Phillips-Johnson

Happy birthday Dr.Ghaly! You are unmatched, truly a gift to us all, a gift to the world!

Violeta Dato Morrison

HAPPY HAPPY BIRTHDAY MY GENIUS KIND DEDICATED HARD WORKING FRIEND . THE BEST NEUROSURGEON PAIN MANAGEMENT PHYSICIAN. MORE BIRTHDAYS AND BLESSINGS TO CELEBRATE

Jennifer L. Johnston Happy Birthday! God had big plans to use you and He did!!! I am so thankful you were born and are a great blessing to many. Have fun celebrating today!!!

Valerie Williams

Happy Birthday Dr Ghaly, you are one of those chosen ppl that you never want to forget. You are such a blessing. I've learned so much from reading this excerpt of your life and through the Grace Of God you still kept your FAITH. You are one of the best.

Norma Jean

Happy Birthday Dr. Ghaly! May God continue to bless you and your hands so that you can continue to do more good and save more lives! Wishing you all the very best!!

Charlene Mentzer Glowaty

You write from your heart, about something you're passionate about. Your heart, your passion, and your emotions are what you share with us. Bless you on your birthday and everday.

Donna Hentsch

Happiest of Birthdays to you Dr. Ghaly!

Thanking all you have done helping people, God has truly given you a gift of being a successful surgeon, you do Good works thru our Lord & Savior

Mike Nutoni

Happy birthday DrGhaly to the best doctor the lord placed on this earth have a great day miss you

Norma Jean

Happy Birthday Dr. Ghaly! May God continue to bless you and your hands so that you can continue to do more good and save more lives! Wishing you all the very best!!

Valerie Williams

Happy Birthday Dr Ghaly, you are one of those chosen ppl that you never want to forget. You are such a blessing. I've learned so much from reading this excerpt of your life and through the Grace Of God you still kept your FAITH. You are one of the best.

Sandi Benedict Crites

Happy birthday my friend $ many many more your work here is far from finished the good lord is gonna keep you here to save many more lives

Jackie Mitchell Martin

Happy Birthday Dr Ghaly! And thank you for your faith that shines like a beacon for the lost

Edwina Bator-Swanson

Happy Birthday Dr Ghaly. May you have many many more years ahead of you. You are loved by so many and you have a large family of friends and many patients that are so grateful for your skills.

Heidi Walker

Happy Birthday Dr. Ghaly!God Bless you and all you do for others

Christie Loftin

Happy Birthday! God has blessed you in so many ways. In turn, it blesses us too!

Arsho Mahserejian

HAPPY BIRTHDAY

Dr. **Ramsis Ghaly**.

Wishing you Always best wishes, and good health.

I always follow your successful stories and I like your spiritual soul, humanitarian heart and clever mind.

Thanks for always sharing your beautiful writings.

Please pray for peace to this world and in the meantime pray for my people and for their land in Armenia .

Thanks and God bless you and your family

Amelia Molina-lucena

Happy birthday Dr. Ghaly . God made you to have the Will power to Help people, God bless

Aldrete

Happy Birthday Ramsis- we love you and are so grateful you are in our lives - you are the most amazing person and doctor and friend and we love you- much love Retta

Judy Conderman

Happy Birthday Dr. Ghaly!! May you enjoy many more healthy happy years. You are a gift from God and the most caring, compassionate, admired and gifted doctor. Our family loves you and appreciates all that you have done for us. Enjoy this beautiful day.

Sarah Popp

Happy birthday to the best doctor

Mammaponio

Compassionate knowledgeable doctor and beautiful soul!

Suzi Hamilton

You are amazing! So glad you pray and wait on God's guidance

Kim Ryan

Love your words—-

As a nurse I love hearing your thankfulness for your patients relief of pain and wonderful outcomes-your not just a surgeon, but a God send to your patients. What a miracle this story is—Thanks so much for sharing!

Kathleen Grace

Ramsis Ghaly Our God is an Awesome and Amazing GOD to bring such miracles for the world to witness through your devoted care, expertise and unfailing faith. Thank you,Dr Ghaly, for all that you do helping all of the world through HIS glorious interventions and Wisdom! Amen Amen Amen

God Bless you in HIS mighty name forever and ever.

We all love you, Dr Ghaly.

Blessings from Egypt

Barbara Carroll

I feel like God helps us every day. You are a true blessing!

Michael Plunkett

Always listen to the voice, Amen ! God works through your hands I have no doubt.

Michelle Lizzethe

Always listen to the voice, Amen ! God works through your hands I have no doubt.

Suzette Jennings

What a wonderful diagnostician and Servant of God you are, Dr. Ghaly.

Cristopher Kladis

Yes, you are used of God and stepping on toes is a part of that. I firmly believe as it is written in the infallible Word of God

“obedience is better than sacrifice “ God bless you Dr. Ghaly and yes listen to that still small voice!

Kathy Everett

Grèat Man and very gallant,*

Judy Kladis

Yes, you are used of God and stepping on toes is a part of that. I firmly believe as it is written in the infallible Word of God

“obedience is better than sacrifice “ God bless you Dr. Ghaly and yes listen to that still small voice!

Holly Davis

I love that you honor the Lord & listen to the Holy Spirit! You are blessed & continue to bless those around you!

Lanette Yingling

I love that you honor the Lord & listen to the Holy Spirit! You are blessed & continue to bless those around you!

Edwina Swanson

God has given you a special gift. With that gift you have saved and enriched many lives of people. You hold a special place in the hearts of your patients and their families.

Brenda Linquist

Oh Dr. Ghaly, you are such a strong and productive branch that is an amazing tribute to our Father. I am privileged to call you an important influence in my life. (I am a sister to one of your past patients-Larry Swarens and an aunt to Wendy Swarens who were helped immensely by your talents.) I wish I lived closer to your location; I have some challenging medical needs.

May God continue to bless you and your work.

Carolyn Rehenan

I've been a nurse for 40 years, still working. I wish so much that today's doctors would drop the attitudes and arrogance and have some actual compassion and care for the patients. The little one I'm working with went to the hospital with status epilepticus. The ER did everything just right. When they got to the floor with the child, the neurologist refused to treat the child. The doctor said the patient is terminal, and had a very, very rare medical problem and refused to treat the child. What kind of Hippocratic Oath did that "so called doctor" swear to? BTW, the child is a full code. This is only one of the situations those parents are facing. The diagnosis is so rare, this is a child on only 9 with this particular gene so these young (compared to me, lol) are arrogant, rude, and actually bully the mother when she tells them what the team of specialists told her was right for this child. It's a disgrace. There is little compassion, understanding or the desire to treat something that may be over their heads. The disease they suffer with is PRIDE. Sorry for the long post, you just made me remember HOW IT'S SUPPOSED TO BE.

Margret Hale

You should take great pride in that. It was a great gift he gave you, in order to help his people to heal & feel good once again. You are a great Dr. And great pride that you are a great servant of the Lord. One of the Best Dr's. Ever!! With a caring & loving that you have for all you work on. I Love your dedication that you put in your work. You have a lot to be proud of in life have a great day.

Lanette Yingling

About 2 weeks ago I woke up with a different kind of back pain. I say "different" because I am no stranger to back pain....have had problems since my early teens. This was very different and continued to worsen to the point of numbness and weakness in my leg! I texted Dr. Ramsis Ghaly the next day when I realized that this was more serious than a pulled muscle. He had me come in 3 days later, ordered an MRI immediately and found a badly herniated disc at L3/4. He talked surgery but tried oral steroids for a week and then injection the following Monday.

However, with my symptoms, Dr. G scheduled surgery for that Friday (yesterday)! He did say it was up to me if I wanted to do it, but had the room scheduled anyway. Boy, am I glad he did!! My pain and weakness continued to worsen this past week and by the time I got to the hospital yesterday at 5:30 am I was miserable!!

Surgery was a success and God was with the doctor. This pain AND strength in my leg is back....praise the Lord Dr. Ghaly has been such a blessing for Jim and I this year! Two surgeries in 4 months!! Oy...pretty sure we are done for now!

Sarah Young

Oh yay!!!! So good to see her picture up and moving. Praise God! Thanks for helping a great person Dr. Ghaly! I'm so happy she will be out of pain!

Julie Annette

Dr, Ghaly is amazing! Hugs and Prayers, Lanette

Linda Andzulis

Dr. Ramsis Ghaly has written several books:

A Christian from Egypt: Life Story of a Neurosurgeon Pursuing the Dreams for Quintuple Certifications

https://www.amazon.com/Christ.../dp/B0793PPF66/ref=sr_1_1...

Touching Stories of My Life in Journey to Christian Holiness and Hands- on Patient Care in a Weeping Healthcare: The Brain of Man of God and the Hand of ... of a Coptic Christian Neurosurgeon

https://www.amazon.com/.../dp/B07XKZ6P7N/ref=sr_1_fkmr0_2...

Christianity and the Brain: Volume I: Faith and Medicine in Neuroscience Care

https://www.amazon.com/.../ref=dbs_a_def_rwt_hsch_vapi...

Christianity and the Brain: Volume II: The Christian Brain and the Journey between Earth and Heaven: 2 by Ramsis Ghaly https://www.amazon.com/.../ref=dbs_a_def_rwt_hsch_vapi...

Christianity and the Brain: Volume III

https://www.amazon.com/.../ref=dbs_a_def_rwt_hsch_vapi...

Christianity and the Brain: Patients Stories: 100 Stories of Hope, Faith and Courage

https://www.amazon.com/.../ref=dbs_a_def_rwt_hsch_vapi...

Cindy Rice

He continues to heal so many! This man is an Angel on earth following the lord as a faithful servant. I owe him everything and I'm forever grateful!

Annette Valtman

Praise God for His healing! And for you Dr Ghaly! You truly are a blessing!

Christie Loftin

God Bless you for all your miracles you perform.

Juli Annette

Dr, Ghaly is amazing! Hugs and Prayers, Lanette

Margaret Agamy

You are the best Dr

Louise Keane

Elle DeLacyDr Ghaly is the best doctor and surgeon!!! I would go back to Dr Ghaly in a heartbeat

Dave Brown

Our lives are better because of what God has done through you, Dr. Ghaly! Thank you, God, and, thank you Dr. Ghaly! Dave & Sue.

Val Aldrete

Great pictures! You patients truly love and appreciate you! Most of your patients are suffering, being misdiagnosed by other doctors, cannot work, most of them don't have any money and they already had bad surgeries and even worst care. You give them hope, restore their dignity and health and they praise the Lord to bless you! And you are Blessed! Val

Spydie Ryider

God bless you Dr. Ghaly!! You are an amazing physician and teacher!! I miss working with you!

Bobi Nordstrom

Praise God! You are a man sent from God. I'll probably never get to meet you but Thank you for all you do for your fellow man. Sincerely.

Mary Nixon

Yes Dr. Ramsis Ghaly is a miracle worker, bless him and you guys fir finding him as I did I'm 2007, my back is better than ever..

Anthony DeVinney

Dr. Ghaly, a unique take on Chicago Violence. I can't imagine what so many MD's, NP's, PA's, and nurses have to go through trying to save the life of others in our trauma centers in Chicago daily. We are all fortunate for these people who are doing God's work every day.

Kathy Hogan

You are such a blessing!

Lanette Yingling

I am also thankful for our surgeon (he did Jim's surgery in May) Dr. Ramsis Ghaly. He is an amazing doctor and surgeon that truly cares for his patients! He always makes sure that recovery is going well by calling us and checking in. God also knew what He was doing when we crossed paths with this doctor!

> Manady Levi
>
> All your love and prayers and sacrifice that you do all your life, I see it and it changed my life, and I know God used you, and I see all the spiritual Riches that you've given to the world to others and how lucky I am to be someone who is included in that! Thank you for calling me Thank you for praying for me even unknowingly God used your beautiful spirit and pure heart to help me
>
> Cindy Rice
>
> Love you Gwen! Dr Ramsis Ghaly never fails to give healing to all he touches! I'm so happy for you!
>
> #HEROESDONTALLWEARCAPES

Someone posted this hashtag and I absolutely loved seeing it! Life is hard and LOVE is the only way to get through it

Dr Ramsis Ghaly I snapped this off your wall of pictures! So thought if you when I seen this hashtag!

Andrew Martin

You are blessed and gifted man

Michelle Lizette

You are a very special man.

Jolanta Krol

Dr Ramsis Ghaly

You are the best doctor and faithful God Worshiper...

We need you in Las Vegas

Dr. Ramsis Ghaly,

God not only blessed you, but also gave you special blessed hands, so you can keep cured people...

May God always keep.blessing you...

Carol Pasteris

It was 22 years ago this month that I had brain tumor surgery. I thank God for keeping me alive for my family & friends. I also thank Dr. Ghaly for doing a fine job during surgery. :)

Cindy Rice

Love you Gwen! Dr Ramsis Ghaly never fails to give healing to all he touches! I'm so happy for you!

Oliver Brandt

Dr.Ghaly, my spine surgeon is guided by a higher power

Lynda Christenman

Gwen, you look wonderful. Love seeing that smile again. Thank you Dr. Ghaly for making that possible.

Charlene Glowaty

You are an amazing doctor and God has truly given you a gift. He blessed you with the knowledge and compassion that you possess as a doctor. May he continue to guide and bless you.

Scott Mitchell

Your the best Dr G!!!

Robin Hellenberg

Your prayer is MIND blowing!!! And you say this while you're operating. I give thanks for your genius. God has given you some amazing gifts. you were so humble about it. You are loved doctor

Cindy Dahl

Thank you so much Ramsis!

I will miss seeing you and sending you off with your coffee and scone to do your amazing work You truly are one of my favorite people to see at Starbucks (and I love seeing your beautiful ties) . I will keep you posted on surgery and see you again in November !

Karen Boland Geheber

You were meant to be a doctor !!!

Lana Wania-Galicia

Continue to be a blessing, Dr. Ghaly! Lifting you up as the Lord God continues to use you as an extension of His healing hands.

Margaret Agamy

Dr Ghaly is a miracle worker

Edwina Swanson

Lucky students. You are the best mentor.

Sandy Shenouda

God bless you Doc ! They are lucky to have you!

Cheryl Glowaty

Thanks for taking great care of us dr Ghaly!

Winnie Patricoski

You are simply the BEST!

Patients Quotes 56

Jan Viano

Dr Ramsis Ghaly You are a gift to this world and to your patients and friends. I sm so thankful for your help and bringing me back to life. Many many blessing I wish for you.

Armen Hart

Our precious Dr Ghaly

You are a Gem

Rick Malina

Sir You are a True Unsung Hero, Thank you for being You

Jim Doyel

Bless you my friend, you are a Godsend to many lucky people.

Rosalyn Abadi

If our country had your devotion to seeking God first, our nation would be strong and respected and healed. God bless you Doctor.

Laurie Kapsalis

A true heart shines bright inside and out. You will always be a beautiful soul. I miss you

Rosalyn Chalfant Abadie

If our country had your devotion to seeking God first, our nation would be strong and respected and healed. God bless you Doctor.

Jim Doyel

Bless you my friend, you are a Godsend to many lucky people.

John DiFiore

Excellent

Charles Putnam

A angel among us. God Bless you my friend.

Michelle Brcik

What an amazing life philosophy to live by!!! Beautiful!!

Tammi Ciciora

You are simply the best Dr Ghaly. You make every patient feel equally important and you are such amazing human! Thank you for all you do for so many

Dr Samuel Kingsley

Really fantastic. You are a real asset to both the surgery and anesthesia programs here. Much appreciated.

Richard J. Fantus, MD, FACS, Professor and Chair, Department of Surgery, Interim Chair, Department of Anesthesia, Medical Director, Trauma, Surgical, and Perioperative Services:

Excellent lecture. I listened to every word. You spoke for an hour straight right after finishing a busy 24 hour call!

Thanks again

Sondra Lynch

You are phenomenal

Mike Nutoni

I can't believe how I looked then to how I look now thanks to you and God what a miracle.You and God are the greatest.

Joshua Prim

I am so grateful for you everyday. I hope you have a great day. We love you and we appreciate everything you have done and do.

Pam Horner

GOD truly blessed you with so much love and compassion for others and then led you to a profession that allowed to to follow in his loving guidance to make people's lives so much better.... You are truly an Angel among us

Michael Nutoni

DRGHALY as always another job well done your the best. Pray for a fast recovery.

Kathy O'BRIEN

Health fast,You had the best s

Jolsanta Karol

You are so fortunate having the best from the best

dr. Ramsis Ghaly ...

We need you in Las Vegas

Dennis

You always work your magic and thank God you're around.

Her son did say they were glad they got you- good day

Kathleen MacGregory Grace

You are a Beautiful ageless soul Inside and out. You always will be for you have that ethereal glow like no others. Shine on Beautiful Soul. Blessings and Love from Egypt

Myrna Macaso

Praying for her healing,Almighty God I trust in you,I hope she will get her miracle just like I did.Dr. Ghaly you you're the best, GodBless

Val Aldrete

Ramsis, her survival is truly miraculous, ALL thanks to your care and devotion. And Thanks to God blessing. Your name should be posted on hospital web site and administration should make all medical staff aware of your incredible skill of saving patients that are left to die. The medial staff should be forced to learn from you. You are my hero!!!!!!!!

Dotti Lopez

The best Doctor ever. I would fly across the world for you. May God continue to bless her and you Dr. Ramsis Ghaly.

Joshua Prim

You are our hero Dr. Ghaly! I'm singing your praises from the rooftops, hoping that anyone who needs it gets a chance to have you as their Doctor/friend

Bobbi Nordstrom

You are our hero Dr. Ghaly! I'm singing your praises from the rooftops, hoping that anyone who needs it gets a chance to have you as their Doctor/friend

Mary Siegel

You bring me closer to Our Lord Jesus with your faith. Thank you.

Linda Williamson

God blessed him by making you his doctor.

Bobbi Nordstrom

God bless you! Such a beautiful soul. You live and love to help people.

Manjeet Batth

Very nice picture Doctor

Thank you so much...You are the best...

Eduardo Gonzalez

Dr Ghaly, you are an amazing physician!

Kathleen McGregor

Ramsis Ghaly HUGE Thank you and Thank GOD for Blessing us with you. Totally fine again. Very Thankful. God Bless you, Ramsis Ghaly!

Christine Secherman

U work miracles!!

Lisa Zizas

THANK YOU ALL so much for all the birthday calls, texts and messages!! It was wonderful to hear from so many of you and it made my day! This birthday was so much better than last year where I spent the day having spinal fusion surgery. So thankful Dr. Ramsis Ghaly was able to fix me and I remain pain free and back to full activity! He is a godsend and I am forever grateful and happy to celebrate this year with my family and friends! Cheers!!

Margret Agamy

You are a miracle worker

Julie Johnson

Dr Ghaly you are truly a gift of God. Ron and Judy Conderman are our neighbors. Steven and Brad are living proof of your gift. Thank you

Kenny Ajedi

Dr Ghaly,

Thank you so much for your mentoring and teaching over these past 3 years. It sure made a difference

Laura Mike

Thank you Dr Ghaly. There is always a lot to learn from you

Michline Rezko

I appreciate your writing because what you said is the truth and made feel good what you have written and I hope continue success in your professional writing God bless you doctor you are the best friend in Facebook I ever I had because the way you put the words together make feel good

You are the brightest shining star among others in the universe of physicians.

I hope you realize how special you are and how important you are to your patients. You are a rarity among doctors. I have seen you fight the insurance compaines when needed for your patients.

You talk to God and love him so much. You tell us a simple stories that illustrate a moral or spiritual lesson. Thank you for being you.God Bless you.

Michael Plunkett

Wow, not only you save people's way of living, to give them a new chance at life without pain or medication. But, you also teach and have taught so many new doctors and medical staff over the years. All of that and you look to God to be on your side in every possible way. Not forgetting your an author of many books. You have touched thousands of lives in positive ways. Awesome human Award Dr Ramsis Ghaly

Charlene Glowaty

You are the brightest shining star among others in the universe of physicians. I hope you realize how special you are and how important you are to your patients. You are a rarity among doctors. I have seen you fight the insurance compaines when needed for your patients. You talk to God and love him so much. You tell us a simple stories that illustrate a moral or spiritual lesson.

Thank you for being you.God Bless you.

Donna Hentsch

You are a Talented and Brilliant man Dr. GHALY, May God Contine to Bless You

Kathie Noller

This should be FRAMED GREAT PHOTO of an AMAZING MAN

Daniel Olzoni

Ramsis Ghaly thx u Dr. Ghaly my back has been really good. If anyone has back problems see him just be ready to wait little bit in waiting room lol! Linda Metheney: Daniel Olznoi he is the best Dan ...

Margret Halle

You are a blessing to many, the lord definitely blessed you with a great talent to help others.

Sebee Michael

You are amazing Dr. GHALY and so dedicated. I have so much respect for you.

Bobby Nordstrom

Bless you and yours! I post stupid stuff while your out there day after day doing your best and doing gods work too! I work all day everyday at Ut southwestern medical center. Great place by the way. But you are such an inspiration. I strive to be more like you. I'll never be like you but I will always do my best like you! I've been doing my job 22 years but I'll never be as good as you. Helping your fellow man. Gosh, I love all you do. You help people.If heaven has a special place you'll be there.I hope to meet you one day. It would be such an honor. A true man of compassion and honor. Sincerely.

Maria Logan

They're so lucky & so blessed to have YOU as their mentor Dr. Ghaly!

Cait Balnous

Ramsis Ghaly Thank Dr. Ghaly! You are a the reason he was standing up right and was able to walk me down the aisle. We are always grateful for you.

Janice Heartfield

Yes you have to father them to be the best for all of God's children on earth and instill the blessings and experience that you are gifted with!!!!

Diana Kay

Thank you Lord for blessing Dr Ghaly with such a tender heart and such miraculous skills and healing skilled hands. Bless him Lord as he blesses others and help Joshua to a full healing and give you glory foe his new lease on life and his wife. In Jesus name amen

Charlene Glowaty

Just amazing what a caring doctor can do .

Wishes for continued recovery for Joshua.

Sandra Crites

your the best dr ghaly

Kathy Hogan

You are a gift from God. Thank you Jesus!

Eileen Myles

The world needs more Dr. Ghaly's that take the time, effort and genuine care to improve lives

Derek Petruci

The man the Myth The legend

Cristina Ruthowski

You are! You are our hero and best doctor ever!!!!

Michael Plunkett

That's worth framing, because you are Superman in so many ways.

Charlene Glowaty

You are my super hero and also that of every patient you ever had and every student you ever taught.

Dotti Lopez

You are Superman. Lol.

Nada Voss

Doctor Ghaly the Super neurosurgeon hero

Kathleen Grace

You're our Beloved Super Hero, no doubt! Best ever! God Bless you, Dr Ramsis Ghaly

The Best International Neurosurgeon & Doctor of Anesthesiology from the world over! Superman doesn't do him justice. A true Blessing from God! Thank you, Dr Ramsis Ghaly for all you do. God Bless you always. Blessings and Love from an American in Egypt. The Basha's Doctor Extraordinaire!

Mike Nutoni

Thank you Dr Ramsis Ghaly ! If it wasn't for you and the Lord I wouldn't be here to see this mile stone.

Sara Curtain

Yep you are definitely a superhero.

Channannair paisanathan

What a wonderful teacher you are! Your program is so lucky to have great teachers. Residents are our future. Investing in our future is the best way forward. Congratulation to all the graduates from IMMC. Hope to join you soon.

Kathleen Grace

Your words make me cry and touch my heart. I thank God daily for all his Blessings and even the ones he did not allow. Thank God for you Dr Ghaly. You are a.true inspiration to the world..the gifted healer. Thank God for you. Blessings from Egypt

Charlene Glowaty

This is beautifully written. This touches my soul and nourishes it

Always a learned lesson from your writings . Blessings

Carol Nelson

Best doctor ever

Danette Meek

You are the Superman of Neurosurgery!

Megha Prasad

thank you so much dr. ghaly!!! and thank you for all of your help and guidance when i worked with you, you will always be my first inspiration to become a doctor!

Mary Nixon

Yes he is awesome. Still going strong since 2008..feel better than ever..thank you and bless you Dr. Ramsis Ghaly

Emily Coley

Had my appt with the amazing Dr Ramsis Ghaly yesterday with my amazing husband Michael. Going back to work soon. Let's be honest, no one ever really wants to go back to work after being off for 3 mos right? But I'm happy that I'm ABLE to return to work. And it'll back to my old routine in no time.

Michael Plunkett

Look like an old Western in the new modern. Your the best Doctor Ramsis Ghaly. May God always be with you, you are always in his light from where I see.

Charlene Glowaty

He is a wonderful doctor and surgeon. He has helped so many people live a pain free life. You certainly have a knack for expressing through your writing. Bless you!

Jolanta Krol

How blessed people are to be patients of Dr Ramsis Ghaly...

Joshua Prim

Good morning, I'm so thankful and blessed for you. Thanks for giving me my life back. We love you. I hope you have a good day and a great weekend.

Emillio Valdez

Happy Fourth of July Dr Ghaly!! I will always cherish those memories, I was very lucky to have had you as my attending. May the Lord continue to bless you and guide your hands

Ivan Radevski

Thank you! Thank you so much! I really appreciate all you do for me.

May God bless you ALLWAYS!

You're an AMAZING human being.

I hope all your dreams come true. Thank you!

Jacki Sujewicz

Hi Dr Ghaly, how are you? This is Jackie. I'm remembering you fondly. I'm hoping you are well. I miss your kindness and working with you. I'm always finding you on LinkedIn but I miss you in person. Your friend always, Jackie

Tabitha Jones

My Dr..... A Godsend. God has blessed this man & his hands…A true genuine person.

Debbie Earles

U are a true blessing

Debbie Millions

Well said Dr. Ghaly you are the Best of the Best

Carmen Einsiedel

U truly r one of a kind Dr Ghaly. U r the diamond. Unique and beautiful! Keep doing what ur doing.

Kathy O'BRIEN

Your the presious stone that reflects unto others, and the best, great picture God bless you always Dr Ghaly

Katie Lindell

This is why you are the best!!!

Maria Logan

You're truly "one of a kind" Dr. Ghaly, a ! !!!

Sam My

I never had a doctor that's been so efficient and quick, don't ever change your ways, keep on doing what you love to do.

Ronald Feeney

That's why I love you so much. God sent you to be our healing Angel.

Greta Paglis

You're a wonderfully blessed man, Dr Ghaly.

Jack Duvick

We never asked why. You made us ask why all the other doctors don't do it. You are amazing and you are our precious jewel.

Suzette Jennings

Your values and trust in God are why you are Dr. Ramsis Ghaly and why we love you. Thank you for all you do for your patients.

I/We hope you are taking good care of yourself, too

Jerry Camille Bever

But these traits are what make you one in a million Dr. Ghaly. This is what makes you the consummate professional. Your patients recognize your dedication to the profession as well as each of us individually as patients. We all know how fortunate we are to have you as our physician!!

Lana Wanis

Indeed. So blessed to have met you, Dr. Ghaly! An honorable man and blessed steward of the Lord!

Scott Mitchell

It's because you have your Superman suit on under your other suit and you are a true Superhero!! Best of the best! And thank you for all you've done and continue to do!! We love ya Doc!!

Kathy Petrucci

You are truly one of a kind as I have never met a more caring doctor let alone do the work that you do! Thank you.

Julie Turecky

You are also just like a diamond one of a kind, wonderful doctor.

Dottie Lopez

The best of all the rest.

Kristine Collins

You are also just like a diamond one of a kind, wonderful doctor.

Louise Keene

Absolutely the best doctor on planet earth! Thank you for all that you do for every one of your patients!!

Eileen Teharine

I love your treatment of patients.

Katherine Schipman

You're doin God's work:)

Lena Walther

You are simply the best!!

Sherry Lee

I LOVE this response. You truly were the answer to prayer when I had all of my back issues, hurt on the job and they wanted to fire me because they said my condition was minor but yet I couldn't even bend to get dressed. That was 11 years ago now! I have my full life back, working full time, I swim, garden, mow the grass, power walk and everything. Due to misdiagnosis (for a whopping 6 months) I will always have some numbness (permemant nerve damage) but it is so much better than the alternative - it could have been so much worse had you not taken me in as a patient!!! And you did it without hesitation, telling me to let you worry about them paying that I only needed to focus on myself and healing. You have helped COUNTLESS people with the gifts God has given you and I for one am so very grateful. Thank you Dr Ghaly

Judy Sargent

You are the most caring doctor love you

Carol Nelson

Love this man. He is a great doctor.

Linda Williamson

God bless you. Wish more doctors had your philosophy.

Joan Pocius

You are an incredible human being and a wonderful doctor. May God bless you abundantly for your ministry both in medicine and life.

Jeff Freeman

Amen. Amen. Amen. Thank you for fulfilling your ministry and calling. I love Dr. Ramsis Ghaly. #PastorJeff90210

Charlene Glowaty

I love love love that you feel that way about your patients! We all love you because you are such a unique doctor unlike any other

Bless you!

Jennifer Nicole

I am so lucky to have been one of those patients!

Dory Melano

Not just an ordinary doctor.he walks extra miles not only for his pstients but family as well .God bless you always Doc.

Aeschylus Bryant

You care about your patients with all of your being!!! I'm living proof! Thank You Dr Ghaly for all you give!

Rita Castillo

Thank you doctor for Takeshi care all your patients like a real diamond, yóu are a rare gen too

Tiffany Lardi Wills

I love you and your "helicopter approach" to diagnosing, repairing and healing your patients! I'm LUCKY AND BLESSED to have been one of your success stories

Dianna Lynn

You amaze me. Where have all the great Doctors gone ? You are one of a kind !

Patients quotes 53

Joshua and Natasha Prim

I don't know how to thank you enough. You are Heaven sent, your incredible mind but more importantly your sincere heart. I will get Josh to stop smoking, and I'll bring all medications. We will be there around 10, see you then

Mor Ben Barak;

Thank you Ghaly for shaping and raising another pumpkins group that will serve this world.Amen

Khalil Mansour

Professor Doctor / Ramses Ghali

Inside Jerusalem of Holies, may God bless your life, service and work.

It is one of Egypt's pyramids in the field of medicine and has many volumes and books that are studied in the city of Chicago in the universities of the Newest State and globally. He is a pride for Egypt and Egyptians thanks

Kathleen McGregor Grace

Sometimes God sends us Angel's disguised as friends.....

So Blessed and Thankful for this Doctor.

Originally from Egypt.

America's Best Neurosurgeon Extraordinaire.

One Man CAN and DOES make a Difference!

The BEST American Doctor, a Neurosurgeon, who took time to assist us when Basha had a sudden fall on the roof, 27 May 2022.

I am so very Thankful to have this Doctor as my friend and brother all of these years even BEFORE I came to live in Egypt.

I can count on my hands how many times, Dr Ramsis Ghaly, has assisted on Consultations when things just didn't seem right.

When sudden surgery left me unable to feel my own legs, here, in a foreign land and

NOW

Basha having a sudden fall that left him in terrible pain with bruises and tears to the Gluteal muscles on one hip. Very Thankful the leg, Mansour's hip, was not broken.

Very VERY THANKFUL FOR

DR. RAMSIS GHALY.

Shokran Khteer

Thank you

Thank you

Thank you

God Bless You Always

Dr Ramsis Ghaly

Thank you for helping Mansour and I when we needed you.

Merci, Dr Ramsis Ghaly.

God only gives the Best

When we believe.

Thank God for Dr Ghaly.

America's Best Neurosurgeon

From Egypt

Orthodox

Speaks English And Arabic

And

My friend Before coming to Egypt.

Thank you, Ramsis Ghaly

Ramsis Ghaly You honour us with your presence, Doctor. YOU show the world that YES! 1 Man CAN and WILL make a difference. YOU ARE the TRUE ANGEL among us all, teaching and sharing your craft with the next generations as we all should. NOT keeping all a secret to be envied and fought over.

WE are so Blessed and Honoured to call you our friend and brother.

I can still remember returning from my own time in a hospital and unable to move my legs properly leaving me to wonder what I could do and afraid again when Basha had his fall 27May 2022.

And GOD answered those prayers as there you were to guide us on these adventures to restored mobility. A True Angel disguised as friend.

I truly cannot ever Thank you enough for the purest heart of Gold and gifted as you are helping from so far away.

I am deeply deeply honored.

Shokran khteer,.Doctor!

Thank you so very very much, Dr Ramsis Ghaly.

George Salib Thank you so much!

I have to Thank God for giving me Dr Ramsis Ghaly, George. Because I could never see me dragging him back down any stairs for more tests and unnecessary things.

We have All we need when we believe. Thank GOD!

Dr Ghaly is an Angel

A true miracle of all the people.

Thank you so much, Dr Ghaly.

George Salib You KNOW he is chomping at the bit being down and out!

He has the VERY BEST DOCTOR/Neurologist from Egypt, too, George, so he can speak quite nicely with him AND the proper care, treatment and medicines to American Standard, George. THANK GOD!

Just need to keep him home..no stairs for awhile yet.

Very Thankful for Dr Ramsis Ghaly in Chicago.

https://www.facebook.com/.../UzpfSVNDOjc0MjYzODEwMzgy.../... — with Mansour Khalil and Ramsis Ghaly.

Brenda Pickeral I am so Blessed and Honoured to have this Doctor in a world that often devalues and negates people as they step on each other to get ahead instead of helping one another as we should.

I can't even imagine where I would be without THIS Doctor as so many times he has guided me here and even when I had a iffy unneccessary procedure that left me unable to walk properly, just to "Keep the peace" and "Fit In." I've since remembered MY Worth and will NEVER do such again or ever allow another to denegrate or devalue me again.

This Doctor is Amazing and I am so grateful to call him my friend and brother.

If you know anyone who needs a wonder Doctor with outstanding skills and chair side manner for even the most delicate brain or spine issues, please send them to Dr. Ramsis Ghaly in Chicago. He is the very Best Neurosurgeon restoring people to their health with his magic hands for over 30 years.

We Love Doctor Ghaly

Thank you, Sis!

Blessings

Tanya Cavanough

Congrats to all! You are such an aspiring doctor and teacher with so much knowledge and I am sure they have benefited from it all and will be amazing in what ever Avenue they choose!

Cindy conn

You are so appreciated by many! You are a blessing to do many!

Karen Boland

ALL your children-how they love and respect you, Dr. Ghaly!

Lanette Yingling

Update on Jim Yingling: after just 4 weeks of recovery post surgery, Jim is back to work! Dr. Ramsis Ghaly is a miracle worker!

Mary Nixon

Yes he is..great news Dr. Ghaly Is the best!!

Carmen Einsiedel

Prayers for you Joshua! U r in the best hands ever with Dr Ghaly! I'm living proof twice.

Margret Agamy

He is the Brst

Kathleen Grace

Praying for Joshua! You're in the Best of Care with Dr Ghaly. My family is proof and I'm almost 7000 miles away. A minor medical procedure left me NOT really walking right...more like a wet noodle and NOT able to really feel my legs. HUGE Thanks to Dr Ghaly for correcting the issue. And my husband having a rather hard fall that Dr Ghaly was consulted on, correctly handling. Huge prayers and Blessings for you that God sent you a very special Angel to us all! God Bless you and rest easy now. God Bless, Dr Ghaly,an Angel disguised as friend. Xoxo

Bravo for our Heroes and Dr Ramsis Ghaly!

I surely don't know where or what I would do without you to rely on and I'm American in Egypt. Even here Medical can be good but little errors make big mistakes! Thank God for Dr Ghaly as I've no doubt I'd be paralyzed or something! Thank God for you, Dr Ghaly!

Charlene Glowaty

Prayers for you Josh. You have the best doctor taking care of you.

Jerry Walter

Dr. Ghaly is truly a miracle worker, he is my hero!

Lanette Yingling

Update on Jim Yingling: after just 4 weeks of recovery post surgery, Jim is back to work! Dr. Ramsis Ghaly is a miracle worker! Ramsis Ghaly we owe it all to you!!

Lisa Johnson

He is pretty amazing! He goes above and beyond any doctor I have been too. He truly cares about his patients!

Lydia Christensen

He certainly is. All of the articles are so fascinating.

He certainly is. All of the articles are so fascinating.

Gwen Favero

Ramsis Ghaly I'll never be able to thank you enough much love Dr. ! All honor and Glory to God for using your hands to do such an incredibly delicate surgery!!!

Zenaida Capul

No one can play the role better than you, You are the best Dr.Ghally.

Kathy O'Brien

Your the best Dr Ghaly, God sent for sure,

Beth Daghfal

You will not find a more honest Dr. and one who cares more for his patients than Dr. Ghaly!!

Sarah Johnson

Oh my...I could cry for him. He must be so happy to have found you and to have new hope!

Marianne Johnson

What a wonderful Doctor.

Donna Hentsch

Dr. GHALY, YOU NEVER FAIL TO AMAZE ME, you are for “WE THE PEOPLE” LOVE YOU DR. GHALY

Terry Mendozza

With firsthand knowledge, I can say that Dr. Ghaly is the kindest and most caring doctor in the USA, and I am thankful every day that I met this wonderful man, who just happens to be the best neurosurgeon ever. If ever God guided a person’s hands, it is Dr. Ramsis Ghaly

Dave Brown

God’s Dr. Ghaly! We are so blessed to have Dr. Ghaly in our lives!! Thank you, Father!!

Nancy Mitchell

Amazing Dr. G!!!!!!

Valerie Willaims

Healing Hand

Sarah Young

Oh my...I could cry for him. He must be so happy to have found you and to have new hope!

Beth Daghfal

You will not find a more honest Dr. and one who cares more for his patients than Dr. Ghaly!!

Arthur Almassy

Bro Ramsis...

You continue to amaze me. You are handsome, accomplished, exceedingly intelligent and very much more. Your waters run deep. Chicago needs you. It's been my great pleasure knowing you!

Bro Arthur

Amelia lucena

The best M.D. .... Fathered patients in giving excellent medical care for many years & counting. Happy Father's day Doc

Joshua and Natasha Prim

Thank you very much. We are so grateful and always thinking of you. 48 hours no pain!!!! 5 years waiting. I can't thank you enough. We are on the right track and you have changed my life in the best way ever. We will call you soon and give you an update. From all of us and especially me

Patients quotes 52

Cindy Rice

So very deserved you are an amazing soul and a one of a kind majestic healer! Divinely guided and beloved by all whom are lucky enough to cross your path! True healer in all senses!

Jim Yingling

Congratulations Dr. Ghaly! You have been such a blessing. Praise God for you!! Words cannot express the gratitude that Lanette and I have for you. Not only your professionalism as an amazing doctor, but also your compassion as a friend. God Bless you Dr Ramsis Ghaly!!

Lanette Yingling

Day 6 of recovery and all is well!! I wish that I could describe how grateful we are, specifically Jim, to have had Dr. Ramsis Ghaly be the one to have performed surgery! He is truly a gifted surgeon that has dedicated his life to helping people. He has not only given Jim hope that his pain has an end, but he has also shown us....again....that God is in control. You see, just 24 days ago, we had no hope for an end to Jim's pain....we were getting nowhere with the doctors that we had been seeing....then we saw Dr. Ghaly. That same day, he scheduled surgery after seeing the MRI reports of a tumor in his sciatic nerve and saw the pain that Jim was in! Thank you so much for your love for people, your love for Jesus and your love the the gift that God has given you! Praise the Lord that the tumor is benign!

Mary Nixon

Yes Dr. Ramsis Ghaly Is amazing.

I tell people all the time how great he is and so glad that you are doing well jim... God is good.

Carolyn Campbell

You're wonderful! You give healing to the hopeless.

Cynthia Schott

Brads doing great!! So thankful to Dr Ghaly!!!

V Aldrete for Jack Jabolski

OMG, what a great doctor, I am sure thanks to your outstanding training and resident leadership. You are following Dr. Aldrete's teachings and dedication to anesthesia education. You are fabulous doctor and I am proud to be your friend. LoveVal

SR and B

OMG! I was just thinking about you. You saved a life. Thank you. GREAT TEAM WORK! I'm grateful you were on tonight-- that was amazing resuscitation!

Bart Smith

Thank you Dr Ghaly … she so appreciated and admired you not just as an incredible doctor but also as a friend. God bless you as you continue your amazing work with peers, students and patients.

Charlene Glowaty

Such wonderful news. You had the best surgeons, Dr Ghaly with the guidance of God. Blessings

Update on my mom… (long post below)

After being in and out of the hospital the last couple weeks and progressively getting worse without many answers. A surgeon hopefully has found the reason why she's been in excruciating pain and why she can hardly walk with a Walker and some days not able to walk at all… He found a mass that's pressing on her spinal cord and causing her to become potentially paralyzed so he will be performing surgery tomorrow morning to remove it. With that being said this surgery is dangerous not only because it could also paralyze her but as well with the state of her lungs it makes going under anesthesia dangerous. We're all hoping and praying that is what my mom needs and that the surgery will be successful without complications. Its hard for us to not have so many mixed emotions and worry about our mom when all of this happened so quickly. On my birthday last month my mom took me shopping and to dinner as if everything was normal besides her having shortness of breath, getting around a little slower than normal and experiencing pain in her legs. To the next day being admitted into the hospital getting released 4 days later then ending right back into the hospital 10 times worse… One minute things seem okay and like she's getting better then the next she can't talk because she's in so much pain. It's hard to understand why all of this is happening to her when she's the most caring and loving person I know but my mom is so strong, she will get through this and come out on top!

All of us girls (her daughters) have been with her as much as we can be with all of us having kids we can't be there as much as we'd like to be. Thankfully my grandma has been by her side every single day doing all that she can to help my mom from taking her to all of her appointments (sometimes multiple in one day) to sitting in the hospital waiting for a room for 10+ hours all 3 of the times she went, to cooking/cleaning and overall just going above and beyond for her daughter while also having her own health struggles and being worn out. Judy Johnson Kladis we can't thank you enough for all that you do for ALL of us, your amazing and we love you more than you'll ever know

Gwen L Favero even though I can't physically be at your surgery just know I'm there with you and im thinking of you wishing I was there! You have a mom, 4 girls and 10 grand babies that all love you most

Prayers for surgery to go as planned and for a good recovery would be greatly appreciated! Also to any of my moms friends that want updates on my mom feel free to message us.

Cindy rice

I do understand. I know her physician personally love! He did my surgery when my spinal cord was collapsing last year, he performed a 12 hour back surgery on my dad! This man will pull your mom through and she will heal!! I believe it with all that I am. I'm here for you sweetheart, please call me if you need me. I'm praying and I have faith in the healing hands of dr Ramsis Ghaly! Love your mom & you so very much!!

Bobby Nordstrom

Amen. Thank you for all you do Dr. Ramsis Ghaly . Thank you for taking such humble pride in healing others. It's people like you that make the difference. You're a blessing.

Christophere Kladis

God be all the Glory, thank you Dr. Ghaly for your faith and skill in Jesus name

Judy Kladis

What a great, Dr. Ramsis Ghaly . Thank you from the bottom of my heart I'm so glad to have you as Gwen's Dr.

Dale Christensen

Thank you my friend, God gave you the ability to help other and you are every patient's blessing.

Lydia Christensen

This post certainly made my day. Thank you Dr. Ghaly for helping my friend. Thank you God for guiding Dr. Ghaly's hands.

Mary Aiadro

Praise God! Dr. Ghaly is his hands!

Edwina Swanson

God-bless you Doctor Ghaly for all you do. The Lord has given you a wonderful gift.

Laura Larsen

Dr Ghaly is amazing! Love that smile!

Sarah Johnson

Ramsis Ghaly thank you for save him so any years ago. I would be lost without him.

Cynthia Rice

Praying for you Gwen and your beautiful family. You are with the very best doctor! Love you!

Charlene Glowaty

Not only did God give you the gift of being a great doctor and surgeon he gave you the ability to be a eloquent writer.

Greg Goldstein

Nice! . You're a true healer …

Matt and Jeanine Cohen

Dr. Ghaly!!! This is her husband, Matt. You are an incredible surgeon and professional! Thank you so much. Oh my goodness...we were so very lucky and blessed to have you overseeing that entire operation. When we spoke and interacted, I had no idea who you were. It is us who were privelidged.

Jeanne is recovering nicely and generally feels well. Thank you again. It was a true Miracle that you and Drs. Darrell & Star were there that evening!!! I don't believe any of you were supposed to be. So very blessed.

Gwen Favero

There are no words to thank you enough for saving me from becoming crippled Dr. Ramsis Ghaly I'm so thankful for you and that you allow God to use you to save people's lives!!! You will forever have a special place in my heart!!! God bless you!!!!

Dale Christensen

Gwen L Favero he truly has been a Miracle Worker to so many.

Colleen Turner

Praise Jesus and Dr. Ramsis Ghaly

Judy Sargent

PRAISE GOD for giving you the knowledge to work the unthinkable. Dr Ghaly, your mind and hands are truly BLESSED

Robert Favero

My amazing wife, Gwen.

Coming home today

Thank you so much Dr. Ramsis Ghaly.

Allie Smith

I'm so happy you went to Dr Ghaly. He is such a special gift from God who takes the best care of his patients. So glad you are feeling better!

Gwen Favero

As I sit here and think of it all I'm just so very thankful to Dr. Ramsis Ghaly before he did surgery I didn't know if I would ever walk or walk normal again or even feel my feet or legs!!! He listened to me, did the correct testing, and allowed God to use his hands to fix me, and I'll forever be so grateful!!!! I'm praising God that the surgery went as perfect as it possibly could have went, and believing that my recovery will go just as well!!!! Thank you Everyone for everything I cannot say enough about how much love I have felt through all of this

Lydia Christensen

That news really made my day. If anyone could remove that tumor with no other problems, it's Dr. Ghaly. Continuing prayers, because you are certainly proof the power of prayer works.

Amy Urban

Thank you dr g! So grateful for you! Thank you for taking such good care of my husband. I rave about you to everyone I know

Dr Daniel Ernestine Chaplain

What a blessing from our Lord and Saviour Jesus Christ! Jesus is yet working miracles today because he did it for Gwen!!! Blessings!!!

Dr. Ernestine Daniels, Chaplain, Light Bearers Ministry, Stroger Hospital of Cook County

Donald, judy and Wittney Sargent

Hi Dr. Ghaly!! Dad asked me to message you and tell you that today is his 1 year anniversary for his back surgery. He said that he has been pain free since the day you finished his surgery. We all want to thank you so very much for everything you did for dad! He is a new man! Dad said he hopes to see you soon!

Violet Morrison

Hello hard working smart genius generous. Best Neurosurgeon of Chicago Illinois thanks a million for your time to greet me on my youthful birthday. Always stay safe. Take care BFF. GOD BLESS. You're the best. Have wonderful time

Cindy Rice

You are exactly what god has sent you here to be! Such an amazing soldier, servant of our dear lord, and above all the most compassionate healing soul I know! Never stope!

Patient Quotes 51

Kellie Coyte

That is amazing. Your hands do God's healing. Amen you were able to free her from the pain. Prayers and blessings on your continued work

Monica De Tore

Doctor Ghaly you are so good, thank God for your life and all the hard work the you always do showing the love in your hard .

God bless you!!!!

Charlene Glowaty

My kind of woman,.love life and her independence. She is lucky by Dr. Ghaly was recommended to her. I remember my first meeting and Dr Ghaly was very kind, listened to everything I said and explained everything so well about my condition. I pray she continues to enjoy her life each and every day. God bless her.

I can't express what an amazing doctor you are.

Healthcare would be better if more doctors were like you.

Look what you did for him and what a wonderful gift he gave you. The Indian arrowhead is such a special gift from the Stoneage.

Bless him.

Ken Walther

You're an amazing man, Ramsis! Your knowledge & strong faith works miracles!

Jerry Bever

Valerie Williams Well said Valerie. You express the sentiments of many of us!! Thank him for you Dr. G.

Uma graduating county surgeon

Thank you Dr. Ghaly! I appreciate your spirit, drive and resolve. I strive to have the same attitude and hopefully as successful of a career as you. Looking forward to helping a few more people together before I go! Have a great day!

Steve Gill

Thanks to you Dr Ghaly I'm here to see my son 28th birthday. You are a true blessing to me!

Donna Hentsch

I'm so Happy for your patient being pain free, and you and your Strong Faith in our God. You are amazing Dr Ghaly

She is truly Blessed Praise God and thank you to you Dr Ghaly, miracles continue thru your God Given Talent

Jolanta Krol

Praise the Lord! Awesome Dr. Ghaly

Most definitely Dr Ramsis Ghaly you are a Miracle Worker.

God Sent to you Special Blessings on your hands, mind and your body...

May Our Loving God

Nancy Hammond

Dr. Ghaly ~ You truly are a blessing to your patients! Thank you for your dedication and passion to sincerely help those of us who have been entrusted to your care.

Valerie Williams

Dr Ghaly you are one of the best HUMAN BEING IVE EVER MEET. GOD IS SO WITH YOU. Thank you for everything

Jane Duvick

Congratulations Cheryl! Great job Dr. Ghaly. You are an amazing doctor! Jane.

Oliver Brandt

Dr. Ghaly is a very smart man and an awesome neurosurgeon….

Cristina Ruthkoski

I wanted to make little tribute to our beloved Dr.Ramsis Ghaly for being a hero on the front lines

fighting COVID 19 and saving many lives. You are an example of love to humanity and inspiration. In the name of all the people THANK YOU SO MUCH and God bless you!!

Jolanta Krol

Super news dr. Ramsis Ghaly

I wish you could come to Las Vegas, and healed us from pain and nerve misery...

May Our Loving God always Blessed You...

Amy Merkel Daly

Dr. Ghaly! Thank you for taking care of my dear brother in Christ, Jim Yingling! You have given he and his wife, Lanette, hope at long last for him to be free of this debilitating pain! Praying God's blessing over you!

Emily Coley

Thank you Dr. Ghaly. You are my real life hero, guardian angel. You are sweetest kindest doctor I've ever encountered. And obviously, extremely skilled & thorough and I don't even know how to thank you enough.

Ric Malina

God bless you Sir ! The Great Dr Ghaly does it again

Katie Lindell

Thank you Dr. Ghaly!!! We love you and are so grateful for all you do for our family and these special guys of ours

Sally Brady

Praise Jesus!! Thank you Dr. Ghaly, you are such a wonderful doctor. Our family is so lucky to have you.

Cynthia Schott

There aren't enough words to express our deep gratitude!! We love you!

Alicia Casanova

The best doctor!

Rick Malina

Speedy recovery Brad I've been here No worries your in good hands with Dr Ghaly and our Lord

Dawn Morrisson

Thank you Dr. Ghaly for all you have done for Brad and for Stephen!!! You have touched our family in the best of ways!

Laurie Malcezwski

Dr.Ghaly you're the Best!!!

Tammy Conderman

Thank you Dr. Ramsis Ghaly for being a faithful servant and using your talents as a blessing for those in need. Our family has been blessed twice and we are so grateful!

Terry Mendozza

God bless you Ramsis. Another miracle performed by you together with Jesus Christ, our Savior

Brenda Dickerson

Doctor, your talent and skill is Blessed by the most high God.

Keep up the good work.

Donna Hentsch

You are an amazing talented surgeon Dr Ghaly. You have a gift from our high God

Sally Brady

So elated for Brad and family. Dr. Ghaly you're the best and know how much our family appreciates you for helping Brad. God bless you!!

Douglas Conderman

Way to go Brad! Thank you so much Dr Ghaly! You are the best

Stephen Polich

Dr Ghaly you are amazing! God Blesses you to heal others

Nancy Jenkins

What a special doctor! You were blessed to have him, Cheryl Burkhart-Esgar .

Lynette Yingling

Oh my goodness!! Thank you so much for these pictures! What a great way to start the day

So very glad that God brought us to you

Kathy O'Obrien

Lord bless him and his family always

You were in the best hands of a wonderful caring doctor, continued heath for you, sir

Jim Yingling

Thank you Dr. Ramsis Ghaly for removing the tumor from Jim with an amazing surgical procedure....done with precision, accuracy and God-given wisdom!! You are a blessing

Carol Nelson

Dr Ghaly is the best. Love him. He actually cares about and loves his patients. He did my first surgery in 1996. He was at Silver Cross Hospital in Joliet at that time.

Jaime Schulz

You tell Dr Ghaly that you know me. I worked with him long time ago. Very compassionate man. I'm glad you have answers and are on the mend.

Mandy Phillips

Dr Ramsis Ghaly is one incredible human! I've never experienced anyone else like him and I only know him through rehabbing some of his patients!

Laynette Yingling

Today is day 1 of recovery....Jim's recovery after a 6 month battle with hip pain. Jim is now sleeping after a very long, complicated and significant surgery yesterday at Central Dupage Hospital with an extremely compassionate and kind neurosurgeon, Dr. Ramsis Ghaly. Jim had been in significant pain for months. He had seen 5 different doctors, had 2 rounds of oral steroids, 2 injections and 5 MRIs to no avail. Then, we found Dr. Ghaly. Without boring everyone with all the details, suffice it to say that God led us to this neurosurgeon! You see, after the 3rd MRI a tumor was discovered in or on Jim's sciatic nerve! We saw Dr. Ghaly last Wednesday (April 27) he saw the significant debilitating pain that Jim was in and he scheduled surgery immediately for May 6th. Yesterday was one of the longest days of my life.

With the delicate nature of this surgery, being at the sciatic nerve, the risks were great. However, Jim and I truly felt God's presence in all of this so we had peace in that🙏

Jim was prepped for surgery at 5:30 am, went under at about 8:30 am and at 10 am, surgery began. Needless to say it was a long day!

When the surgical nurse at CDH texted me at 2 pm that the tumor was out, I lost it! All of the stress of Jim's pain, the difficulty of seeing him suffer and the unknown regarding the location of the tumor was released. I thanked God for 10 minutes..... for everything. Words cannot describe the emotions that I felt at that moment!

At 6pm, Jim finally made it to a room, a little loopy to say the least and now (Saturday) he is home and ready to recover!

Turns out the tumor was IN the sciatic nerve, not next to it! And was the size of my thumb! God surely directed Dr. Ghaly's hands in removing the mass

Thank you to all of our friends and family that have been supportive throughout this process, helpful in helping with ru ning of the business, taking care of our home and dogs, providing food and medical supplies and, of course, prayers! We are grateful for all of you and especially Dr. Ghaly who, in my estimation, performed a miracle!!

Gary Chandler

Dr Ramsis Ghaly #1!

Bobby Nordstrom

Thank you for helping so many people. Amen.

Diana Nelson

You have a wonderful talent Dr.

Jim Yingling

Thank you Dr. Ramsis Ghaly for removing the tumor from Jim with an amazing surgical procedure....done with precision, accuracy and God-given wisdom!! You are a blessing

Susan Smith Jim YinglingGod has certainly blessed Dr Gahly with amazing talent and skills.

Diane Nelson You have a wonderful talent Dr.

Cristina Batelli You are the best.

Amy Merkel Daly Praising God with you! So thankful for Ramsis Ghaly!!!

Gary Chandler GC, Dr Ramsis Ghaly #1!

Jamie Riffell Schultz

You tell Dr Ghaly that you know me. I worked with him long time ago. Very compassionate man. I'm glad you have answers and are on the mend.

Rhea Hagar Lumsden

Thank God for Dr. Ghaly! Praying for an uneventful and complete recovery for Jim. This is what those vows mean Lanette...for better or worse and in sickness and health. You were there for Jim as he would be for you. That strengthens your relationship! Love you

Mandy Phillips

Dr Ramsis Ghaly is one incredible human! I've never experienced anyone else like him and I only know him through rehabbing some of his patients!

Mary Nixon

Omg wow, that is just amazing. And yes Dr. Ramsis Ghaly Is an amazing surgeon, he did my back surgery, in 2008 and it's been amazing what a difference it is to not be in pain anymore..he is a miracle worker, and we love him..when you see him for follow up please tell him mark and Mary Nixon said hi!! So glad Jim is doing well

Jennifer Daly Petrucci

Sending prayers for your husbands recovery. Dr. Ramsis Ghaly is truly the best and you are all in the best hands.

Carol Nelson

Dr Ghaly is the best. Love him. He actually cares about and loves his patients. He did my first surgery in 1996. He was at Silver Cross Hospital in Joliet at that time.

Stacia Robinson Little Dr. Ghaly is the most skilled doctor! He performed back surgery on my dad years ago. I truly believe he was sent here from God almighty to be a healer for his people.

Patti Stiegleiter

What a testimony! Yes, God sent you to the best doctor. Dr. Ghaly was the instrument for my nephew and a dear friend. Both needed a miracle. Thank you God for your intervention and the talents and compassionate Dr. Gahly possesses. Praying for healing and comfort.

Lanette Sellers Yingling Dr. Ghaly's post this morning! I swear this man doesn't sleep!!

Ll, Wow. I'm amazed at the surgeons words. Just how rare this was and how he not only relied on his own skill but also prayed for the surgery. you Jesus!

Lk, Dr. Ghaly did my surgery 2 years ago. I would go back to him in a heartbeat. He is truly a miracle doctor!

Jim YinglingGod has certainly blessed Dr Ghaly with amazing talent and skills.

Joan Pocius

They are positive but asymptomatic

Lynn Swanson

So glad you found Dr Ghaly. He is the best. He will take very good care of your husband. My husband has had surgeries with him. Speedy recovery.

Lynn Menth

So wonderful for both of the special men in your life to be in much greater comfort. Hope Jim's recovery is uneventful. Hugs to you

Mary Nixon

Omg wow, that is just amazing. And yes Dr. Ramsis Ghaly Is an amazing surgeon, he did my back surgery, in 2008 and it's been amazing what a difference it is to not be in pain anymore..he is a miracle worker, and we love him..when you see him for follow up please tell him mark and Mary Nixon said hi!! So glad Jim is doing well

Jillian Overman

Dr Ramsis Ghaly is a man of faith and his hands work as God's tools. There is no doubt. He's my neurosurgeon and I wouldn't trust anyone else.

Dave Brown

PRAISE GOD!!! THANK YOU Dr. Ghaly!! Praying Jim and Lynette for Jim's recovery! And so thankful that He brought Jim and Dr. Ghaly together!!

Dave Brown

Again, thank you Dr. Ghaly and good to be back on line with you. Sue continues to be doing great with her back! We are so blessed to have you in our life! Praise God!

Michael DeCilla

God Bless you Dr. Ghaly you are truly a God sent to restore peoples lives. You are an amazing caring doctor sharing your remarkable talents to cure people.

Lena Withers

Dear Ramsis, You are a miracle worker!!

Kathleen Grace

In Jesus Name we Pray. Thank you, Dr Ramsis Ghaly for all you do. You are a wondrous inspiration to the whole world and a Beautiful Gift from God to All. GOD BLESS YOU ALWAYS. Love from Egypt

Cindy Rice

Very touching you are in gods hands Dr Ghaly is a true Angel on this earth!

Connie Forsythe

Well Judy you took her to the right Dr. Prayers for a speedy recovery

Charlene Glowaty

Congratulations! You work so hard every day to achieve this accomplishment, and I can't think of anyone who deserves it more. .You set an amazing example for other doctors and your students

Lena Withers

Dear Ramsis, You are a miracle worker!!

Kathleen Grace

In Jesus Name we Pray. Thank you, Dr Ramsis Ghaly for all you do. You are a wondrous inspiration to the whole world and a Beautiful Gift from God to All. GOD BLESS YOU ALWAYS. Love from Egypt

Be sure, when I need surgery one day on my back..You are the ONLY Doctor I'll trust to do it. Congratulations and God Bless you! A true Hero to all! Sending love from Egypt

Cindy Rice

Very touching you are in gods hands Dr Ghaly is a true Angel on this earth!

Connie Forsythe

Well Judy you took her to the right Dr. Prayers for a speedy recovery

Brenda Linquist

You are amazing in the medical field and equally amazing and beautiful as an accomplished, dedicated, loving, human being.

CONGRATULATIONS Dr Ramsis Ghaly!

Sarah Marcus

Dang!!!!

My favoritest peeps on the earth are Coptic Brain Surgeons!!!!!

And he's my top fan!

Yay, Dr. Ramsis Ghaly!!!

Mark Nugyn

You truly are a wonderfully gifted surgeon Dr. Ghaly.

I wouldn't trust anyone else to work on me.

I'm back to work thanks to you.

Sally Brady

Wonderful honor for a great doctor. Congrats, Dr. Ghaly

Elizabeth Oliver

Congratulations. You are a blessed man as you have honored our Lord and your profession to bless all who are in your care. Have a wonderful day.

Melinda Withers

What a wonderful gift you are to all of us. You have the biggest heart I've ever seen in my life

Sharon Ledbetter

Well done

Well deserved

May God continue to bless the work of your hands all for His Glory

Diana Swanson

You are the best Dr.Ghaly,Congratulations.

Karen boland

You are top shelf, Dr. Ghaly!

Zenaida Capul

You are the best Dr.Ghaly,Congratulations.

Dina Arvanitakis

Blessed to know Dr Ghaly and to call him my friend. Congratulations Dr. Ramsis Ghaly !!!!!! You are doing God's work and healing and restoring many people.

Emily Linn

My Neurosurgeon. My Hero.

If you need a neurosurgeon, this is the man you want to see. He's Quadruple Board certified: NeuroSurgery, Neuro-Critical Care, Anesthesiology & Pain Management. And the accomplishments only just start there. His bedside manner is one that I've never experienced in my life & I've been a nurse for 17 years. He cares.

• Sebee Michael

You are amazing Dr. GHALY! I might be needing you soon after all these years of nursing.

Charlene Mentzer Glowaty

You are truly a great doctor and surgeon. You are personable, great listener, and empathetic to the concerns of your patients. God has truly blessed your patients when they found you

Michael Plunkett

You are an Angel Doctor of the Lord with the heart and soul in the right place. Awesome story, and looks like the airway is not impinged any longer and those vertebra are spaced and not crunching nerves making inflammation. You fixed it!

Cristina Rojas-Rutkowski

OMG!!!! So happy for you my favorite doctor!!!! You leave traces of love on every single patient's hearts!!!!!

CONGRATULATIONS

!!!

Christie Loftin Well deserved! You perform God's Miracles!

Jillianne Renee Overman·

Dr Ramsis Ghaly is a man of faith and his hands work as God's tools. There is no doubt. He's my neurosurgeon and I wouldn't trust anyone else.

Patient Quotes 50

James Talbot

Thank you Dr.Ghaly and yes I am still working because what God and you Did for me September 15th 1997 when I had brain surgery and three mini strokes with a 20 % chance of coming off the operating table and if I did,then I could be a vegtable .

Michael Plunkett

Love the Tie, you wear it well. Special gifts like this I am sure really touch your heart. I know you have many patients thankful, you remove pain and restore the part of life they were missing. You are special as a Dr. That you also Pray, I think that could be one of the major reasons, you and God are working together through Jesus. It's the way I see it. Kellie Coyte This is Dr. Ghaly, chief neurologist surgeon, and medical teacher to the interns. This Dr. Is a special God's healer. Amazing story here about removing nerve pain. I have witnessed many patients cured with life debilitating problems, some unable to walk or stand or sit. I wish there was some way you could see Dr. Ghaly. He is not in Florida, he is licensed as a Dr. In several States. He is an author of many books too. Kellie Coyte I do believe he has a connection through Jesus. Follow him and see what he post. One after the other, he has restored peoples lives, got them off pain killers, changed their worlds. Removed their pain.

Charlene Glowaty

Always learning to better help your patients.

Blessings

Nimit shah

What an excellent and apt lecture it was on EVD management Dr Ghaly today. Thank you so much for this. I hope to carry all your neuroanesthesia teachings to Ohio with me as they will be immensely helpful to me.

Nimit shah

Good morning Dr Ghaly,

Once again you demonstrated exemplary teachings in our call. Thank you so much for everything you do for us.

Bretonya Johnson

Congrats you deserve to be praised for all that you do and sacrifice for the medical field! It's good to see your passion has not went unnoticed

Louise Engert

Thank you Dr Ghaly. I will never forget you coming to UIC to see if we had opened the floor up for Neurosurgery patients yet.

San Yoon

Great call last yesterday Dr. Ghaly. Thank you for teaching me some things last night

Cindy Rice

Ramsis Ghaly you are an amazing light and this poem you wrote brought me to tears! My family is everything to me, love them all so very much! You have touched my family with your healing hands to give us our lives back. I am so forever grateful, we are all so very grateful for you THANK YOU FROM THE BOTYOM OF MY HEART!

Flor Andocutin

Ramsis Ghaly once again thank you for all your support Dr Ghaly the Surgeon with a heart of gold

Betty Markel

God Bless you always for your love and beliefs. You have touched so many life's!

Diana Swanstorm

Thanks so much Dr. Ghaly. Love your posts. xx

Valerie Williams

Congratulations THE BEST NEUROSURGEON DOCTOR EVER! Love you Dr Ghaly

Kathryn O'Brion

Congratulations to this couple

Dr Ghaly, you are remarkable surgeon God bless you always

Debbie Anderson

Dr. Ghaly is a fantastic dr! He took care of my son many years ago when he was suffering with a spine problem. No one else did what he did! So thankful for him! So happy you found him, too!

Brenda Linquist

Dr Ramsis Ghaly you are a life changer and loved so much!

Valerie Williams

Dr Ghaly, God sure gave us "ALL" a blessing when you came into this world. You are not only the best neurosurgeon but you are the best a person can be. You care. You laugh with your patients. You remember us all. My eyes water up how great and amazing you are. I don't with this type of surgery on anyone but if you do please and I mean please on see Dr Ghaly. You mean the world to me and I appreciate you for everything you have done for me and my husband. I thank you for everything. You made my burdens lighter

Edwina Bator-Swanson

She was and is in the hands of an amazing doctor. Thank you Dr G for helping so many. The Lord has given you a great gift.

Myrna Burgos Gustafson

God bless you Doc abundantly!

Mary Siegel

What an inspiration to all of us. Thank you for the beautiful words. It's really good to hear things like this.b

Jennifer Campin You're a champion Ramsis Ghaly

Michael Plunket, Praise the Lord, Dr Ghaly works through Jesus, Amen.

Jolanta Krol

She looks great.

dr. Ramsis Ghaly you are walking angel.

I could used your blessings.

I am in hospital, and have problem to sta

Linda Andzulis

Gloria Gaither expresses precisely what Dr. Ramsis Ghaly refers to as the two secrets full of mystery, holiness and blessings to those taking part in both!

For a moment - just for a moment the door flap between here and eternity opens and the angel dust of eternity gets on you and for a moment life gets real, and you are transformed, and you're never the same again.

Listen to Gloria here

https://youtu.be/Dr2mrGnap7E?t=1006

My Blessed Miracle Patient Two Decades Ago A True Story of Bob Wals !

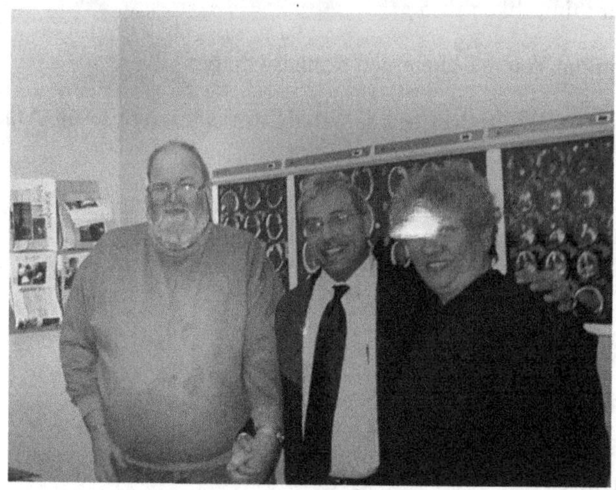

Twenty years ago, I stood against the establishment and I declared Bob wasn't in Coma but the world around him was: Bob has always been alive and man shall not take his life away against God's will!

Almost two decades ago, a patient was placed on hospice to die because he was in a permenant coma and vegetative state as a result of inoperable brain tumor transferred from downtown hospital after three brain surgeries to Joliet hospital.

Patient' family were very attentive to the patient and were so loving . The wife Ginny Wals spend day and night with her dying husband following the doctors recommendation that he was suffering from inoperable brain tumor and he is in Permenant coma and will never wake up!

However, the wife noticed that her husband Bob has life in himself and did purposeful movements at night and was sleeping and snoring in the morning when physicians made their rounds!

Day after day in the hospital, her husband wasn't dying and she refused to allow the doctors and nurses to give him sedatives or to dehydrate him and starve him to death!

The wife was telling the nurses and doctors tgat her husband wasn't in coma but rather he was sleeping and his routine sleep during the day and awoke at night! No one listened to wife and thought she was emotionally irrational!

One day after she gave up in the doctors and nurses telling them their observations, to have a second opinion and at that time my reputation was just starting!

I remember when I was called for second opinion, I was asked to agree with the current plans and the wife was being unrealistic!

I went to see the patient and I met the wife and looked at the films. My first look at Bob, I felt shivering in my body and I felt life in him and he wasn't in coma as they were told and forced to believe and the brain did not look terminal. I saw a man wanted to live and God didn't want him to die. I saw that his time wasn't over yet and doctors we're taking his life away! I felt as if someone was suffocating him! I leaned at his shoulder and I told him Bob, "we love you, Lord Jesus has a mission for you and want you to live for it before He take you to Him and I will take care of you and tomorrow you will be home" I saw the tears were running from his eyes. It angered my soul to see how can hospitals allow lives to be taken away so soon and playing God! I immediately agreed with the wife and disagreed with the world around her!

I declared that Bob wasn't in Coma but the world around him was: Bob has always been alive and man shall not take his life away against God's will!!

I took Bob to surgery and I cared for him afterwards. Bob made the best recovery, wake up from sleep, enjoyed his family and his grand daughter that he was so attached to her until he died five years later!

Ginny his wife what an angel! She never gave up in her husband despite everyone around her said she was crazy to have me do Bob fourth brain surgery and gave him chance to live! She was told after all, you were going to disagree with downtown professors and agree with Dr Ghaly, graduated three years after residency and had no experience!

The story astonished the community and was written in Chicago Tribune June 10, 2001 as featured article by Mary Daniel, Tribune Staff Reporter, May her soul be comforted entitled: "A Miracle Worker" https://www.chicagotribune.com/.../ct-xpm-2001-06-10...

The picture below was by a Chicago tribune photographer was sent to make sure and the reporter interviewed so many tines Ginny to confirm the story and the miracle!

I wonder how many patients, we let them go so soon and we okay God to them and their families that otherwise should have been alive like Bobs!

O man who are you to okay God and take the life of innocent patients away!

I visited him and his family many times until Bob passed away five years later. Since then, Bob and his family in my heart and prayers!

Thank you Ginny and family and may Bob loved memory for ever alive!

https://www.chicagotribune.com/.../ct-xpm-2001-06-10...

COMMENTS

DM, Sir there is no question that God has given you surgical abilities that are stellar and a faith in him that is unwavering!! You have given life to two of my family members and we are so blessed by your hands!! Stephen Schott and Brad Conderman

SP, They were such a wonderful family

JK, Been there i fully understand!!!

DL, How Blessed !

DE, Thank you for sharing your incredible story

CR, So beautiful

Our Angel Richard Fuesz Experience!

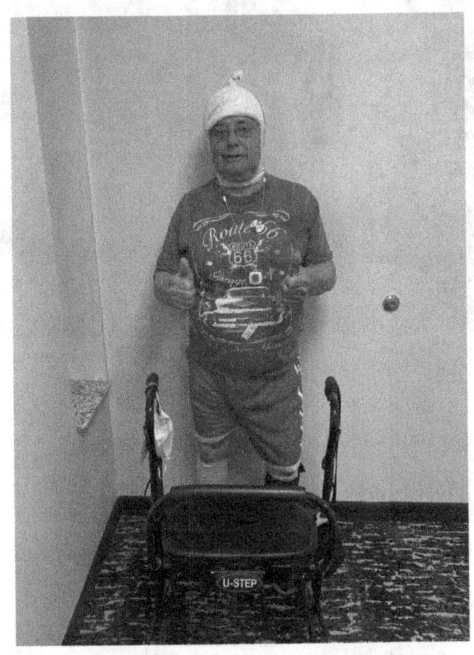

I know Richard since 2001 and his family! What a blessed angel!

Richard is recovering well after the major brain surgery praise our Lord Jesus and intercession of Archangel Michael. Rounding early and here he is fully awake and ready for full recovery. Already all the staff love this man and rank him high among all patients in the unit!

We pray for speed recovery!

Amen

Ramsis Ghaly

Www.ghalyneurosurgeon.com

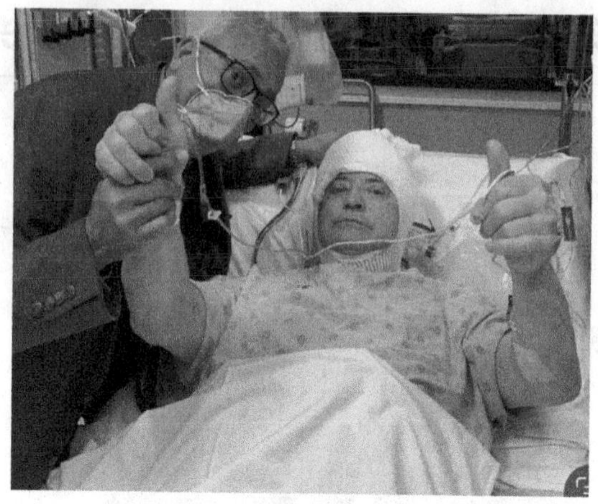

JK, Prayers ...

What a huge success thanks to Dr Ramsis Ghaly..

LM, Glory to You, OH Lord.

CG, Praying that God will heal you and you will have a speedy recovery.

DL, God bless you both.

MN, Richard I pray for a fast recovery the Lord Jesus sent you the right doctor to perform the surgery I know DrGhaly was there to do major brain surgery on me I had a fast recovery and here to talk about praise the Lord Jesus for you Richard.

CC, Speedy recovery

BCD, God Bless you. Amen

BNM, raying for Richard to have a speedy recovery. Praise God our Lord and Savior!

MH, You are an awesome & an amazing Dr. Love how many you heal each year. You are truly blessed to have such an amazing talent. Have a very bless day sir.

MS, God chose you to do this work for sure. God bless you both.b

JS, Praise the LORD for a great recovery

BL, God is good always and forever. Dr. **Ramsis Ghaly** He works His miracles through you.

RC, Speed recovery. Blessings for pacient and doctor

LR, God bless you!

AL, Amén

DN, You are awesome you get nothing but great reviews

AP, Praying for a speedy recovery

Our angel going home today sweet home after major brain surgery two days ago. Praise our Lord Jesus. Amen to His glorious Name and Healing. Speed recovery our angel. Our archangel Michael all around us.

Ramsis Ghaly

Www.ghalyneurosurgeon.com

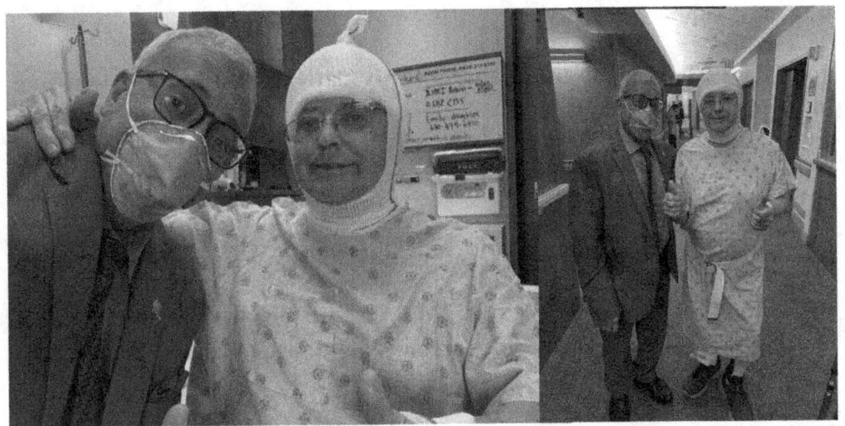

AL, Gracias al señor

CG, May the peace and comfort of God surround you during your time of recovery.

JW, May He lay His healing hands all around ur body & may find peace & comfort during this time. Amen. God is good all the time.

All the time, God is good

Sometimes we have endure things that we don't want too but then u have to look at the positive. God is refining you. It doesn't feel food at the time but when you get to the other side, things become clear.

I always leave out words. Read between the lines

KB, Sending prayers

RM, God Bless

JD, May GOD give you a restful recovery

DL, Amén.

AB, Praise God

MS, Thank you for sharing things. It's so important. To know you and God are there.

Tf, Prayers

Rc, Praises in the name of god. Good vibes!

Touching, Inspiring and uplifting!

Ramsis Ghaly

Four days after major brain surgery, My patient send me this touching, inspiring and uplifting!

He is already pushing himself at home and he is walking In the condo floor hallway 800 feet!

It is a Picture of endurance, perseverance and determination to never give up!

Regardless of the tine of the day, Walking, sitting, sleeping, he is always looking positive and ready to overcome the down thoughts and negative energy and doubts!

Yes Amen to Patient empowerment with faith in our Savior and Lord Hod!

Bless his heart and his faith! Praise our lord Jesus speed recovery !

"So I say to you, ask, and it will be given to you; seek, and you will find; knock, and it will be opened to you. For everyone who asks, receives; and he who seeks, finds; and to him who knocks, it will be opened."

Luke 11:9-10

Ramsis Ghaly

Www.ghalyneurosurgeon.com

Inspiring and uplifting

Our angel at home performing an evening hallway 800 feet walk before bedtime. Bless his heart and his faith! Praise our lord Jesus speed recovery !

Ramsis Ghaly

Www.ghalyneurosurgeon.com

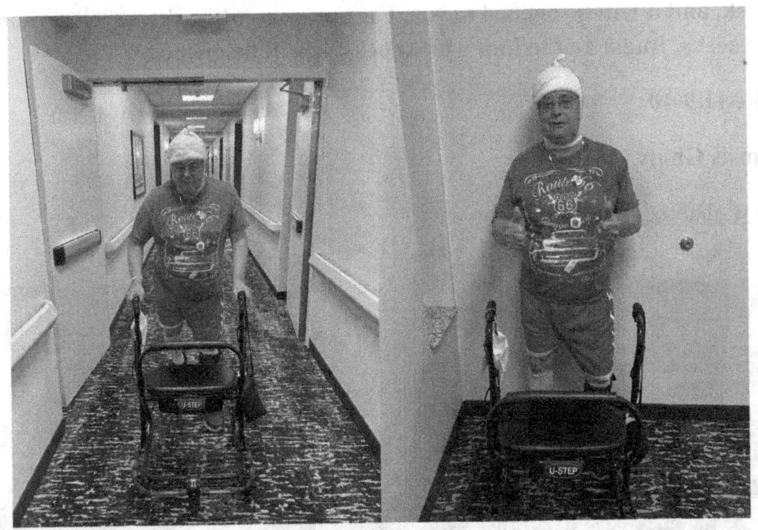

KO, Good heath to you sir, praise the Lord for your great surgeon

CG, You have the best surgeon who along with God is by your side during your recovery.

LM, You are truly a man of God.

Touching, Inspiring and uplifting!

Ramsis Ghaly

Four days after major brain surgery, My patient send me this touching, inspiring and uplifting!

He is already pushing himself at home and he is walking In the condo floor hallway 800 feet!

It is a Picture of endurance, perseverance and determination to never give up!

Regardless of the tine of the day, Walking, sitting, sleeping, he is always looking positive and ready to overcome the down thoughts and negative energy and doubts!

Yes Amen to Patient empowerment with faith in our Savior and Lord Hod!

Bless his heart and his faith! Praise our lord Jesus speed recovery !

"So I say to you, ask, and it will be given to you; seek, and you will find; knock, and it will be opened to you. For everyone who asks, receives; and he who seeks, finds; and to him who knocks, it will be opened."

Luke 11:9-10

Ramsis Ghaly

Www.ghalyneurosurgeon.com

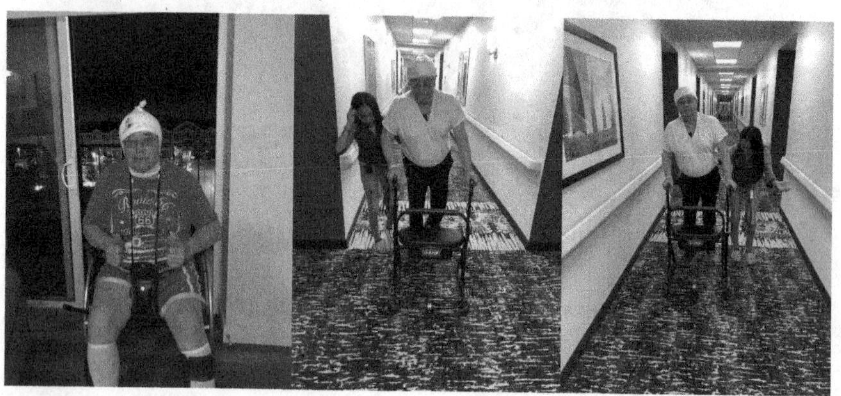

AP, Amen

LY, Amen!!!

LW, God works miracles thru you.

SS, Gloria a Dio a suo figlio Gesù e allo Santo Spirito Amen

JT, healing prayers

jm, Congratulations

"Wish You A Speedy Total Recovery